Promoting Health in Children and Young People

The Role of the Nurse

Promoting Health in Children and Young People

The Role of the Nurse

Edited by

Karen Moyse
MSc, BSc, RGN, RSCN, RHV, PGDAE (Hons)
Psychology and Independent Nurse Prescriber

WILEY-BLACKWELL

A John Wiley & Sons, Ltd., Publication

This edition first published 2009
© 2009 Blackwell Publishing Ltd

Blackwell Publishing was acquired by John Wiley & Sons in February 2007. Blackwell's publishing programme has been merged with Wiley's global Scientific, Technical, and Medical business to form Wiley-Blackwell.

Registered office
John Wiley & Sons Ltd, The Atrium, Southern Gate, Chichester, West Sussex, PO19 8SQ, United Kingdom

Editorial offices
9600 Garsington Road, Oxford, OX4 2DQ, United Kingdom
2121 State Avenue, Ames, Iowa 50014-8300, USA

For details of our global editorial offices, for customer services and for information about how to apply for permission to reuse the copyright material in this book please see our website at www.wiley.com/wiley-blackwell.

Library of Congress Cataloging-in-Publication Data

Promoting health in children/young people : the role of the nurse / edited by Karen Moyse.
    p. ; cm.
  Includes bibliographical references and index.
  ISBN 978-1-4051-5800-8 (pbk. : alk. paper) 1. Pediatric nursing. 2. Health promotion. I. Moyse, Karen.
  [DNLM: 1. Health Promotion. 2. Pediatric Nursing–methods. 3. Adolescent. 4. Child. 5. Nurse's Role.
WY 159 P965 2009]
  RJ245.P77 2009
  618.92'00231–dc22
                2008026135

A catalogue record for this book is available from the British Library.

Set in 9.5/11.5pt Palatino by Aptara® Inc., New Delhi, India
Printed in Malaysia by KHL Printing Co Sdn Bhd

1 2009

Contents

Contributors   viii

Foreword   xv
Fiona Smith

Acknowledgements   xvii

Introduction   xix
Karen Moyse

Theme 1   Foundations of Health Promotion with Children/Young People   **1**

1   Reducing Health Inequalities   3
Roderick P. M. Thomson

2   Planning for Health Promotion   11
Karen Moyse

3   Creativity   25
Claire Daniel

4   Government Policy   33
Janet Badcock

Theme 2   Child Development   **43**

5   Child Development   45
*Karen Moyse, Janet Savage, Alison Price,
Carole Taylor and Mary Hill*

6   Health for All Children   58
Janet Badcock

Theme 3   Everyday Health Issues for Children/Young People   **67**

7   Preventing Childhood Obesity   69
*Ros Parkinson, Diane Jewkes,
Vicky Grayson, Karen Moyse,
Cheryl Sheard, Liz Whelan,
Fenella Lindsell, Jackie Butler
and Janet Savage*

8   Dental Health Promotion   83
Karen Moyse, Sue Toon and Helen Fowler

9   Skin Cancer Prevention   96
Lesley Strazds

10   Accident Prevention   101
Karen Moyse

Theme 4   Promoting Health in Minor Illness and Minor Injury   **113**

11   Sure Start Community Children's
Nursing Service – Developing a Minor
Illness/Injury Service   115
Karen Moyse and Zo'e Ellis

12 Fever Management in Young Children
   (0–5 Years)   124
   Karen Moyse

13 Health Promotion in Young Children's
   Minor Illnesses   134
   Karen Moyse

14 Health Promotion in Minor Injuries   144
   Karen Moyse and Chrissie Bousfield

**Theme 5   Children/Young People in
Hospital**   **153**

15 Health Promotion for Pre- and
   Postoperative Care   155
   Julie Spice and Annette Dearmun

16 Surgical Wound Healing and Health
   Promotion   163
   Elaine Salmons

17 Planning Hospital Discharge   169
   Jane Houghton

**Theme 6   Promoting Health in
Chronic Illness**   **179**

18 Asthma Management   181
   Annie Wing

19 Managing Children's Skin Conditions   192
   Elizabeth Barrett

20 Health Promotion for Children/Young
   People with Cancer   202
   Louise Soanes

21 Constipation   209
   Ali Wright

22 Health Promotion in Childhood Diabetes   220
   Helen Thornton

23 Children/Young People with
   Disabilities and Complex Health
   Care Needs   228
   Sarah V. Wilcock

Theme 7   Medicines Management   **233**

24 Medicines Management   235
   Roger Kirkbride

Theme 8   Pain Management   **247**

25 Pain Management   249
   Elizabeth Bruce

**Theme 9   Promoting Emotional
Health**   **257**

26 Baby Massage and Baby Yoga   259
   *Karen Moyse, Helen Surguy and
   Liz Whelan*

27 Health Promotion Course: Living
   with Babies   266
   Helen Surguy and Karen Moyse

28 Baby Play   272
   Jane Blenkinsop

29 Baby Club   281
   Kate Hawksworth

30 Positive Parenting   287
   Karen Moyse

31 Promoting Children's Mental Health –
   Focus Bullying   293
   Karen Moyse

32 Safeguarding Children (Health Promotion) 301
   Karen Moyse

33 The Health of Children/Young People
   in Care   307
   Cathy Sheehan

Theme 10   Teenage Health Issues   **313**

34 Health Promotion Course – Living with
   Teenagers   315
   Joanna Livingstone

35 Promoting Sexual Health to Young People 325
    Barbara Richardson-Todd

36 Preventing and Managing Substance
    Misuse   337
    *P. C. John Graham, Janet Savage, Karen
    Moyse, Jimi Poyser and Donnamarie
    Donnelly*

37 Smoking Cessation   346
    Roger Kirkbride

**Theme 11   Evaluating Health
Promotion   351**

38 Evaluating Health Promotion   353
    Karen Moyse

**Theme 12   Health Promotion in
Context   365**

39 Health Promotion in Context   367
    Vicky Grayson

Theme 13   National Perspectives   379

40 National Perspectives   381
    *Carolyn Neill, Kate McPake, Susan Anne
    Jones, Nicola Lewis and Karen Moyse*

Index   399

Contributors

Janet Badcock. MSc, BA, RGN, RSCN, RHV, CPT. Janet has worked with children in both hospital and community settings, including Sure Start areas. Other experience includes teaching, management and service development projects. At the time of writing Janet worked for Derbyshire County Primary Care Trust, but has now moved on to a new area. She is a mother to her son Matthew.

Elizabeth Barrett. MB, BCh, BA, D.Obstet, MRCGP, FPCert. Dermatology hospital practitioner, family planning and GP trainer. Elizabeth Barrett qualified in 1977. She is a general practitioner in Derbyshire and also works as a hospital practitioner in dermatology. She has written health information articles for the local newspaper for several years, and has a special interest in patient involvement in health care, at all levels.

Jane Blenkinsop. NNEB Diploma in Nursery Nursing. Jane has worked as a nursery nurse for 14 years. After beginning her career in the private sector, Jane moved on to work with health visiting teams within Sure Start. During her time with Sure Start, Jane gained extensive experience of working with children and families in group situations and also home visiting. She has facilitated baby play groups, baby massage courses and worked to the portage model with preschool children. Jane is currently working as an inclusion officer, supporting childcare providers in meeting the additional needs of children/young adults. Jane has an interest in the emotional development of children, particularly the attachment between children and their parents.

Chrissie Bousfield. MSc, BSc (Hons), PGDAE, RN. Formerly Clinical Nurse Specialist, Burns Unit, Nottingham, and currently Lecturer, School of Nursing, University of Nottingham. Since qualifying Chrissie has devoted her career, both clinically and academically, to the speciality of burn trauma, plastic/reconstructive surgery and tissue viability. In 1992 she achieved a scholarship to the Shriners Burn Institute in Boston, Massachusetts, USA. Chrissie has published books on burns trauma management, and worked as a Nurse Consultant at the Harley Street Clinic, London, specialising in tissue viability. Chrissie continues to act as an expert witness within her speciality, and is also contributing to a teaching programme on trauma in a children's hospital in Gwalior, India, as part of a UK charity event.

Elizabeth Bruce. MSc, BSc (Hons), RGN, RSCN. Liz is a clinical nurse specialist with the Pain Control Service at Great Ormond Street Hospital for Children. She is also an honorary research fellow at the Institute of Child Health, London. Her main research interests are in pain assessment and the management of procedural pain. Liz coordinated the children's pain assessment project, which involved developing a website to disseminate information about children's pain assessment. Liz is a member of the RCN Pain in Children Group. She has been involved in workshops to develop pain management guidelines with the International Society for Paediatric Oncology and the development of nursing competencies for pain management with the British Pain Society.

Jackie Butler. Once Jackie's children started school, she became a swimming teacher through the Swimming Teacher's Association, and found that she absolutely loved it. Jackie is a fully qualified swimming instructor and continues to attend courses to keep up to date. She has been teaching swimming for about 15 years and teaches at all levels. She also trains swimming teachers. Jackie finds her job crosses all walks of life. She says that it is immensely satisfying and often challenging.

Claire Daniel. BA (Hons) Textiles, PGCE Art and Design. Claire followed her degree by working as a visual merchandiser for Jigsaw and then moved into the television and film industry where she gained experience in photography and graphic design. Following on from her teaching position in London, Claire has assisted in several schools and exclusion programmes within the East Midlands. She has two beautiful daughters, Jessica and Scarlet, and a son, Alexander.

Annette Dearmun. PhD, BSc (Hons), RSCN, RGN, DN, DNE (RNT), ITEC. Annette has worked in children's nursing for over 25 years. For her PhD she studied the experience of newly qualified children's nurses. Annette is Chair of the RCN Children's Surgical Nursing Forum and is a member of the Royal College of Surgeons Children's Forum. Annette was formerly Chair of the RCN Children's/Young Person's Field of Practice. Annette has published many articles in children's nursing. Annette is currently Associate Director of Children's Nursing, Oxford Radcliffe Hospital, and Lecturer, Oxford Brookes University.

Donnamarie Donnelly. Post Graduate Diploma in Drama therapy. Donnamarie is a registered mental health nurse and has worked in both forensic and acute mental health settings. She has been working in the substance misuse field since 1992, first with adult service users and then with young people. Donnamarie has been the manager of *Face It* Young Person's Drug and Alcohol Service since 2000. She has also trained as a drama therapist.

Zo'e Ellis. CIMA (Certified Institute of Management Accountants), HND in Business and Finance. Zo'e has lived in Langwith/Whaley Thorns all her life and so too have previous generations of her family. Zo'e is a member of the Children's Centre Advisory Group in Langwith/Whaley Thorns, and is also a parent governor at Whaley Thorns Primary School. Zo'e is married, with three wonderful boys, ages 9, 8 and 3 years.

Helen Fowler. BSc (Hons) Social Policy and Sociology, Diploma Nursing, RN (Child Branch). Helen has been working as a children's nurse since qualifying in 1998. She has experience in acute paediatric medicine and currently works as a surgical nurse for the hospital trust in Derbyshire. She has published research in paediatric nursing. Helen is married, with a young son, age 3 years.

P.C. John Graham. John joined the Nottinghamshire Police Force in 1967. He has worked as a foot patrol officer (when policemen covered their neighbourhoods on foot) and patrol car officer. In 1972 he joined the Traffic Department at Worksop, where he sometimes dealt with serious road accidents. Whilst at that department he trained in firearms and was often in an armed response vehicle. In 2001, after 34 years in the service he retired. Never one to be still, he went on to join the DARE programme, which he has been involved in for the last 7 years. John feels that his role at DARE is totally different from operational work, but thoroughly enjoyable and worthwhile. The DARE programme is thought very highly of by pupils, teachers and parents alike.

Vicky Grayson. BA (Hons) Nursing Studies (Children), Independent Nurse Prescriber, Certificates in Caring for the Critically Ill Child, and Mentoring Students. Following qualifying as a children's nurse from Sheffield Hallam University, Vicky worked on a general paediatric surgical and medical ward for 4 years, where she obtained a senior staff nurse position. In 2005 she began to work alongside Karen Moyse as a community children's nurse, caring for children with minor injuries and illnesses. In 2006 she was appointed to take on this role and further develop the community children's nursing service, which Karen had initiated. Vicky is currently on maternity leave following the birth of her son.

Kate Hawksworth. BA (Hons) Community Health (Specialist Practitioner), Health Visiting, Diploma in Health Care Practice, RGN, Nurse Prescriber. Kate has 28 years experience as a qualified nurse both in the primary care and in the acute sector. Her community nursing experience has involved working as a team leader in a disadvantaged inner-city area. As a health visitor she has worked within a Sure Start team, based also in an area of social and economic disadvantage. Kate believes reducing social exclusion in the most isolated families is challenging and very rewarding. Kate was involved with other health visitors and community nursery nurses within Sure Start in setting up a *Living with Babies* course, for which they received an award from the local primary care trust. Outside work, Kate is married, with three lovely grown-up children.

Mary Hill. NNEB, HPSET, C&G 7307/1 and 7307/2. Mary is a play specialist at the University Hospital of Nottingham, where she has worked for over 16 years. For the last 5 years, she has worked on a busy 23-bedded children's ward. Mary is also a qualified tutor in adult education. She has worked in various colleges and establishments in the Nottingham area, providing courses to young people (16+ years).

Jane Houghton. MSc, RGN, RSCN, DN Certificate. Jane qualified in 1982 in Manchester. She has worked in several nursing roles: staff nurse, then sister on a paediatric regional burns unit, children's community nurse, diabetes nurse in Manchester and paediatric diabetes clinical nurse specialist in Bradford, then nurse consultant child health at Lancashire Teaching Hospitals NHS Foundation Trust. At the same time she also worked as a bank nurse in a children's accident and emergency department for many years. Jane has been Chair of the RCN Children's Diabetes Group and Chair of the RCN Children's Ambulatory Care Forum. This work has led to her being involved in several national working parties and policies, such as NICE guidelines and technical appraisals, Skills for Health, CEMACH, BNFC and MHRA.

Diane Jewkes. RGN, RM, Diploma in Counselling, Health Promotion Certificate, Independent Nurse Prescriber, La Leche Peer Counsellor Programme Administrator. Diane is married, with four children (all breastfed), and five grandchildren (four out of five breastfed). Diane has worked as a midwife for 20 years, in both hospital and community practice. She has also worked as a midwife for Sure Start, setting many health promotion groups for parents. Diane has always worked in areas with high deprivation scores. She is currently working as a sexual health practitioner.

Susan Anne Jones. BSc (Hons) Community Health Studies (Specialist Practice) School Nursing, SRN, SCM, Qualified Nurse Prescriber. Sue began her nursing career in 1972. Following a career break of 6 years, she returned to the NHS in 1986 to work as a community-based school/clinic nurse. In 1999 her employing NHS trust set up a dedicated school health nurse team and in April 2000 she progressed to school health nurse manager, which is her current role. In 2006 after studying part-time over 2 years, she achieved the BSc (Hons) Community Health Studies (Specialist Practice) School Nursing, with first class honours from the University of Wales, Swansea. Sue is passionate about children's/young people's rights. Sue is excited about taking the school health nurse role forward in Wales.

Roger Kirkbride. BPharm, MRPharmS, CDipAF, MBA. Roger became a member of the Royal Pharmaceutical Society in 1982. After working in a number of community pharmacy positions, he moved to Boots Head Office where he undertook a variety of roles in marketing and property before moving on to strategy development. During this time he gained a finance qualification and a Master of Business Administration (MBA) from Nottingham University. Roger left Boots in 2004 to pursue a career as an independent pharmacy consultant, working with the NHS, the pharmacy industry, and others to promote the integration of pharmacy into the NHS and its use as a point of access to health care. During this time he has written and presented extensively on the use of point-of-care testing and has contributed to a number of CPD modules for pharmacy publications. Roger is married to a theatre sister and has two (supposedly) adult children.

Nicola Lewis. BSc (Hons) Community Health (Specialist Practitioner), CCN, RGN, RSCN. Nicola has been a community children's nurse (CCN) since October 2000. She is currently CCN Team

Leader for Abertawe Bro-Morgannwg University NHS Trust, South Wales. Her background in children's nursing includes general paediatric inpatient care at East Glamorgan Hospital NHS Trust and the Princess of Wales Hospital NHS Trust. Nicola gained her RSCN in 1995 at Birmingham Children's Hospital. Following this she specialised in paediatric oncology and haematology at the Welsh regional unit at Llandough Hospital in Cardiff, gaining relevant clinical and theoretical qualifications. Nicola achieved her BSc in Community Health, CCN pathway, at the University of Wales, Swansea, in July 2001. Her area of professional interest is to develop an acute CCN service separate from the respite service her team predominantly provides.

Fenella Lindsell. Fenella Lindsell is mother of four children and director and co-founder of YogaBugs Ltd. She started practising yoga when she was 25 following a visit to India. Inspired by what she learned there, she returned, married Rob and set up a large complementary health and yoga centre in SW London (The Art of Health). Fenella trained as a yoga teacher originally with the British Wheel of Yoga and then went on to practise extensively with Lyengar, Astanga and Jivamukti teachers. YogaBugs hatched at The Art of Health in 1996 and in 2003; Fenella joined forces with her sister in law, Lara Goodbody, and together with two other directors, they have grown the company to become the largest provider of children's yoga in the world.

Joanna Livingstone. BSc Community Health (Specialist Practitioner) Public Health Nurse, RGN, Registered Nurse (Child Branch), Health Promotion Certificate. Joanna has worked for 6 years as a health visitor in Derbyshire. During this time she undertook a 3-year secondment to the *Living with Children/Teenagers Programme*, where she was involved in organising and delivering parenting courses. Joanna has many years experience in both general and paediatric nursing. She has three children – one of whom is a teenager.

Kate McPake. BA (Hons) RN, HV, PGCE. Kate is currently employed as a public health nurse in Edinburgh. She has served as the RCN representative on the Children's/Young People's Committee in the Scottish Parliament for the last 3 years. Prior to this she was a curriculum leader in Health Care in Further Education. Kate has also been the principal assessor on the SQA marking team for Care Practice Higher and continues to be involved with the marking team.

Karen Moyse. MSc, BSc (Hons) Psychology, RGN, RSCN, RHV, PGDAE, Health Promotion Certificate and Independent Nurse Prescriber. Other certificates include Baby Massage, Positive Parenting and Minor Illness/Injury Management. Karen has worked with children for many years as a children's nurse, health visitor and more recently as a community children's nurse. She has also worked as a lecturer in health at Nottingham University, where she developed a postregistration course in Community Children's Nursing. Karen has an interest in child development, particularly promoting children's emotional development, and has written several articles in this area. She has an interest in children's minor illnesses/injuries management, as well as parenting. Karen has a daughter, Lucy.

Carolyn Neill. M.Phil, BSc (Hons) Nursing Studies, Diploma in Research Methods, RGN, RSCN. Carolyn has previously worked as a staff nurse on an adult orthopaedic unit and on a children's burns and plastics ward. She has been employed as quality coordinator at the Royal Belfast Hospital for Sick Children for the past 14 years. This wide-ranging role includes undertaking audit and benchmarking projects, developing quality initiatives and devising policies. Carolyn completed her M.Phil in 2003, which focused on investigating the lived experience of the paediatric clinical nurse specialist. Her key interests are care of young people, development of parent information materials and user involvement.

Ros Parkinson. RGN, RSCN, ENB 998, Asthma Diploma, Diploma Module in the Management of Diabetes. At the time of writing, Ros was employed as a children's diabetes nurse, based at Lincoln County Hospital. Ros has previously worked as a senior practice nurse, specialising in chronic disease management, based in Nottinghamshire. She has also worked as a community children's nurse with the Lifetime Service in Bath. Health promotion for the entire family has always been important to Ros in all her nursing roles.

Jimi Poyser. Jimi has spent most of his adult working life as a mechanical engineer, part of which was spent as a mining mechanic. Jimi left the mining industry in 1989 and took up voluntary youth work, working in a few local youth clubs. He gained his youth work qualification in 1992. Jimi is a drugs and alcohol worker for young people at *Face It* in Nottinghamshire, where he has worked for the last 10 years. Jimi has also management experience, and has been a DJ.

Alison Price. NNEB, HPS. Alison has worked as a play specialist for 18 years. She has worked on a children's orthopaedic ward, children's medical ward, and is currently working in the Children's Outpatient's Department, Queen's Medical Centre, University Hospital of Nottingham.

Barbara Richardson-Todd. BSc (Hons), RGN, Cert. Ed, RSCPHN (School Nursing), Dip. N. Practice, Health Ed. Cert. Barbara has been a school nurse since 1987. She has been active locally and nationally in promoting school nursing. Barbara has presented papers throughout the UK and at the First School Health Conference in Abu Dhabi. She has been involved in the Chief Nursing Officer's Stakeholder group and subgroups, looking at modernising the school nursing role. Barbara is a member of the RCN National School Nursing Forum and a member of the School and Public Health Nurses Association. Barbara has five children between the ages of 32 and 16 years, as well as two grandchildren. Barbara is a school nurse coordinator and practice teacher for Suffolk PCT.

Elaine Salmons. BSc (Hons) Health Studies, BSc (Hons) Advanced Professional Practice (ENB Higher Award) Community Children's Nursing Pathway, RGN, RSCN, ENB 998, ENB R62. Elaine has worked in both hospital and community settings with children and their families. She worked as a children's nurse at the University Hospital Nottingham for 20 years, gaining experience in a number of different areas, including general surgery, plastic surgery and community children's nursing. She is currently working at Birmingham Children's Hospital as a senior specialist nurse for inherited metabolic disorders and newborn screening. Elaine has previously been a member of the RCN Community Children's Nurse Forum.

Janet Savage. BSc Community Health – School Nurse, RGN, RSCN, Community Practice Teacher. Janet has worked as a staff nurse, senior staff nurse and ward sister in children's nursing. In 1998 she became a school nurse in Birmingham, where she later worked as a school

nurse team leader. At present Janet is working as school nurse/community practice teacher in Erdington, Birmingham.

Cheryl Sheard. Personal Trainer, Qualified YogaBugs Teacher. Cheryl has been a coach and personal trainer for 26 years. She teaches all forms of fitness to all ages from toddlers to pensioners, athletes to the physically disabled. Cheryl teaches YogaBugs and physical education at local schools. Her fitness company Kynetik also delivers relaxation talks and fitness seminars to health care trusts, schools and colleges.

Cathy Sheehan. BSc (Hons) Advanced Professional Practice (ENB Higher Award) Community Children's Nursing Pathway, RGN, RSCN, Certificate in Caring for the Critically Ill Child. Cathy is a designated nurse for Children in Care and Adoption and has been in this position for the past 3 years. Her experience to date has been in children's nursing and Cathy has a wealth of experience in this field. Cathy has worked in general paediatrics, as a school nurse for children with special needs, a paediatric intensive care nurse and as a community children's nurse. Cathy qualified as an RSCN/RGN in 1989 following completion of an integrated course at Great Ormond Street Hospital for Sick Children. She is currently undertaking an MSc in Organisational Leadership in Health and Social Care. Cathy is a wife, mother to three teenage children, and stepmother to five children, so she has a busy but happy household.

Louise Soanes. MSc, BSc, RGN, RSCN. Louise has worked in paediatric oncology since 1988. During that time she has worked on four paediatric oncology centres in London, both in clinical and educational posts. She has also worked at London South Bank University as a senior lecturer in children's and adolescent cancer nursing. She is currently a senior sister for children's services at the Royal Marsden Hospital in Surrey.

Julie Spice. BSc (Hons) Children's Nursing, SRN, RSCN, RHV. Julie has spent the majority of her nursing career working with children and families in both hospital and community settings. For the last 13 years she has worked on a paediatric elective ward at Ipswich Hospital, where she is currently ward manager. The focus of her dissertation for her degree in Children's Nursing was developing the preoperative assessment of children undergoing elective surgery. Julie has been a member of the RCN Children's Surgical Nursing Forum since 2007. She is married, with three children.

Lesley Strazds. Lesley began her nursing career in 1975. She has experience in both gynaecology and ophthalmic outpatients at Kings Mill Hospital, Nottinghamshire. Lesley joined the dermatology team as a junior member in 1991. Through personal interest and study, her role progressed to the position of dermatology nurse specialist in 1999. She has enjoyed learning and developing skills within dermatology over the years and has a professional interest in both skin cancer and paediatric dermatology.

Helen Surguy. BA (Nursing), BSc Community Health (Specialist Practitioner) Health Visiting, RGN, ENB 100 (Intensive Care Nursing), City and Guilds 7307 (teaching), Independent Nurse Prescriber, Advanced Life Support Certificate, Intermediate Life Support Instructor, and Baby Massage Certificate, and is a Member of the Guild of Infant and Child Massage. Helen has been nursing for just over 20 years. She has worked in both intensive care nursing and health visiting. More recently, she has worked within Sure Start, developing teaching programmes for mothers and their babies. Helen led the development of the *Living with Babies* course, which received an award from the local primary care trust. Helen has recently become a mother to daughter Amy.

Carole Taylor. Hospital Play Specialist (HPSEB). Carole is a qualified nursery nurse. She has previously worked as a nanny in Paris, and then went to Great Ormond Street Hospital for 4 years as a nursery nurse, before moving to Nottingham. Carole now works in PICU at University Hospital Nottingham as a qualified hospital play specialist. She is married, with a 6-year-old daughter.

Roderick P.M. Thomson. FRCN, FFPH, M.Ed, MSc, Dip. Ad. Ed, Dip. HV, RMN, RGN, RHV. Rod is a consultant in public health for Sefton Primary Care Trust in the UK. Rod is also a Visiting Professor at John Moores University, Liverpool. His nursing career spans mental and physical health care in hospital and community settings. His role includes the leadership for community safety programmes, such as infection control, emergency planning and substance misuse.

Rod has worked in Cuba and Lithuania as well as presented papers in Australia, Canada, Japan, Taiwan and Europe on a range of nursing and public health topics. He is an active member of the Royal College of Nursing, and achieved its highest award, a Fellowship, in recognition of his exceptional contribution to the art and science of nursing.

Helen Thornton. BSc, RGN, RSCN, OND, ENB 928, ENB 998, Health Promotion Certificate, Independent and Supplementary Nurse Prescriber, and has attended multiple courses and conferences on diabetes. Helen has been a paediatric diabetes specialist nurse for over 18 years and has presented at regional, national and international conferences. Currently, Helen has strategic responsibility within her hospital department for implementation of the Diabetes NSF and is the editor of the paediatric supplement of the *Journal of Diabetes Nursing*. Helen's initial training was in ophthalmology, where she first encountered caring for people with diabetes. After Paediatric and General Nurse training and whilst staffing on a paediatric medical unit, Helen's interest in diabetes was rekindled by the number of adolescents who continuously required readmission. After having had the opportunity to attend the Youth Diabetes Project's medical weekend at Firbush, she met a breed of nurse called *diabetes specialist nurse* and was hooked. In 1989 she took up a part-time post at her current hospital and has subsequently developed, with colleagues, a comprehensive paediatric diabetes service.

Sue Toon. RGN, RN (Child Branch). Sue's lifelong ambition was always to be a nurse. From the age of 5 years she would role-play being a nurse with her younger siblings. The dream came true when she was accepted to do her General Nurse training at Nottingham in 1973. After qualifying she staffed on the burns and plastics unit in Nottingham. She later moved to Derby where she continued to work with adults. However, she was asked to help on a children's ward and was thus inspired to work with children. She went on to complete her Children's Nurse training, and is currently working on a children's ward in Derby.

Liz Whelan. Diplomas in Baby Yoga, YogaBugs ($2\frac{1}{2}$ to 5 years) and Yoga'd Up (8 to 12 years). Liz started practising baby yoga when she was pregnant with her daughter. Her daughter suffered from colic; she wanted to find something to help comfort her. Liz teaches yoga to children in nurseries and schools across South Yorkshire and Derbyshire.

Sarah V. Wilcock. B.Med Sc Nursing Studies, Ad. Diploma Nursing (Child Branch). Sarah has been a qualified nurse for 8 years. She manages a children's continuing care service in the East Midlands. Sarah has worked in the community since 2001. She is currently studying part-time for an MSc in Organisational Leadership in Health and Social Care.

Annie Wing. MA, BA (Hons), PG. Cert, RGN, RSCN, RHV. Annie is a children's nurse by background with a special interest in community nursing services and respiratory disease. Her career pathway developed within the field of education, and she now works at Education for Health, a leading education and research charity for health professionals, accredited by the Open University. Education for Health provides a comprehensive and innovative approach to health professional training across the fields of respiratory and cardiovascular disease, allergic conditions and diabetes. Annie is an assistant director of education at Education for Health.

Ali Wright. SRN, RSCN. Ali is currently working as a specialist children's nurse in stoma care, gastrostomy and ACE (antegrade continence enema) care for Children's Services at the Nottingham University Hospitals NHS Trust. Ali has also worked as a ward manager, senior sister and gastroenterology nurse specialist, before taking up her current post in 2004. She has an interest in children's continence and has organised hospital and community-based nurse-led clinics in childhood constipation. Ali is married and has a daughter called Beth.

Foreword

I am delighted to write the foreword to this much-needed text which brings together many different aspects and issues in relation to health promotion. This is undoubtedly a practical textbook, applying theory to case study examples arising from day-to-day nursing practice. The role of the nurse, health visitor and midwife in this field is even more critical today than ever before.

Good health is vital if children/young people are to enjoy their childhood and achieve their full potential. Mortality and morbidity have substantially reduced over the last century along with the introduction of clean drinking water and improved sanitation. Medical advances along with the inception of the NHS have also contributed, with increased understanding, knowledge and public health-based initiatives. For example, the national immunisation programme is a key preventative measure in reducing illness and death from vaccine-preventable diseases in young children and in other risk groups. Infant mortality is a good indicator of the overall health of a society, and while the latter rates are at an all time low, and falling, there are widening variations among social groups. The UK is lagging behind other European countries in respect of infant mortality, appearing 15th on the European Union league table.

The promotion of health for children/young people is one of the Government's top priorities and the focus of many initiatives across the four countries of the UK. We can see why when one compares the UK with Europe only to find that we have poorer outcomes for young people. For example, the UK has the highest rate of sexually transmitted infection rates in teenagers across Western Europe. Many of the Government targets are focused on tackling the underlying determinants of poor health and health inequalities, including poverty and access to good nutrition.

All practitioners have a responsibility to promote health. This book will increase understanding of the key determinants of health, disease prevention and health promotion so that practitioners are able to empower children/young people, as well as families, to make healthy lifestyle choices. Key issues featuring in today's press are covered such as binge drinking, smoking, teenage sexual health, obesity and the increasing rate of emotional and mental health problems amongst young people. Helpful tips, strategies and techniques are provided throughout for practitioners to consider when teaching and engaging children/young people in discussions about their health and the impact of their behaviours.

Written for students and practitioners, the subject matter (health promotion) of this book can clearly be seen as integral part of everyday nursing practice regardless of the setting in which one works with children, young people and their families. Congratulations to all the chapter authors, and the editor who have created a textbook that will, I am sure, be a standard reference for all child health nursing students, as well as those seeking to specialise in the field of health promotion and public health.

Fiona Smith
Adviser in Children/Young People's Nursing
Royal College of Nursing.

Acknowledgements

A special thank you to several individuals and organisations whose help has been invaluable – thank you.

Accident prevention

Karen thanks Dr Mike Hayes (Projects Director) and Katrina Phillips (Chief Executive) at the Child Accident Prevention Trust.

Baby play

Christine Coombes, Health Visitor
Derbyshire County PCT (formerly North Eastern Derbyshire PCT)
Sure Start: Creswell, Langwith/Whaley Thorns and Shirebrook

Child development

Sally Shearer, Senior Nurse, University Hospital Nottingham

Children/young people with disabilities and complex health care needs

Sarah Wilcock thanks her team – C.A.R.I.N 4 Families (continuing care and respite in Nottingham) for their support.

Health promotion in childhood diabetes

Helen thanks Dr Cynthia Woodhall, colleague and friend. Helen has found her dedication to paediatric and adolescent diabetes inspiring. Helen also thanks the fantastic children, young people and their families she has worked with.

Living with teenagers

For their part in the development of the Living with Teenagers (LWT) programme, the following key personnel should be acknowledged:
North Eastern Derbyshire (NED) PCT, and High Peak and Dales PCT for funding the initial LWT

pilot courses and for ongoing support in continuation of the programme.

The LWT team, particularly facilitators and participants for their part in delivering and shaping the programme.

Mandy Chambers (Assistant Director of Public Health) NED PCT for her continued support and encouragement.

Rosie Brown – freelance public health consultant for her part in devising the original LWT training materials.

NED Health Promotion for their part in developing and piloting of the original LWT materials.

The design and print team of NED East Derbyshire District Council.

All agencies that support the programme in any way, thank you.

National perspectives

Wales
Karen Healey, formerly Senior Nurse Children's services, Bro Morgannwg NHS Trust
Carwen Earles, Academic Lead for Public Health and Primary Care at Swansea University

Preventing childhood obesity

Cheryl and Liz thank Fenella Lindsell, Director of YogaBugs Ltd.

Preventing substance misuse

Richard Goad, DARE, UK

Sure Start community children's nursing service

Janet Badcock,
Christine Barber,
Zo'e Ellis,
Jo Kirk,
Trisha Owen,
Vanessa Roberts,
Hilary Saunders,
Derbyshire County PCT (formerly North Eastern Derbyshire PCT)
Sure Start: Creswell, Langwith/Whaley Thorns and Shirebrook (children's centre)

Reducing deaths and inequalities in childhood

Roderick Thomson thanks Professor Mark Bellis and Dr Karen Tocque from the North West Public Health Observatory, the Association of Public Health Observatories and the Department of Public Health Sefton PCT for their assistance.

Finally, thanks to Roger Kirkbride (Pharmacist) and Ali Wright (Nurse Specialist, University Hospital Nottingham) for all their help and support. Thank you also to Fiona Smith (RCN Adviser in Children's/Young People's Nursing) for her help during the initial stages of the book.

Special thanks to Derbyshire County PCT who have given kind permission for many examples of their good practice to be shared.

Derbyshire County NHS
Primary Care Trust

Thank you also to my family, Simon and Lucy, for their patience.

Introduction

Welcome to *Promoting Health in Children/Young People: The Role of the Nurse*. This is a practical textbook designed for nurses working with children, young people and their families. Other practitioners may find it useful too, such as nursery nurses and teachers.

The book covers a wide range of health issues within its 13 themes. Each theme contains a number of chapters, or simply one chapter. Each chapter focuses on a key health issue, as well as different teaching methods to promote the health of children/young people. Each chapter provides its own references list, and some chapters provide details of additional resources that the reader may find useful.

Many different health issues have been presented in this book. Too many perhaps, but children/young people find themselves in all kinds of situations, from minor health issues to much more serious situations. All these health issues require some kind of health promotion input. Nurses have an important health promotion role to play in each and every one of these situations.

The National Service Frameworks (NSFs) for children, young people and maternity services (Education and Skills, Department of Health, 2004) provide an important foundation for the basis of this book; featured at the beginning of most chapters is a link with the NSFs. Clear links are thus provided for the reader on how recommendations contained within the NSFs can be associated with practice.

It is important to think about the NSFs for Northern Ireland, Scotland, Wales and England, as they provide an essential foundation for the future development of health services for children/young people in the United Kingdom (UK). Dr Sheila Shribman recently highlighted that although good progress is being made in line with the NSFs, there is still much to be achieved for children/young people (Shribman, 2007). This book may provide you with some ideas.

The purpose of this book

The intention of this textbook is to provide a practical approach to health promotion. This book looks at theory, as many health promotion textbooks do, but the subtle difference is that strong links are made with working examples from practice. The book hopefully demonstrates to nurses how health promotion is and can be incorporated as part of normal everyday nursing practice.

It was felt by many contributing to this book that health promotion is an implicit part of practice. However, sometimes nurses do not realise this, particularly when they first begin to practice. Health promotion may seem complex, yet it is easier than some sources portray. This book hopefully demonstrates that health promotion can be quite fun, interesting and not altogether too complex, especially when working with children/young people.

Many of the chapters are written by nurses who are very experienced within their own field for which they have provided a contribution to the book. Contributions have been received from a variety of other professions too, such as teaching, general practice, pharmacy, nursery nursing and organisations who work alongside health professionals. I have learnt a great deal myself from reading their contributions, and hope you will find them equally interesting and useful in your health promotion practice.

Change

Change is a constant theme that emerges in health care. This book therefore has to be viewed in light of the context it was written in. Political influences obviously have an important bearing on health. The book was written at a time when much policy activity had just taken place for children/young people. This included the NSFs for children, young people and maternity services (Education and Skills, Department of Health, 2004) and Every Child Matters (Education and Skills, 2003/4), not to forget the Children Act (2004).

Undertaking health promotion with children/young people

When putting together your own health promotion activity, on a specific health promotion subject, different resources will need to be examined. The use of books, journals and recently published reports, related to your subject, will all be essential resources. The internet can provide rapid access to some materials, and introduce you to organisations, such as charity organisations, that can provide really useful information, as well as ideas for health promotion activities.

Once you have that information, you need to think about what you might do with it, based on an understanding of health promotion. So what is health promotion all about for children/young people? The following outlines some insights.

Hall and Elliman (2003) describe health promotion as any planned activity which is designed to improve physical or mental health, and prevent disease, disability or premature death. There are many and varied descriptions of health promotion, which provide slightly different interpretations of the term. In this context the above serves us well. Fundamentally, health promotion is about helping children/young people to take an interest in improving their own health now and for their future well-being. For young children, much health promotion activity is invested in parents and carers; encouraging them to create a healthy start for their children.

Health promotion is thus about working with individuals – children, young people and their families. It is also about working with groups in local communities and participating in national campaigns to improve health. Health promotion may take place in communities and hospitals, as well as other settings. It is also about collaborating with other practitioners to create better services for families.

The *determinants* of health are factors which can influence children's/young people's health. They can have a significant impact. The following have been highlighted by the Government in recent reports as key determinants of health (Department of Health, 2004, 2006):

- Socio-economic and geographical location.
- Smoking, including second-hand smoke, which impacts on children's health.
- Obesity.
- Sexual health, involving risk-taking behaviours.
- Mental/emotional health, which can also influence physical health.
- Alcohol consumption.

These determinants may have an impact on health in the short-term. Crucially, they can be storing up health problems for later.

Activity

You might want to think about some of the determinants of health in your own life. Looking at these determinants of health in your own life can help you to understand how different factors impact on the lives of children/young people.

There are different *dimensions* to health that need considering too. Ewles and Simnett (2005) outline these different dimensions to health:

- Physical health (body).
- Mental and emotional health (thoughts and emotions).
- Social (interactions with others).
- Spiritual (beliefs).
- Societal (health of the society in which the individual lives).

With the dimension *societal health*, for example, children living in a country where war and famine exist may be unhealthy, due to the situation which is happening around them.

Disease prevention is often associated with health promotion. Disease prevention is sometimes considered in terms of *primary, secondary* and *tertiary prevention* (Hall and Elliman, 2003). The aim here is to generally prevent a specific disease or group of diseases (Hall and Elliman, 2003). Primary prevention could include reducing the incidence of a disease through immunisation or health promotion. Secondary prevention can involve the detection of disease through screening tests, thus reducing the impact of the disease through early detection. Tertiary prevention is about limiting the impact of a disease once it is present.

Once you have an understanding of health promotion, along with your subject information, what do you need to consider in relation to presenting? To present health promotion successfully with children/young people and their families, nurses must have an understanding about the following:

- Child development.
- Communication.
- Children learning and teaching children.

An understanding of *child development* is essential. Nurses must have some understanding about what to expect from children/young people at different ages. For example, nurses need to know how children/young people think, their emotions, and what to expect behaviourally from them. Of course, their development does not remain static; it is constantly changing, moving on. Significantly too, children/young people are not all functioning in the same way, at a similar age; children will differ. This book considers children from birth right through to the end of adolescence.

Communication is a really essential issue for nurses if they want their health promotion activities to have an impact. If nurses are not able to communicate with individuals effectively, no matter what they do or say, it will fail to impact positively. Care always needs to be taken.

It is very easy for messages to be misunderstood or misinterpreted, particularly in situations that might be stressful or emotional. For instance, when a child or young person is ill in hospital, parents/carers will be very concerned. Messages delivered with empathy and sensitivity can make such a difference.

It is useful for nurses to reflect upon their interactions with families, and consider how their communication skills can be improved. Hall and Elliman (2003) agree that for health promotion to be successful a practitioner's interpersonal skills should be developed to a very high level. No matter how experienced a nurse becomes, it is valuable to continue to reflect upon one's communications with families. The book discusses communication in a number of different chapters.

To help ensure health promotion messages have a successful impact, different *teaching* methods can be used, which will add variety. Nurses also need to have some understanding about how children/young people learn, so appropriate *learning* strategies can be applied to health promotion activities. The book explores teaching and learning, particularly in the chapters on planning health promotion, and child development.

When presenting health promotion activities, the issues of child development, communication, learning and teaching all come together, as well as knowledge of health promotion itself. Communications need to be appropriate for children's/young people's age and ability. Information should be presented in different ways, essentially in ways that will enable children/young people to understand. For example, young children will prefer pictures and limited amounts of information to aid their understanding. Conversely, teenagers will require more detail and discussion to enable them to explore different viewpoints. The book considers delivering health promotion information to different age groups, using different teaching methods.

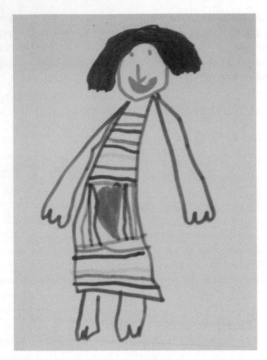

Figure 1   Feeling healthy by Lucy Bee.

With young children, for example, drawings can be useful to find out what they have learnt from the activities that you have undertaken with them. Figure 1 depicts a child's drawing following a health promotion activity about feeling healthy.

Health promotion thus involves a variety of different knowledge and skills, coming together, in the delivery of health promotion practice. This book provides some of that knowledge, as well as maybe the inspiration for nurses to go on to develop their skills.

Childhood in a contemporary context

Childhood in Britain today brings with it generally better lifestyles, but some limitations compared to several decades ago. Due to parental fears about child safety from traffic problems and wariness of strangers, for example, bringing what Brooks (2006) describes as *containment*. Children do not have the same freedoms that we might associate with several decades ago. It is not so easy for children to play in their local neighbourhoods as it once was.

Containment can impact upon health. Travelling to school by car, for example, is a normal way of life for many children. Yet, it places limitations on children's opportunities for exercise and social interaction. Children are not able to experience the physical benefits of walking to school. They also miss out on social interactions that might naturally occur en route to school. Parents may not always realise the limitations that driving to school imposes, in an effort to safeguard their children. However, there may be no realistic alternative.

E-communications have a significant influence on young people in today's Britain. E-mail communications and the ability to access so much information via the internet has profoundly influenced the way we live. Young people especially love their mobile phones, particularly *texting*, which has become skill, an art all of its own. Yet, dangers can present themselves here too. Information can spread very quickly, messages that may be unkind or untrue. Young people may find that they are not communicating with the person they think. The Government is currently looking into what can be done to protect children/young people from dangers imposed by e-communications.

Children's/young people's health, at the beginning of the twenty-first century, shows improvements, but there are also some persistent problems, as well as the development of new health issues. There are improvements in infant mortality rates. There are improvements too with child poverty, but this problem still persists. There is a reduction in deaths and serious injuries from road accidents. However, childhood obesity has crept upon us and brings with it many health promotion challenges.

There are a number of targets that have been set by the Government to improve health in the UK. These targets relate to adults as well as children/young people. *Choosing Health* identifies six public health priorities (Department of Health, 2004). These include the following:

(1) Tackling inequalities (child poverty)
(2) Reducing the number people who smoke
(3) Reducing obesity
(4) Improving sexual health
(5) Improving mental health
(6) Reducing harm and sensible drinking

Behaviour impacts on health – drinking, smoking, eating in excess, as the targets illustrate. Health promotion activities are one way to tackle these priorities, which nurses need to consider. Crucially, nurses always need to work hard to understand the perspective of children, young people and their families. Nurses must not assume that the health behaviours outlined are easy to change.

A final thought

Although there may be many challenges ahead, it does not mean that they cannot be tackled in a positive, fun way, especially when working with children/young people.

My final comment has to be from children themselves. We will hear from a little group of children I know well. Three little girls (ages 7, 7 and 4 years) who are very fond of each other, and when they are happy their laughter is captivating. What do you like to do best, I asked? *Play, have fun and laugh together* was their response.

Some of these words are echoed in the work of Roald Dahl who knows how to captivate children. Dahl (2001) wrote in his book *Matilda* that children really love to laugh; they are not nearly as serious as adults. This thought, I believe, is one that you should take with you in your health promotion activities with children. So whatever health promo-

tion activities you are taking part in, try to make children laugh – they will love it, and may learn something from it too. You will undoubtedly help to make the experience a more memorable one for them. Enjoy!

Karen Moyse

References

Brooks, L. (2006) *The Story of Childhood, Growing Up in Modern Britain*. London: Bloomsbury Publishing Plc.

Children Act (2004) London: Crown Copyright.

Dahl, R. (2001) *Matilda*. London: Puffin books.

Department of Health (2004) *Choosing Health: Making Healthy Choices*. London: Crown Copyright.

Department of Health (2006) *Health Profile for England*. London: Crown Copyright.

Education and Skills (Department of) (2003/4) *Every Child Matters*. London: Crown Copyright.

Education and Skills (Department of), Department of Health (2004) *National Service Framework for Children, Young People and Maternity Services*. London: Crown Copyright.

Ewles, L., Simnett, I. (2005) *Promoting Health*. Edinburgh: Baillière Tindall.

Hall, D., Elliman, D. (ed.) (2003) *Health for All Children*, 4th edn. Oxford: Oxford University Press.

Shribman, S. (2007) *Children's Health, Our Future. A Review of Progress Against the National Service Framework for Children, Young People and Maternity Service 2004*. Department of Health. London: Crown Copyright.

Theme 1

Foundations of Health Promotion with Children/Young People

Chapter 1   Reducing Health Inequalities

Chapter 2   Planning for Health Promotion

Chapter 3   Creativity

Chapter 4   Government Policy

1

Reducing Health Inequalities

Roderick P. M. Thomson

NSF

The aim of the National Service Frameworks (NSFs) for children, young people and maternity services (Education and Skills, Department of Health, 2004) is about setting standards that will help to tackle inequalities, addressing the particular needs of children, their families and communities, who are likely to achieve poor outcomes.

Introduction

In most cultures children/young people are seen as special and held in high regard by their families, the local community and the state. As children/young people are the future of a family and a nation, children and child welfare are often the topic of political debate and policy. The United Kingdom (UK) could be held up as an example of this; child and young people focused, as an examination of the political party manifestos over the past 30 years will show. Whether it is education in schools, the reform of the Child Support Agency or the development of new safeguarding arrangements following a child abuse inquiry, the health and well-being of children/young people are topics that strike a cord with parents, politicians and the population at large.

In this chapter the interlinked topics of *health inequalities* and *childhood deaths* are explored. In the first section of this chapter, patterns and causal factors of health inequalities are considered. The second section looks at how national policies can be translated into local action by the National Health Service (NHS) and its partner agencies. Interventions are illustrated by examining one part of North West England.

National perspective

Health inequalities

In 2003 the UK Government published its action plan for tackling health inequalities (Department of Health, 2003). Tony Blair in his foreword to this publication stated: 'Our society remains scarred by inequalities. Whole communities remain cut off from the greater wealth and opportunities that others take for granted', and he went on to say, 'We have to start to tackle this health gap' (Department of Health, 2003, p. 1).

The plan sets out the complex social and economic factors that were the causes of these inequalities. The Government's aim was to reduce health inequalities by looking at the wider determinants of health – poverty, poor educational outcomes, unemployment – and the problems of disadvantaged communities.

In the UK, deaths of children/young people are unusual events, but sadly they do occur. In a review of child health by the Association of Public Health Observatories (APHO, 2006), over 16 500 deaths were recorded between 2002 and 2004 for children/young people under the age of 20 years in the UK:

- This equates to over 5500 deaths per year on average.
- The largest single-age group was children aged less than 1 year, accounting for 56% of the registered deaths.
- The second largest group consisted of young people aged 15–19 years, accounting for 21% of the registered deaths in this 3-year period.

So what are these health inequalities and what effect do they have on the life chances of children/young people? In its report on the patterns of health inequalities within the North West region of England, the North West Public Health Observatory highlights: 'A baby boy from Manchester has the lowest life expectancy in England, at 72.3 years compared to 80.8 years in East Dorset, a difference of 8.5 years', and 'A baby girl from Blackburn with Darwen can expect to live until 77.9 in comparison to 85.8 years of a girl born in Kensington and Chelsea, a difference of 7.9 years' (Wood et al., 2006).

Both of these examples illustrate a fundamental point that even in the UK, one of the wealthiest nations on the planet, there are differences in the life chances of children born in different parts of the country. Two reports originally published in the 1980s identified the health gap between the richest and poorest communities within the UK. In 1980 the Black Report was produced by an independent working group to highlight that whilst the overall health of the population had improved, there was a growing gap between the least and most affluent in the country (Townsend and Davidson, 1992). These findings were reiterated in 1987 in the *Health Divide* (Whitehead, 1992).

These reports have become key reference tools to public health practitioners in the UK. Arguably, their value to health practitioners and the public at large was not that the publications highlighted a new discovery. The authors demonstrated clearly what most people knew instinctively, namely, that the more affluent you were, the greater the likelihood that you would live a longer and healthier life.

The Black Report was endorsed by Acheson (1998) in his *Independent Inquiry into Inequalities in Health Report*. This in itself has become a significant document, advocating effective interventions to tackle the wider influences on health inequalities.

In the context of child health, it was not just that a baby boy from Manchester would die at 72 years rather than 80 years. These independent reports confirmed that infant and child mortality rates were not just higher in the most deprived communities, but the gaps in the infant and child mortality rates for the least affluent and most affluent were widening.

To illustrate this point, consider three statistics listed by the Department of Health:

(1) The infant mortality rate among children in social class V in 1998–2000 was double that for social class I.
(2) Children in social class V are five times as likely to suffer accidental death than their peers in social class I.
(3) The risk of residential fire death for children is much greater for those in social class V.

It can be seen from these examples that the difference between infant mortality rates in social class I and social class V is significant. Infant mortality rates for social classes III and IV, whilst lower than Class V, are higher than social class I. One of the causes for this variation in life chances becomes apparent from studying the other two statistics presented. Statistics 2 and 3 reveal the higher risk to children in lower social classes from accidents. The causes of infant and child mortality are explored later in the chapter.

Defining social classes

As shown above, researchers have subdivided the UK population into several categories based on occupation. Although some of the occupations have changed over the years to reflect technological changes, the basic classification has essentially remained unchanged. The five classes are as follows (Drever and Whitehead, 1997):

(I)   Professional occupations
(II) Managerial and technical occupations
(III) Skilled occupations – non-manual and manual
(IV) Partly skilled occupations
(V)   Unskilled occupations

Government targets

To address these inequalities, the Government tasked the NHS with achieving significant changes in the life chances of local communities. In 2003 the Government's inter-departmental document, *Tackling Health Inequalities: A Programme for Action*, sets out the public service agreement targets to reduce key inequalities (Department of Health, 2003, p. 7):

- Public service agreement target: By 2010 to reduce inequalities in health outcomes by 10% as measured by infant mortality and life expectancy at birth.

This target has two objectives. Starting with children under 1 year, the Government wants to reduce, by at least 10%, the gap in mortality between manual groups and the population as a whole, to be achieved by 2010. The second objective is for local authorities to reduce, again by 10%, the gap between the fifth of areas with the lowest life expectancy at birth and the population as a whole, by 2010.

The UK Government also identified a target in relation to road traffic accidents. By 2010 it wants to see a reduction in the number of people killed in road accidents by 40% and the number of children killed or seriously injured reduced by 50%, compared with the average for 1994–1998 (Department of Transport PSA5, 2006).

Causes of death in different age groups

The following provides details on the causes of death amongst children/young people. Data have been obtained from the APHO (2006). It relates specifically to 2002–2004 for England, but there are similarities with other parts of the UK. The original source for some of the data reported by the APHO (2006) was sought from the Office of National Statistics, annual death extracts – http://www.statistics.gov.uk

Infant mortality

Definition – number of deaths at ages under 1 year per thousand of live births (APHO, 2006).

For children from birth to 1 year, the majority of deaths were due to immaturity and congenital abnormalities. Approximately 37% of the deaths were linked to immaturity with congenital abnormalities responsible for around 16% of deaths (APHO, 2006).

For immature babies with birthweight of under 1500 g, the mortality rates are 104 times higher than normal-birthweight babies. For babies over 1500 g but below 2500 g, the mortality rate is still 22 times higher than normal-birthweight infants (APHO, 2006). The APHO (2006) review of child health indicators also noted that low-birthweight babies were at greater risk of sudden infant death syndrome when compared to normal-birthweight children. The evidence suggests that they are four times more likely to suffer sudden infant death syndrome than those babies of normal birthweight.

Ethnicity was also identified as factor in infant mortality by the APHO (2006). Their analysis of the data points out that low-birthweight babies were more common amongst Asian mothers than other cultural groups.

Infant mortality data are commonly classified under two main headings: those occurring from live birth to 27 days and then from 28 days until 1 year of age. The APHO (2006) maintains that two-thirds of infant deaths occurred in the 0- to 27-day period, known as the neonatal period.

Causes of mortality in children and young people

Causes of mortality – in children aged 1–4 years per 100 000 of the population and in persons under 20 years per 100 000 of the population (APHO, 2006).

For children aged from 1 to 10 years, the commonest causes of death were unintentional injury, congenital abnormalities, cancer and diseases of the nervous system (APHO, 2006). As highlighted above, accidental injury was the greatest cause of childhood death, which includes transport accidents, drowning, choking, suffocation and fire. The highest figures of unintentional injury were reported amongst the most disadvantaged groups in the population.

As the causes of these deaths were accidental then they were potentially preventable. It should be remembered that as well as causing deaths, accidents are also a cause of non-fatal injuries amongst more children. Interventions, therefore, that reduce the number of deaths are also likely to reduce the number and severity of such injuries too.

Most deaths due to congenital abnormalities were more common in the first year of life; however, 15% of deaths in 1- to 4-year-olds were also due to congenital abnormalities. Cancer, as a cause of death in childhood, is a relatively rare factor, accounting for approximately 14% of deaths in children aged 1–4 years (APHO, 2006). Conditions affecting the nervous system accounted for another 14% of deaths amongst this age group. Particularly important amongst these diseases in terms of prevention are meningitis and encephalitis.

For children/young people in the 5- to 14-year-old age group, around 26% of the deaths were due to injury, with a further 25% of deaths due to neoplasm. Just over 30% of the childhood cancers were due to leukaemia. Brain and spinal tumours account for a further 25% of childhood cancers. In the case of injury, road traffic accidents were the cause of approximately half of the deaths. Most of the serious injuries or deaths occurred when children/young people were pedestrians. Cycling accounted for almost 15% of serious or fatal injuries in children.

Ethnicity would also seem to have a bearing in relation to road accidents. There have been some studies which suggest that there may be a higher rate of child pedestrian accidents amongst minority ethnic communities (APHO, 2006).

Amongst young people in the 15- to 19-year age group, injuries accounted for 56% of deaths. Most of these were related to transport injuries. Other leading causes of death included self-harm 18% and neoplasms 13%. The marked rise in deaths from accidents in this age group compared to the other age groups, along with deaths from self-harming behaviour, highlights the increase in risk-taking behaviour associated with this age group.

It can be seen that there are a range of factors which have a bearing on the life chances of children and young people. The second section of this chapter explores how some of these factors can be tackled by local initiatives.

Local interventions

The following will outline some health initiatives that have taken place in Sefton. Just north of Liverpool, in the North West England, is the metropolitan borough of Sefton. Its total population is almost 290 000. Almost 25% of the population is under the age of 20 years. In the south of Sefton there are higher levels of deprivation, with several parts of this area falling within the 20% of least deprived electoral wards in England (Sefton Health, 2004). Deaths in children (birth – 14 years) have been decreasing from a rate of 4.1 per 100 000 in 1994–1996 to 1.13 in 1997–1999.

Reviewing their accident prevention policy in 2003, the local primary care trusts and the local authority took stock of their plans to reduce accidents in the light of a new report, *Preventing Accidental Injury – Priorities for Action* (Department of Health, 2002). This report highlighted the following short-term priority areas:

- Falls at or near home.
- Road accidents.
- Dwelling fires.
- Play and recreation.

In response to the new guidance, a Sefton Injury Prevention Strategy was launched in 2003. The 5-year strategy focused on the development of projects and schemes to reduce accidents, affecting children in the home, school and community. Sometimes described as a *settings approach* to a public health issue, the strategy aimed to use local accident data to influence changes in these settings.

Set out over leaf are the main settings identified by agencies where accidents occurred in Sefton. Also included are the specific priority areas they believed needed to be addressed to reduce serious injury or death amongst children/young people.

It is easy to see how the strategy could call upon the knowledge and skills of local health visitors and school nurses to play a part in accident prevention. However, the strategy was not going to be limited to these branches of nursing. For example, district nurses, whilst home visiting, were being called upon to provide advice to elderly patients and their carers. Although the main focus of their advice was towards reducing accidents amongst older people, there was also the opportunity to provide advice for grandchildren if any were present in the home.

Practice nurses or nurses staffing walk-in centres or accident and emergency departments were also in a position to provide advice to parents/carers, children/young people. This type of prevention would, of course, be a secondary prevention message, as the child/young person or parent/carer was attending the surgery or department as a result of an injury. Nonetheless, there was a clear opportunity to discuss how to prevent further injuries occurring to the patient, as well as other members of the family.

The information below identifies the key settings and priorities for local action.

Setting	Priority Area
● School/college	Risk taking behaviour Environmental risk Policy and practice
● Home	Physical home safety Safety awareness
● Neighbourhood	Reducing injuries to child pedestrians Drivers exceeding speed limits Use of seat belts Safe play areas Development of derelict sites and void properties

The settings approach to health promotion has been described by Ashton and Seymour (1993) in their book, *The New Public Health*.

Sure Start

To help improve the health of children in Sefton and to reduce accidents, the borough partners welcomed the opportunity provided by the Government to create Sure Start centres, in several of the most deprived electoral wards in the borough. Sure Start is a UK Government programme which aims to achieve better outcomes for children, particularly

those under 4 years of age. It also aims to help parents/carers and communities by the following:

● Increasing the availability of childcare for all children.
● Improving health and emotional development of younger children.
● Supporting parents/carers in their aspirations towards employment.

Three overarching aims underpinned these developments:

(1) Better outcomes for all children, particularly closing the gap in outcomes between children living with a single parent/carer and the wider child population
(2) Better outcomes for all parents/carers, increased opportunity to participate effectively in the labour market, ensuring pathways out of poverty and strengthen families and communities
(3) Better outcomes for communities, including less crime, higher productivity, a stronger labour market and the building of a civic society

Further information can be found on these aims by accessing the Sure Start website – http://www.surestart.gov.uk

Writing in the borough's public health report for 2004, Linda Turner, the lead officer for accident prevention, described how the local accident prevention strategy was developing and the key role Sure Start was playing (Sefton Health, 2004). Turner (Sefton Health, 2004) highlighted that injury data had shown a high level of risk to children living in deprived communities. Sure Start centres were used as focal points for developing new skills and knowledge amongst parents/carers and children/young people.

For preschool children, who were unable to assess risk for themselves, the focus of the accident prevention campaign was their parents/carers. A programme called *Beany Bump* was provided. It includes training for parents/carers, a resource pack containing useful information and checklists, as well as a starter pack with safety devices. A safety equipment scheme enabled parents/carers to purchase larger items such as safety gates and fireguards at cost price. Initial findings suggest that there has been a slight decrease in the number of accidents to children under five, which may be linked to these interventions.

Road safety

For children/young people of school age, the injury prevention programme switched its focus to the children/young people themselves. With this programme the aim was to reduce risk-taking behaviour. It focused on locations frequented by children/young people. The campaign known as *Think On* publicised its risk-reduction messages at bus stops, in schools and youth clubs, and in other places used by young people. The campaign also targeted road safety as many of the accidents to children were related to traffic.

Children from low-income households are more likely to live near main roads, more likely to play by or in roads (due to the lack of safe places to play) and to walk rather than travel by car. It is not surprising then that four out of every five pedestrian or cycle accidents involving children/young people can occur within 1 km of their home. Led by the borough council, efforts were made to create safer play areas closer to the communities where most children lived. A range of other measures were introduced to reduce accidents, including the following:

- Traffic calming and pedestrian crossings.
- Marked pedestrian and cycle routes to improve access.
- Improved lighting.
- Education and training initiatives.

Key players in all these local initiatives have been nurses. In some cases they have played leading roles in the development of programmes. The primary care trusts in Sefton took the innovative step several years ago to invest in a Public Health Neighbourhood Nursing scheme. Community nurses from a range of backgrounds were freed up from some of their clinical caseload duties to enable them to work more closely with small local communities. The new responsibilities of the neighbourhood nurses

included carrying out local needs assessments and leading health promotion programmes on such issues as accident prevention, positive parenting and healthy eating.

Needs assessments have taken two forms: the first focuses on assessing the needs of a community, whilst the second focuses on assessing the needs of individual children/young people. Techniques such as health equity audits can be used to assess the vulnerable groups, particularly how they access health services within a community. As part of *Every Child Matters* (Education and Skills, 2003), the Government published a new tool for assessing the needs of an individual child or young person. Known as the common assessment framework (Education and Skills, 2006), this tool enables a wide range of practitioners to carry out a holistic needs assessment of an individual child, taking into account family and environmental factors.

One of the local health promotion initiatives on healthy eating and accident prevention included in the Neighbourhood Nursing scheme was *Health Sac*. A public health neighbourhood nurse adapted a scheme used by a primary school in her area to incorporate health promotion material. The material was provided in such a way that the school children and their parents/carers could share learning about health issues such as *5 a Day* (Department of Health, 2004), first aid and injury prevention. The scheme was very popular with all concerned and has been extended to all the neighbourhood regeneration areas of Sefton.

Tackling lifestyle factors

In another initiative the neighbourhood nurses took part in a survey which explored the views of local children/young people about their knowledge on a range of lifestyle issues. Known as *Rampworx*, the information from the survey has informed health promotion programmes, ensuring that they run in partnership with children/young people. Themes include avoiding/reducing use of alcohol, smoking and preventing sexual health problems. The aim of these health promotion programmes is to equip young people with age-appropriate knowledge and skills to safeguard their future health and well-being.

Reducing smoking amongst young women was felt to be important. It can have a long-term impact on infant mortality as nearly two-thirds of teenage mothers smoke before pregnancy and around 50% smoked during it. Of the modifiable risk factors in relation to preventing low-birthweight babies, reducing smoking is seen as a key area for nurses to intervene either to prevent young women from taking up smoking or helping them to stop. Combined with initiatives such as the *Back to Sleep* campaign (Department of Health, 2007), smoking cessation programmes have helped to reduce the number of cases of sudden infant deaths significantly.

The examples above illustrate the coordinated and multi-layered approach that is needed to reduce the factors that could injure or kill children/young people. These health promotion activities need to be sustained in order to protect each child and young person as they grow.

Conclusion

The causes of health inequalities are complex and deep rooted. Health inequalities affect the life chances of children/young people in terms of early death or in life years lost in adulthood. Such inequalities have been linked to poverty and social class. These variations in health opportunities can be seen across the UK. Both the causes and the effects of such inequalities can be altered by concerted action at national and local levels. In the UK, the Government has set targets for the NHS and other statutory agencies to reduce health inequalities. At local level, nurses can make a major contribution to improving the health chances of children/young people through health promotion initiatives. To maximise their contribution, nurses need to have knowledge about the causes of health inequalities and their potential impact on the health of children and young people. Nurses also need knowledge of the health promotion techniques that can be used to assist children/young people and their parents/cares to reduce the chances of serious injury, illness or even death. The role of nurses in caring for children/young people must begin with pre-vention. As the largest group of health care practitioners, nurses are well placed to make a significant difference to the life chances of children/young people.

Resources

http://www.apho.org.uk
http://www.dft.gov.uk
http://www.everychildmatters.gov.uk
http://www.isdscotland.org/isd/4339.html
http://www.nwpho.org.uk
http://www.statistics.gov.uk

References

Acheson, D. (1998) *Independent Inquiry into Inequalities in Health Report*. London: TSO.

Ashton, J., Seymour, H. (1993) *The New Public Health*. Milton Keynes: Open University Press.

Association of Public Health Observatories (APHO) (2006) *Indications of Public Health in the English Regions 5: Child Health*. York: Yorkshire and Humber Public Health Observatory.

Department of Health (2002) *Preventing Accidental Injury – Priorities for Action*. London: TSO.

Department of Health (2003) *Tackling Health Inequalities: A Programme for Action*. London: TSO.

Department of Health (2004) *5 a Day*. London: Crown Copyright.

Department of Health (2007) *Reducing the Risk of Cot Death*. London: Crown Copyright.

Department of Transport. Public Service Agreement (PSA) 5 (2006). In: Association of Public Health Observatories (APHO) *Indications of Public Health in the English Regions 5: Child Health*. York: Yorkshire and Humber Public Health Observatory

Drever, F., Whitehead, M. (1997) (eds) *Health Inequalities*. Decennial supplement: DS Series No. 15. London: TSO.

Education and Skills (Department of) (2003) *Every Child Matters*. London: Crown Copyright.

Education and Skills (Department of) (2006) *The Common Assessment Framework for Children and Young People: Practitioners' Guidance*. London: TSO.

Education and Skills (Department of), Department of Health (2004) *National Service Framework for Children, Young People and Maternity Services*. London: Crown Copyright.

Sefton Health (2004) *Annual Report of the Directors of Public Health*. Sefton, Merseyside: Sefton Primary Care Trusts.

Townsend, P., Davidson, N. (1992) The Black Report. In: Townsend, P., Whitehead, M., Davidson, N. (eds) *Inequalities in Health: The Black Report and the Health Divide*, 2nd edn. London: Penguin Books.

Whitehead, M. (1992) The Health Divide. In: Townsend, P., Whitehead, M., Davidson, N. (eds) *Inequalities in Health: The Black Report and the Health Divide*, 2nd edn. London: Penguin Books.

Wood, J., Hennell, T., Jones, A., Hooper, J., Tocque, K., Bellis, M. (2006) *Where Wealth Means Health*. Liverpool: North West Public Health Observatory.

2 Planning for Health Promotion

Karen Moyse

Introduction

Unexpectedly, you have been asked to present a health promotion session to a group of mothers on promoting young children's dental health. How are you going to do this? You know your subject, but are unsure how best to present it, in a way that the mothers will find both interesting and informative. This chapter provides a useful guide on how to plan for health promotion, so that you can competently develop such a session. The chapter includes details on *teaching methods* you might use as well as *resources* that might help. In addition, the chapter explores *learning strategies* that need to be considered when planning for others to learn new knowledge and skills.

Positive health behaviours

The purpose of health promotion with children/ young people is to encourage positive health behaviours. This is not only in the short-term during childhood, but long-term into adulthood too. Hopefully, laying the foundations for the rest of children's lives; attempting to establish attitudes and behaviours that will lead to healthier lifestyles. However, adopting a healthy lifestyle means change, which some children/young people might not want to consider.

For example, my young daughter is passionate about chocolate. Why does she love it so much? For the sheer pleasure of the taste, she tells me. What are the long-term consequences of her continuing to eat chocolate? Severe toothache and not such a pretty smile, at the very least I would suspect. She usually likes to have chocolate at the weekend, and more often if she can persuade me to buy it. How can I help her to change this habit?

I need to replace some of the chocolate with an alternative, such as fruit or cheese. She loves fruit, and cheese can be really great protection from tooth decay. Others, friends and family, give her chocolate too. I will also need to advise them of our new approach on *limited chocolate*, which I am not sure will go down too well. So in my efforts to improve her health, I will undoubtedly upset my daughter and other family members. To make this change, it is going to cost in my relationships with others and my daughter having to eat less of something she really enjoys. Do I really want to take up this challenge?

My example is only a very simple one. Nonetheless, to change behaviour costs, but at the same time it can also cost in terms of poor health if one fails to change behaviour. It is useful to think about our own health behaviours, as it can help us in understanding the situation for others. Certainly, for the children/young people we are working with, it may not be so simple to change behaviour. Changing behaviour can impact on all kinds of things in their lives, such as relationships with others, activities and routines.

Health promotion activities as learning events

It is useful to remember that health promotion activities are new learning events for those we are working with; new knowledge and skills, which may in some cases take time to learn. There is a need for patience and understanding with the giving and receiving of health promotion information, just as we would with any aspect of nursing. As practitioners we are the teachers or facilitators of those new learning events for children/young people and their families.

For ease of discussion within this chapter, those we undertake health promotion activities with, either on a one-to-one basis or in groups, will be called participants.

Empowerment

Empowerment is a term that is used frequently in relation to health promotion. Naidoo and Wills (1994) describe *empowerment* as an approach that is taken in health promotion to help individuals and communities to meet their own perceived needs.

Historically, approaches to health promotion have been quite directive. They have been expert-led, expecting participants to be passive and conforming (Naidoo and Wills, 1994). In more

Box 2.1 Your health behaviours.

- List your positive health behaviours.
- List your negative health behaviours.
- What do you need to change in terms of lifestyle in order to make yourself healthier?
- Consider the consequences to your health of not changing these negative behaviours.

recent years approaches to health promotion have been more empowerment driven. Here, there is much more negotiation and networking among all those involved (Naidoo and Wills, 1994). The facilitator of health promotion is less directive, and the group works together to reach agreed aims. The empowerment approach means that health promotion activities are delivered on more equal terms, allowing greater collaboration among all those involved.

If participants are expected to change their behaviour, as is often the aim of health promotion, it is better that everyone works together to achieve that aim. Telling participants that they need to change their behaviour will not necessarily achieve what you are hoping.

Social psychologists advocate that with behaviour change there is a need to examine participants' attitudes towards a specific behaviour (Ajzen and Fishbein, 1980). Attitudes are about participants' positive or negative feelings on an issue (Lloyd et al., 1984). An empowerment approach may help the development of positive attitudes amongst your participants, allowing them to explore their thoughts and feelings, rather than directing them.

Sometimes changing attitudes may stimulate a change in behaviour (Naidoo and Wills, 1994). Nonetheless, do not always expect a change in attitude to come about quickly, as attitudes are often built up over many years.

Learning involves three main psychological processes (Naidoo and Wills, 1994):

(1) Cognitive (thinking)
(2) Affect (feelings)
(3) Behavioural (doing).

The cognitive aspect incorporates a person's knowledge and information. The affective aspect is associated with emotions and feelings. Finally, the behavioural aspect is concerned with a person's skill (what she/he can do) (Naidoo and Wills, 1994). Attitudes can be changed by providing information or by increasing an individual's skills or by changing an individual's feelings on an issue.

With the empowerment approach the nurse works as the catalyst of change (Naidoo and Wills, 1994). The practitioner acts as the facilitator, getting things going and then withdrawing from the situation, allowing individuals to take over for themselves. As in the case of a home nursing service, the nurse gives information and support to help parents/carers with their sick child. Then the nurse withdraws at the point where parents/carers feel confident to manage the care of their sick child themselves.

Historical influences on the empowerment approach stem from the work of Freire (1972). He talks about abandoning the goals of purely depositing individuals with information. In its place Freire (1972) suggests an active dialogue among all group members, everyone becoming jointly responsible for the processes that occur together, discussing and sharing ideas.

Lawson (1979) highlights a cautionary note about the empowerment approach. If participants fail to put their thoughts into words, either because they do not want to, or are unable to do so, then it becomes difficult for the facilitator to progress with the empowerment approach. Some participants may therefore need encouragement to share their thoughts and ideas.

There are many health promotion models which provide ideas and explanations about heath-related behaviours and how to encourage positive changes in health. It is not the remit of this book to look at models of health promotion. The reason for this is that many health promotion texts already do this. However, providing details about the empowerment approach will be a valuable starting point in learning about health promotion.

Elements of planning and preparation

Planning and preparation are key components of the health promotion process (Daines et al., 1993). Good planning can make all the difference between success and failure of a health promotion activity or session. The following provides details on how you might plan for a session with parents/carers or older children.

Once it has been decided that you are going to be responsible for delivering a health promotion session, you need to consider the *what*, *when* and *where* – as they may need to be booked early:

- What – exactly what are you going to deliver, or do you need any outside speakers?
- When – date, time.
- Where – book a venue.

In relation to the time and venue, it is important to find out what are the best times for your participants and where are the most accessible locations. Not giving these issues sufficient consideration could result in very few participants turning up.

Developing publicity literature

There is a need to *publicise* your session so that potential participants are aware that it is happening. A leaflet or small poster can be produced quite simply. It will need to contain basic details. These can include the following:

- Course title.
- Something about the course.
- Who might find it useful.
- Venue, dates and timings.
- Who to contact for further information and where.
- Is there anything participants need to bring?
- Availability of refreshments.

The design needs to be eye-catching. Let simplicity be your golden rule – not too much information, not too many different pictures and colours. With the use of computer programmes, interesting designs can be created.

The content of the material can be developed in consultation with potential participants from the local community. Kai (1996) maintains that information is invariably defined by practitioners, with little or no consultation with parents/carers. Simple oversights can be avoided by involving participants in your design.

Perhaps participants can also be involved in the planning and preparation of your health promotion session. They could play a part in your planning meetings or perhaps help to inform the local community about your health promotion session. They might even be willing to help distribute some of the leaflets for you.

Publicise the session in local centres, such as general practitioner surgeries, shops, library and village hall. It can also be distributed at key local events. Remember before you put up any posters, you will need to seek permission. You do not want to upset anyone by putting up posters in a place where members of the local community feel they may be inappropriate.

Elements of planning

Daines et al. (1993) maintain that there are certain key elements to planning a session, which are outlined below:

- Needs.
- Aims.
- Objectives or outcomes.
- Content.
- Methods and resources.
- Evaluation, including assessment.

Needs

Ewles and Simnett (2005) have described several different types of need, which are outlined below:

- Normative need – this is based on the value judgements of practitioners. Falling short of this standard means that there is a need. Some normative needs can be expressed by law.
- Felt need – felt by the individual.
- Expressed need – what individuals say that they need. Expressed need can potentially conflict with the judgement of practitioners.
- Comparative need – a need identified by making a comparison between similar groups.

When considering need it is not only about individual need, or the need of a group of individuals, but can be considered in terms of community need.

Community profiling is as a tool used by practitioners for community development work (Hawtin et al., 1998). When undertaking a community profile, practitioners are required to carefully identify the needs, usually health needs, of their local community (Hawtin et al., 1998). Through community profiling practitioners can then investigate the best ways to meet those needs, which may be the introduction of new services or the modernisation of existing ones. Community consultation is an essential part of the profiling process (Hawtin et al., 1998). Here, practitioners can find out what the community feel their needs actually are.

Considering needs in relation to a specific health promotion session, as we are here, explore with your participants what content and teaching methods they would like to see included that will help to meet their learning needs. This can be undertaken during your first session together, or if possible, in advance of coming together as a group.

Aims and objectives or outcomes

It is important that both participants and those teaching them are clear about what needs to be achieved (Daines et al., 1993). This can be discussed with the group assisted with the use of an aim (or aims) and objectives/outcomes.

The aim outlines the purpose of what needs to be achieved and can be used as a statement of intent (Daines et al., 1993). The aim is about where you are going with your participants in your health promotion work together. The aim is usually expressed in general terms.

Objectives/outcomes are different to aims. Objectives/outcomes are about how participants will get to where they are going. They are the stepping stones that lead towards the aim (Daines et al., 1993). Objectives/outcomes are very specific and say exactly what will be achieved.

Daines et al. (1993) express objectives/outcomes in terms of the following:

- Think (cognition).
- Feel (affect).
- Do (behaviour).

This reflects the different psychological processes involved in learning, as discussed earlier in the chapter.

Objectives/outcomes are expressed as verbs. Some of which might include the following:

- Think – compare, criticise.
- Feel – to be more aware of.
- Do – demonstrate, perform.

Other verbs that you might find useful include the following:

- Explain.
- Select.
- Identify.
- Recognise.

It is helpful to start writing a list of objectives/outcomes in the following way, *participants will be*

Box 2.2 Aim and objectives/outcomes for a dental health session.

Group: A group of 7-year-old children in school (10). Aim: To raise children's awareness about dental health, so children are able to competently care for their own teeth.

Participants will be able to do the following:

Objective 1: Explain different ways they can care for their teeth and why it is important.

Objective 2: Identify foods that are good and bad for teeth.

Objective 3: Demonstrate how to brush their teeth correctly.

able to, and then state exactly what you expect of them. Examine Box 2.2 for an example of presenting an aim and objectives/outcomes.

Daines et al. (1993) maintain that objectives/outcomes can help not only with planning, but also with evaluation. In relation to their use for evaluation purposes, consult Chapter 38.

It is useful to be able to talk through your objectives/outcomes, as well as aims, with your participants. This enables them to know what to expect. Importantly, present this information in language they can understand.

Remember that participants need time to digest this information. All too frequently objectives/outcomes, as well as aims, are written in ways that participants cannot understand. They are presented on a screen and then whisked away before participants have really had the time to digest them. They were not written in 2 minutes, which means participants need more than several seconds to digest them. Participants need time to think about them, particularly as they are going to be expected to achieve them. Perhaps go one better, and involve them in setting the aims and objectives/outcomes for your session.

Content

As already highlighted earlier in this chapter, provide your participants with the opportunity to discuss what they would like to see included in the session. Is there anything they would really like to know that will help them in the future?

With the content it is very tempting to provide lots of detail. Nevertheless, try to restrain yourself from doing so. As Daines et al. (1993) recommend, avoid giving out too much information. Your participants do not need to know everything on the subject. It is better to provide key information only. Consider what they really need to know in relation to the aim and the objectives/outcomes of the session.

Remember to define what you are talking about. Go on to present the content in a logical way, as this will help their learning. Give your session a beginning, middle and end. It may help to reiterate points and check understanding as you go along. If someone does not understand, try explaining in a different way. Remember to always provide opportunities for questions and comments. Finally, sum up at the end.

Think of interesting and fun ways to present your content. You do not have to be the only presenter, use outside speakers, specialists in different areas of practice, for example. Furthermore, provide members of the group, who may be specialists in their own area, with the opportunity to contribute something, if they are keen.

Teaching methods

There are lots of different teaching methods that you can use. It is not the remit of this book to provide an exhaustive list. However, a few of the main teaching methods will be discussed here. If you would like to know more about different teaching methods, there are specialist books available in this area. They can usually be located at university libraries in the teaching section. Daines et al. (1993) provide comprehensive information in their book. Rogers (1992) provides details in her book too. There are also teaching packages that can be obtained from your local health promotion library that will provide ideas on different teaching methods that can be used with children/young people.

The teaching methods that you opt for will depend on a number of different factors. These include the participants you are working with. In addition, the setting in which you are working is going to influence what you can and cannot achieve with your participants.

It is useful, and probably much more interesting for your participants, to opt for a small selection of different teaching methods during the same health promotion session. By using a combination of different teaching methods, the process can be more fun for everyone.

Daines et al. (1993) discuss teaching methods under three domains:

- Presentation – simply presenting information.
- Interaction – where knowledge and experiences are shared, such as discussions and questioning techniques.
- Search – where learners explore and discover information themselves. This can include individual case studies or collaborative tasks, for example.

Lectures/talks and demonstrations are presented here under *presentation*. With lectures/talks, information is presented by a speaker. Daines et al. (1993) maintain that there are a number of characteristics associated with a good lecture/talk. These include the following:

- Clarity/clear presentation.
- Logical organisation.
- Interest for participants.
- Emphasis on the important points.
- Involvement of listeners.
- Appropriate resources.

It is useful to remember that whatever the age of your participants some will find it difficult to concentrate for long periods. This is particularly true for young children. Importantly too, do not forget to bring interaction into your lecture/talk. Again this will make it more fun and interesting for everyone and help with attention. Interaction helps participants to learn from each other.

Demonstrations are another method. Daines et al. (1993) talk about two types of demonstration: *show* (I show you) or *do it with me* (we all do it together).

Be clear about what you are going to demonstrate and break it down into manageable chunks (Daines et al., 1993). Demonstration requires skill. You need to be talking to your participants whilst demonstrat-

ing, rather like the TV chefs, as they make their wonderful exotic dishes. Some practice with a friend may be a useful starting point.

Recently, I demonstrated bandaging techniques to a group of children. The children, a group of 8-year-olds, had a great time bandaging each other, under close supervision obviously. Occasionally they managed to tie each other in knots.

Interestingly, by asking your participants to have a go, you develop a clear understanding of their learning so far. Demonstration could perhaps be used as a basis for assessment, if you need to include one.

Some of the best teaching methods that can be used are *interactive* ones. You could perhaps try injecting interactive methods within your lecture/talk to spice it up a bit. Some interactive methods include the following:

- Discussion.
- Questioning techniques and quizzes.
- Role-play.
- Small group work.

Discussions are about meeting with others to share ideas and information. They can help participants reach a more in-depth understanding of health issues. As Rogers (1992) states, participants are exploring meanings together.

Rogers (1992) believes that discussion allows participants to respect the views of others, as well as to articulate their own views. However, not everyone will be happy to share their views and opinions. Daines et al. (1993) point out that not everyone is necessarily confident enough to join in a discussion.

From the experience of working in communities, where participants are not always confident to join in, it can be quite a delicate process drawing them into discussion. Think about ways of involving them, subjects that interest them perhaps. In minor illness sessions, for example, parents'/carers' experiences of caring for their children when sick would be a common way of drawing them into discussions. It needs to be voluntary; however, participants should never be made to feel that they have to say something. Willingness to join in usually comes as confidence grows, both individually and as a member of the group.

It is important to thank everyone for their involvement in discussions. Try to be particularly encouraging of those who do not regularly participate and have done so for the first time.

To trigger discussion initially, you may want to present information, such as a video featuring a case study perhaps. Daines et al. (1993) maintain that you can then structure your discussion with the use of various questions.

Remember room layout is important for a successful discussion. Participants need to be able to see each other and to feel that they can openly engage with one another. They need to be able to see the expressions on each others' faces. Non-verbal communications are as important as verbal ones, as the work of Argyle (1983) has demonstrated.

Questioning techniques are another interactive teaching method. They are really useful as they can be incorporated into anything you are teaching. Remember to ask your questions clearly, so participants understand what you are asking, which may involve repeating the question or writing it down. Also ensure that the actual answers to any questions are provided, and do not become lost in discussion. Answers can also be provided in written form, such as handouts.

A quiz is a really fun way of asking questions and ensures active participation. For participants who enjoy a touch of competition, try putting them into teams and see which team gets the most correct answers, and give them a prize. A quiz can also be used at the end of a course as a form of assessment. It can be a way of finding out how much your participants have learnt.

Role-play is another good teaching method; it can be fun as well as helpful for increasing understanding. Role-play is the acting out of a specific situation where individuals assume specific roles (Daines et al., 1993). It helps participants to understand situations from the perspective of others.

Care needs to be taken with role-play however. Some participants may be really keen to have a go, and do not mind how they appear. Others may be a little more apprehensive and might not wish to play the part of another character. It is important that as you are sensitive to how your participants feel.

Allow discussion to follow the role-play to help provide a greater understanding. Rogers (1992) believes that it is the most valuable method to use where behavioural skills are being taught.

In community practice I have used role-play to help children's nurses with behavioural skills, particularly communication skills. The focus taken was in relation to communicating health promotion messages to families in the home. We examined undesirable ways to communicate and then more appropriate ways to communicate the same message to families. Children's nurses were able to see the impact of their interactions on others, through the use of role-play.

Small group work is another teaching method that provides important scope for learning. Small groups carry out a specific task or activity together, where they can learn from each other (Daines et al., 1993).

Small group activities can be particularly useful where you have a large group. Being part of a really large group will inhibit some participants from communicating. However, if participants are given the opportunity to join in with small group activities, they will do so more readily.

Pairs activities can be really useful for taking an idea discussed in the main group onto a new level. Pairs activities, where two participants talk together using a worksheet to jot down their thoughts and ideas, are quite a useful addition to a lecture/talk. You will need to ensure that participants are discussing what is on the agenda however, and that not too much digressing is occurring. It can be quite enlightening nonetheless, when participants report back to the main group with many different opinions on the same health promotion issue, as well as opinions on issues you were not expecting.

The final category discussed by Daines et al. (1993) is *search*. This is where, following initial guidance from yourself, participants seek out information. They can either do this individually or in groups together.

Examples of search methods include case studies, diary accounts and visits. Case studies are able to bring health promotion issues alive (Daines et al., 1993). With the use of a diary, for example, participants can write down what they have experienced, reflect upon this, and bring it back to the main group for discussion (if they feel okay about sharing it).

Visits are another really interesting way to bring health promotion alive for your participants. They can go out as a group to a venue that is relevant to the subject being explored. For example, taking children preoperatively along to their local hospital for a visit may help to ease some of their apprehensions. For a small group of adolescents a trip to the local health promotion unit, to locate resources for project work, may be of interest. In both cases obviously seeking appropriate permissions first is going to be essential.

A variety of teaching methods have been suggested. A couple of extra points to consider before you opt for whatever methods you feel are the most suitable. Importantly, consider your own skills and abilities in managing your chosen teaching methods. In addition, remember to vary your teaching methods, do not stick to one method. Variety helps to keep your participants interested.

Resources

There are lots of different resources that you can use. As with teaching methods, it is not the aim to talk about them all here. What this section does is to provide an overview of some resources that can be used and where you might be able to seek them out, when putting a session together.

Devising your own resource is one approach that you might have considered. You may find the points made earlier about developing publicity leaflets useful. Putting together a simple handout or poster for a health promotion activity could be fun and interesting to do.

If you are thinking of developing a health promotion leaflet for use with families, this may be a little more demanding and time-consuming. It will have to be checked for appropriateness and quality, not only by potential users of such material, but also by other practitioners, managers, and the primary care trust clinical governance group, all of which takes time.

There are lots of ready prepared resources that you can access and use. Some places to go for resources include the local health promotion unit, websites, the children's section of your local library, as well as contacting specific charitable organisations that produce leaflets of their own.

Some resources to use include the following:

- Posters.
- Leaflets.
- Displays.
- Models.
- Books.
- Video clips/CD or DVD extracts.

- Games.
- Specialist equipment.
- Toys.

It is useful to have your own resource box, as suggested by Daines et al. (1993), within which you can keep all sorts of things you might need. If you keep the box with you at all times, then you have everything at hand when you need it.

The box might include the following:

- Art materials – labels, paper, pens, small card.
- Dressing up clothes.
- Hats.
- Music.
- Posters (something to stick them on with).
- Stickers/rewards.

Where to go for appropriate resources may need some consideration. See what you already have stored away or are there any monies needed to purchase additional materials. Some organisations may give you a certain number of leaflets free of charge.

Visit your local health promotion resource unit as they have resources that can be loaned out, if you are eligible to join their library. They also have lots of sources of information that you can consult. The health promotion unit can provide leaflets on a variety of health promotion issues, such as immunisation, accident prevention and sexual health, to name but a few. Your local community primary care trust will be able to provide contact details of your nearest health promotion resource unit.

Downloading resources from the internet is another alternative. The NHS Clinical Knowledge summaries website is a fantastic resource. It provides up-to-date evidence-based information on health. It has been developed to support health care practitioners, as well as patients, to be able to make informed decisions about health (NHS Institute for Innovation and Improvement, 2008), and can be accessed via http://www.cks.library.nhs.uk. In addition, it produces some excellent patient information leaflets, which are presented on a wide range of health conditions. Look under the category of child health. Some of the conditions in this category are outlined in Box 2.3.

Another useful internet resource is the NHS National Electronic Library for Health, where child health information can be located. This can be accessed through the following website – http://www.nelh.nhs.uk/.

The library provides access to a wide range of topics related to the health and well-being of children/young people (NHS National Library for Health, 2006). It is mainly aimed at health practitioners. Parts of the library can only be accessed if you are an Athens user. You will need to provide your Athens account details to access these areas (NHS National Library for Health, 2006).

Another useful website is NHS Direct online – http://www.nhsdirect.nhs.uk. It is a self-help guide for patients and their families. NHS Direct (2006) states that it covers the most common symptoms that people who call them ask for advice on. It takes a condition and provides a small amount of information in relation to that condition (see Box 2.4).

The selected links at the end of their lists are quite useful, as they take the reader on to other websites for further information.

Local libraries are a source you might not have thought about. The children's section may be quite useful. Here you might find a variety of different books for children about specific health issues. During one of my recent trips, I found books on asthma, eczema, infectious diseases and children

going into hospital for minor operations, which children would be able to read themselves.

Once you have all your resources, and know what content you plan to present, you will need to consider how you are going to *present* it. There are a variety of multimedia sources that can be used:

- Acetates – coloured acetates, coloured typefaces, different typefaces and images.
- Flip charts.
- Photographs.
- Powerpoint.
- Video.
- Whiteboard – incorporates multimedia.

Think about how you can use these multimedia resources. If you are unsure how to use a particular resource, learn how.

The way you use resources is important. For example, you might want to use a video that is 40 minutes long. This may be too long to play continuously for your group. Break it up into sections. Ask your participants to look out for specific things in each section. Different groups of participants could be looking for different things. Then, in between each section have a discussion about what they have identified.

Evaluation, including assessment

The final aspect to consider in relation to Daines et al.'s (1993) elements of planning is evaluating your session. The process of evaluation is about finding out if your health promotion session has achieved all it set out to achieve. *Did participants learn what they needed to know? Did they find the session interesting? What were their feelings generally about it?*

It is essential to evaluate as it informs you as the facilitator what has worked well, and what needs modifying. The process of evaluation will provide ideas about what can be included in future health promotion activities.

A typical way to evaluate with older children and adults, who are able to read, is to provide your participants with a form to complete, which asks a series of questions about your health promotion session. Participants do not need to identify who they are on the form. This enables participants to write how they feel without having to identify themselves. Following this, a discussion can take place with the group as a whole, where participants can talk about any specific points. With children, a much simpler approach needs to be taken. Just spend a few minutes exploring with them, if they liked it. Children will give you an honest answer. Perhaps get them to draw a simple picture about how they felt, using facial expressions.

Armed with participants' verbal, written and drawn responses, you are then able to put together a report, which can be presented to your management team. The management team will then have a clear idea about how your health promotion session was viewed by participants, which will influence their decision about further funding.

Having considered how to evaluate your health promotion session, you may want to also consider *assessment*. The process of assessment is about finding out exactly what your participants have learnt. This can be undertaken in a variety of ways, such as a quiz or a question and answer session, or a small piece of homework perhaps. Depending on the nature of your health promotion session, it may not be appropriate to include an assessment. Assessment strategies are further discussed in Chapter 38.

Teaching plans

All the elements that Daines et al. (1993) discuss for the planning process can be concisely included in a teaching plan. The teaching plan does not need to be in great depth, but should just include sufficient information to provide yourself, and any other interested parties, insight into what you have planned. Box 2.5 provides an example.

Cognitive processes and learning strategies

Psychology is the study of human behaviour (Lefrançois, 1994). Developmental psychology is concerned with how behaviour changes over the passage of time (Lefrançois, 1994); studying how children/young people grow and develop as they become older. As practitioners much of our time is spent interacting with children/young people,

helping them to learn about positive health behaviours. Our approach needs to change according to the age group we are working with. In addition, we are supporting and working with their parents/carers. Not only do we have the learning needs of children/young people to consider, but also their parents/carers too.

This section of the chapter focuses on *learning strategies* that may be common to all ages. The cognitive processes that underlie these learning strategies will be considered. Being aware of these cognitive processes and learning strategies will enable you to be more effective in the delivery of health promotion. Chapter 5 provides more detail, specifically in relation to the cognitive processes of children/young people.

The following processes will be considered:

- Motivations.
- Senses.
- Attention.
- Memory.
- Communication – rewards and praise.

Motivations

Consideration must first be given to what motivates your participants. Their motivation, or lack of it, will impact upon how they will approach your health promotion session. For instance, whether participants feel they need or want to know about it.

Motivation will vary according to circumstances. For example, a mother who is caring for a young child unwell at home with a high temperature and unsure what to do is likely to be motivated to know more. She will want to learn what can be done to bring her child's temperature down. Conversely, a very experienced mother with an older child may not need this information, as she knows and feels competent already to manage the situation.

Motivation can vary on a day-to-day basis. Feelings on a particular day can impact on your participants' motivation levels. A tired child, for example, may not feel motivated to learn on the day you are working with her. A lack of sleep can affect how she responds to your health promotion session. Working with the child on a different day, after a good night's sleep, she may well feel very different and really motivated to learn.

Box 2.5 Teaching plan.

Session: Children's play.

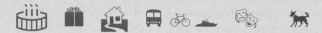

Group: A group of ten parents/carers.

Aim: To raise parental/carer awareness on the value of play for young children (0–5 years), so they will seek out more play opportunities for their children.

Objectives/outcomes

Parents/carers will be able to the following:

- Identify different aspects of playful behaviour, and types of play, in young children.
- Recognise play as a valuable part of child development.
- Demonstrate a new game that they have recently started playing with their child.

Content:

- Different types of play and how it exhibits itself in young children's behaviour.
- The benefits of play.
- Various games that can be played with young children.

Methods:

- A talk, with participation from the group.
- Small group discussions.
- Practical demonstrations by participants.

Resources:

- Handouts, pens and paper, Powerpoint, toys and videos.

Evaluation:

- Small questionnaire.
- The demonstration could be used for assessing parents'/carers' learning.

Senses

To learn, your participants need to be able to hear what is being said as well as being able to see what is being demonstrated. Your job is to ensure that participants can hear and see. There are certain things that you can do to help. For example, make sure that your own voice is loud enough, and that any resources being played are at a sufficient volume so that everyone can hear. Seating arrangements and lighting options will enable participants to see more clearly what is going on. It is also useful to check periodically that participants can see and hear effectively. Sometimes participants may be reluctant to highlight their difficulties.

If you have any participants with visual or hearing problems, then it is useful to find this out before they come. You are then able to make any necessary provision for them.

These all may seem obvious issues to consider, but sometimes they can be overlooked. By being aware of them can help to improve learning for your participants. It will help them to engage more effectively in the events that are happening during your health promotion session.

Attention

Attending is essential in the learning process. Attending is the means by which information is transferred from the senses to memory (Lefrançois, 1994). If your participants are motivated, there is a good chance they will attend and learn.

It is necessary that you encourage participants to attend; otherwise, they will fail to learn. This does not necessarily mean by directly telling them to attend, but by varying what is happening. This might include using different teaching methods, as previously discussed, or changing your focus, or encouraging participants to do something themselves as part of the session.

Do not expect your participants to fully attend at all points, no matter how good it might be. You need to be aware that there are limitations to attention. Participants' attention will naturally wander at certain points. Children's abilities to attend can be fairly limited, particularly when young.

Memory theories

It is essential for participants to be able to remember what they have learnt. They need to remember so that they can turn their new knowledge into actions – positive health behaviours.

Psychologists talk about *short-term memory* and *long-term memory* (Baddeley, 1982). Short-term memory is described as what is happening within our immediate consciousness at any given moment in time, and is sometimes referred to as working

> **Box 2.6** The cognitive processes involved in learning.
> - Senses.
> - Attending.
> - Short-term memory.
> - Long-term memory.

memory (Baddeley, 1982). Working memory could be described as what we are working on in our mind at any given moment in time. Long-term memory is the stable information or knowledge that we have (Lefrançois, 1994). Information has moved on from short-term memory, and has become knowledge embedded within long-term memory, and can be drawn upon when needed (Box 2.6).

An important factor to consider about short-term memory is that it has limited capacity; only a small number of items can be considered at any one time. Miller (1956) in his famous work on short-term memory concluded that most people can hold 7 ± 2 items. Any more than this forgetting begins to occur.

Careful consideration needs to be given to the amount of information we provide to participants. Too much information and they will start to feel overloaded, and difficulties are likely to occur in being able to attend. Baddeley (1982) points out that the ability to learn can be disrupted due to more and more inputs of information being received, and so reducing clarity of the original piece of information given. The more information we provide could result in less information being remembered.

Without rehearsal and effort, information can quickly disappear from short-term memory too (Peterson and Peterson, 1959). This suggests the more our participants do with the health promotion information provided, the better they will be at remembering it.

Rehearsal can be really important to learning. Do not assume that because your participants have heard something once that they will remember it. Try to repeat points, or summarise issues, to help participants remember. It is essential to do this with the really salient points, particularly at the beginning and again at the end of your session. Ley (1988) has explored the giving of health information to patients, and maintains that it helps with memory if important information is given at the beginning and then repeated again at the end.

The abilities of short-term memory can be improved with the use of a strategy called chunking. Chunking information, or grouping together a number of similar or related items, can greatly assist the remembering process (Lefrançois, 1994). For example, when working with children during a healthy eating activity, ask them to group together healthy foods and then group unhealthy foods. Actually, use the foods themselves, so that the situation has an interesting visual and tactile component.

The transfer of information from short-term memory to long-term memory involves deriving meaning from the experiences that we have (Lefrançois, 1994). This can be influenced by how deeply we think about that information (Lefrançois, 1994). The more deeply information is thought about, the more likely it will be remembered (Craik and Lockhart, 1972).

Perhaps providing your participants with an activity to do, based on the information you have discussed, will help the information to become more meaningful to them, and thus more likely to be remembered. Returning to the healthy eating example, children can identify their favourite healthy food and seek out a dish which includes it. Then under adult supervision, they could have a go at making the dish.

Communication – rewards and praise

How we communicate with our participants is going to make a difference to what they learn. Communication is an enormous subject. This section will focus on one aspect of communication – rewards and praise, as they can make a significant difference to learning.

Your communications with participants should be *encouraging* and *rewarding*, as advocated by Daines et al. (1993) and Sutton (2000). This helps participants to feel relaxed about sharing information and positive about any behaviour changes they might be making. Take time to listen to what they have to say.

Lefrançois (1994) maintains that *praise* is verbal confirmation that an individual has undertaken something well. Daines et al. (1993) have devised a list of words that can be used when praising participants:

- Congratulations.
- Keep it up.
- That's a good idea.
- That's great.
- Smashing.
- Well look at you.
- Wow!

Behaviour followed by praise is likely to encourage any new behaviour (Sutton, 2000).

A reward is about giving an individual a treat perhaps, when they have undertaken something well. Sutton (2000) asserts that *rewards* are highly individual. Whatever reward that you use in promoting health, it has to be one that your participants will find rewarding. Gold stars might motivate a 6-year-old, but will not necessarily impress a 16-year-old.

Sutton (2000) discusses rewards across the lifespan. For children she suggests stickers and outings, for example. Sutton (2000) maintains for young people, however, the focus of reward is very much about social rewards – friendships. These rewards may include inviting friends over or going out to a special event. In the health promotion context, it is not always possible to provide these kinds of rewards. Nevertheless, working with parents/carers, who are able to, is a useful starting point. Do not forget that parents/carers should also be praised for their efforts in helping to promote their children's health.

Some of the cognitive processes involved in learning new information have been touched upon. Learning strategies that might help your participants learn, in line with these cognitive processes, have been suggested. Remember when communicating with your participants, praise them for their learning, particularly where there are positive changes in health behaviour.

Summary

This chapter has focused on the planning of health promotion. The chapter provides the reader with details of all the different elements of planning that need to be considered when putting together a health promotion session. It has also examined the value of empowerment in learning about health promotion.

For learning to be effective there are a number of different cognitive processes and learning strategies that need to be considered. This chapter has provided details on some of these. Communication skills are especially important in nursing, and certainly so when teaching health promotion; therefore, the use of praise and rewards has been considered in helping to support changes in health behaviour.

A wealth of information has been covered within this chapter. It might appear daunting, but you may find that only certain aspects of this chapter are pertinent to your needs, as you read through. Over time, much of this information will become second nature in its application to your health promotion sessions. This chapter may simply become the resource that initially sent you on your way.

References

Ajzen, I., Fishbein, M. (1980) *Understanding Attitudes and Predicting Social Behaviour*. Englewood Cliffs: Prentice Hall.

Argyle, M. (1983) *The Psychology of Interpersonal Behaviour*. Middlesex: Penguin Books.

Baddeley, A. (1982) *Your Memory: A User's Guide*. London: Penguin Books.

Craik, F., Lockhart, R. (1972) Levels of processing. *Journal of Verbal Learning and Verbal Behaviour* 11: 671–684.

Daines, J., Daines, C., Graham, B. (1993) *Adult Learning, Adult Teaching*, 3rd edn. Nottingham: Department of Adult Education.

Ewles, L., Simnett, I. (2005) *Promoting Health: A Practical Guide to Health Education*. Edinburgh: Baillière Tindall.

Freire, P. (1972) *Pedagogy of the Oppressed*. Middlesex: Penguin.

Hawtin, M., Hughes, G., Percy-Smith, J. (1998) *Community Profiling, Auditing Social Needs*. Buckingham: Open University Press.

Kai, J. (1996) Parents' difficulties and information needs in coping with acute illness in preschool children: a qualitative study. *British Medical Journal* 313: 987–990.

Lawson, K. (1979) *Philosophical Concepts and Values in Adult Education*. Milton Keynes: Open University Press.

Lefrançois, G. (1994) *Psychology for Teaching*. California: Wadsworth Publishing Company.

Ley, P. (1988) *Communicating with Patients*. London: Croom Helm.

Lloyd, P., Mayes, A., Manstead, A., Meudell, P., Wagner, H. (1984) *Introduction to Psychology: An Integrated Approach*. London: Fontana Paperbacks.

Miller, G. (1956) The magical number seven plus or minus two. *Psychological Review* 63: 81–97.

Naidoo, J., Wills, J. (1994) *Health Promotion, Foundations for Practice*. London: Baillière Tindall.

NHS Direct. (2006) *NHS Direct Self-Help Guide*. Available at: http://www.nhsdirect.nhs.uk (accessed 20 September 2006).

NHS Institute for Innovation and Improvement (2008). *CKS Safe Practical Answers Fast*. Available at: http://www.cks.library.nhs.uk (accessed 20 September 2006).

NHS National Library for Health. (2006) *National Electronic Library for Health*. Available at: http://www.nelh.nhs.uk/ (accessed 20 September 2006).

Peterson, L., Peterson, M. (1959) Short term retention of individual items. *Journal of Experimental Psychology* 58: 193–198.

Rogers, J. (1992) *Adults Learning*. Buckingham: Open University Press.

Sutton, C. (2000) *Helping Families with Troubled Children: A Preventive Approach*. Chichester: John Wiley & Sons.

3 Creativity

Claire Daniel

Introduction

The heart of this chapter is about creativity and how it can help you. It is my intention to highlight how creativity can be nurtured within human development. Hopefully, this will enable you to illuminate health promotion information in digestible forms to children/young people.

The importance of nurturing creativity in the care and education of young children has been formally recognised. It is endorsed by the Government in its framework *Birth to Three Matters* (Sure Start Unit, 2003).

Creativity is an essential tool within us; it aids our thinking as we push and pull materials, explore ideas and entertain new ways of seeing, hearing, touching and doing. Creativity is the part of us that nurtures self-expression and reflects our thought processes. It is not a unique gift; we all have it. It is tangible, it can be taught, objectified and vilified, if not measured. It is unrestrained and assists our literary as well as visual language. Creativity helps us to engage with the world around us and those within it. Creativity produces new ideas for the individual concerned, which may potentially influence others. Creativity may flow through all thinking processes as well as artistic pursuits.

If we accept this idea of creativity, then we can move onto thinking how best to utilise creativity to deliver messages of health promotion for children/young people.

Creativity can take place in all kinds of human activity from cookery to chemistry. It requires inventiveness, curiosity, risk-taking and imagination. The arts can have a strong role in developing creativity in babies and young children. They can offer opportunities for sensory development, exploration and discovery, for experimentation, for asking *What if?* Creativity can also be useful for practising different types of communication (Bruce, 2004).

Adults are central in helping children/young people find out how to be creative through the arts. They can introduce new materials, words, stories, movement and music, as well as building stimulating environments and displays (Bruce, 2004).

Skills to teach health promotion

To assist yourself in teaching others, think about how you learn yourself. Do you listen well, what grabs your attention? Do you colour coordinate your notes? Is a video an effective learning tool for you? What methods do you already employ without thinking about them, and how can they be helpful when informing children/young people in your care?

Activity

Take 5 minutes now and write down all your best learning experiences. Think about why they were the best.

In addition, note down the organisational tools you use in your everyday life to help you learn and remember.

Think about your hobbies and interests, and how these may be employed; a keen reader can easily become a keen storyteller. Delicious tales work wonders at captivating children's listening skills.

Demonstrations are the cornerstone of all good teaching practices; medical appliances and diagrams will obviously be vital to your health promotion activities. These may be supported by encouraging children/young people to then demonstrate their understanding of them in a visual manner too.

Children preparing to enter hospital, for example, could be assisted with the use of puppets, dolls and a set of bandages. Perhaps you can help them to draw their fears and expectations with the use of a series of faces demonstrating different expressions and emotions. Exploring their feelings with you may help them to see you as a friendly and caring figure at a scary and unsettling time.

Outlined below is a six-point plan including key skills that could assist teaching. Consider your health promotion subject and note down ideas for relating this subject to children/young people in your care. Remember that they need to be able to personally relate to your subject:

- Be secure in your subject knowledge. It is important to know what you are teaching.
- Choose age-appropriate language and visual aids to help engage and explain your health promotion material.
- Ask open-ended questions and play games where knowledge can be learned, applied and tested by them.
- Use age-appropriate illustrations and demonstrations, analogy and metaphor. This will broaden and deepen children's and young people's understanding.
- Use diverse materials that include ideas from other countries. Address gender bias in materials, and promote multicultural awareness.

- Critical assessment of your efforts – always try to record how your presentation went. It will help to reflect and make changes to teaching methods. This should mean that when the activity or session is undertaken again, it will be better and more successful. Allow opportunities for your children/young people to do the same; this will strengthen their understanding of the health promotion subject.

Reflection is really important in nursing. Learning to be a reflective practitioner can help to develop practice. Schon (1983) has talked about the importance of practitioners reflecting upon their experiences to take practice forward.

The term *age-appropriate* is a term that frequently pops up. But what if to date you have limited experience with children/young people? How will you know what is age-appropriate? Textbooks will obviously provide guidance, but go beyond these. Investigate popular culture. For instance, children identify strongly with their favourite television characters. Do not forget to watch the advertisements in between the programmes too, for the latest desired products. Toy and craft shops can supply a wealth of physical material, including puppets, play dough, crayons and well-known toy characters.

How we learn

Psychologists have discussed different ways in which people learn. There is evidence to suggest that one way in which people learn about the world can be categorised into different modalities:

- Visual – the observer who learns new things by seeing.
- Auditory – information learnt through the spoken word.
- Kinaesthetic – becoming physically involved.

Shaw and Hawes (1998) have discussed these different modes of learning, and believe they can work together to enable experiences to be more memorable.

However, some children/young people may have a preference for a particular mode of learning; they may prefer learning by kinaesthetic means, rather than auditory, for example. With children, this may mean setting up a make-believe scenario in school perhaps, so that they can become involved. Learning to cross the road safely, for example, may be a relevant topic. Children can act out what they need to do, thus learning appropriate and safe ways to cross the road.

A useful explanation on learning modalities has been outlined by Verster (2007) on the website – http://www.teachingenglish.org.uk/. The website provides examples for each modality. Included in Verster's explanation is an additional modality, those who prefer learning through tactile means. Below are some examples for each of the modalities.

Those who prefer a visual learning style will do many of the following:

- Look at the teacher's face intently.
- Enjoy looking at wall displays and books.
- Use lists to organise their thoughts.
- Recall information by remembering how it is set out on the page.

Those who prefer an auditory learning style will prefer the following:

- Like the teacher to provide verbal instructions.
- Like dialogues, discussions and plays.
- Solve problems by talking about them.
- Use rhythm and sound as memory aids.

Those who prefer a kinaesthetic learning style will prefer doing the following:

- Learn best when they are involved or active.
- Find it difficult to sit still for long periods.
- Use movement as a memory aid.

Those who prefer a tactile learning style will want to touch the following:

- Use writing and drawing as memory aids.
- Learn well with hands-on activities, such as demonstrations.

Previous experiences are also important when learning new information. A child's/young person's learning style is determined by previous learning experiences and the culture and the society in which they live. Find out what children know already. Use drawings and discuss the drawings together, as a way of finding out.

Role models are another important way in which children learn. Bandura (1977) has explored the influence of role models in learning. A role model is someone that an individual holds in high esteem. Young children enjoy characters featured in books, television programmes and films. A television character can happily instruct young children, who see the character as a relevant role model. Perhaps a new slant on a familiar story or nursery rhyme could be made into a suitable teaching aid, helping young children's learning in a creative and fun way.

Style and rapport

How a health promotion activity is delivered can have a significant influence on learning. If you have an effective delivery style, which actively engages your audience, this will be an important asset in children's learning. In addition, the rapport you develop with them is going to make way for easy responsive discussions.

During a training exercise a group of student teachers were asked to present their new scheme of work to a class of 30 young people, aged 13. The student teachers were given 5 minutes, and once documents and notes were prepared, it was announced the proceedings would be videoed. The students had focused on the content of their work and the provision of quality learning outcomes, but many had forgotten the art of delivery. When viewing their performances, nervous tension was broken by raucous laughter and astonishment at their own behaviours. The students were amazed to hear the pitch of their own voices, some shaky, some shrill and others trailing off into inaudibility.

If you are not a natural performer, then you will need to rehearse. The more you do this, the more your delivery style will be strengthened. This will work dividends when faced with the interruptions that so often happen when delivering health promotion in classrooms or children's centres.

Try looking in a mirror, using a video camera or asking a colleague or friend to provide feedback.

I have listed some pointers here that will act as a guide. They may only be small gestures, but combined they can make a powerful, positive impact:

- When in a classroom or children's centre, it would be advisable to greet everyone at the door. An introductory nod and hello can initiate a warm response.
- Think about your position when you teach. If you are going to stand, how and where are you going to do this in the room? With small children it is fundamental that you physically try getting down to their level. If borrowing a classroom, you should not stand behind the desk; this can be divisive. It would be better to carefully rest yourself in front of it or join small children on a chair the same size as their own.
- When dealing with a group, try to remember the names of those you are working with. To help with this, start with circle time – throw a ball to each other and shout out your name. Make badges with older children of reading age.
- If there is a board available, use it to write keywords and concepts for your discussion. It will aid you as a prompt and provide a visual stimulus for those you are talking to.
- Ensure that your sentences do not trail off into inaudibility. Do not speak too fast and try not to be monotone. If you want others to be excited by what you are saying, make it sound exciting.
- Smiling and laughing are important. Use good eye contact with everyone you are talking to.
- Gestures are important too, as they can be very descriptive, helping to emphasise points. If you struggle, try holding your hands loosely in your lap.

Differentiation

Children's psychological and physiological needs differ from adults. Children should be considered as individuals. The following outlines some specific points in relation to children/young people with special needs.

Children/young people with special needs may have specific communication requirements. It is important to engage with their individual strengths. As Warnock (1978) has recognised, it is children's/young people's needs, not their disabilities that should be acknowledged when differentiating strategies for learning.

Children with special needs may benefit from touching, handling materials before a discussion can take place. The combination of senses in conjunction with listening and speaking often connects their learning.

Visually impaired children, for example, will benefit from increased dialogue, large lettering, bold contrasting colours and the availability of tactile learning materials. To find out more about children with visual impairments, access http://www.direct.gov.uk/ and the National Blind Children's Society, http://www.nbcs.org.uk/.

Similarly, children with dyslexia will benefit from some of the learning aids highlighted. *Dyslexia* is a term used to describe children/ young people who have an impaired ability to read with comprehension, but their intelligence is unimpaired (Blackwell's Nursing Dictionary, 2005). To find out more, access the British Dyslexia Association website http://www.bda-dyslexia.org.uk/, and the association for Scotland http://www.dyslexiascotland.org.uk.

These conditions do not prevent high achievements and should not be seen as a barrier to learning, rather they need awareness and understanding. I would urge you to engage in further reading, if and when appropriate, for the teaching of health promotion.

For those children/young people with a natural artistic nature, they may need appropriate extension tasks. As with any group, some children/young people will finish first, whilst others take their time. It will help you to manage a group if you can provide leverage in the form of well-planned extension exercises.

Girls and boys can coexist within an education framework. Many projects and suggestions will be effective for both sexes. However preferences exist, typically girls will prefer to talk and draw, boys usually enjoy making things.

Importantly, although this may sound obvious, but when working with children it always needs considering – think about the size and abilities of those you are going to be working with. Young children are going to be small; they need to be able to work with materials that they can physically handle. Their gross and fine motor skills will need to be considered. Are they physically able to do the tasks that you are expecting of them? Putting materials high up, for example, they are going to be too small to reach them. Consider their abilities and size.

Practical guidance

The following provides some practical ideas for activities that might be useful when teaching health promotion. Remember you will need to consider the parents'/carers' wishes and include them in your action plan.

Babies and toddlers

- They love bright contrasting colours, and black and white geometrical designs. They respond best to the human face and to sounds. By 3 months, babies can see differences in hue as well as colour, respond to facial expressions and distinguish pitch and volume of sound.
- Babies are not passive, but active learners.
- Babies love lights, patterns and shapes. Different mobiles might be useful, which can captivate babies. Try them, particularly when babies and toddlers need distracting, such as when an injection needs to be given or blood is being taken. Bubbles can also be a great distraction.
- Older babies love paints, water and sand. Two- to three-year-olds adore play dough. You could use the play dough to shape the implements that will be used in their treatment. Make it a fun learning and naming exercise. By playing, the real implements may not seem so scary.

Preschool (3- to 5-year-olds)

- Smaller children love anything with a surprise. Pulling something from a bag will cause much more excitement than placing an object on a table for them to look at, especially if that object is in a velvet bag. Use magic words to let it escape. Use a fairy wand for girls or a magician's wand for boys. Let them take turns themselves.
- Role-play – imaginative play is excellent.

- When creating your health promotion material, beware of colouring in exercises, as they can sometimes be a little limiting for children's imaginations.
- Drawings – drawn results only need to be an effective learning tool, which children can see and describe. They do not have to look beautiful to us.
- When children are being creative, try interrupting on occasion with leading questions. For example, *what else might you find at the dentist?*
- Use a treasure box. Encourage children to make/decorate a box (an old shoe box, for example) and they can keep their new knowledge inside it. Constructing and making are crucial skills for children's development, so save all your old cartons and use junk modelling to illustrate your topic.
- CDs are easily portable. Children learn well and respond to music and actions. It means too that the learning will not stop when you leave. So make up rhymes and basic songs to illustrate your health topic. Build in actions and see how easily they copy you.
- Children love incentives; encouragement is simple when you give them stickers. Try giving away a star chart for them to complete at home. This will extend the learning and involve parents/carers. If you are working with a child on a repeated basis, she/he can bring it back for a further reward on her/his next visit.

Junior school children (5–7 years)

- Ask children to examine and discuss their drawings around the health topic you have selected.
- Role-play – for example, the teacher (or other adult) adopts the role of the old woman who lives in a shoe; she needs help from the children, who are expert carers and who can advise her on how to keep her many offspring out of trouble. At this stage, children enjoy sharing their make-believe and play-making with others (Arts Council, 2003). Using your health promotion publications, for example, pretend to be a character in the leaflet, ask the children to act out characters, thoughts and feelings. Help the children to engage with the publications by asking leading questions. *Where do the*

children live? How do they like to spend their free time?

- An old family favourite of ours is the *memory game*; take a collection of objects and view them together. Now cover with a tea towel and without the children looking, take an object away. See if they can tell you what objects are missing? This could work as a lovely starter game to introducing the implements needed to teach a health topic.
- If developing health promotion based on *healthy eating*, try a little culinary wizardry. Make faces with the food. Ask leading questions. *What fruit travelled the furthest to be on your plate today? Which fruit has the strongest smell?* Introduce tasting sessions, but ensure that you have parents'/carers' permission first, and also check for any allergies the children might have, so you know what foods to avoid (see Figure 3.1).
- It is still age-appropriate to use treasure boxes, music, storytelling and reward charts.

Middle years (8–11 years)

Teamwork, working in pairs, can be useful at this age. Try to engage children in finding answers to questions together – *how high can you jump?* Get them to record in pairs how high they did jump. Then, get them to think about which parts of the body were involved in doing the jumping.

Leading questions are paramount to making the mind work and providing you with an opportunity to praise them when they are right. Much of the games, role-play and suggestions from the previous age group can be amended with more sophisticated leading questions.

Some examples for the 8- to 11-year age group are outlined:

- Materials that they blow might be useful as a starting point for a discussion about breathing.
- *When I'm 64* – I chose to work with a group of children examining where their lifestyle choices may lead them in later life, the effects of which will literally be etched on their faces. Ask them to look in a mirror and draw themselves at 64. Introduce leading questions. *If you smoke what might happen to your skin? If you never brush your teeth, will you have any left?*

- A friend of mine made a fabulous jelly sculpture. A simple display will really stimulate children of this age. Working with a group of school children you can ask the teacher to assist you. Have the children bring in objects around your topic from home and then create a sculpture as a focal point for discussion. Art does not need to be permanent, look to Anthony Gormley's sand art for inspiration. You could make a sculpture of the human body. Or try making models of parts of the body. Make a model of the respiratory system using cardboard tubing and sponges, for instance.

Young people (11–16 years)

At 11–16 years young people have experiences which they can draw upon that are useful for discussions and debates on health. They also have opinions of their own, sometimes strong opinions. If using discussions and debates, be aware that some may not be confident to join in. Think about ways you can encourage those less confident to become involved. Some examples for 11–16 year olds are outlined:

- Role-play – produce an advert for a health promotion topic. Think about developing a short drama perhaps. Role-play allows young people to participate as a character, and as such they may be more open to sharing their views. Role-play can also help young people to see the views of others. Smaller groups will work best.
- Draw from imagination and memory. Remember that young people can be heavily influenced by their peers.
- It is often useful with 11- to 16-year-olds to invite participation early. Then you can assess what they know and add to their knowledge. It also gives them the opportunity to talk. It can rid them of some energy before you proceed. It works well for a group. However, manage the time spent on this well; a big loud alarm clock may help.
- Digital imagery and video can be useful. Videos/DVDs can lend themselves well to form the visual and audio components of teaching.

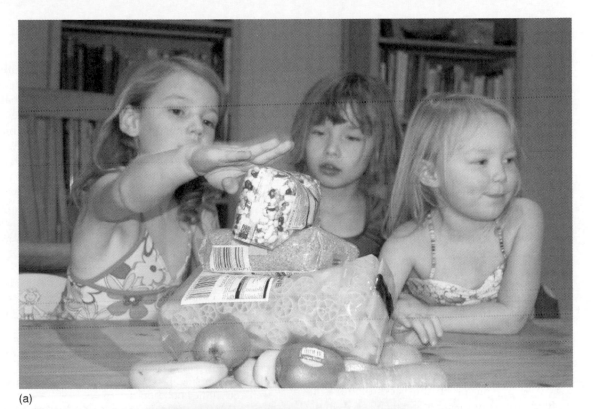

(a)

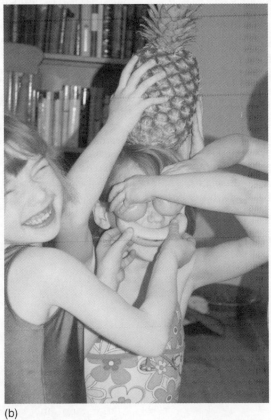

(b)

Figure 3.1 (a), (b) Children playing with fruits and vegetables.

They look professional, can raise many issues and are valuable for stimulating discussion. However, young people may miss the information you wish them to have, so stop the tape and highlight what you want them to note down for discussion. This will help them stay focused.

- Case studies – these are useful for 13-year-olds upwards. Case studies help young people develop their analytical and thinking skills. Topics can be explored in depth and can be particularly helpful for complex issues. Think about how you can relate case studies to young people's own personal experiences.
- Ordered antics – the game where you find out what you need to know and are learning about, by working as a team, literally reading from each other. In a group we used this teaching method to assist young people in learning how to put a condom on correctly. Type a list of instructions that relate to your health topic in large bold letters. Then chop this up into smaller portions, ready to pin pieces on the backs of those involved. Ask your group to get themselves in the right order. Ordered antics then pursue.

There are many more creative practical ideas that can be used with different age groups. The above simply provides you with a starting point.

Conclusion

This chapter has looked at creativity. It has examined how creativity is important in human development, and how it can help with health promotion activities. Some practical ideas have been provided which can be used when working with children/young people of different ages.

I hope the chapter leaves you with a sense that creativity can be fun. It can certainly help to engage children/young people in the process of learning about health promotion in a fun and innovative way. Possibly, this chapter has demonstrated that being creative is perhaps not as difficult as you first thought. Have a go and see where it takes you.

References

Arts Council, England (2003) *Drama in Schools*, 2nd edn. England: Arts Council.

Bandura, A. (1977) *Social Learning Theory*. New Jersey: General Learning Press.

Bruce, T. (2004) Cultivating creativity in babies, toddlers, and young children. In: *Reflect and Review: The Arts and Creativity in Early Years*. England: Arts Council.

Blackwell's Nursing Dictionary (2005) Oxford: Blackwell's Scientific Publications.

Schon, D. (1983) *The Reflective Practitioner*. New York: Basic Books.

Shaw, S., Hawes, T. (1998) *Effective Teaching and Learning in the Primary Classroom*. Leicester: Optimal-Learning.net.

Sure Start Unit (2003) *Birth to Three Matters, A Framework to Support Children in the Early Years*. London: Sure Start Unit, Education and Skills.

Verster, C. (2007) *Learning Styles and Teaching*. BBC British Council Teaching English. Available at: http://www.teachingenglish.org.uk/think/methodology/learning_style.shtml (accessed 13 November 2007).

Warnock, M. (1978) (2000) In Addison, N., Burgess, L. (eds) *Learning to Teach Art and Design in Secondary School. A Companion to School Experience*. London: Routledge Falmer.

4

Government Policy

Janet Badcock

Introduction

Policy making is a government's translation of their political vision into programmes and actions to deliver outcomes, desired changes to life in the real world (Cabinet Office, 1999a,b).

Policy is the cornerstone of care, particularly as it serves to protect the public against poor practice, improves equity by ensuring common standards across relevant agencies and services, and provides specialist specific information. It does this by changing the way organisations work, think and connect with each other (Bullock et al., 2001).

Although there have been long-standing policies on child social care, it is really only a relatively recent achievement that such policy has been written, which is directly relevant to children's nursing and child health care. Rather sadly, the catalyst for such policy has often arisen from tragedies in which children have died or been subjected to serious harm, such as the death of Victoria Climbié and the outcome of children receiving complex heart surgery at Bristol Royal Infirmary between 1984 and 1995. Both highlight the inadequacies in our health and social care systems. They are discussed more fully later in this chapter.

Understanding the Government policy

Often the mass of the Government documentation can feel difficult to negotiate. Nonetheless, there is logic behind the production of the Government policy. Major guidance, such as the National Service Frameworks (NSFs) (Education and Skills, Department of Health, 2004) for children, young people and maternity services, are an overview of policy. Usually, they have additional paperwork to support them; for instance, the NSF section on *Promoting Health* has a sister policy entitled *Choosing Health: Making Healthy Choices Easier* (Department of Health, 2004). This additional documentation provides greater depth with practice examples that can be put into action.

Government documentation and policy usually go through a variety of different stages, and a single topic will have a range of green and white papers which will inform the content of a subsequent Bill and Act of Parliament. Green papers are usually consultation documents, and are designed to be able to gather views from professionals and service users on the particular topic under scrutiny.

From these consultation rounds, the final white paper is developed, which is the definitive guidance. This enables the ideas and comments generated in the green paper – consultation – to be incorporated into the final document, the white paper. Most Government guidance also includes an executive summary which provides a brief background to the main paper. If you are carrying out a literature search, it is often a good idea to look at the executive summary first to see if it contains what you are looking for, before dipping into the main white paper for more depth on the issue.

A white paper is not always backed by law to make it a legal requirement to act upon it. A Bill is a proposal of how services will change to meet new plans or policies by developing new regulations. It acts as a draft law. Before a Bill becomes an Act, it needs to go through five stages in both the House of Commons and the House of Lords before receiving Royal Assent. An Act is a legislative spine onto which reforms for children will be built upon and dictates some of the superstructures that are required to ensure standards are being met.

The background to recent child-related Government policy

In February 2000, the death of Victoria Climbié shocked the nation and shook the Government into developing some far reaching reforms that would alter the way children's/young people's services would be delivered in the future. Victoria was a child who died as a result of violent and long-standing abuse at the hands of relatives, with whom she was living. What was most concerning about this case was that in the 9 months between coming to live in this country and her death, Victoria had passed through many social services departments, two hospital visits, and the family had been in contact with four separate housing authorities (Laming, 2003).

Despite concerns being raised on a number of occasions, opportunities were missed where interventions could have saved her life. She finally died with a total of 128 separate injuries (Laming, 2003). The fact that current systems were not adequately working together to protect children from harm or poor care was clear. Work began on reforming the child protection system even before the official report was released concerning the case. It was announced

in 2001 that the Department of Health would develop a new NSF for children/young people which would set clear standards of care for practitioners to follow.

The urgency for such reforms was compounded by the publication of a report written by Professor Ian Kennedy (Kennedy, 2001) following a public enquiry into the care received by children undergoing heart surgery at the Bristol Royal Infirmary during the period of 1984–1995. This report identified that a number of children were dying as a result of surgery received at that hospital, more than would normally be expected. The report highlighted the need for high-quality, safe services that were geared towards the needs of children.

Lord Laming's report on Victoria's death detailed 108 recommendations to attempt to prevent such a tragedy from occurring again. Many of the recommendations centred around communication such as *not listening to the child*, poor recording of events, poor communication between staff within and between agencies and the inability of people to recognise the signs of abuse. It recognised gross failure of a system and lack of good practice. It centred heavily on how children's hospital services, primary care, social services and other services failed in their duty to protect this child. The inquiry prompted the production of the green paper – *Every Child Matters* (Education and Skills, 2003).

Every Child Matters proposed a range of measures to reform and improve the ability of services to safeguard children/young people and formed the basis of the subsequent white paper – *Every Child Matters: Next Steps* (Education and Skills, 2004). The release of the white paper coincided with the introduction of the *Children Bill* to Parliament, which sets out how the Government were intending to make children's reforms far-reaching and obligatory. The Bill received Royal Assent in November 2004, thereby becoming an Act of Parliament. This provided the Government with the legal underpinning required to undertake the desired reforms. The new Children Act (2004) detailed the intention to appoint a children's commissioner to champion the views and interests of children/young people, and set out clearly the duties of agencies in safeguarding children/young people, especially those in highly vulnerable circumstances. It also detailed how an integrated inspection framework would review progress of the children's agenda.

The complete NSF for children, young people and maternity services was finally released in November 2004, coming under the umbrella of the Every Child Matters: Change for Children agenda. Since then there have been a number of documents released that add extra depth to guidance, also coming under the Every Child Matters: Change for Children mark.

The first Minister of State for Children was appointed in 2003. Based in the Department for Education and Skills, the minister was responsible for children's services, childcare, provision for under 5 years, family policy and the major reform agenda for children identified as being at risk. Responsibility for children's social services was brought into the remit of Department for Education and Skills, with the aim of bringing greater integration and cohesion of services together. This formed the basis of one of the most far-reaching organisational changes to bring all of children's services under one remit.

The Department of Education and Skills has since divided into two parts. Within Education and Skills, there is now the Department of Children, Schools and Families. This Department is overseen by the Secretary of State for Children.

Every Child Matters

As discussed in the section above, Every Child Matters (Education and Skills, 2003) was concerned with safeguarding children/young people's interests and well-being. It would be impossible, here, to cover the vast array of policy that has arisen from this piece of work. The website http://www.everychildmatters.gov.uk gives access to all the different aspects of the documentation. At the cornerstone of all these documents and guidance produced, are the findings of a Government-led widespread public consultation. This has ensured that the people most involved in the services under reform were involved in any new developments. Table 4.1 describes some of the different aspects of children's/young people's lives, which they wanted to be considered in Every Child Matters. It also looks at what these might mean in more depth.

The NSFs for children, young people and maternity services are widely regarded as the guidance that enables the *be healthy* component to be realised; although, all the outcomes of Every Child Matters

Table 4.1   Every Child Matters five outcomes.

Be healthy	Physically healthy
	Emotionally healthy
	Parents and carers promote health
Stay safe	Safe from neglect
	Safe from accidental injury
	Safe from bullying and discrimination
	Parents, carers and families provide safe homes and stability
Enjoy and achieve	Ready for school
	Attend and enjoy school
	Achieve stretching national educational standards at school
	Achieve personal and social development, and enjoy recreation
Make a positive contribution	Engage in decision-making and support the community and environment
	Engage in positive behaviour
	Develop positive relationships
	Develop self-confidence
	Develop enterprising behaviour
	Parents, carers and families promote positive behaviour
Achieve economic well-being	Engage in further education and employment or training on leaving school
	Ready for employment
	Live in decent homes and sustainable communities
	Live in households free from low income
	Parents/carers and families are supported to be economically active.

have implications for any service that provides care for children.

The NSFs for children, young people and maternity services

The NSFs for children, young people and maternity services (NSFs, Education and Skills, Department of Health, 2004) form one of a number of frameworks which aim to provide standardisation of care to an area of speciality. NSFs also exist for cancer care, older people, coronary heart disease, diabetes, long-term conditions and mental health.

The main purpose of an NSF is to provide a structure for all relevant services to ensure consistency, quality and equity, thus avoiding the *post code lottery* approach to standards in health care. The NSFs for children, young people and maternity services are the first major health-related documentation that considers the special needs of children/young people from preconception through to 19 years. It is concerned with the holistic care of children/young people that live in the community and who may only use hospital-based care on brief occasions, as well as those children with more complex needs, and those with acute medical needs. It considers the impact that family, housing, education and community amenities have on children's well-being, in a way that has been hitherto unexplored.

Some aspects of the NSFs for children are a 10-year programme during which time the Government intend to make long-term improvements in children's/young people's health. The aim is to integrate services to ensure fair, high-quality and integrated health and social care. By 2014, it will be expected that health, social and educational services will meet standards set out in the NSFs.

The NSFs purport a cultural shift that will ensure services are designed around the needs of children, young people and their families. They have a very strong preventative element to enable intervention at the earliest stage, and therefore hopefully prevent needs escalating to a higher level of concern. When considering public health, most guidance has, until recently, concentrated on those activities that are more obviously health related, such as good nutrition and the damage of smoke-filled environments. However, the growing realisation that play and general development have a bearing on good health, has meant that they are now being included in a list of health promotion activities that every nurse working with children should adopt (Chief Nursing Officer, 2004). This trend away from a medically modelled approach towards a social and public health-based model of child health is perhaps the most significant change in the way that health promotion is now being delivered.

The NSFs centre around 11 standards, each one considering a key aspect of health care. Each

standard has been written to cover seven main themes that will ensure high-quality coordinated service delivery. These themes are as follows:

- Early identification of needs using a new Child Health Promotion Programme and the common assessment framework (CAF).
- Effective intervention to meet any identified needs. This will include the availability of parent/carer and child/young person information and support systems, as well as access to specialist intervention programmes.
- Prevention of ill health.
- Multi-agency partnerships to improve coordination of care that will effectively safeguard children/young people from harm.
- Effective commissioning of services to ensure quality and equity of service delivery, especially in areas where health inequalities exist.
- Listening to children/young people and families, not only in the planning of their own care, but also in the planning of new services or current service redesign.
- Appropriately skilled staff with appropriate training.

Standard 1: Promoting health and well-being, identifying needs and intervening early

This standard is based around the findings of *Health for All Children* (Hall and Elliman, 2003), which highlighted the social and environmental context in which children/young people grow up. Recommendations from this document support the view that the child surveillance programme was too narrow and not necessarily effective. There was a need to move to a more broad-based health promotion programme. This new programme includes the following:

- Each child will have a comprehensive assessment of need by the age of 1 year, to include the child's physical, emotional and developmental needs, to identify families who may require additional services, and ensure parents/carers have sufficient support to carry out their parenting role. This assessment will start before birth

Box 4.1 Implications for children's nurses.

- If you are concerned about a child's developmental progress, do report this and ensure action is taken.
- If you recognise that a child's immunisation status is not up to date, then arrange for immunisations to be completed.
- Any nurse contact can be an opportunity to discuss aspects of health promotion.

Box 4.2 Implications for children's nurses.

- Consider all contacts with a child/young person and their family as an opportunity to assess or review needs and offer relevant basic advice.
- Ensure all health promotion advice is evidence based and consistent with that given by other members of the hospital/primary health care team.
- Should the information conflict with what the parent/carer has already been given, spend some time explaining why you have given that specific information.
- Back up verbal information with written information, but be aware of difficulties some families might have with reading.

and will be reviewed at various points throughout the child's life.

- The provision of evidence-based health promotion advice.
- Childhood screening such as the identification of visual or hearing difficulties, thyroid deficiency, cystic fibrosis, growth and weight problems.
- Against preventable infectious diseases. This programme is continually expanding, and an update of the current immunisation schedule is available on http://www.immunisation.nhs.uk.
- Early intervention to address identified needs.

The full implication of *Health for All Children* (Hall and Elliman, 2003) is detailed in greater depth later in this book. Box 4.1 provides some points about its implications for children's nurses.

Each of the following sections will provide specific details, in table form, for children's nurses about the standard under discussion.

Standard 2: supporting parents/carers

This standard was set to ensure that mothers, fathers and carers are confident and able to bring up their children and teenagers in a way that promotes positive health, development and emotional wellbeing. This will be achieved by ensuring there is easily accessible, consistent evidence-based information available. Access to practitioners as well as parent-to-parent support will be available. The standard sets out many ways in which support may be achieved. Special consideration needs to be given to families who have difficulty in accessing services,

either due to lack of confidence, language, learning difficulty or geography.

The standard gives particular emphasis to supporting fathers and foster parents. It includes information on healthy lifestyle choices, positive parenting, management of minor illness and the emotional impact of parenting. It also considers support during the transitional stages of growing up, from child to adolescence and adolescence to adulthood. It considers how to promote independence, communication and boundary setting. Parents/carers should have access to variety of support including one to one, written and group advice (Box 4.2).

Standard 3: child/young person and family-centred services

This standard is concerned with the way practitioners and services communicate with and involve children, young people and their families in their own care and in the development of their own services. It asks for practitioners to see the world through children/young people's eyes. This will mean listening and developing services which are responsive to individual needs and preferences. The standard calls for a range of services in settings that are accessible to the client group being served. This might involve taking services out of traditional medical or social care institutions and providing them in places where children, young people and families more frequently congregate. Such places might include nurseries, children's centres, sports centres, schools and community centres.

Standard 3 includes issues surrounding informed decision-making, confidentiality and consent. Informed decision-making is the need for individuals to be able to make decisions having been presented with the evidence. For example, in giving advice on the risks of smoking, the individual might still choose to smoke, but at least they are in possession of all the evidence-based information and choose to take that risk.

Confidentiality is the need to keep all information given by an individual safe and not divulge it to others without the individual's permission. This is the cornerstone of gaining trust. Consent is the agreement of the individual to undertake a certain procedure or treatment. This will include referrals and letters made to others. In order for an individual to give consent, it is important that they are able to make informed decisions, as described above.

The standard fully explains the concept of child/young person-centred services, which considers the whole child – not just the illness presented, and with the overall experience of the child/young person and family in mind. It advocates the use of the CAF in assessing the needs of a child/young person and their family. The CAF views the child/young person within the three domains of need: the child's developmental needs, parenting capacity and family and environmental factors. The eight main characteristics of a child/young person-centred service are as follows:

- Listen to children, young people and their families.
- Respect their voice, opinions and confidentiality.
- Accurate information to be given.
- Informed consent.
- Easy access to services.
- Integrated services to avoid duplication, multiple appointments or disjointed delivery.
- An holistic assessment of need.
- A quality-based service with its roots firmly based within effective clinical governance and quality assurance.

Box 4.3 outlines some ways children's nurses can help to ensure that services are child/young person focused.

Box 4.3 Implications for children's nurses.

- Learn how to listen to children and their parents/carers; try to view experiences through their eyes.
- Ensure the environment is suitable for developmental ages and stages.
- Ensure children/young people and parents/carers are involved in the care, planning and evaluation of any new service initiatives.
- Ensure consent is obtained and confidentiality is respected at all times and evidence-based information is given to allow for informed decision-making.

Standard 4: growing up into adulthood

Standard 4 details how all young people will have access to age-appropriate services which are responsive to their specific needs as they grow into adulthood. This is with the view that they will make the transition into adulthood and achieve their maximum potential in terms of education, health, development and well-being. There is also a desire to ensure young people take responsibility for their own health, making their own informed choices and decisions. This also includes the engagement of young people in the delivery of their own health care.

Assurance of confidentiality and *ease of access* are the two areas young people have reported are the greatest influence in the uptake of services by them. As a young person moves from child to adult services, effective multidisciplinary planning is required in cases of complex medical or social need.

The NSFs highlight five key target areas for promoting health in young people. These are as follows:

- Nutrition, including diet and physical exercise.
- Sexual and reproductive health, including access to contraception, reducing teenage pregnancies and sexually transmitted diseases.
- Mental health, including psychosis, anorexia nervosa and self-harm.
- Injury.
- Substance misuse, including smoking, alcohol misuse.

Box 4.4 Implications for children's nurses.

- Avoid overly childish terminology or activities, but be aware that they will need careful explanations of their condition or situation.
- Ensure the young person has an up-to-date view of what is happening to them; many adolescents with chronic conditions may be still working on explanations given to them as a 4-year-old.
- Encourage independence.
- Respect dignity and privacy. If in hospital, and a teenage unit is not available, try and provide a side ward if possible, or a bed next to another young person.
- Ensure consent is obtained before carrying out procedures. Ensure you have documented that consent has been asked for and given.
- Give the young person an opportunity to ask questions without their parents/carers being there. Often young people with a long-standing illness are used to their parents/carers asking the questions.

Box 4.5 Implications for children's nurses.

- If you suspect a child/young person is being abused, always report your concerns to your line manager. Be aware of your responsibilities.
- Always listen to what the children say.
- Document exactly what you heard the child/young person say or saw. Date, time and sign your entry into the child's/young person's records.
- Do not assume the situation has resolved – check out what has happened with your line manager.
- Remember, you are not the only person dealing with the child/young person, communicate with others who need to know, but ensure the family know that you are doing so and that you are ensuring confidentiality of the information.
- Keep yourself regularly updated in the field of safeguarding children.
- If you feel you need to talk to somebody about a situation you have seen a child/young person go through, this is only natural, do speak to your line manager or safeguarding nurse to debrief.
- Be aware of the impact the abuse may have on the child's/young person's development.

Box 4.4 outlines the implications for children's nurses.

Standard 5: safeguarding and promoting the welfare of children/young people

This standard is concerned with ensuring that all children/young people are safeguarded from harm, so they are able to fulfil their potential. It calls for all agencies to work together to properly identify children/young people at risk of harm. It calls for appropriate action to be taken if a child/young person is identified as being at harm.

The Area Child Protection Committees, which are multi-agency groups ensuring policies and standards are met locally, have been replaced with Local Safeguarding Children's Board. This NSF standard, as well as Every Child Matters (2003), identified the need that all staff at all levels should understand their roles and responsibilities. It should be recognised that Lord Laming's report on the Victoria Climbié's case (Laming, 2003) presented a number of areas where concerns had been identified, but not followed up. Assumptions had been made that other people were dealing with an issue (Box 4.5).

Standard 6: the ill child

This standard is concerned with the care of children/young people who are ill, mainly in the community setting. It highlights the need to develop *Local Children's Clinical Networks* that bring together local and specialist services. This will include common procedures, greater communication and improved joint planning. The basis of this standard is that children/young people receive care that is evidence based. They should be cared for by appropriately skilled staff. Care should be given as close to home as possible. Parents/carers, as well as children/young people themselves, should be provided with adequate information which will allow them to manage minor illnesses and chronic conditions. Continuity of care is of key concern, with information flowing between primary care, hospital settings, school and social settings when

Box 4.6 Implications for children's nurses.

- Give clear explanations of any care that you are giving.
- Provide opportunities for families to expand their knowledge of general health issues.
- Do not assume knowledge. For example, many families do not know what a normal temperature is, or how to use a thermometer.
- With newly acquired knowledge, start to promote independence and confidence in parents/carers to mange their own illnesses.
- Always ensure you communicate with the relevant practitioners who will be working with the families, ensuring consent has been given for information sharing first.
- There are new opportunities arising for children's nurse skills in the community setting. This book includes a description of how an acute community children's nursing service was set up in Derbyshire.

Box 4.7 Implications for children's nurses.

- Consider the child/young person as a whole person.
- Consider the context where the child/young person has come from (home/school/social life, community) and that is where she/he will be returning.
- Conserve dignity and privacy, and ensure informed consent is sought.
- Care and services should be planned in partnership with children/young people and their families.
- Ensure you are appropriately skilled in all areas of care you are involved in.
- Ensure the setting, food and activities are safe and appropriate to the developmental needs of the child/young person.
- Communication with community staff is essential, particularly as they will be involved in the child's/young person's care following discharge.
- Report any concerns you might have over a child's/young person's safety and ensure it is followed up. Do not assume other people are aware.

appropriate, whilst at the same time maintaining confidentiality. The standard strongly advocates the use of children's nurses more widely both in the management of chronic illness and in the realm of minor and acute illness care. Services should be accessible and flexible (Box 4.6).

Standard 7: children in hospital

Children/young people should receive high-quality, evidence-based care that has been developed through clinical governance (systems set up to ensure safety and quality). This standard concerns the delivery of child-centred hospital services, the quality and safety of care, and the quality of the setting and environment (Box 4.7).

Standard 8: disabled children/young people and those with complex health needs

This standard is concerned with those children/young people who are disabled, or who have complex health needs. This standard advocates that

they be provided with coordinated, high-quality, child/young person and family-centred care. Their needs should be appropriately assessed. Joint care plans should be made with their involvement, as well as the involvement of relevant family members. Social inclusion should be strived for. Services and care should be provided that will, whenever possible, enable children/young people and their families to live ordinary lives. Early identification and intervention, as well as appropriate family support, are key messages within this standard (Box 4.8).

Standard 9: the mental health and psychological well-being of children/young people

This standard calls for timely, integrated and high-quality multidisciplinary health care for children/young people suffering from mental health problems. It recognises the need for good preventative mental health care and early

Box 4.8 Implications for children's nurses.

- Remember that these families are often in contact with many other services. Ensure good communication to improve continuity of care.
- Holistic care should be given at all time.
- Encourage independence.
- Give consideration around your own learning needs; how are going to communicate with the child/young person with limited speech? What additional training might you need?

intervention. It calls for the effective assessment treatment and support for families who are experiencing early signs of mental health disorders in their child/teenager, so as to prevent deterioration. Mental health promotion is an as important message to impart to parents/carers as is physical health promotion (Box 4.9).

Box 4.9 Implications for children's nurses.

- Consider the emotional and psychological impact of care given, as well as the physical impact.
- Be aware of the extra level of support that families may require.
- Always report if you consider a child/young person's mental health is being compromised.
- Often the smallest things can make the difference to preventing mental health issues:

- Clear explanations.
- Referring on to support services.
- Trying to fit treatment plans into daily routines for the family.
- Listening to concerns.

Standard 10: medicines management for children/young people

The special requirements for children/young people involved in prescribing and administering medicines is of key importance here. As a result of the NSFs, the British National Formulary for Children (BNFC) was published in 2005. It should be

Box 4.10 Implications for children's nurses.

- Always ensure you review the child's/young person's medication.
- Explain to parents/carers what might be expected in terms of side effects in taking any medicine, and advise how quickly the medication might take to work.
- Always ensure the child/young person is discharged with enough medication to last until the family are able to order more supplies.
- Ensure sugar-free preparations are given.
- Oral medicine syringes can be used for administration, where and when it is helpful for babies and young children.
- Clearly record the weight and age of the child/young person, so that correct dosage may be prescribed. Document all dosages given clearly.

available on all paediatric units and in primary care settings.

The BNFC (2005) calls for the correct dosage of medicine to be made based on the weight and age of the child/young person. Oral syringes designed for medicine application should be used to provide more accurate dosage. Sugar-free solutions should also be prescribed, if possible, to prevent dental caries. Families should be fully informed of any benefits or side effects of taking medication to enable them to make informed decisions over treatment choices, and to improve concordance in taking up the treatment planned. Medicines provided to children/young people should be reviewed regularly to ensure they are still required and are not resulting in adverse effects. As a child/young person grows, changes need to be made to dosage so that it remains effective. Accurate recording of drug information is required to ensure that new prescriptions do not interact or overdose a child/young person. Allergies and adverse effects need to be recorded. This is all important in ensuring safety for the child/young person (Box 4.10).

Standard 11: maternity services

This standard calls for women to have access to supportive, high-quality maternity services that are designed around their own needs and those of their babies. It highlights the need for coordinated services, improved health promotion and early parenting advice to women and their partners. This standard is particularly targeted at maternity and neonatal services.

Conclusion

The development of recent Government policy carries great relevance to the modern children's nurse. When caring for children/young people in hospital, it can be easy to consider their illness in isolation of what else might be happening to them in their lives. A nurse needs to have an enquiring mind, getting to know the context in which children/young people live within their community, in order to provide care that is meaningful and safe. There is also a need to remember that although families usually work within a network of other practitioners, the in-patient nurse often has a unique opportunity to observe interactions, dynamics, developmental patterns and behaviours that other practitioners do not have the opportunity to see, in brief contacts with families.

The purpose of public enquiries into serious events, such as Victoria Climbié's death (Laming, 2003) or the Bristol Heart Inquiry (Kennedy, 2001), is to ensure that lessons are learnt from errors of the past. In addition, to ensure safe procedures are followed in the future to prevent others suffering. One message that comes out clearly from the Laming and Kennedy is that, as a practitioner, if there is something that is concerning, whether about the safety or well-being of a child/young person, or the quality of care given by another practitioner, do not assume that others have noticed and taken action. Although poor professional practice or parenting is relatively rare, it can happen in anybody's work environment.

Considering that the life of a child/young person might be at stake, it is everybody's responsibility to sensitively check the situation with other practitioners or agencies. Document what has been observed, inform others if concerns remain and ensure action is taken. Anybody who still needs convincing should read Lord Laming's report (2003) in full. It does not make comfortable reading.

References

British National Formulary for Children (BNFC) (2005) London: BMJ Publishing Group Ltd.

Bullock, H., Mountford, J., Stanley, R. (2001) *Better Policy Making*. London: Centre for the Management of Policy Standards.

Cabinet Office (1999a) *Modernising Government White paper*. London: HMSO.

Cabinet Office (1999b) *Professional Policy Making for the 21st Century*. London: Cabinet Office.

Chief Nursing Officer (2004) *The Chief Nursing Officer's Review of the Nursing, Midwifery and Health Visiting Contribution to Vulnerable Children/Young People*. London: The Stationary Office.

Children Act (2004) London: The Stationery Office.

Department of Health (2004) *Choosing Health: Making Healthy Choices Easier*. London: The Stationery Office.

Education and Skills (Department of) (2003) *Every Child Matters – Green Paper*. London: The Stationery Office.

Education and Skills (Department of) (2004) *Every Child Matters – Next Steps*. London: Education and Skills.

Education and Skills (Department of), Department of Health (2004) *National Service Frameworks for Children, Young People and Maternity Services*. London: Crown Copyright.

Hall, D., Elliman, D. (eds) (2003) *Health for All Children*, 4th edn. Oxford: HMSO.

Kennedy, I. (2001) *The Inquiry into the Management of Care of Children Receiving Complex Heart Surgery at Bristol Royal Infirmary 1984–1995*, Command Paper CM5207. London: Crown Publishing. Available at: http://www.bristol-inquiry.org.uk/final_report.

Laming, L. (2003) *The Victoria Climbié Inquiry: Report of an Inquiry*. London: Crown Publishing. Available at: http://www.victoria-climbie-inquiry.org.uk.

Theme 2

Child Development

Chapter 5   Child Development
Chapter 6   Health for All Children

5 Child Development

Karen Moyse, Janet Savage, Alison Price, Carole Taylor and Mary Hill

NSFs

Practitioners should meet the needs of the *whole child*. Children should receive care that is coordinated around their needs (Department of Health 2003).

Introduction

Children are delightful. They are just wonderful to watch and listen to. They can be fascinated by the simplest of things. Children's development is an interesting subject. No matter how many years you may spend observing children and reading about them, there is always something new to learn and capture your interest.

For nurses to be able to effectively meet the needs of the whole child, which includes health promotion, they must develop an understanding about children's development, how children think and learn. Studying child development will help nurses interact more effectively with them. Importantly, remember children's development is not static, but progressive; it constantly changes.

This chapter examines theories about children's development, particularly *cognitive* development (thinking) as well as looking carefully at how children *learn*. In addition, communicating with children is considered. *Play* can be an effective way of communicating with children and promoting their health. A group of play specialists from the University Hospital Nottingham will highlight how they use play and other activities to help children/young people when they are receiving care in hospital.

Child development theories

This section looks at psychological theories on child development through the work of particular theorists. It considers how these child development theories might be applied in practice. In addition, this section will provide you with the opportunity to link theory and practice.

As you study child development, view language as a reflection of children's thinking. Through their behaviour during play, for example, children demonstrate their understanding of the world around them.

The three theorists that will be studied include the following:

- Jean Piaget.
- Lev Vygotsky.
- Erik Erikson.

Jean Piaget (1896–1980)

Piaget was interested in children's cognitive development. Cognition has been described as the process by which knowledge is acquired (Collins English Dictionary, 1998). Piaget researched children's thoughts and how they developed language, as well as the importance of play in children's cognitive development.

Piaget's work enjoyed great acclaim during the 1950s and 1960s. Since that time some of his work has been further evaluated. He was born in Switzerland. In his early career Piaget worked on intelligence testing (Smith et al., 2003).

Piaget wanted to understand why children did things in the way that they did. A technique was developed by Piaget to find this out, known as the clinical interview. He trained other researchers in his technique. The clinical interview involved asking children open-ended questions. He was looking for an explanation of how children came to understand the world around them (Smith et al., 2003). Piaget concluded that the essence of knowledge was *activity*.

Piaget identified four different stages of cognitive development:

- Sensorimotor stage (0–2 years).
- Pre-operational stage (2–7 years).
- Concrete operational stage (7–12 years).
- Formal operational stage (12+ years).

The word *operation* features prominently within his stages of development. By term Piaget meant *operation mental activity* (Cole et al., 2005). Piaget placed mental activity (operations) into different stages of cognitive development.

The *sensorimotor stage* is the first of Piaget's cognitive stages. He discusses how babies learn about the world around them through sensory actions (Cole et al., 2005). This can involve babies handling objects or putting objects into their mouths. *A baby boy picks up a toy brick and puts it in his mouth. He moves it around, feeling its different surfaces with his tongue and lips.*

The *pre-operational stage* is about symbolic action (Cole et al., 2005). The child learns through the use of language. Words act as symbols to represent objects, actions and thoughts. *A little boy points to an object and appropriately calls it a train. The shape of the object*

and actions made by the object when handled have come to be recognised by him as a train. His use of the word in the correct context has been reinforced by those around him, allowing him to associate the word with the object. Reinforcement and association are key elements in language development.

At this time (2–7 years) the symbolic use of play also emerges (Cole et al., 2005). Children use objects and toys to represent everyday items. *A girl plays with some stones that she lays out in a regular fashion. A group of dolls are placed around the stones. The stones are used to represent everyday objects – cups and plates. The girl imagines that the dolls are having tea together.*

Children use play as a way of trying to understand the meaning of events they have experienced in their lives. *The girl has been taken out to tea on many occasions. With the dolls she is enacting some of those previous experiences.*

Piaget considered that children before the age of 8 years were not able to engage in true mental operations. He felt that they tended to focus their attention on single items. A basic characteristic of children before 8 years of age was, he felt, *egocentrism*. By this term Piaget did not mean they were selfish, but they experienced difficulty seeing the perspective of others (Cole et al., 2005). However, Donaldson (1990) has argued that some children can begin to understand the perspective of others before this age.

Considering children's behaviour before 8 years of age, particularly the behaviour of toddlers, they are very much trying to assert their own will, seeing things from their own perspective. Interacting with young children, however, you may find that some can see the perspectives of others before the age of 8 years, as Donaldson (1990) claims.

Interacting with her 4-year-old, a mother tries to offer her some juice. The mother is rushing, and keeps spilling the juice. The mother is angry with herself for being so clumsy. The child observes this activity and asks her mother if she is alright, and gives her a hug. The child is showing that she can understand how her mother is feeling and even tries to comfort her. Quite a mature understanding is demonstrated by the child.

The age from birth to 7 years is a period where the baby grows and matures into a child. The period is full of so much change. The child's personality really comes to the fore. Perhaps this is the point, Apted (1999) was trying to make in the *7 up series – Give me the child until he is 7, and I will show you the*

Activity

Interact with young children and see what con-
clusions you draw yourself on egocentric behaviour. Perhaps egocentric behaviour depends on
the context of the situation and the child's previous
experiences in that context. Read some of Piaget's
and Donaldson's works more closely, and see what
you think.

man. Do we now see the signs of the future adult
emerging at 7 years?

The *concrete operational stage* develops around
7 years of age. Piaget believed that this was the stage
where true mental actions were beginning, with logical thought processes developing (Cole et al., 2005).

Activity

Have a conversation with a child of 7 or 8 years of
age. You will find it interesting to follow the child's
thought processes and witness the simple logic of the
child's.

When teaching health promotion, consider that
children in the concrete operational stage are able
to follow games with rules and their ability to create
categories increases (Cole et al., 2005).

Activity

Think how you might incorporate these cognitive
abilities (games with rules, categorization) into any
health promotion activities you are planning. For example, you could find out what matters to these children in relation to their health. Present them with a
range of health issues, ask them to place these into
categorises (1–5) based on how important they are to
them. The health issues could be physical, but also
emotional and social too.

Piaget's final stage of cognitive development is
the *formal operational stage*. This stage begins to
emerge from 12 years of age onwards. Piaget believed that this was the highest level of thinking. At
this stage a new level of logical thinking emerges

(Cole et al., 2005). The young person is able to undertake much more complex problem-solving activities.

The young person is now leaving childhood behind and becoming an adult. Observe not only the
physical changes that we commonly associate with
adolescence, but also changes in thinking. When undertaking health promotion activities with young
people, remember they are capable of quite complex
thinking. They also have previous life experiences
to draw upon, which may help in the development
of new knowledge.

Activity

Try undertaking a health promotion session with a
group of teenagers. You may find that they are not always ready to accept your opinion, but may want to
question what you have to offer. This may be based
on their own experiences. Be prepared for this. As
Cole et al. (2005) state, teenagers can be quite questioning of authority.

Piaget's theories on cognitive development provide some interesting insights into how chil-
dren/young people are changing and developing
in their thinking. His theories can be helpful when
putting together health promotion sessions, as they
provide nurses with an understanding of how children's/young people's minds work at different
ages.

Lev Vygotsky (1896–1934)

Another important theorist to look at is Vygotsky.
He was a Russian developmental psychologist. His
educational background was literature and cultural
history (Smith et al., 2003). Vygotsky saw culture
and social organisation (how we organise groups) as
having an important influence on the child's mind
(Vygotsky, 1934).

Similar to Piaget, Vygotsky saw the child as active
in the construction of knowledge and understanding (Smith et al., 2003). However, Vygotsky's focus
was more on the direct intervention of more knowledgeable others in the child's learning.

Through social interaction with more knowledgeable others, the child acquires the tools of thinking and learning. It is through the process of mutual engagement in an activity with another that the child is able to become more knowledgeable (Vygotsky, 1934).

A child is thus able to learn more effectively if she/he undertakes activities with someone more experienced than herself/himself – *a young boy undertaking golf instruction regularly with his father, for example, may go on to swiftly develop in this sport. Through this process of joint activity the boy begins to understand what he needs to do.*

An adult working with a child regularly on a one-to-one basis will help the child become more knowledgeable. *Kerry (6 years old) sits down with her mother each evening to read. Kerry's mother helps her with this activity. Kerry's reading is developing really well.*

An important aspect of Vygotsky's theory is that the person the child is working with needs to be more able than the child, helping and guiding the child. It may be an adult, but equally it could also be a young person, such as an older sibling. Nurses, therefore, through their interactions with children/young people, particularly at an individual level, can help to take children's/young people's knowledge forward.

Vygotsky also saw the use of language as important to the child's development. The child is able to reflect upon her/his own thoughts through the use of language, which will help the child to see things in new ways (Vygotsky, 1934).

Erik Erikson (1902–1994)

Our third theorist is Eric Erikson who, like Vygotsky, was interested in the involvement of others in children's lives. Erikson was keen to know how children/young people develop their social identity. Erikson (1963) believed that an individual's social identity developed through their interactions with others, the relationship between self and the social world.

Erikson (1963) believed that the formation of an individual's identity was a lifelong process, which takes the individual through many different stages. Throughout life the individual asks themselves who they are. At each stage of life they reach a different answer. He proposed that social development has eight stages. Each stage involves a crisis that the individual must resolve in order to move on to the next stage. At each stage the individual is exposed to new possibilities.

For children prior to 7 years of age Erikson (1963) proposed the following stages:

- Trust/mistrust (1st year) – the infant learns to trust those who meet her/his basic needs.
- Autonomy versus shame and doubt (2nd year) – the child learns to exercise her/his will and ability to control herself/himself. If not, the child can become uncertain about herself/himself.
- Initiative versus guilt (3–6 years) – the child learns to initiate her/his own activities. If the child is *not* encouraged to do this, she/he may feel guilty for attempts to do so.

Erikson (1982) believed that a mother creates a sense of *trust* in her child based on the relationship she generates. How sensitively the mother undertakes the child's care, and responds to the child's needs, can form the basis of a sense of developing identity for the child. As the child grows, the mother will guide her/him, providing a sense of meaning to her/his achievements. This is an important foundation in the development of identity.

As nurses, this theory provides us with insights into why the mother/child relationship is so vital for the long-term development and health of children. *A mother is developing a close bond with her child. She sensitively undertakes baby massage. Conversely, a mother who is experiencing difficulties with that bond can be taught the same skill, to help strengthen the relationship with her baby.*

A mother's interactions with her child can be seen as influential in the child, developing a sense of self-confidence. In fact, Erikson (1982) did draw parallels with his ideas about the child developing trust, with the work of other researchers who talked about the child developing confidence, such as Benedek.

Erikson's (1963) second stage, *autonomy versus shame and doubt* (2nd year), refers to the child becoming more independent. The child needs to be supported in her/his attempts to be more independent, if not the child may feel shame for doing so. Further, the child may go on to doubt what she/he is trying to achieve, if not supported. Erikson's ideas about this stage were recognised by Bowlby (1969).

Erikson's third stage involves the child making further attempts to become more independent during the stage of *initiative versus guilt* (3–6 years). Erikson (1963) points out that once again, if the child is not supported, she/he then begins to feel guilty for attempts to do so.

During this time, when children are developing a sense of independence, it is important that parents and carers support them. However, independence has to be within the realms of what is safe to do so. If you go on to use these theories and apply them in your practice with parents and carers, point out any safety aspects that might need to be considered too.

There are two further stages in Erikson's theory of social development that affect children/young people. These include the following:

- Industry versus inferiority (from 7 years through to puberty) – children learn to be competent at activities valued by adults.
- Identity versus role confusion (adolescents) – the young person develops a sense of personal identity as part of her/his social group. If not, the young person becomes confused about who she/he is and what to do in life.

Erikson (1982) described *industry versus inferiority* as the stage which sets the child up for her/his entrance into life. But life, he stated, must first begin at school. The child needs to start to become a worker at school and learn to win recognition by producing things. There is a danger, Erikson goes on to say, that the child can develop a sense of inferiority if she/he experiences difficulties working at school. This may discourage the child from identifying with other children.

Hopefully, the child establishes a good initial relationship with the social world through school. Puberty then develops and childhood comes to an end (Erikson, 1982). The next stage of social development is *identity versus role confusion*. The young person needs to develop further her/his sense of identity development or will go on to have doubts about herself/himself. Erikson (1982) asserts that in many instances where young people fail to settle on an occupational identity, this will disturb them and cause role confusion. *Kerry, who we met earlier in the chapter, is doing well at school she knows what she wants to be when she leaves school. She is about to take her ex-ams, which if successful will take her on to university and a career in nursing.*

Erikson's theory can provide useful insights into social development that not only help nurses to understand children/young people, but also the foundations of adult behaviour. Adolescence is a fascinating stage, which we will look at a little further.

Adolescence

Piaget described adolescence as a time when adult roles are being taken on. Young people begin to plan ahead (Cole et al., 2005). As discussed, Erikson (1968) sees adolescence as the time when identity becomes important; the young person develops a set of beliefs about themselves.

There are huge physical changes happening to young people at this time too. Young people's bodies are changing from that of a child into an adult. Young people may have concerns about these changes and wish to discuss them. Nurses can be especially supportive.

A useful text you might want to look at young people that studies puberty and other health-related matters is *What's Happening to Me* by Meredith (2006).

Puberty, using drama techniques

Puberty can be defined as the stage of adolescence in which the sex glands become functional and secondary sexual characteristics emerge (Collins English Dictionary, 1998). The young person becomes physiologically capable of sexual reproduction. To help young people understand about this new stage in their lives, drama techniques can be used.

A health promotion class was undertaken in school with a group of pupils on the subject of puberty. The technique of hot seating was used, where questions are put to the person in the hot seat. A character was developed for the hot seat. The character was 2 years older than the pupil group. Pupils then directed their questions to the character.

Questions included the following:

- Where can I go in school to get a sanitary pad if I need one?
- Can I still have a bath if I have a period?

Still images were used for scenarios that pupils had developed earlier in the lesson. A still image is the creation of an image using a group of people to capture a particular moment, much like a video freeze-frame. The scenarios included asking a member of staff for a sanitary towel and telling a friend that they had body odour problems.

Thought tracking was then used with the still images to further explore how and what each of these characters may be thinking and feeling. Thought tracking involves the nurse asking the person in the still image what their character is thinking or feeling at the moment in time in which the picture is frozen.

Pupils enjoy using these techniques; it can give them an opportunity to ask questions, share their knowledge and gain insights into how their words and actions can impact on others. The interactive techniques used in the lesson encourage full involvement of all pupils.

Learning theories

This chapter has so far provided some insights into the cognitive processes involved in acquiring knowledge and developing a sense of social identity. The next stage is to consider how nurses can help children/young people learn. Learning theories will be briefly examined which might help in your teaching. This section provides a brief overview on learning specifically related to children; however, Chapter 2 provides more in-depth information, which is also related to adults.

When children are learning a new task, Siegler (1998) suggests that there is a period of change. Importantly, the role of the nurse is to encourage and support them through this change.

Attention

The following sums up some of the main points to consider in relation to child attending. To learn children need to attend in the first instance. Young children only attend for short periods. Vurpillot's (1968) work demonstrates the difficulties young children have in attending, but shows that their ability to attend improves with age.

Try some of the following strategies to help children attend:

- Always vary your activities as this can help to maintain children's interest.
- Make activities interactive; being actively involved can help to sustain children's attention.
- Importantly, always build in time for breaks. This will help children's learning as they will not feel too overloaded.
- Do not expect children to concentrate for long periods.

Memory

Young children first begin to remember faces and words for objects and people they recognise. Campbell and Coulter (1976) found that it takes them longer to remember particular events. Memories of particular events are called episodic memories, which develop around 4 years of age. Think about your earliest memories from childhood, a particular event that happened, for example. At what age were you first able to recall such an event?

From about 2 years of age, children are able to start to generate very simple categories (Cole et al., 2005). Obviously, categorisation becomes a little more complex as they become older. When working with young children of 4 to 5 years old, for example, start to use categories in your health promotion practice. Categorisation can help increase memory as Collins and Quillian (1969) have found.

When talking about healthy eating, for example, generate a traffic light category system for children to identify healthy foods, unhealthy foods and those foods which might fall somewhere in the middle:

- Green – healthy foods.
- Yellow – other foods.
- Red – unhealthy foods.

Another important point in relation to memory relates to the amount of information young children can remember; like adults there is a limit to the amount they can recall. Research on short-term memory has shown that adults can commonly remember seven items from a list (Miller, 1956). However, 6-year-olds are more likely to remember only 2/3 items from a list (Lefrancois, 1994). It has been suggested that sometimes young children are not able to keep enough relevant information in mind (Siegler, 1989/1994). In view of this, take care with the amount of information you provide.

Rewards and praise

Children, as they learn new skills, need lots of encouragement (Sutton, 2000). Rewards and praise are so important in learning. Praise can help an individual feel she/he really making progress. Children love being praised when they have completed a task well. Watch their face light up in delight when you give praise them. It can help with their self-confidence too.

Rewards can provide an incentive for children to participate in an activity, and also help children to attend. Think about the kind of things that your age group would find rewarding. You might need to check if your reward will be acceptable to parents/carers.

Activity

You have been asked to undertake a health promotion session with a small group of young children. Think about the age of your group. Plan your session thinking about learning theories in your design. For example, what activities might you include? How long would these activities last for (work out your timings)? How would you encourage children in their learning?

Communication

How we communicate with children/young people is vital. The following outlines some general points in relation to communicating with children/young people.

Special time

Putting aside time for children/young people is really important; a time that they know is theirs, where they can communicate with you directly. This is known as the *special times* approach, which was developed by Rachel Pinney for children with special needs. Petrie (1997) advocates this approach, and believes it can be particularly useful when getting to know a new child.

For a young child the technique begins by an adult letting the child know she/he will have time together, when she/he can play. The adult gives the child her/his undivided attention (Petrie, 1997). Play is completely directed by the child; the adult has to do as the child says, no suggestions at all must come from the adult. (If you have not done this before, it can be quite hard to hold back from directing the child.)

Importantly, the adult needs to give the child feedback, so the child knows that she/he has been understood (Petrie, 1997). The adult obviously needs to ensure that the environment is safe for the child too. Have a go, see how you get on. The approach provides the child with the opportunity to express herself/himself, as well as providing the nurse with insights into how the child is thinking.

Listening to children/young people

Nurses spend a lot of their time giving advice to children/young people. Yet, sometimes all they might want is to be listened to. *Listening* to children/young people is essential. The nurse might be the one person who the child/young person feels will listen. In the busy working environment it is not always easy to find time. However, listening should always be an important priority in children's/young people's care.

Petrie (1997) provides advice on how to be an encouraging listener:

- Give children/young people your attention.
- Listen.
- Do not interrupt, at least at first.
- Let them know you are listening, through the use of body language and facial expressions.
- Reflect back, letting them know you have heard and understood.

Once the child has expressed her/his thoughts then it will be more appropriate to ask questions and provide advice.

Many nurses already think that they are good listeners. Yet, it is always worth taking time out every now and again, reflecting upon your communications with children/young people. Or ask one or two of your colleagues to observe you, and see what they suggest.

Petrie (1997) suggests getting down to the child's level when interacting. This is a really good point. Often when people are speaking with a child, they fail to do this and they speak over the child's head. All that the child can then see is a set of knees. Have a go and see what it feels like. How much of the communication seems to get lost when the face of the other person cannot be seen? The positions of one's body and the facial expressions used have a crucial impact on communication too. Argyle (1983) has written extensively on non-verbal communications and what messages they convey.

The National Society for the Prevention of Cruelty to Children (NSPCC, 1996) produce a useful leaflet on listening to children/young people. Simply called *Listening to Children*, available direct from the NSPCC, it is designed for parents/carers but nurses will find it useful too.

Asking questions

Children are naturally curious and want to know. Morris (2005) talks about curiosity as an important characteristic associated with the young of species. Children, when they feel confident enough, will ask questions. Sadly, some adults feel that children asking questions is a bit off putting, and will only tolerate it up to a point.

Children should be encouraged to ask questions. When responding to their questions, answer in a way that they will understand; use language they are familiar with.

To be able to effectively provide care, the nurse will need to ask questions of the child, for example, to find out how the child is feeling. There are different ways of approaching questions. Petrie (1997) discusses the use of closed and open questions, as a way of finding out how a child feels.

Closed questions may only yield a one-word answer in response, which may not be enough. However, the response received may be as much as the child is prepared to give. Example is as follows:

Nurse: How do you feel?
Child: OK.

Open questions can be more enlightening, if the child feels up to it. Example is as follows:

Nurse: How does the new dressing feel compared to the old one?
Child: A bit tight. Can you make it less tight?

The second question and response enables the nurse to really know how the child feels.

If communicating with a child is difficult, always ask the parents/carers for help. Communicating through parents/carers can ease many a difficult situation. A favourite toy can often help too. Ask about the toy or perhaps use the toy (with child's permission) to demonstrate an aspect of care.

Be aware that asking too many questions, particularly if the child is not feeling well, is not a good idea (Petrie, 1997). Supportive comments may suffice.

Becoming independent

As children become older they start to become more independent. They begin to do more for themselves and others too. At around 7/8 years, Brewer and Cutting (2001) maintain that children start to feel personally responsible for their own actions, including their actions towards others. Example is as follows:

Lucy (7 years old): I have got to help Claire feed Alex, I promised I would help.

In terms of health promotion work, particularly during sessions and activities, nurses can ask children to do things for themselves. Or perhaps ask them to complete a task before the next session, such as completing a chart on how many times they have cleaned their teeth during a week.

Brewer and Cutting (2001) also maintain that children of this age start to develop strong opinions about what is right and wrong. Speak to a child of 7/8 years about smoking, for example, and see what kind of response you receive. Example is as follows:

Lucy: Duncan, why do you smoke? It is not good for you. I am going to hide your smoke packet.
Mother (later): Why did you say that to Duncan?
Lucy: I did not want him to smoke because it is not good for him. And I am right.

In terms of health promotion they are interested in the messages provided, and form opinions about what is right and wrong from an early age.

This section of the chapter has taken a brief look at ways that may help when communicating with children. The following section looks at play and interacting with children in hospital.

Play in hospital

Play and interacting thoughtfully with children/young people can be really important for communication. Thoughtful communications will enable the nurse to find out what children/young people are feeling.

Play is really valuable to children, and its value should never be underestimated. Many theorists have studied children's play, notably Erikson and Piaget. Too little play can deprive children of important learning opportunities. Smith et al. (2003) report that play is beneficial for children's development. It is important to expose them to a wide range of resources and allow them to be creative. Watch children at play and see what you think.

Play can particularly help children come to terms with different life experiences. Mussen et al. (1990) suggest that play helps children deal with any anxieties they may have experienced. Play may therefore help children come to terms with problems of ill health, for example.

For information about children's play contact the Children's Play Information Service (2008) (http://www.ncb.org.uk/). It holds an extensive collection of reference material on the subject of play and is based at the National Children's Bureau library. The National Association of Hospital Play Staff (2007) website is useful for information on hospital play (http://www.nahps.org.uk/).

The following provides nurses with insights into play and interacting with children/young people in hospital, as discussed by the play specialists from University Hospital Nottingham.

Children's outpatient department

Children's outpatient's department, QMC campus, is a large area with 12 consulting rooms and an open plan seated waiting area. Children/young people come for consultation on a wide range of specialities including orthopaedic, surgical, neonatal, medical, dermatology and gastroenterology.

My role, as a hospital play specialist, is non-clinical and a key part of it involves building a rapport with children/young people and their families. The basis of my work is about establishing trust and providing explanations. Samantha Thorpe recognised this in her interview with me recently when she said, 'Building a rapport with individual patients is clearly fundamental to the success of the work carried out by play specialists' (Thorpe, 2006, pp. 20–21).

Children/young people will present in clinic with a variety of previous experiences, expectations and preconceived ideas. The work that I do involves trying to break down these thoughts and feelings into manageable pieces, so that their real fears and anxieties can be addressed in a supportive way.

Referrals can take many forms but are often initiated from observing children/young people in the waiting area or treatment room. I assess a child's/young person's behaviour and attempt to meet her/his needs with age-appropriate specialised play techniques.

Specialised play can be divided into preparation, distraction and post-procedural play. I use especially adapted dolls, photo stories and an ability to focus purely on the child/young person and what they say or communicate. Play offers them an opportunity to express their feelings before, during and after a procedure. They all have very different needs and therefore play programmes can be tailored accordingly.

Distraction is an important technique, and can take many forms, from looking in a magazine whilst having a blood test, to counting games or using visual aids. Each situation will be different and unique to each child/young person. Barry (2000) explains that the work of play specialist is diverse and certainly requires imagination.

For example, Peter (his name has been changed in line with confidentiality guidance; Nursing and Midwifery Council, 2004) aged 10, a chronically ill patient, would always be tearful in clinic. Before our sessions he appeared to accept being fearful and upset as part of the hospital experience, almost as though it was an agreed side effect.

After several preparation sessions and lengthy discussions, I learnt that Peter was frightened of not being able to cope with the blood tests. Peter felt that he had already coped with so much, in medical terms, and that he was no longer capable of dealing with the thought of having further blood tests. Peter needed to feel empowered and to be equipped with coping skills. He was not frightened by the procedure but more the thought of not coping. It was really important to recognise that Peter had just come to the end of his tether with medical procedures.

It had been difficult for Peter to communicate his thoughts to others, so it was part of my role to voice his concerns. Clough (2005) states helping a child express and deal with her/his feelings constructively and positively is probably one of the most important things an adult can do to help. Through encouragement and by learning positive thought techniques, Peter learnt that he could cope with the blood tests.

In children's outpatients I have a unique opportunity to offer play programmes outside the clinic appointment. This means that if a child/young person requires further input, a date and a time can be arranged for them to see me. This is particularly useful and important for those who become distressed and cannot cope with any further intervention during their clinic appointment. As most blood test procedures are routine, there is less of a time constraint and indeed doctors are usually happy to wait 4 weeks for the results, thus giving the programme time to work. A large part of making these programmes a success is liaising effectively with staff and family members, so that the child or young person's behaviour is not misunderstood and they receive appropriate support.

Probably the most important aspect of my role is to be an advocate for the child/young person. The play specialist is someone who is able to consider the child's/young person's view and how the best outcome for the child/young person can be achieved, in a fun and informal way. The play specialist can change the negative perception of a hospital visit into a less frightening one.

PICU

A paediatric intensive care unit (PICU) is not the most obvious area where you would expect to find play being used to promote children's health. Play, in this setting, is however a very useful and powerful tool.

Acutely sick babies sometimes require some form of assisted ventilation and use intensive care beds.

Typically, they have a very short stay before being well enough to return to the ward. However, more and more we are seeing babies requiring long-term ventilation, often from birth or early infancy. These are the babies and families who are able to benefit most from play, as a way of promoting emotional health.

Long-term babies and their families have more time and energy. They are an ideal group to work with on promoting health through play, as well as discussing child health promotion topics. Once a baby, who requires long-term ventilation becomes stable (often having a tracheostomy and therefore a safe airway) they are receptive to play.

Play is primarily used to help a baby develop a sense of normality and to help them reach their developmental milestones, as far as they are able. The play specialist needs to know the diagnosis of each individual baby. Working closely with families, particularly mothers, the play specialist along with the named nurses is able to develop good working relationships and trust. Many families who have a baby requiring long-term care on PICU are young and need lots of reassurance and teaching. We are, in effect, promoting good health on a daily basis often without realising it.

Hospitals should be healthy settings and being in hospital should not jeopardise the health of a baby or child; instead the hospital can often be an ideal environment in which to introduce health promotion and day-to-day routines.

A typical example of this was with a baby who had been on PICU since he was 7 weeks old and was ventilator dependant. A good relationship had been developed with the family. We agreed on a daily routine for the baby. Together the mother and I used play activities to promote the baby's development and discussed general baby care. His mother was very young and although very competent, she actively looked and asked for guidance on all areas of his specialist care and normal baby care.

Play was the tool that enabled this mother to be relaxed with her son. It almost gave her the permission to touch, hold and feel him, without worrying about all his medical problems. It enabled her to care for him and feel needed and to do what all *normal* mothers do. For a short time she was able to forget that this was a clinical environment. Play sessions, whenever possible, would happen with mother and baby on the floor, with the use of a special play mat. Health promotion topics were discussed in an informal way. It was rather like a coffee morning or a chat with the health visitor. All the experiences that most mothers usually take for granted are often not possible for a mother whose baby is in hospital for long term. They do not get an opportunity to meet other mothers and thus do not build up the same support networks, which can be so vital.

The initial aims of a play session are to promote normal stages of development and to offer some form of normality and fun. It can, however, offer much more to a family with a long-term ventilated baby. The play specialist in an intensive care environment is often seen to be the most approachable member of the multidisciplinary team as she is perceived as the one person who is least busy, and can be more easily called upon. The help of a play specialist can be utilized in this context to help promote children's health, as well as family health.

Adolescents

Adolescents, teenagers, young people, whatever title we give them, they often do not know who they are or where they fit, in the no man's land we call a children's ward. As they are neither adult nor child, they can find themselves in the midst of hospital life, with all the ups, downs and dramas that can come with it. Understandably, they sometimes find it hard to cope. Many of them watch the hospital dramas on the television, and this can give them a very unrealistic view of what hospital life is about.

Young people can often feel that the environment on the ward is too babyish, but the alternative of being cared for on an adult ward alongside elderly, very sick or dying patients, is too scary for them to contemplate. On adult wards there are also restrictions on visiting times and no facilities for parents/carers to stay overnight.

My experiences have taught me that although we do not provide play activities as such for this age group, they still need input and support, occasionally even more than some of the younger children. With planning, consideration and flexibility, we can give appropriate care to young people on the ward. Compromise is definitely the key when dealing with this age group.

There are many factors that can affect a young person when in hospital which need to be handled with care and sensitivity. These factors can include separation from family and friends, a fear of pain and the loss of freedom and control. Further, changes in body image such as potential scarring from surgery or mobility issues from a plaster cast, crutches or even a wheelchair can impact on their schooling and social life. Frequently, fear or anxiety can be covered by bravado and non-compliance, yet underneath this behaviour is a frightened and confused young person.

The main aspect of my role as play specialist is to act as an advocate for the young person. In order to do this I form a relationship with them, usually by talking, eliciting their likes and dislikes, hobbies and interests. Some of the strongest relationships I have formed were initiated by asking a very simple question – *who is on the front of the magazine you are reading?* My interest is not just in their medical condition but how they feel emotionally. I therefore support them and assess how they are coping with their treatment, ensuring that they are prepared and informed regarding their admission.

It is vital to understand the issues behind any fears. One 15-year-old girl left the consulting room in tears after a pre-admission check for elective surgery. When I spoke to her, she was not frightened about her admission, but upset because she would need to remove her new acrylic nail extensions before surgery. This is a big deal when you are 15 years of age. The problem was resolved by my promise to give her a French manicure upon return from theatre.

The play specialist is often seen as a safe person, as we are not doctors or nurses, who they sometimes see as a little threatening. Obviously, we liaise and work closely with other practitioners involved in their care. We try to facilitate compromise and boundaries if required. If you start a battle with this age group you can be sure of retaliation.

Finally, health promotion on discouraging smoking, drug misuse, self-harm and eating disorders is relevant to this age group. Young people vary in their maturity and their method of dealing with problems, but we support them in any way we can, even if it is just to provide a listening ear. Trust and mutual respect are essential when working with young people.

Sometimes young people just need to be reassured that it is OK to be scared or that even if they cry, they are still doing well. The fact that they have held my hand until it is numb and sobbed through fear in the anaesthetic room will always remain a closely guarded secret between the two of us.

Children's play and interacting with young people in supportive ways can turn potentially frightening experiences in hospital into situations where children, young people and their families cope really well. Play specialists are undoubtedly an essential asset.

Conclusion

This chapter on child development has examined some theories on cognitive development and social development, as well as learning and communication. It is important for nurses to understand how children/young people function (think and feel) at different stages in their lives, so nurses can meet their needs effectively.

Children/young people's development is constantly changing. When undertaking health promotion with different age groups, an understanding of child development will enable the nurse to provide activities that are age-appropriate, which hopefully they will enjoy, and will enhance their health.

Playing with children and interacting with young people in hospital has been explored through the work of play specialists. Three different approaches to play in the hospital environment have been presented. The play specialists from University Hospital Nottingham have provided some really interesting and moving insights. Their work is vital in helping children/young people to understand their own health needs.

Play specialists help children's/young people's physical health by primarily supporting their emotional health. One cannot be achieved without the other – caring for the whole child/young person.

References

Apted, M. (1999) *7 Up, a Book of the Acclaimed TV Series*. London: Random House.

Argyle, M. (1983) *The Psychology of Interpersonal Behaviour*. Middlesex: Penguin Books.

Barry, P. (2000) *A Child's Recollection of Hospital*. National Association of Hospital Play Staff. Available at: http://www.nahps.org.uk/Childsrecollection.htm (accessed September 2008).

Bowlby, J. (1969) *Attachment and Loss*. London: Hogarth Press.

Brewer, S., Cutting, A. (2001) *A Child's World, a Unique Insight into How Children Think*. London: Headline Book Publishing.

Campbell, B., Coulter, X. (1976) In Rosenzweig, M., Leiman, A. (1989) *Physiological Psychology*. New York: Random House.

Children's Play Information Service. (2008) National Children's Bureau Library. Available at: http://www.ncb.org.uk/ (accessed September 2008).

Clough, J. (2005) Using books to prepare children for surgery. *Paediatric Nursing* 17: 28.

Cole, M., Cole, S., Lightfoot, C. (2005) *The Development of Children*, 5th edn. New York: Worth Publishers.

Collins English Dictionary (1998) Glasgow: Harper Collins Publishers.

Collins, A., Quillian, M. (1969) Retrieval time from semantic memory. *Journal of Verbal Learning and Verbal Behaviour* 8: 244.

Department of Health (2003) *Standard for Hospital Services. National Service Framework for Children, Young People and Maternity Services*. London: Crown Copyright.

Donaldson, M. (1990) *Children's Minds*. London: Fontana Press.

Erikson, E. (1963) *Childhood and Society*. New York: Norton.

Erikson, E. (1968) *Identity, Youth and Crisis*. London: Faber.

Erikson, E. (1982) In: Jenks, C. (ed.) *The Sociology of Childhood*. London: Batsford Academic and Educational Limited.

Lefrancois, G. (1994) *Psychology for Teaching*. California: Wadsworth Publishing Co.

Meredith, S. (2006) *What's Happening to Me?* London: Usborne Publishing Ltd.

Miller, G. (1956) The magical number seven plus or minus two. *Psychological Review* 63: 81–97.

Morris, D. (2005) *The Naked Ape: A Zoologist's Study of the Human Animal*. London: Vintage Books.

Mussen, P., Conger, J., Kagan, J., Huston, A. (1990) *Child Development and Personality*. New York: Harper Collins Publishers.

National Society for the Prevention of Cruelty to Children. (1996) *Listening to Children, a Guide for Parents*. London: NSPCC.

Nursing and Midwifery Council (2004) *The NMC Code of Professional Conduct*. London: Nursing and Midwifery Council.

Petrie, P. (1997) *Communicating with Children and Adults, Interpersonal Skills for Early Years and Play Work*. London: Arnold.

Siegler, R. (1989/1994) In Lefrancois, G. (ed.) *Psychology for Teaching*. California: Wadsworth Publishing Company.

Siegler, R. (1998) *Children's Thinking*. Englerwood Cliffs, NJ: Prentice Hall, Erlbaum.

Smith, P., Cowie, H., Blades, M. (2003) *Understanding Children's Development*. Oxford: Blackwell Publishing.

Sutton, C. (2000) *Helping Families with Troubled Children*. Chichester: John Wiley & Sons.

The National Association of Hospital Play Staff. (2007) Available at: http://www.nahps.org.uk/ (accessed November 2007).

Thorpe, S. (2006) The power of play. *Children Now Journal*, 30 August–5 September, p. 20–21.

Vurpillot, E. (1968) The development of scanning strategies and their relation to visual differentiation. *Journal of Experimental Child Psychology* 6: 632–650.

Vygotsky, L. (1934) *Thought and Language*. Cambridge MA: MIT Press.

6 Health for All Children

Janet Badcock

NSF

The National Service Framework for children, young people and maternity services (NSF, Education and Skills, Department of Health 2004) maintains that the health of all children should be promoted and delivered through a coordinated plan of action. The importance of prevention and early intervention is emphasised. *Health for All Children's* provides such a plan for all children.

Introduction

Health for All Children provides a coordinated programme for the promotion of children's/young people's health (Hall and Elliman, 2003). It helps to facilitate prevention and early intervention for children, where needed.

Health for All Children is a cornerstone document that acts as a key reference point for any practitioner wishing to improve children's health. Its importance is such that it forms one of the building blocks for the *National Service Frameworks for Children, Young People and Maternity Services* (NSFs, Education and Skills, Department of Health, 2004).

There have been many editions of *Health for All Children*, which is a testament to both its success and changing times. It demonstrates how child health is working to keep up with emerging new evidence. Essentially, *Health for All Children* is concerned with the prevention and early detection of illness and developmental disorders so that they may be treated earlier to avoid unnecessary complications. The book has a number of different contributors from the field of child health.

Prior to the publication of this fourth edition, there had been strong emphasis on a stringent Child Health Surveillance programme, whereby all children were offered a screening programme. *Health for All Children* argued that such a programme was not based on good evidence, besides being costly and ineffective to run. The Child Health Surveillance programme contained the vaccination schedule and some aspects of health promotion.

The fourth edition systematically reviewed the Child Health Surveillance programme and concluded that there were only certain elements of the old programme that should remain. In its place a new programme was introduced based more heavily on the promotion of good health, with a much more streamlined system for the screening of certain childhood conditions. The majority of recommendations in the 4th edition were subsequently approved by the NSF working party (see Chapter 4).

Major issues that the *Health for All Children* team considered in developing the fourth edition were the following:

- What should be available to all families?
- What would be targeted to those families in need?

They identified that all children should have access to an immunisation programme. In addition, opportunities within a child's first 2 years of life to pick up on abnormalities and provide information on child rearing and parenting issues were to be given.

They noted that a significant amount of time was spent by community practitioners on assessing children in whom it was clear that they were developing within expected norms. This left limited time and resources available to provide intensive support to those families who really needed it. To ensure effective use of resources, it was important that additional support should be available to those families that were most vulnerable. Assessment of family need thus became a key element of the proposed new Child Health Promotion Programme (Hall and Elliman, 2003). In addition, assessment of family need forms a key element within the NSFs.

Needs assessments are broadly based on the known key determinants of ill health and are used as a general marker when meeting families. Although it is known, for example, that poverty can be a key determinant of poor health, not all families on low incomes necessarily live unhealthily or have poor coping strategies. Caution needs to be taken. Each family should be assessed on their own merits. Equally, it should not be assumed that just because a family is affluent, they do not have any health needs. Indeed, the majority of families welcome support on parenting and health promotion information at key points in their child's life.

What might differ is the manner in which some people will receive health promotion information. Some may feel confident to ask health practitioners, read books or access the internet for information. However, other families will require a more hands-on approach. Individual families should be assessed based on their own unique set of circumstances, which includes their understanding and knowledge about health and child rearing. Additionally, their access to healthy food, safe housing,

education, social networks and their own coping strategies should be considered. To this end, *Health for All Children* advises that by the age of 1 year all children and their families will have received a comprehensive assessment of their needs so that plans can be put in place for future care.

Health promotion

Health promotion and the absence of ill health

As described above, the new programme is largely based on the promotion of health. Health promotion comes under the umbrella of Public Health. *Health for All Children* defines health promotion as: 'Any planned and informed intervention that is designed to improve physical or mental health or prevent disease, disability and premature death' (Hall and Elliman, 2003, p. 6).

Hall and Elliman (2003) are clear that although parents/carers have a responsibility for their children's health, society has also a role in ensuring children's rights and needs are met and protected. *Health for All Children* outlines the importance of using an *empowerment* model in promoting the health of children to enable parents/carers to achieve responsibility for their children's health. Hall and Elliman (2003) believe this can be achieved by working both at an individual level and a community level. The book you are currently reading contains many examples of where the promotion of children's health has been achieved, using an empowerment approach with good effect.

Whose responsibility is child health promotion?

Whose responsibility is the promotion of children's health? The simple answer to this question is that it is the responsibility of all practitioners. In the community, face-to-face contacts largely involve general practitioners (GPs), practice nurses, health visitors, community nursery nurses, school nurses, midwives, community children's nurses, pharmacists and community psychiatric nurses. They often deliver services in extended schools, Sure Start centres, children's centres, in people's homes, surgeries and other community settings. There has also been a move towards the use of lay people, who have undergone specific training, to provide healthy living advice. Often these are people who live in the community they are serving.

In addition to the above, there are many unseen hands supporting health promotion work, often coming under the remit of the Public Health department. These individuals are involved in the setting up of new initiatives, along with often forming strong alliances with statutory and non-statutory organisations to develop new services. New initiatives might include safety equipment schemes, parenting courses, healthy living centres and healthy eating initiatives, for example.

Most health organisations have a health promotion department from where health promotion leaflets and other teaching materials can be borrowed, and are ideal to use when wanting to get a health promotion message across. Each NHS organisation is arranged slightly differently, and staff will use different work titles. Contact the local Public Health department and find out exactly what resources are in your area.

Ensuring consistency

When providing health information to parents/carers, always ensure you know what their prior knowledge is on the subject. This will help when trying to pitch information at the right level and will ensure you can deal with any apparent contradictions in advice that may have been given from others sensitively. When appropriate, back up your information with printed literature. This may mean written or largely pictorial leaflets, depending on the literacy level of families. Do avoid overloading them with too much written information unless they have asked for more in-depth details. Sometimes it will not get read, especially when they are busy dealing with an ill child. Choose something that puts the message across simply.

When choosing a leaflet to back up information, be cautious of those which have been written or sponsored by a manufacturer, however research-based they may seem. Many quote statistics from their own research trials. Even the unhealthiest of foods can manage to look healthy in some manufacturer's leaflets. Instead, look for up-to-date leaflets

that have been produced by organisations such as the Department Health or specialist professional bodies, as they will ensure less bias. These leaflets will be based on established evidence, and will not contain advertising. This will ensure that the information you are giving will be consistent with the Government message.

Many leaflets are now available in a variety of languages. Your Health Promotion department will be able to help accessing these materials.

The scope of child health promotion

Traditionally, health promotion has covered the more obvious aspects of healthy diet and nutrition, drug, alcohol and cigarette misuse. However, the scope of health promotion within Child Health is becoming increasingly broader and now includes mental health promotion and the child development, which includes communication skills and play skills (Chief Nursing Officer, 2004).

In addition, *Health for All Children* (Hall and Elliman, 2003) covers the following aspects of children's health:

- Physical examination.
- Growth monitoring and nutrition.
- Laboratory and radiological screening tests.
- Iron deficiency.
- Hearing and vision defects.
- Developmental and behavioural problems.
- Child protection (safeguarding).
- Children in special circumstances.

This chapter explores three themes from *Health for All Children*: children's communication, children's growth monitoring and iron deficiency anaemia.

Children's communication

Communication is considered an important aspect of care. For the child its importance lies in the need to be understood and to interact with others.

Communication is not just in the acquisition of words. It is found in gesture, whether through informal gesture or formal sign language, body language and in facial expressions (Education and Skills, 2002).

Often it can be difficult to know when a child is ill, or in unfamiliar surroundings, whether an inability to communicate is due to the new surroundings of the hospital environment, for example, or due to a communication delay in development. However, once the child has settled into any hospital setting, the child should start to open up and communicate.

Communication is a key aspect of the human experience. Older children, like adults, communicate using both verbal and non-verbal methods, but babies and toddlers predominantly use the latter. Socialisation skills are very closely linked with communication, and often when one of these is impaired, the other experiences a knock-on effect. Children who are unable to communicate effectively are often prone to temper tantrums and crying outbursts, as they cannot make their needs understood and find it difficult to get on with other children (I Can, 2007).

Communication, like child development, can be open to wide variations of normal. However, the key difference in knowing if a child has a communication difficulty is not just in the child's ability or inability to reel off words accurately. Other factors come into play, such as whether the child is able to understand language, able to follow age-appropriate instructions and is able to make her/his needs clear, using verbal and non-verbal means (I Can, 2007).

When children are ill or they are in unfamiliar surroundings, they are less likely to act normally. Once children have settled and are feeling better, they should be able to communicate effectively with their parents/carers, even if they clam up as soon as the nurse arrives. Find out from parents/carers about their child's communication skills. Gaining insights into how the child communicates at home may provide an indication of how well the child is coping with being in hospital.

It is possible to have a communication difficulty and otherwise have age-appropriate development, although communication difficulties may also exist with a general delay in the child's development. If you do have concerns that a child in your care has a communication difficulty, then alert the paediatrician and indicate any observations you have made. Any action taken should be detailed in your discharge letter to the health visitor/GP, so that they are aware of any concerns and can follow them

through. A useful website for information on communication is http://www.ican.org.uk.

Hall and Elliman (2003) stress the need to assess the hearing of any child who has language problem, as hearing and language are strongly associated; if a child is unable to hear, the child will have difficulty communicating.

Hall and Elliman (2003) point out that language difficulties can be associated with academic problems later, such as delays in reading. Communication and language difficulties are explored in their chapter on identifying children with developmental problems (Chapter 13).

Always, find out if parents/carers have any concerns about their child's language.

Children's growth monitoring

Children's growth monitoring involves the accurate measurement of height, weight and head circumference. Hall and Elliman (2003) examine this issue in Chapter 8 of their book.

The monitoring of growth is important as it is a way of detecting signs of underlying diseases and problems. Most parents/carers are very interested in how well their child is growing, but it can evoke great emotion, possibly because it is an affirmation about how well they are nurturing their child.

If a child is not growing well, parents/carers can become anxious. Understandably so, as they may feel responsible and are concerned about their child's health. Parents/carers may even feel that practitioners are questioning their parenting skills. For these reasons, measurements of growth need to be taken accurately and dealt with sensitively in order to prevent undue alarm.

Measurement techniques

There are a number of areas that need to be considered when measuring, recording and interpreting results. The following explores some of these issues.

Weight

Hall and Elliman (2003) advise that children should be weighed on self-zeroing scales, which are placed on a firm surface. Scales need to be regularly calibrated to ensure accuracy.

Babies should be weighed naked and toddlers with vest and pants. Children should be weighed in light clothing, unless otherwise directed.

Poor weight gain can be a sign of underlying acute or chronic disease, inadequate nutrition or neglect. However, in these instances, there are usually other signs and symptoms present. Equally, the overweight child is now becoming more of a medical and social issue for child health. Overweight needs to be handled very sensitively, so meaningful help can be provided.

A useful time to undertake a weight check is when a child attends for immunisation. Hall and Elliman (2003) also suggest that scales can be available in clinics, so that parents/carers have the opportunity to weigh their child themselves, particularly if there are no concerns.

Length and Height

Hall and Elliman (2003) advise that supine length should be measured. Once the child is 2 years of age, height measurements can then be undertaken.

Supine length measurements can be undertaken with a suitable measuring mat. Two practitioners trained in the correct technique should be involved to help ensure accuracy.

From the age of 2 upwards an appropriate standing measurement tool should be used, such as the Leicester height measure. For younger children, it is advisable to have two people carrying out the measurement; again this will help with accuracy.

Abnormalities in length and height can indicate underlying disease processes such as the following:

- Hypothyroidism.
- Growth hormone insufficiency.
- Turner's syndrome.
- Bone dysplasia.
- Idiopathic short stature.
- Psycho-social short stature – this is usually the result of abuse.
- Excessively tall stature – which might indicate a range of syndromes.
- Growth impairment.

Importantly, a single measurement will not identify a problem. A series of measurements will need to be recorded to identify if there is a problem.

Head circumference

Head circumference can be measured using a reusable lasso plastic tape. The measurement should be taken at the largest circumference point of the head.

Hall and Elliman (2003) outline the conditions that can be identified through monitoring of head circumference. These include the following:

- Hydrocephalus.
- Microcephaly.
- Subdural effusion.
- Haematoma.

Recording and plotting

Suitable growth charts should be used to accurately plot and interpret results. With children for whom growth is developing normally, use the charts filed in the personal child health record. For a child whose growth appears to be faltering, a more detailed growth-monitoring chart developed by the Royal College of Paediatrics and Child Health should be used as the basis for recording. Care should always be taken with plotting measurement results on growth charts to avoid errors. Check the child's age before plotting. Not only plot the measurement, but also note it down in the child's record, in figures, dated and signed. It is essential that practitioners are able to interpret growth charts correctly, so they are able to explain results appropriately to parents/carers.

Interpreting results

Weight can be a short-term measure of well-being, while height tends to be a longer term measurement. A child might dramatically lose weight in the period of a week, for example, due to an acute illness such as gastroenteritis. Problems with height will be detected over time, whether due to physical or psychological causes. Weight can also be a measure of long-term health. A slow trend up or down may only be visible over time, indicating difficulty of a more chronic nature.

With head circumference Hall and Elliman (2003) maintain that after 8 weeks of age, if there are no concerns about a baby's head circumference, it need not be recorded. However, if concerns about a baby's growth, health or development do arise, then it needs recording.

When giving health promotion advice to parents/carers, be certain to give advice that is relevant to their lifestyle and find out what methods that might have already been tried. It is important to develop a rapport with families so that their child's growth may be properly monitored. Should growth be faltering, it is important to ensure that the child is referred to a paediatrician.

Iron deficiency anaemia

Health for All Children identified that iron deficiency anaemia (IDA) is a common nutrition-based disorder of childhood. Its prevalence can vary from 5 to 40%, which will be rather dependent on the demographic make-up of specific areas. IDA can span the social divides, and the correlation between deficiency and socio-economic status is not clear (Hall and Elliman, 2003).

Younas and Prakash (2006) indicate that the prevalence is higher in certain ethnic minorities such as Chinese, African Caribbean and particularly in children from the British, Pakistani, Bangladeshi and Indian populations. Children who are being fed vegan or vegetarian diets also need particular monitoring to ensure they are receiving both sufficient iron and calories (British Dietetic Association (2007; http://www.bda.uk.com).

IDA is identified by the World Health Organization as a haemoglobin count of less than 11 gdL. However, readings in transferrin saturation, serum iron and zinc protoporphyrin level, as well as total iron binding capacity, are also often used to identify IDA (Hall and Elliman, 2003).

The effects of IDA

IDA has long been associated with slowing of the intellectual faculties and overall development of the child. It is known that these effects are largely reversible once corrected with iron supplements; although such children who have been available for long-term follow-up have been found to have some minor residual effects on intellect. It is unclear if this is due to the effects of the previous anaemia or environmental factors, which may have led them to becoming iron deficient in the first place (Hall and Elliman, 2003).

As well as having effects on intellect, Younas and Prakash (2006) cite the following signs and symptoms which may be associated with IDA:

- Breathlessness and lethargy.
- Reduced activity, tiring easily.
- Pica – the child has an increased appetite for non-foodstuffs (paper, paint).
- Pallor.
- Spoon-shaped finger nails and ridging of nail surfaces.
- Scaling at the corners of mouth.
- Changes to hair.
- Some splenomegaly.

The causes of IDA

The reasons for such a high incidence of IDA are felt to be due to variety of causes. Some of the causes are felt to be the early introduction of cow's milk, cultural reasons and premature birth, for example.

The early introduction of unmodified cow's milk, which is low in iron, is felt to be a major cause. It has been identified that children who drink large amounts of cow's milk before the age of 1 have a lower iron status (Younas and Prakash, 2006).

Cultural differences in diet may also be a major cause that predisposes certain Asian groups to a low iron status. Younas and Prakash (2006) identify that the area of origin of the birth mother is a significant factor. Asian mothers tend to start their babies on cow's milk earlier and delay the introduction of solids later, compared to the rest of the British population.

Iron deficiency has been long associated with premature birth and low birthweight. Premature babies are now routinely provided with iron and vitamin supplements.

Early cord clamping at birth has also been identified with lower levels of iron in the blood. There are some other less common causes too, which you may wish to explore.

Any child that has been prescribed iron supplements should be advised that it may cause constipation, and information should be given on how to avoid this. They should also be advised about the dangers of overdose. The safe storage of medicines should be discussed too.

In the United Kingdom (UK), iron supplements are not routinely given or advised for the population as a whole as a preventative measure, although all infant formula milk in the UK is fortified with iron. IDA is a preventable condition and in addition to giving foods rich in iron, suitable for the child's age, the following advice should also be given to parents/carers. This advice is pertinent to babies and young children. For exact recommendations in relation to these age groups, check current dietary guidelines. Hall and Elliman (2003) advise the following:

- Breast milk, although it has a low level of iron, it is taken up easily by the body, so that its iron resources are well absorbed. This should be the milk of choice. Breastfeeding mothers themselves need to ensure that they are having an adequate dietary iron intake.
- Unmodified cow's milk (doorstep milk) should not be given to babies (under 1 year) as their main drink/feed.
- Weaning should commence at 6 months, so that babies can obtain iron from other food sources.
- Iron found in meat is the most easily absorbed type of iron. Iron found in vegetables is less easily absorbed, but still an important source of iron.
- Provide a source of vitamin C (vitamin drops: vitamins ACD), a diluted fruit drink or piece of fruit, depending on the child's age, check current guidelines). Vitamin C helps to improve the bio-availability of consumed iron.
- Tannin in tea can block the absorption of iron, avoid it.

Specially formulated baby milk, fortified with iron, has been available free to families on the Welfare Food system for some time. Until recently this involved the allocation of tokens that could only be exchanged for baby milk at health clinics. The system presented difficulties for some families in relation to access, particularly in rural areas, where the milk services would only be available once a week or fortnightly. It would be easy for these families to run out of milk.

In 2006, the Welfare Food system changed and now eligible parents/carers are able to use vouchers in wide variety of commercial settings that ease the difficulty of geographical access. Commercial settings are also open more regularly.

Hall and Elliman (2003) explore IDA in Chapter 10 of their book. If IDA is suspected in a child who is anaemic, then this concern should be raised with the child's paediatrician or GP.

Sure Start

Sure Start centres and children's centres actively advise families about their young children's health and development. Nutritional advice and communication skills are two areas of health promotion that they regularly explore.

IDA, as discussed, is one area of dietary concern. Recently, however, there have been growing concerns about children's diets generally and how to help improve the health of young children, so they do not become unhealthy or obese. Obviously, providing parents/carers with knowledge about healthy eating needs to be encouraged, but there are other health promotion methods that can be used. For some families learning new cookery skills has been beneficial. The teaching of cookery skills to young families has become an important part of the work undertaken by Sure Start.

Sure Start identified that many young families had not previously been given the opportunity to develop their cookery skills. This may be due, in part, to the decrease experienced during the 1980s and 1990s in cookery classes at school, along with the increase in commercially available processed foods.

Thankfully, this trend is now being reversed, as its effects have been realised. With recent campaigns and evolving the Government policy, children's learning about food and its preparation are now being taken more seriously in schools. In addition, cookery courses form part of parent education programmes in many Sure Start centres and children's centres to help readdress the balance.

It is important that any information given to parents/carers surrounding nutrition is relevant to the family's circumstances in terms of skills, access to food and finances. For example, some parents/carers have poor cooking skills and they rely on processed foods. Others may not have access to proper cooking facilities if living in bed and breakfast accommodation, or experience difficulty accessing to shops, if living in some rural villages. For those living in rural areas there may only be the local corner shop, which does not sell a wide range of products, and some of those that are sold may be overpriced. It is only by making advice specific to the families that you are working with, will they be able to make the necessary changes to their lives. Eating healthily is such a crucial part of staying healthy.

Earlier in the chapter, children's communication skills were explored, in line with *Health for All Children* (Hall and Elliman, 2003). Sure Start has a key role to play here too, helping young children to develop their language skills, through group activities, for example. Where children are identified as having a language delay, not only the groups are helpful in providing opportunities for children to expand their language skills, but in some centres language therapists are available to provide advice and support.

Conclusion

This chapter has explored some of the recommendations contained within *Health for All Children* (Hall and Elliman, 2003). The chapter has particularly focused on children's communication, children's growth and IDA. *Health for All Children* provides an important framework from which children's health can be promoted at different ages. Sure Start centres and children's centres are helping to achieve the recommendations contained within Health for All for children's health.

To help promote a healthy childhood and prevent ill health, opportunities must be taken to provide families with information on healthy lifestyle choices. This includes providing opportunities for promotion at individual, group and community levels. Children's nurses in both hospital and community settings have a professional responsibility to provide health promotion advice, as advocated within the NSF (Education and Skills, Department of Health, 2004). If a child has been admitted to hospital with a lifestyle-related illness, this is often the time when parents/carers will truly understand the significance of health promotion information.

References

British Dietetic Association (2007) Available at: http://www.bda.uk.com (accessed May 2007).

Chief Nursing Officer (2004) *The Chief Nursing Officer's Review of the Nursing, Midwifery and Health Visiting Contribution to Vulnerable Children and Young People*. London: Department of Health.

Education and Skills (Department of) (2002) *Birth to Three Matters: A Framework to Support Children in Their Earlliest Years*. Nottingham: Education and Skills.

Education and Skills (Department of), Department of Health (2004) *National Service Frameworks for Children, Young People and Maternity Services*. London: Department of Health.

Hall, D., Elliman, D. (eds) (2003) *Health for All Children*, 4th edn. Oxford: Oxford University Press.

I Can (2007) Available at: http://www.ican.org.uk (accessed September 2007).

Younas, S., Prakash, N. (2006) Is it enough? *Student British Medical Journal* 14: 1–44.

Theme 3

Everyday Health Issues for Children/Young People

Chapter 7   Preventing Childhood Obesity

Chapter 8   Dental Health Promotion

Chapter 9   Skin Cancer Prevention

Chapter 10   Accident Prevention

7 Preventing Childhood Obesity

Ros Parkinson, Diane Jewkes, Vicky Grayson, Karen Moyse, Cheryl Sheard, Liz Whelan, Fenella Lindsell, Jackie Butler and Janet Savage

NSF

The National Service Framework (NSF) highlights the importance of a healthy diet and exercise for the future health of children and young people (Education and Skills, Department of Health, 2004a).

Introduction

Reading so much material related to children's health, without doubt the issue of concern currently is childhood obesity. There has been a dramatic rise in childhood obesity during recent years. Childcare experts are very concerned. Targets and initiatives have been put forward by the Government to reduce the problem.

Obesity is a condition of excess body fat associated with increased risks of diabetes, cardiovascular disease and other diseases (Campbell and Haslam, 2005). If current trends continue, nearly one-third of boys and girls under 11 years of age will be obese or overweight by 2010, in England, for example (Department of Health, 2006a).

A study on the beliefs and attitudes of nurses in primary care on the management of obesity demonstrated that most nurses had received very little specific training on obesity management (Brown et al., 2007). With concerns about childhood obesity

mounting, this needs to change. Nurses need to be thinking about ways they can improve their own education, so they are effectively equipped to help children and young people.

The purpose of this chapter is to help raise awareness about the issue of childhood obesity and the risks it can bring to health. The essence of this chapter is about providing nurses with ideas on how to help prevent childhood obesity through the encouragement of positive health behaviours – healthy diet and exercise. In the coming years nurses will have an important role in preventing childhood obesity; this chapter provides knowledge that will help to inform health promotion practice.

Childhood obesity

Ros outlines some of the evidence on childhood obesity from current literature sources.

Decades ago one would never have thought that we would have to devote a whole chapter to the topic of obesity in children. However, the problem is significant and rising at an alarming rate within the United Kingdom (UK) (International Obesity Taskforce, 2004a). Studies indicate that there has been a marked increase in obesity figures in children since the 1980s. Worldwide there is growing concern about the health and future health of our children and young people; the World Health

Organization (WHO, 1998) has stated that obesity in general terms has become a *global epidemic*.

Throughout the world there are approximately 22 million children under the age of 5 who are severely overweight and, staggeringly, approximately 155 million school-aged children overweight (International Obesity Taskforce, 2004b). The numbers are rising, particularly in the developed world. In the UK itself there are probably a million obese individuals under 16 years of age – one of the highest prevalence rates within Europe (Educari, 2004).

Nurses need to address this major and growing problem – we owe it to children and young people. For this reason we need to look at current *lifestyles, eating habits, education* and *resources*, which will all help to ensure healthier lives for future generations (British Medical Association, 1999). It is well documented and proven that poor health in childhood will lead to poor health outcomes as adults, and will make those individuals prone to major health complications and diseases, such as type 2 diabetes, coronary heart disease and cancers, to name but a few (WHO, 2003).

Defining childhood obesity

Obesity is much easier to determine in adults. Standard body mass index (BMI) measure, used in adults, is not sufficient in children, as it will not take into consideration variables such as growth, and periods of body change, for example (Scottish Intercollegiate Guidelines, 2003). However, there needs to be some form of easily measurable assessment in children/young people, if practitioners are to be able to address the problems and advise on lifestyle changes appropriately (Cole et al., 2000). Age and gender-specific BMI percentile charts have been produced and designed by the Child Growth Foundation, and these have become a useful assessment tool (WHO, 2007). Using these charts we can define obese children as those with a BMI higher than the 98th percentile of the UK 1990 reference chart for age and sex. Overweight children are those with a BMI over the 91st percentile.

Another useful measure to take into account would be waist circumference. Central obesity is a major problem, often seen as a significant warning sign for long-term health complications (McCarthy et al., 2001). Waist circumference provides a more accurate measure of adiposity, but of course there may be various barriers to this being used as an assessment tool. The procedure could be seen as too personal or invasive. Looking at trends in British teenagers, waist circumference seems to have increased dramatically between 1987 and 1997. This would mean central obesity in our young people has increased faster than BMI in general (McCarthy et al., 2003).

Prevention and what needs to be achieved

Unfortunately, the problem of obesity is not going to disappear soon. The Government is, of course, concerned and during the last few years various reports have tried to address underlying problems and made recommendations.

Choosing Health (Department of Health, 2004a), the Government document, showed a commitment to fighting the problem. The Government has vowed to halt the year-on-year rise in childhood obesity. The document looked at the grass roots and came up with various measures to tackle the prime causes, concentrating on schools and working closely with local authorities and primary care trusts (PCTs) (Department of Health, 2006a).

The National Healthy Schools programme was introduced with four aims, two of which were aimed at healthy eating and physical activity (Healthy Schools, 2007). PCTs were asked to work in *partnership* with education and the family. From September 2006 a national programme to record height and weight in all children in year 6 and reception was introduced, and continues nationwide, coordinated by PCTs.

Obesity has become a prominent feature in many child health reports over the past few years, which have looked more widely at safeguarding and meeting the needs of our children/young people. These reports have highlighted the need to support and include the family at every step in child health. *Every Child Matters* (Education and Skills, 2003/4) simply states that in healthy children, how big they are depends on three key factors, namely:

- The shape children inherit from their parents.
- What children eat.
- How active children are.

This might make you think that the problem is easily solved, by focusing upon the second and third factors mentioned – diet and exercise. But there are many underlying factors to take into account. In order to adjust these successfully, and for the long-term, nurses need to work closely with the family and wider community to change traditions, beliefs, lifestyles and behaviour. Not an easy task!

The NSF (Education and Skills, Department of Health, 2004b) has set national standards which as nurses we must strive to achieve, if the children/ young people are to be healthy. These standards focus on health promotion and supporting the family with suitable education and resources. From conception through to adulthood, the standards ask for high-quality care to promote and safeguard the health and welfare of all children/young people. Early intervention and working in partnership with other practitioners is fundamental to ensuring these standards are put into practice. However, resources must be available to support the family on an individual and wider community basis. Midwives, specialist nurses, health visitors, community nurses and general practitioners all need to become more involved through their regular contacts with families.

The National Institute of Clinical Excellence (NICE, 2006) has published guidelines on the prevention, identification, assessment and management of overweight and obesity. Children are specifically mentioned in these guidelines. The guidelines recommend that obesity prevention remains a priority for the Government, and partnerships are essential to implementing locally based strategies (NICE, 2006).

Nurses need to provide sensitive advice and lifestyle education at every opportunity and with each contact. Nurses need to spend enough time with families in order to establish where they may be going wrong with nutrition, mealtimes, physical activities and health matters. We are then in an ideal situation to suggest and use health promotion tools and education for the family as a whole.

The Department of Health (2006b) wants nurses to lead the way for a healthier nation of children and young people. It recognises that we need to be *sensitive*, show empathy and be non-judgemental with families when dealing with this delicate subject. It is a lot to ask of children and families to change their whole way of life. Progress can be very slow and can prove frustrating for all concerned. Media involvement can be seen as a barrier to making these life changes, as families will be susceptible to various clever advertising mechanisms promoting less healthy activities.

The following sections provide some ideas on ways to prevent childhood obesity, with the use of health promotion.

Breastfeeding

The NSF maintains that the best long-term approach to tackling obesity is prevention, particularly during childhood. Action needs to be taken from birth. Breastfeeding is the best nutrition for babies, as it is associated with better health outcomes (Education and Skills, Department of Health, 2004a). Breastfeeding, therefore, will be our first health promotion topic in relation to preventing obesity. Breastfeeding can provide children with the best start in life.

Breastfeeding is the natural way for a mother to feed her baby. Advances in science have meant that formula milk is safe for babies. Unfortunately, advertising by formula milk companies and endorsement by practitioners has led to large numbers of mothers choosing to use formula milk in preference to breastfeeding. In some parts of the country very few mothers breastfeed, thus the tradition, knowledge and experience of breastfeeding is becoming lost.

Breast milk is an extremely complex substance which contains everything the baby needs for its growth and development. It contains valuable antibodies from the mother which give the baby immunity from disease. Breast milk has long-term immunological effects, which last well into adulthood. Breastfed babies are therefore much less likely to have infections. Breast milk contains human fatty acids and protein. Breast milk is the perfect food for human babies.

In contrast, formula milk can in no way replicate the complex nature of breast milk. It is not possible to add to formula milk the substances that we know are in breast milk. An example of this can be illustrated in relation to iron content. Breast milk contains very little iron but it also contains lactoferrin, which facilitates absorption of iron; therefore, all the iron in breast milk is utilised by the baby. Formula milk contains much higher levels of iron, but because it does not contain lactoferrin, very little is absorbed. This leaves high levels of iron in the gut, which can increase the risk of gastroenteritis.

Breast milk is highly concentrated and varies according to age of the baby, time of day and the particular feed. Breastfed babies actually take around the same volume of milk each day from around 2 weeks of age, until they are weaned. Conversely, formula-fed babies need to keep increasing the amount of milk they take and may need to change their milk to one which has higher protein content, in order to satisfy their needs.

Formula-fed babies are often introduced to solids far earlier than their breastfed counterparts. Consequently, formula-fed babies are more at risk to obesity than breastfed babies. Practitioners know the benefits of breastfeeding, but sadly do not know the full long-term risks of formula feeding. Stanway (2005) discusses the fact that formula feeding in infancy can increase the long-term risks of coronary heart disease.

Benefits in brief

Some of the benefits of breastfeeding compared to formula feeding are outlined below, as discussed by Minchin (1998):

- Breastfed babies are less likely to have gastroenteritis, urinary tract infections, chest and ear infections.
- Breastfed babies are less likely to be obese.
- They are less likely to have asthma or eczema.
- There is a reduced risk of cot death associated with breastfeeding.

Support

Whole generations of women have lost the art of breastfeeding, and in consequence they may need much support and encouragement to breastfeed successfully. Women would learn breastfeeding from their mothers and relations. It was once an integral and accepted part of family life. It was expected that mothers would breastfeed their babies. In today's society it is not unusual to have whole families where no baby has been breastfed for generations. Often unsuccessful attempts to breastfeed by mothers and grandmothers has led to the im-

pression that breastfeeding is difficult, painful and not worth even attempting. It is vital for the health of our society that this trend is reversed. Indeed, there are signs that breastfeeding rates are increasing, albeit slowly.

Within the NSF (Education and skills, Department of Health, 2004a), the need for promotion and protection of breastfeeding is highlighted in standards 1 and 2.

NSF standards

Standard 1 Promoting health and well-being
Standard 2 Supporting parenting

Practice

Health promotion initiatives can play an enormous part in helping more mothers to start breastfeeding. As a Sure Start midwife in Derbyshire my role was to promote breastfeeding. The following outlines some of the health promotion initiatives that we developed.

An important Sure Start target for us was to increase breastfeeding rates in an area where less than 30% of women actually initiated breastfeeding. There was a need to increase the initiation of breastfeeding by 2% each year (Sure Start, 2007). In the first 3 years, breastfeeding initiation rates in our area increased dramatically to 50% (Kirk and Sure Start: Creswell, Langwith/Whaley Thorns and Shirebrook, 2005).

One of the first initiatives was to start the *Bumps and Babes* groups. These were aimed at pregnant women and new mothers. The groups offered different activities, which included arts and crafts, pamper sessions and health promotion information, as well as refreshments. The idea was to replicate the support that would have been received from family and friends in the past. We wanted to raise participants' self-esteem, enabling them to have more confidence in themselves as mothers, obviously encouraging and supporting breastfeeding as part of this process.

Before starting such a group, it is vital to canvass local women to determine the best day, time and venue for them. These issues impact greatly on the likelihood of achieving good attendance rates.

The Bumps and Babes groups proved to be very popular. From the first group Sure Start recruited ten ladies to be *peer counsellors*. Peer counsellors act as support to expectant and new mothers, as highlighted by Ingram et al. (2005). They are ideally women who have experienced some success at breastfeeding and who wish to share their knowledge and skills with other mothers.

It is important that peer counsellors are trained for their role. Sure Start trained their peer counsellors through the *La Leche* organisation. The La Leche Breastfeeding Answer Book (Mohrbacher and Stock, 2003) proved a useful resource in their learning.

Peer counsellors learn the importance of correct positioning of the baby at the breast, along with knowledge about the common problems of breastfeeding and how to avoid them. Following their training our peer counsellors were given a graduation ceremony and received certificates and badges. Members of the local press were invited along, which in turn generated more publicity for breastfeeding.

The peer counsellors provided local, culturally sensitive support at times when practitioners, like midwives and health visitors, were unavailable. If a mother had problems breastfeeding, for example, a peer counsellor would visit and provide support and would understand when to refer on to a doctor or midwife. The counsellor would generally listen and respond to mothers' needs.

A further initiative was a *mother and baby drop-in group*, which was organised by a local health visitor, a community psychiatric nurse and myself. The group provided mothers with the opportunity to come along for a chat and discuss any health and family concerns. Breastfeeding support was provided as needed. It was recognised that breastfeeding problems were often linked to difficulties in other areas of a mother's life, thus providing a mother with the opportunity to discuss her concerns might help with breastfeeding.

During *National Breastfeeding Week*, which is held annually each May, we tried different fun activities each year to promote breastfeeding. One year we held pamper sessions in local village halls. A local beauty retail outlet was invited and they provided free makeovers for mothers. A masseuse offered free neck and back massages, our peer counsellors offered foot massages, and a nail artist gave free manicures. Free refreshments and play activities for children were also available. The halls were decorated with breastfeeding posters, and a sim-

ple quiz with prizes was organised. Our activities gained lots of publicity locally for breastfeeding.

Hospitals have their part to play too in the promotion of breastfeeding. In hospitals breastfeeding is encouraged and actively promoted. The UNICEF Baby Friendly Initiative (UNICEF, 2007) outlines ten steps that hospitals (and community practice) need to achieve in order to become *baby friendly*. These include having clear policies, trained staff, and education for pregnant and new mothers on all aspects of breastfeeding. There should also be support available for breastfeeding mothers. In gaining this award hospitals are showing their commitment to breastfeeding. Baby-friendly status has been shown to improve breastfeeding rates dramatically.

I found that my role as a midwife within Sure Start, talking to pregnant women about breastfeeding and discussing its importance for their baby's health, really did encourage more mothers to try breastfeeding. Many of the different health promotion initiatives on breastfeeding that were put into practice at Sure Start, similar ideas have been highlighted by NICE (2005).

Nutrition and growth

Children/young people need a healthy well-balanced diet. Without this they will not grow and develop normally. Parents/carers, as well as schools, have an important role to play through the foods they offer and the health messages they provide. The Government has put into place a number of different health promotion campaigns to encourage healthy eating both in schools and for the benefit of families too. Our second look at health promotion ideas in this chapter focuses on nutrition and growth.

Food campaigns

5 a Day and food in schools

The Government has responded to the rising concern of Britain's obesity problems by launching the *5 a Day* campaign (Department of Health, 2004b). The campaign is aimed at everyone and encourages children/young people and adults to eat five portions of fruit and vegetables each day. Having five portions of fruit and vegetables daily helps the body stay looking and feeling healthy in many ways. Fruit and vegetables contain essential nutrients and vitamins that are important for the body to remain healthy. Fruit and vegetables help to maintain a healthy weight and they provide lots of fibre and antioxidants (Department of Health, 2004b). Antioxidants are important as defence mechanisms to prevent diseases such as cancer and heart disease.

From experience, children/young people and their families perceive incorporating the five portions of fruit and vegetables a day as difficult. A banana or a handful of grapes or a tablespoon of peas all classify as one portion. The 5 a Day campaign has produced several posters and leaflets which detail what is classified as a portion of fruit or vegetables. Tinned and dried fruits can also be included. A 5 a Day website has been established (http://www.5aday.co.uk) which gives further information and recipes for incorporating fruit and vegetables into daily diets.

The Welfare Food scheme has incorporated fruit, vegetables and vitamins within this scheme. Families would previously obtain baby milk from baby clinics and chemists; however, the scheme has now changed. Milk can now only be purchased from specified shops where fresh fruit and vegetables are sold (Department of Health, 2005). The vouchers are issued on a weekly basis so families have to go to the shop at least once a week, which encourages the purchase of fresh produce.

A primary school in the South West England promotes the 5 a Day campaign by selling fresh fruit snacks and fruit smoothies at its tuck shop. The children help run the shop with support from parents. The school has found that children's attitudes towards eating fruit are much more positive since introducing this new approach (Health Development Agency, 2006).

Dinner menu

In 2005, Jamie Oliver, television celebrity chef, highlighted concerns about school dinners. Jamie set up a campaign to get junk food out of school canteens and introduce healthier foods. Channel 4, which ran the series of programmes, sponsored the campaign. Jamie changed the menu of schools he visited and discussed with canteen staff how to cook and care for fresh and healthy foods. The series was a success with high audience ratings and support for his campaign. As a result, the Government was pressured to act. New standards for school menus were introduced (Johnson, 2006).

The Government's National Food Standards for school lunches and other school foods are outlined below (Johnson, 2006):

- High-quality meat, poultry or oily fish should regularly be available on pupil menus.
- Serve pupils at least two portions of fruit and vegetables with every meal.
- Limit deep-fried foods to no more than two portions per week.
- Remove fizzy drinks, crisps, chocolate and other confectioneries from school meals and vending machines.

A secondary school in the East of England aimed to improve the knowledge and health of their pupils by introducing a traffic light system into the canteen:

- Red – representing foods that were high in fat and sugar (poor nutritional value).
- Green – representing foods such as fruit and vegetables (healthy options).

The meals in the canteen were examined and alternative ways of producing foods that pupils would eat were gradually developed. Chips were still available on the menu, but only once a week. Better snack options became available which included fruit salads. Drinks machines, instead of containing unhealthy drinks, contained water, milk and fruit juices (Health Development Agency, 2006).

Resources

There are many different resources that nurses can use with children/young people to promote messages about healthy eating. Health promotion units will be able to provide details about the full range of resources available.

Toolkits

A very useful toolkit has been designed by the Child Growth Foundation to help prevent obesity, called the *Glugs*. It is aimed at very young children, with appropriate teaching methods and resources for this age group. Tam Fry (2007), chairman of the Child Growth Foundation, explains that the Glugs are animated cartoon characters that are part of a health promotion programme to prevent obesity. The toolkit presents stories, recipes and games with rewards for children. The hope is that it will develop into a national resource.

Books

There are many useful books that can be used to promote young children's interest in healthy foods. *Oliver's Vegetables* by French and Bartlett (1995) is a fun and colourful book to read with young children. Oliver's favourite food is his beloved chips, but he soon learns that growing vegetable involves more than potatoes; other vegetables can be tasty too.

Children's TV programmes

Some children's television programmes can be quite a good way of promoting positive health messages. For example, a television programme that has become very popular with children recently, certainly amongst 7 and 8 years old, is *Lazy Town*, created by Magnus Scheving (Lazy Town, 2008; http://www.lazytown.com). Positive health messages are clearly evident within this lively programme, featuring a mixture of puppets and real characters. Messages about healthy eating, the prevention of tooth decay and the importance of exercise are all put across in a captivating way for children. *Sports candy*, better known to us as fruit, is frequently recommended.

Parents/carers can help to take their children's knowledge on healthy eating a little further by watching such programmes with their children and discussing the health promotion messages.

Cookery lessons

The practical side of healthy eating is a must for exploration – shopping and cooking. At home young people may like to become involved in shopping and cooking to help develop a more practical side to their knowledge on healthy eating.

Schools are soon going to be playing a bigger role in teaching cooking skills to young people. It has recently been announced by the Government that cookery lessons will be introduced into schools

for children 11- to 14-year-olds. School nurses could find that they have a role here helping to encourage healthy eating.

Whilst shopping for healthy eating, young people may find reading some of the food labels enlightening. Health promotion activities can be developed, encouraging young people to explore the sugar and fat content of particular foods, for example. Foods with a low fat content could be encouraged and interesting ways they can be prepared explored.

Adolescence is a particularly influential age, when young people are beginning to form opinions of their own, and perhaps making some important decisions about nutrition and their diets. They are able to understand the impact of what they eat and how it might affect their health. Young people may be keen on burgers and chips, for example, but too many will soon impact on their waistlines, preventing them from staying slim, which girls will particularly become concerned about. Some young people may opt to become vegetarian and give up meat altogether. If so, remind girls of the importance of having a high enough iron content in their diets, particularly once they start their periods. Low intakes of iron can cause anaemia. Signs of low iron intake include tiredness and fainting (Tassoni, 2007).

Different resources for different age groups have been explored in an effort to promote healthy eating.

Activities

There are many different activities children/young people can be involved in that will teach them about healthy eating. Below some ideas are presented. Children/young people may find them fun and interesting, depending on the relevance to their age group:

- Menu planning.
- Displays on healthy eating.
- Devising a healthy eating game.
- Talk about favourite foods.
- Drawing activities.
- Trying new tastes (ask about allergies first).
- Identifying the different food groups.
- Making healthy snacks – sandwiches, smoothies.
- Poems about foods or tastes they like.
- Growing fruit and vegetables at home or in school.

Growth

As Ros mentioned earlier, trends in children's growth are being monitored closely. In England the *National Child Measurement Programme* has now begun (Department of Health, 2006c). This involves a huge data collection exercise across the country on children's heights and weights by health staff in schools. The exercise will help PCTs by informing their local planning needs. PCT health staff will measure children in their reception year (4- and 5-year-olds), and those in year 6 (10- and 11-year-olds) (Department of Health, 2006c).

The Department of Health (2007a) has produced guidance for PCTs on the scheme. Information is also available for parents in the form of a leaflet – *Why Your Child's Weight Matters* (Department of Health, 2007b, available from http://www.dh.gov.uk/healthyliving).

The leaflet, as well as providing information about the measurement exercise, also outlines details on encouraging healthy lifestyles for children through diet and exercise. Some of the healthy habits they encourage include the following:

- Sitting down together as a family to eat a meal.
- Switching the television off when families are eating.
- Eating healthy foods and being positive about these foods.
- Praising good eating habits, instead of nagging.
- Involving children in food preparation.

In addition, useful ideas are provided on physical activities that can be undertaken together as a family. Further information sources include websites on nutrition and exercise. These are as follows:

http://www.eatwell.gov.uk/agesandstages/children
http://www.parentlineplus.org.uk
http://www.playgroundfun.org.uk
http://www.activeplaces.com

The leaflet is really useful and one that perhaps could be amended and made available to more parents.

Changes may be made to children's growth charts. A report published recently highlighted a need for the UK to adopt WHO child growth standards (Department of Health, 2007c). Current UK growth charts are based mainly on formula-fed babies, while the WHO charts are based on how children should grow under optimum circumstances, including those that are exclusively breastfed (Department of Health, 2007c). Historically, there has been a problem for some mothers who have breastfed their babies; these babies perform differently in relation to the UK growth charts. In some cases this might have caused mothers unnecessary anxiety about their babies' growth.

The feeling is that if more babies are breastfed in the early months, this can prevent obesity problems in later life (Department of Health, 2007c). The recommendation is that the WHO charts could be used from 2 weeks of age, through to 2 years, and then practitioners refer back to the UK charts. The idea will be considered by the Government for piloting (Department of Health, 2007c). A copy of the report is available from Scientific Advisory Committee on Nutrition – http://www.sacn.gov.uk (SACN/RCPCH, 2007).

Physical activity

The importance of physical activity for the health of children and young people cannot be underestimated. The Government wants to enhance the uptake of sporting opportunities. The Government feels, downward trend in physical activity undertaken by children and young people witnessed in recent years that the needs to be reversed (Department of Health, 2006c). The promotion of physical activity will be our next focus, in the battle against childhood obesity.

The NSF maintains that there are lifelong benefits of being active (Education and Skills, Department of Health, 2004c). If children are active while they are young and continue to be active as adults, this will have benefits for their long-term health. The Government wants to reduce the risk of major chronic diseases, which can be increased by individuals failing to be active. Currently, the UK population is not active enough; rates of walking, as well as cycling, have fallen over the last 25 years (Department of Health, 2004a).

There are concerns about the current generation of children leading lifestyles that are too sedentary and not being active enough. Further, there are concerns that children/young people are spending too much time engaged in computer games, television and junk food, which childcare experts believe could result in the development of behavioural problems, mental health problems (Clark, 2007), as well as problems associated with obesity.

The NSF (Education and Skills, Department of Health, 2004c) has set two targets. Initially, to increase the uptake of physical activity to at least 30 minutes three times a week in all children/young people under 16 years. The second target is to increase the opportunities for children/young people to undertake sporting activities, within and beyond the school curriculum.

This section of the chapter presents some ideas on how children and young people can participate in gentle exercise, as well as more energetic exercise. These forms of exercise not only have benefits for physical health, but may also have benefits for psychological health. There are lots of different forms of sport and exercise children/young people can participate in, football, netball, dancing, tennis and cross country, to name simply a few. Here yoga, a relatively new addition to the exercise repertoire for children, will be examined, as well as a long-established favourite – swimming.

Yoga for young children (2$\frac{1}{2}$–7 years)

Yoga, as a discipline for adults, is more relevant than ever. It can be an important part of people's daily lives, which seem to be increasingly driven by deadlines, decisions, targets and challenges.

Whether yoga is chosen first as a form of exercise, or required for its philosophy to help make sense of life, individuals who take yoga classes begin a journey of discovery. Physically and psychologically yoga can bring an inner peace, a confidence to cope with all that life brings.

There are many styles of yoga which all help to strengthen the body, encourage correct breathing, enhance balance and encourage peace of mind. Given all this, how wonderful for children to be able to harness this power, to begin life with a sense of confidence in their own physical abilities, an idea of how to bring a little calm into their lives.

Children need to be physically active, and exercise should be fun with a series of free-flowing natural easy movements. Children overheat more easily and dehydrate more quickly than adults; therefore, the ideal exercise for early years children is

something not too structured, in the form of games involving running and jumping. This makes yoga ideal for children. Already with a fantastic sense of mimicry and wonderful imaginations, children copy animals, head off on adventures and create fantasy worlds. Without realising it, children are pushing their own boundaries. With yoga they explore their capabilities in a fun, non-competitive way.

Our world provides all of us all with major hurdles. Children, in particular, are often ill prepared to deal with the day-to-day changes that take place in their lives, starting nursery, moving house and changes in family and peer group structures. As our own lives take their course, so our children get caught up in what is happening. In addition, the Government State School system demands that we test our children at regular intervals. Whilst some individuals agree with this, the inevitable outcome it places on children outside school means they too are losing precious time just to talk, vent feelings or simply play. As children get older, there is less emphasis on physical activity in schools, leading to more sedentary lifestyles.

YogaBugs is an organisation addressing these issues. YogaBugs was originally the idea of Fenella Lindsell, a yoga teacher, who with her husband Robert, set up The Art of Health in January 1996 (along with three other directors). The idea for YogaBugs came when Robert's son wanted to join him and Fenella in their yoga practice. It became a family environment where he felt safe, familiar and able to cope with any anxieties. Lara Goodbody joined Fenella in 2003 to further expand the business, which has gone from strength to strength.

YogaBugs as an organisation is now considered a leading authority on yoga for children and currently has over 1200 teachers in the UK. Classes are delivered in the form of YogaBugs for 2$\frac{1}{2}$ to 7-year-olds and Yoga'dUp for 8-year-old to teens. YogaBugs has a network of teachers who go into nurseries, preschools, health centres and schools. They also work with Brownies, Rainbows and after-school clubs.

YogaBugs teachers instruct a session which uses stories, songs, adventures and games to children who have no preconception of what yoga is about. Children come to play, to escape into imaginary worlds, to sing and have fun. It is remarkable for teachers to see the effect that yoga has. Even the shyest of children will have a go. For example, the child who usually sits silently will chuckle whilst pretending to be a grumpy crab on the beach, the child with autistic tendencies who after just a few sessions can meet your gaze confidently whilst being a scary lion, and the selective mute who cannot find a voice because all situations are so nerve-racking, but can speak when she becomes a mermaid.

Not only are children discovering how good and natural it feels to have an active brain and body, but these sessions provide messages about healthy eating, staying safe and anti-bullying. The sessions can reinforce acceptable and non-acceptable behaviour in a non-threatening, subtle way.

From experience, yoga may provide some of the following benefits:

- Breathing exercises which help to improve concentration and energy levels.
- Relaxation techniques that help to clear the mind.
- Postures that can help strengthen the body.
- Posture work which helps to tone the body (which will help to reduce the rising levels of childhood obesity).
- Yoga helps the development of creativity and self-expression.
- The practice of yoga improves coordination and balance.
- It promotes healthy sleeping patterns.
- Allows children to explore their intuitive nature and spirituality.
- Yoga maintains a child's natural flexibility.
- Yoga improves self-confidence through vocalisation techniques and postures that are designed to release day-to-day anxieties.

Yoga is a complete form of exercise in a safe and non-competitive environment.

At the end of the session, which lasts between 30 and 45 minutes, children have the opportunity to lie down and relax. The session may have led them on a journey through a tropical rainforest, a far-away mountain, or that magic land under their beds.

Relaxation is an important part of the session, as children learn how to relax completely and let go. Children close their eyes and float away, often to soothing music. Their breathing slows and calms. They are learning for themselves how to find a little inner peace, something we all need from time to time. Perhaps yoga provides a place to escape to, where computer games and glorified graphics does not even come close.

Yoga for older children (from 8 years of age)

What will yoga do for the pre-teens? Yoga is a form of complete exercise that can be offered to all children/young people because it develops physical stamina, emotional balance, and intellectual and creative skills, which all help to contribute to a happier, more grounded individual.

At a time when their bodies are growing and changing, yoga gives children/young people energy and strength. It helps them to deal with situations which can make them very angry and frustrated. Children/young people feel anger very strongly, certain postures can help them deal with angry outbursts, and rather than repressing these feelings, they can let them out in a controlled manner.

Prior to the age of 8 years, children tend to play in a world of fantasy and imagination, but as children develop, they benefit from a more structured approach both in terms of discipline and concentration. Yoga, therefore, becomes a natural choice as it helps to develop their abilities to the fullest extent, whilst enabling them to develop successful, useful and fulfilled lives.

At the age of 8 breathing exercises are ideally introduced. Breathing exercises help to maintain healthy cardiovascular and respiratory systems, as well as improving energy levels.

Yoga seems to help in different ways psychologically. Yoga for this age group allows them to develop their own imaginations, powers of visualisation, vocalisation and therefore cultivation of their own personalities. Children may also find that yoga helps them to cope with transitions in their lives; as they change from a child into a young person. Children/young people, who are withdrawn, or who are physically not so strong or confident, are able to benefit from taking part in yoga classes with their fellow classmates. Yoga is a non-competitive activity, which helps to put them at ease.

Yoga can give children/young people confidence to deal with the pressures of schoolwork by helping to reduce symptoms of anxiety and stress. Through simple breathing and relaxation techniques, children/young people can be taught to deal with concerns they have for their work or friends. If a child is not stressed they will naturally be able to learn more and remember what they have learned. Children's/young people's concentration levels can benefit too, by undertaking postures that focus the mind. Balancing poses are particularly helpful for improving concentration skills.

There may also be a variety of physical benefits. Yoga for this age group can help to develop stamina and agility in sporting activities. Posture work creates balance, which can particularly help in competitive sports such as hockey, netball and football. Yoga can also be beneficial for those who are not so sporty by helping to improve coordination, balance and developing areas of low muscle tone.

Boys tend to benefit from yoga because their muscles get stronger and remain more flexible, and this helps with other sporting activities. It can help girls to strengthen their upper bodies, as well as helping them through some of the discomfort they might experience during menstruation. In addition, yoga helps children/young people tend to sleep better as they are more relaxed and calm.

As an activity a yoga class is all inclusive, noncompetitive and a fun way of bringing a group of children/young people together. They can have the chance to enjoy breathing and posture work in a fun-themed format, which will challenge and enable them to work together. There is also time to enjoy the benefits of relaxation and visualization techniques. Children/young people may be able to find stillness and a sense of self worth at a time when their lives can be quite demanding.

Some recommended reading:

- *The One Bug Your Kids Should Catch* (Lindsell, 2008).
- *Yoga for Kids* (Gibbs, 2006).
- *The Complete Idiots Guide to Yoga with Kids* (Komitor and Adamson, 2000).

Swimming

Swimming can be an important activity for children and young people, helping them to keep fit, stay healthy and learn to be safe in water. Some of the health benefits of swimming are discussed in this section.

Swimming may come easily to some children, but not others. The main reason for this is that water is not a natural environment. Children need to learn how to use water for their own benefit. Not everyone, for various reasons, has the opportunity to learn to swim as a child. After childhood, learning to swim can be difficult. The safest place for children to learn is in a swimming pool with lifeguards present.

Swimming offers some real health benefits. It is recognised as one of the best all round exercises for most people. It can work all the muscle groups, provided all the strokes are used. Swimming exercises the heart and the lungs (cardiovascular fitness), as well as improving flexibility, and it can help to control weight. Another factor in its favour is that very few injuries can be sustained from swimming, compared with some other sports.

Swimming can also be seen as a relaxing exercise; it gives children and young people a feel-good factor afterwards. It can have social benefits too; children and young people becoming involved in water-based activities through schools and clubs.

Interestingly, swimming has been shown to improve certain health conditions, such as asthma, disabilities, and can help those recovering from injury. It can be particularly helpful in obesity, where children will be trying to keep their weight down. Water can also create massaging effects because of its hydrostatic pressure. This can be responsible for lowering blood pressure, improving circulation, as well as being relaxing and soothing.

The first step is for children not to be afraid of water. Baby and toddler swimming are now very popular. The idea here is that children learn to swim naturally at an early age. The water begins to feel very natural to them and so they do not develop a fear of water.

Once children are about 5 years old, they might be swimming confidently. They can then go on to develop strokes that will enable them to become stronger swimmers. As children become older, to help improve their fitness, they can go on to swim distances.

Sometimes as teenagers they may lose interest in swimming. Hopefully, however, due to a childhood of regular swimming, they will go on to develop an enjoyment of the sport and exercise in general. Swimming can give them a basic all-round fitness that can be applied to other sports and activities.

A vital part of any sport, including swimming, is the *fun* element. Learning to swim should always be seen as fun. Races and games can be encouraged with supervision. It is important to bear in mind that children are individuals, with their own character and preferences. Some children will prefer swimming, whilst other children will prefer different sports. There are plenty of sporting activities to choose from.

Water is a unique environment however; there is nothing else quite like it. It can be fun and help to burn off calories. Children can go swimming together and exercise at their own level of fitness. It is always important to ensure that it is safe to swim, with good supervision available.

Details about children's swimming lessons can be found by contacting local leisure and sports centres. Once children have learnt to swim they may want to become members of swimming clubs or take on various swimming challenges and awards, in their attempts to stay fit and healthy.

Books are a really useful way to talk with children about first experiences. There are a variety of books which young children can read, encouraging them to take an interest in swimming. For example, the Oxford Reading Tree, in its series of books on first experiences, produces a book called *At the Pool* (Hunt and Brychta, 2007). Aimed at primary school children, the story describes different activities that can help children learn to swim safely. A picture and vocabulary section also feature.

Resources for parents/carers are important too. A book that may be of interest to parents/carers:

- *Acquatic Readiness, Developing Water Competence in Young Children* (Langendorfer and Bruya, 1994).

Websites can provide further information:

http://www.humankinetics.com
http://www.sta.co.uk

This section has explored ways children and young people might find physical activity fun, as well as its potential health benefits. Nurses may want to explore the fun and health benefits of exercise with children and young people, as a starting point for change in developing a healthy lifestyle and preventing obesity.

Teaching methods

Teaching methods used can help to convey messages of positive health, in a way that is both fun and interesting for children and young people. Janet illustrates how drama was used to convey messages about healthy eating with children/young people. Equally, drama can be used for teaching about the physical and psychological benefits of physical activity.

Healthy eating

A lesson on healthy eating was developed using drama as the teaching method. The National Curriculum (2008) (http://www.direct.gov.uk) specifically mentions the use of drama in education, and yet many school nurses have limited or no experience of how to do it. Teaching about health through drama can provide nurses with an interesting and powerful tool for helping children/young people to learn about health.

Drama example – the lesson was aimed at the 10- to 12-year age group. The drama itself had two teenage characters, one of whom was overweight (the main character). The friends meet at a local burger bar and discuss the possible health benefits of eating burgers and chips. This can contain off the wall ideas such as the pickle on the burger counts towards one of your five portions of fruit and vegetables a day. The wilder the statements the better, as it lightens the atmosphere and allows pupils to think of ways healthy eating messages can be easily misconstrued.

A pupil can play the part of the first young person (main character). The school nurse can play the part of the second teenage character. A further character is introduced into the drama, which is that of the main character's mother. The school nurse can play two parts: that of the mother, as well as the second teenage character. These parts can be differentiated with the use of props, a scarf for the second young person and an apron for the mother perhaps.

The concept of diary pages can be introduced to pupils, looking at the main character's diary pages to allow pupils to have more background information, as well as insights into her/his thoughts and feelings. The diary pages are written in such a way that the information contained within the pages allows the drama to progress and can be used for follow-up lessons.

Theatre in education techniques can be used, which include *hot seating*; where pupils interview the characters. This allows pupils to ask questions and find out more about what motivates the characters, particularly in relation to the main character; what motivates her/him to overeat and her/his feelings towards being overweight.

Still images can be used in conjunction with *thought tracking* to further explore how others within the drama relate to healthy eating and obesity. Still images are the creation of an image using a group of people to capture a particular moment, much like a photograph or a video freeze-frame. Thought tracking links in with still images. After the pupils have created a realistic image, the nurse asks them, whilst they are still *frozen*, what their character is thinking about. The aim of this is to reinforce an understanding of the created image.

Forum theatre can be used to demonstrate conflict between parents and children. Forum theatre is a technique where the drama can be stopped at certain points and the audience can dictate how they would behave differently if they were the characters involved. To gain maximum benefit from this, a pupil can take on the part of the mother perhaps at differing points within the drama. This process can help pupils to learn how to deal with conflict and prepare them for putting across their views within a safe environment.

There are no particular answers to any questions within this drama. However, the drama provides an opportunity for pupils to further explore the issues – their thoughts and feelings towards healthy eating and obesity.

For further details about using drama as a teaching method and the use of particular drama techniques, consult The Play House (2007) (http://www.theplayhouse.org.uk).

Conclusion

This extensive chapter has provided some ideas on preventing childhood obesity. It has examined the extent of the problem and reviewed some key Government documents on recommendations for changing current trends. Health promotion messages on healthy eating and physical activity have been examined. Education and resources have been explored too. The nurse has an important role in helping the future health of children, young people and their families. However, there are signifi-

cant barriers to overcome; lifestyle changes are not easy to make, there are so many different factors involved. The nurse needs to convey messages sensitively to influence change. Partnership working, with children, young people, families and other agencies is essential to help the future generation become healthy, stay healthy and avoid ill health by preventing obesity.

References

British Medical Association (1999) *Growing Up in Britain: Ensuring a Healthy Future for Our Children*. London: BMA.

Brown, I., Stride, C., Psarou, A., Brewins, L., Thompson, J. (2007) Management of obesity in primary care: nurses' practices, beliefs and attitudes. *Journal of Advanced Nursing* 59(4): 329–341.

Campbell, I., Haslam, D. (2005) *Obesity: Your Questions Answered*. Edinburgh: Churchill Livingstone.

Clark, L. (2007) Let them go out to play. *Daily Mail*, 10 September.

Cole, T., Bellizzi, M., Flegal, K., Dietz, W. (2000) Establishing a standard definition for child overweight and obesity worldwide: international survey. *BMJ* 320: 1240–1243.

Department of Health (2004a) *Choosing Health: Making Healthy Choices Easier*. London: Crown Copyright.

Department of Health (2004b) *5 a Day*. London: Crown Copyright.

Department of Health (2005) *Healthy Start*. Available at: http://www.healthystart.nhs.uk (accessed 4 December 2006).

Department of Health (2006a) *Health Profile of England*. London: Crown Copyright.

Department of Health (2006b) *Raising the Issue of Weight in Children and Young People*. Available at: http://www.dh.gov.uk (accessed September 2007).

Department of Health (2006c) *Measuring Childhood Obesity: Guidance to Primary Care Trusts*. London: Department of Health.

Department of Health (2007a) *Supporting Healthy Lifestyles: The National Child Measurement Programme*. London: Crown Copyright.

Department of Health (2007b) *Why Your Child's Weight Matters*. London: Crown Copyright. Available at: http://www.dh.gov.uk/healthyliving (accessed April 2007).

Department of Health (2007c) *New Report on Child Growth Standards Welcome*. London: Crown copyright.

Educari (2004) *Children, Young People and Health Related Decisions: A Review of the Research Literature and Discussion of the Implications for Health Education of*

Children and Young People. Roehampton: University of Surrey.

Education and Skills (Department of) (2003/4) *Every Child Matters*. London: Crown Copyright.

Education and Skills (Department of), Department of Health (2004a) *National Service Framework for Children, Young People and Maternity Services: Core Standards*. London: Crown copyright.

Education and Skills (Department of), Department of Health (2004b) *National Service Framework for Children, Young People and Maternity Services, Standards 1 – Promoting Health and Well-being, Identifying Needs and Intervening Early, Standard 2 – Supporting Parents*. London: Crown Copyright.

Education and Skills (Department of), Department of Health (2004c) *National Service Framework for Children, Young People and Maternity Services*. London: Education and Skills, Department of Health.

French, V., Bartlett, A. (1995) *Oliver's Vegetables*. London: Hodder Children's Books.

Fry, T. (2007) Meet the Glugs. *Community Practitioner* 80(1): 15–16.

Gibbs, B. (2006) *Yoga for Kids. Fun and Easy Stretching Exercises for Children Aged Three to Eleven Years*. UK: Southwater.

Health Development Agency (2006) *Case Studies by Theme*. Wired for Health Website. Available at: http://www. wiredforhealth.gov.uk (accessed 15 September 2006).

Healthy Schools (2007) *Healthier Living and Learning (National Programme)*. Available at: http://www. healthyschools.gov.uk (accessed September 2007).

Hunt, R., Brychta, A. (2007) *At the Pool*. Oxford Reading Tree Series. Oxford: Oxford University Press.

Ingram, J., Rosser, J., Jackson, D. (2005) Breastfeeding peer supports and a community support group: evaluating their effectiveness. *Maternal and Child Health* 1(2): 111–118.

International Obesity Taskforce (2004a) *Obesity in Children and Young People, a Crisis in Public Health*. Available at: http://www.iotf.org (accessed September 2007).

International Obesity Taskforce (2004b) *Childhood Obesity Estimates*. European Congress on Obesity, Prague, 30 May 2004. Available at: http://www.iotf.org (accessed September 2007).

Johnson, A. (2006) *Setting the Standard for School Food*. Department for Education and Employment. Available at: http://www.dfes.gov.uk (accessed 19 September 2006).

Kirk, J. and Sure Start: Creswell, Langwith/Whaley Thorns and Shirebrook (2005) *Monitoring and Evaluation Report*. Derbyshire: Sure Start: Creswell, Langwith/Whaley Thorns and Shirebrook.

Komitor, J., Adamson, E. (2000) *The Complete Idiots Guide to Yoga with Kids*. New York: Penguin Books (USA) Inc.

Langendorfer, S., Bruya, L. (1994) *Acquatic Readiness, Developing Water Competence in Young Children*. Leeds: Human Kinetics Europe Ltd.

Lazy Town. (2008) Available at: http://www.lazytown. com (accessed January 2008).

Lindsell, F. (2008) *The One Bug Your Kids Should Catch*. London: Virgin Publishing.

McCarthy, H., Ellis, S., Cole, T. (2003) Central overweight and obesity in British youth aged 11 to 16 years: cross-sectional surveys of waist circumference. *BMJ* 326(7390): 624.

McCarthy, H., Jarrett, K., Crawley, H. (2001) The development of waist circumference percentiles in British children aged 5.0 to 16.9 years. *European Journal of Clinical Nutrition* 55(10): 902–907.

Minchin, M. (1998) *Artificial Feeding: Risky for Any Baby?* Australia: Alma Publications.

Mohrbacher, N., Stock, J. (2003) *Breastfeeding Answer Book*, 3rd edn. Nottingham: La Leche League of Great Britain.

National Curriculum (2008) Available at: http://www. direct.gov.uk (accessed January 2008).

NICE (2005) *Promotion of Breast Feeding: Initiation and Duration. Evidence into Practice Briefing*. London: National Institute of Clinical Excellence.

NICE (2006) *Guidance on the Prevention, Identification, Assessment and Management of Overweight and Obesity in Adults and Children*. Available at: http://www.nice. org.uk (accessed September 2007).

Scientific Advisory Committee on Nutrition (SACN) and the Royal College of Paediatrics and Child Health (RCPCH). (2007) *Children's Growth Standards*. Available at: http://www.sacn.gov.uk (accessed August 2007).

Scottish Intercollegiate Guidelines (2003) *Management of Obesity in Children and Young People*. Edinburgh: SIGN.

Stanway, P. (2005) *Breast Is Best*, 5th edn. London: Pan-Macmillan.

Sure Start (2007) *Sure Start Targets*. Available at: http:// www.surestart.gov.uk (accessed 19 April 2007).

Tassoni, P. (2007) *Child Development, 6–16 years*. Oxford: Heinemann From Harcourt.

The Play House (2007) *Welcome to the Play House*. Available at: http://www.theplayhouse.org.uk (accessed 3 May 2007).

UNICEF (2007) *UNICEF Baby Friendly Initiative*. Available at: http://www.unicef.org.uk (accessed 13 April 2007).

WHO (1998) *Preventing and Managing the Global Epidemic*. Geneva: WHO.

WHO (2003) *Diet, Nutrition and the Prevention of Chronic Diseases*. WHO Technical Report Series. Geneva: WHO.

WHO (2007) *Child Growth Standards: Methods and Development*. Geneva: WHO. Available at: http://www. who.int (accessed September 2007).

8 Dental Health Promotion

Karen Moyse, Sue Toon and Helen Fowler

NSF

The National Service Framework (NSF) (Education and Skills, Department of Health, 2004) advises that the oral health needs of children/young people are identified within local health promotion programmes.

Introduction

What is better than a beautiful smile, as evidenced through a happy smiling child with well cared for teeth. The trick is to keep teeth that way. Undoubtedly, as any parent/carer knows, this is a hard task but well worth the effort. There are so many different delicious delights out there to tempt children: sweets, chocolate, sugary drinks. How can they all be kept to an absolute minimum, so that children do not damage their teeth? An interesting dilemma for any parent or carer, but one which nurses can help through health promotion.

For children there are developmental processes going on that can impact on dental health; new teeth erupting and dietary transitions taking place (Harris et al., 2004). With these issues in mind Seow (1998) maintains that they present as unique risk factors associated with dental decay in young children. Encouraging children to take good care of their teeth is important. Developing positive oral health behaviours while children are young may help to prevent dental health problems later in life. This chapter discusses how to promote positive oral behaviours. Sue and Helen present insights into community and hospital practice.

Definition of terms

Box 8.1 provides definitions of key terms associated with dental health.

Development of teeth

The purpose of teeth is to enable us to eat through the processes of biting and chewing food. Teeth also help with speech, as well as being part of our smile.

Structure of teeth

Teeth, situated within the upper and lower jaws of the mouth, are made up of several layers. The British Dental Health Foundation (2007) outlines the structure of teeth (Box 8.2).

The development of children's teeth

Children's teeth are more vulnerable than those of adults, because they are still developing. Children

Box 8.1 Definitions.

Dental caries – tooth decay. This is when holes form in the enamel of the tooth (Prodigy, 2005).

Dental plaque – soft deposits form on the surface of the teeth. These contain many types of bacteria. Good oral hygiene will remove plaque (Prodigy, 2005). When the plaque becomes hardened it is called tartar. It sticks firmly to the teeth. Tartar can only be removed by a dentist or dental hygienist, with special instruments (Prodigy, 2005).

Gum disease (periodontal disease) – inflammation or infection of the tissues that surround the tooth (Prodigy, 2005). Gum disease is a common reason for loss of teeth in adulthood.

have two sets of teeth, initially their primary or milk teeth. These are then followed by permanent teeth.

It is important that children are helped to care for their primary teeth, as these teeth hold the space for permanent teeth. Occasionally, young children can be seen with their primary teeth in a poor state: brown, missing teeth or sometimes simply stumps.

The primary teeth usually begin to erupt when a baby is about 6–8 months of age (Wisdom, 1999). By the time a child is $2\frac{1}{2}$ years of age, most of the 20 primary teeth will be present (Wisdom, 1999). At approximately 6/7 years of age the permanent teeth will begin to erupt. The primary teeth become wobbly, and are pushed out of the way by the permanent teeth, eventually falling out.

Children feel it is a special time when they begin to lose their primary teeth. They become excited and love to show off to their friends at school. The tooth fairy usually comes, bringing money to spend on something special. I have been reliably informed, by those who really know, that the going rate is

Box 8.2 Structure of teeth.

Enamel – it is the hard protective outer coating of the tooth. It does not contain any nerves or blood vessels.

Dentine – the dentine layer lies under the enamel. It can be very sensitive to pain. Dentine covers the central pulp of the tooth.

Pulp – it is the soft tissue which contains blood vessels and nerves and is located in the middle part of the tooth.

£2–5 per tooth. (I doubt the tooth fairy in our house will extend to such extravagance.)

All the permanent teeth should be in place by the time the child is 13 years of age (British Dental Health Foundation, 2007), with the exception of wisdom teeth, which come through between 18 and 25 years of age (British Dental Health Foundation, 2007). A full complement of teeth is 32.

Dental tips for young people

Young people need to take good care of their teeth, as they will have to last them for the rest of their lives. The American Academy of Family Physicians (2000–2005) suggests the following tips to maintain teeth in good health:

- Brush teeth twice a day with fluoride toothpaste.
- Avoid smoking as it stains the teeth.
- Protect the mouth when playing sport.
- See a dentist for regular check-ups and cleaning.

Flossing of teeth is not recommended until young people are older. Further information that may be useful for young people to know is as follows:

- Young women, if pregnant, may experience inflammation of their gums.
- Those who suffer from asthma have a tendency to breathe through their mouths when asleep. This can cause a dry mouth, which will increase plaque formation (Albert, 2005).

Health needs

Having a healthy mouth is all part of general good health (Audit Commission, 2002). However, evidence shows that certain geographical areas and certain social groups in the United Kingdom (UK) suffer from poor dental health.

Figures

A survey undertaken in 2003 on children's dental health in the UK provides some important and reliable evidence. The survey was conducted by the Office of National Statistics (ONS, 2004) on behalf of the four UK health departments (England,

Northern Ireland, Scotland and Wales). A sample of over 10 000 children/young people participated, between the ages of 5 and 15 years of age. This survey takes place every 10 years, so comparisons can be made. Survey results for 2003 are listed below:

- The decay in permanent teeth had decreased since 1983.
- There were particular improvements in the teeth of 15-year-olds.
- The proportion of 5- to 8-year-olds with filled primary teeth had fallen since 1983.
- There were no significant changes between the 1993 and 2003 figures on the proportion of 5- and 8-year-olds with obvious decay experience in their primary teeth.
- The lowest levels of decayed teeth were in England.
- The highest levels of decayed teeth were in Northern Ireland.

(Children's Dental Health survey (ONS, 2004).)

The survey also sought evidence on children's decay experience:

- Amongst 5-year-olds 43% had obvious decay experience with their primary teeth.
- Amongst 8-year-olds 57% had obvious decay experience with their primary teeth.
- Amongst 12-year-olds 62% were free from decay experience (permanent teeth).
- Amongst 15-year-olds 50% were free from decay experience (permanent teeth).

Hall and Elliman (2003) state that tooth decay, which they identify as having the greatest impact on dental health throughout adult life, has demonstrated a decline during the past two to three decades. However, they go on to state that there is a bottoming out of these improvements for young children, while improvements for older children are continuing.

Population variations

Deprivation

Evidence highlights that children living in deprived areas have more problems with their teeth than those living in other areas. Within the Acheson (1998) report, for example, children living in the North of England had more decayed teeth than those living in the Midlands and the South. The Audit Commission (2002) maintains that there is considerable variation between geographical areas in the amount of tooth decay, with the poorer, more deprived areas showing greater levels of decay, both in number and severity. Children living in poverty seem to have the highest levels of tooth decay (National Alliance for Equity in Dental Health, 2001). A report – *The Dental Caries Experience of 5-Year-Old Children in Great Britain* – revealed that children in Glasgow had some of the worst rates of decayed teeth in children under 5 years. Glasgow's 5-year-olds were found to have an average of $3\frac{1}{2}$ decayed, missing or filled teeth (Pitts et al., 2001).

Culture

There are also ethnic variations. Hall and Elliman (2003) mentioned that in the UK, Asian children have more decayed teeth than white children. The beginnings of these differences may occur during the weaning period, when some families may be unsure what to give their children. In an effort to stay as close as possible to the diet of cultural origin, some families try to seek products which do not contain meat and may thus opt for more sugary products (Department of Health, 1988).

Children/young people with special needs

Certain groups within the population need specific attention. As the NSF (Education and Skills, Department of Health, 2004) maintains, children/young people who are vulnerable need particular consideration when it comes to dental health.

Children/young people with special needs are sometimes more vulnerable to dental health problems. They may suffer from certain physical or mental health problems which make them more vulnerable (British Fluoridation Society, 2007). Sometimes they are not able to care for their own teeth, and need help. Or they may be on long-term medication which makes them more prone to developing dental caries. It is important that sugar-free medications are encouraged (Education and Skill, Department of Health, 2004) which help to lessen the risk of dental caries.

Dental problems

The four main dental problems highlighted in the NSF (Education and Skills, Department of Health, 2004) include the following:

- Tooth decay/dental caries.
- Dental erosion.
- Gum disease/periodontal disease.
- Unintentional injury, causing a tooth to be lost or fracture.

Hall and Elliman (2003) point out that the first three are largely preventable.

Dental decay

Dental decay can be a real problem. The wide availability and ease with which children can purchase products that are harmful to their teeth is not helpful. Sweets and sugary drinks are so easily obtainable. Children/young people and their parents/carers may not always be fully aware of the harm some of these sugary products can do. Not only do they damage children's early teeth, but also contribute to dental health problems in later life.

In the early stages of decay there are no symptoms. However, a dentist may be able to observe a cavity with the use of an X-ray. Once a cavity reaches the dentine of the tooth, it may become sensitive and toothache develops (British Dental Health Foundation, 2007). Children/young people should be encouraged to visit the dentist regularly and immediately if toothache presents.

Dental erosion

Dental erosion, Hall and Elliman (2003) point out, is experienced by over one-half of 5-year-olds. It begins as loss of enamel from the teeth. It results from a chemical action on the teeth related to acidic drinks, usually caused by either pure fruit juices or fizzy drinks.

Gum disease

Hall and Elliman (2003) highlight that just over one-fourth of 5-year-olds have unhealthy gums due to poor cleaning habits. Brushing with low-dose fluoride toothpaste is recommended. This can help to prevent gum disease.

Injury

Injuries to teeth can occur due to accidental damage. Small children can injure their teeth while playing or even when doing everyday activities. Young people tend to injure their teeth whilst undertaking sporting activities. Sadowsky (2005) says dentists estimate that up to almost 39% of dental injuries occur while teenagers are playing sports. Front teeth are more likely to suffer as a result of a sports injury. Chips and cracks of the teeth can be repaired. Mouthguards or protectors can provide useful protection for teeth and surrounding soft tissues (Sadowsky, 2005). Mouthguards or protectors are able to cushion a blow to the face (American Dental Association, 2007).

There are several types of mouthguard or protector available. However, Brodie (2006) along with other dentists recommends a custom-made protector.

Government policy to address need

The Government is keen to seek improvements in oral health, particularly in reducing the amount of tooth decay in children (Audit Commission, 2002). The Government is also keen to encourage new ways of working within practice (Audit Commission, 2002).

With the highest need evident in the more deprived areas, this should be a key focus of policy. The British Dental Association (BDA, 2002) believes that tackling inequalities in oral health is essential. Children with dental decay go on to experience discomfort, which can lead to dental extractions (BDA, 2002).

The BDA (2002) is in support of the initiatives that Government have so far undertaken. These include the following:

- England – *Brushing for Life* (free dental packs).
- Scotland – caries prevention scheme for 6- to 7-year-olds.
- Wales – fissure sealant scheme.
- NI – specific initiates (see national perspectives).

The NSF (Education and Skills, Department of Health, 2004) in its recommendations urges adequate service provision for children/young people. It also advises that dental health promotion should be provided as part of the Child Health Promotion Programme by local practitioners. They suggest that more intense and targeted health promotion is needed for dental health.

Key health promotion messages

The NSF (Education and Skills, Department of Health, 2004) maintains that dental decay is preventable. Children can be encouraged to care for their teeth from an early age, with parental/carer help and assistance. These positive health behaviours can then become well-established habits.

There are several ways that children/young people can be encouraged to care for their teeth. The following outlines several health promotion behaviours:

- Regular tooth brushing.
- Fluoride.
- Diet.
- Avoiding certain drinks.
- Regular dental check ups.

Regular tooth brushing

Tooth brushing with toothpaste is one of the most effective ways to remove plaque (Wisdom, 1999). From practice experience young children sometimes do not like the taste of regular toothpaste. Children's toothpastes can be used. As Brodie (2006) states, children's toothpastes tend to have milder flavours, and are better tolerated by children than regular toothpastes.

Brodie (2006) also advises that it is better to continue supervising children with the cleaning of their teeth up to the age of 6 or 7 years. From practice observation, young children do not always clean their teeth properly. They try to do the job as quickly as they can. This can result in children failing to access all areas of the mouth. Or they forget to do the job at all. Assisting children can be a great reminder and a good way of establishing a regular tooth brushing routine.

Use of a mirror can help so children can see what they are doing when cleaning their teeth. Cleaning teeth when the parent/carer is doing the same job may help. Children often want to copy and do the same actions as others.

It is particularly important not to miss the bedtime brushing routine. If missed, bacteria and sugar will build up over night and cause harm. There is less saliva available at night to clean the mouth (Wisdom, 1999). It is essential to always brush before bedtime, a habit that children really need to establish.

The routine of tooth brushing needs to happen at least twice a day, importantly too, spending at least 2 minutes brushing on each occasion. The brushing technique should consist of inner, outer, chewing and biting surfaces of each tooth (Prodigy, 2005). Do not forget the gums and tongue too. The technique with tooth brushing is to use circular movements (British Dental Health Foundation, 2007).

A toothbrush needs to be changed every 3 months (British Dental Health Foundation, 2007). There are many interesting, varied and colourful toothbrushes available for children. Some are even available as particular Disney characters, such as Tigger and Micky Mouse. These novelty toothbrushes can be a way of encouraging children to be interested in cleaning their teeth.

Electric toothbrushes are available and they can do a good job. An electric toothbrush has a vibrating head, which provides a large amount of cleaning action (British Dental Health Foundation, 2007). Children may also find them interesting and fun.

Baby's teeth should be cleaned. Wisdom (1999) recommends that a soft clean cloth can be used initially, and then move onto a soft-bristled toothbrush. A small amount of toothpaste to be used, a pea-sized amount is recommended (Brodie, 2006).

Fluoride

Fluoride is a compound used as an additive to drinking water to prevent dental decay (Blackwell's Nursing Dictionary, 2005). Fluoride is also contained within children's toothpaste, as well as regular toothpaste. Some of the improvements in children's teeth have been attributed to fluoride toothpaste (Audit Commission, 2002).

Improvements in children's teeth have also been attributed to adding fluoride to water supplies (Audit Commission, 2002). Fluoridation of public water has been shown to reduce tooth decay, especially amongst socially deprived communities. However, decisions about adding fluoride to the water supply lie locally, and many areas have decided not to add it.

In *Our Healthier Nation* (Secretary of State for Health, 1998), the Government highlighted the importance of fluoride in local water supplies. The Government asserted that fluoridation of water supplies to the optimum level can substantially reduce the amount of tooth decay in children.

Fluoride is naturally present in water supplies in varying concentrations (British Fluoridation Society, 2007). Many areas of the UK do not have fluoride added to their water supply. Areas of the UK that have added fluoride include the West Midlands and the North East England (British Fluoridation Society, 2007).

Different arguments and debates exist about the issue of water fluoridation. Some sources have doubts about adding fluoride to public water supplies, due to concerns about its overall impact on health. Nonetheless, there is a large body of opinion that supports its use. As well as the Government, there have been other reports that point out the benefits of adding fluoride to water supplies. Acheson (1998) recommends fluoridation, suggesting that it can decrease inequalities in dental health. The National Alliance for Equity in Dental Health (2001) maintains that young children in areas where the water supply is fluoridated have less tooth decay.

The British Fluoridation Society can provide more information on this subject. Detailed information can be obtained from their website – http://www.bfsweb.org/. The aim of this organisation is to improve dental health by helping to encourage optimum fluoride content of water supplies (British Fluoridation Society, 2007).

Diet

Improvements in children's teeth have also been attributed to improvements in children's diets (Audit Commission, 2002). Eating a healthy balanced diet can be really good for children's/young people's dental health. Conversely, too much sugar in the diet can cause severe problems. Harris et al.'s (2004) systematic review on the risk factors associated with dental caries in children found clear evidence that the consumption of sugar, either in amounts, frequency or timings, was risk factor for poor dental health.

If a child snacks frequently on foods which contain sugar, this can cause problems for their teeth. Each time a child eats food which contains sugar, plaque will form in the mouth and combine with the sugar to produce acid (Wisdom, 1999). The acid then causes problems for the teeth, attacking the teeth. Repeated acid attacks in the mouth, due to frequent snacking, can lead to dental caries.

Wisdom (1999) has produced some tips on snacking:

- Cut down on sugary snacks.
- Have snacks that are low in sugar, such as cheese and vegetables.
- Avoid sugar-rich foods which stay in the mouth for prolonged periods, such as hard sweets and lollipops.
- Avoid sticky sweets which lodge on tooth surfaces, such as toffees.
- If giving children sweets, serve them with meals.

Sticky foods are retained in the mouth for longer than other foods. The acid which destroys teeth is thus around for longer in the mouth, resulting in prolonged acid attacks on teeth (Wisdom, 1999).

Importantly, the value of cheese and other foods that are rich in calcium will help to keep bones and teeth strong. More details about such foods can be obtained via the Dairy Council (Dairy Council, 2007; http://www.milk.co.uk). Cheese is especially good for teeth. Eating cheese as a snack after meals neutralises acids in the mouth, which can help to prevent tooth decay (British Dental Health Foundation, 2007).

Avoiding certain drinks

Fizzy drinks can be harmful for children's/young people's teeth. Jamie Oliver's campaign on school dinners has recently highlighted the harmful effects of fizzy drinks.

Children as young as 4 years old already need to have their teeth filled due to damage caused by fizzy drinks (Yaqoob, 2002). Acid contained within these drinks causes the enamel on the surface of teeth to erode. The acid causes generalised erosion all over the tooth.

It is not just fizzy drinks that can cause these problems. Families think that giving fruit juices is a healthy option. However fruit juices too can cause similar problems, especially if these drinks are given in a bottle.

Tooth enamel is quite a hard coating, but when the enamel is worn away the dentine beneath is exposed (British Dental Health Foundation, 2007). Teeth start to become sensitive to hot and cold and sweet foods (British Dental Health Foundation, 2007). Eventually damage to the tooth can cause pain.

The advice given on children's drinks is as follows:

- Give water or milk to drink.
- If children insist on having fruit drinks, these should be limited to mealtimes.
- If giving fruit juice, this should be diluted.

Do not brush immediately after having a fruit juice. In fact, the British Dental Health Foundation (2007) recommends leaving at least 1 hour after eating or drinking anything acidic, so teeth can build their mineral content back up again. The danger is that by brushing too soon erosion to the tooth's enamel can be caused.

Dental check-ups

It is important to have a dental check at least once a year (Prodigy, 2005). The dentist is able to detect any potential dental problems that might be developing. It is also an opportunity to report any problems that children/young people may be having with their teeth and gums.

Dental health checks can begin from an early age. Young children can attend the dentist when parents/carers go for their usual check-ups. After a couple of visits they can then begin to have appointments of their own. Apparently, more children are now visiting the dentist at an earlier age (ONS, 2004). Dentists and their nurses try to make the experience of going to the dentist a positive one. Providing young children with the opportunity to watch television, whilst in the dentist's chair, and

the provision of badges and stickers all help to make children feel more at ease.

Some Sure Start centres/children's centres have their own dental health practices attached to the centre, which are especially for young children. This enables young children living in deprived areas to get improved access to dental health checks.

More recently, however, within parts of the UK some parents/carers have experienced difficulties accessing a dentist for their child. They have been unable to register their child with a National Health Service (NHS) dentist (Marsh, 2002). Where parents/carers are not able to register with an NHS dentist, the choices open to them are either registering with a private dentist, or they go without a dentist for their child. Obviously, not having the opportunity to attend the dentist cannot be good for a child's teeth.

Health promotion resources

This section focuses on some of the *resources* that nurses can use to make your health promotion activities more fun and interesting for children/young people.

Before you decide which resources to opt for, it is worth spending a little time thinking about the developmental needs and abilities of your target group – the children/young people you will be working with. This will help in the selection of suitable resources.

Health promotion campaigns

National campaigns are an important way to promote dental health messages to children/young people. National campaigns involve special events undertaken at certain points during the year, with usually a particular focus or theme. Consider what activities you could undertake locally in line with a national campaign.

National Smile Month

National Smile Month is a campaign organised each year by the British Dental Health Foundation. The campaign is usually held in mid-May until mid-June. Each campaign has a theme. The 2007 campaign focused on teeth cleaning – *two minutes twice a day* – promoting the message that children should clean their teeth on two occasions each day and for 2 minutes on each occasion.

Books

Books are a great learning resource. There are lots of interesting books out there on dental health that can be read with young children.

Sitting with a child going through a book can be a great opportunity to teach them about caring for their teeth. There are audio books, magical tooth fairy books and interactive books. *Len Lion's Wobbly Tooth* by Abby Irvine and Pippa Young, for example, is a good story and comes with its own magical tooth bag especially for wobbly teeth.

Books with well-known children's characters are often a good starting point, for example:

- The Little Princess: *I Want My Tooth* by Tony Ross.
- Maisy: *Maisy, Charley and the Wobbly Tooth* by Lucy Cousins.

Books in preparation for the first visit to the dentist are often useful too.

Design your own book on dental health

If you are particularly good at art and design, or good at making up stories, design your own book for children. Make the book interactive, so children not only listen to the story but also actively do something with the characters involved. Children's own actions then begin to impact on the story.

Young children love characters. You only need to think about the characters that Disney has created and how they captivate children. Develop your own character perhaps, which may help to capture their attention.

Here are some ideas as starting points for your story:

- The naughty bunny that ate so many chocolates that his teeth fell out.
- The bunny with the beautiful smile, who always brushed his teeth.

Models

Local health promotion units often have models of teeth to assist with health promotion activities. For example, a giant tooth and giant toothbrush may come in useful when demonstrating tooth brushing techniques.

A three-dimensional model of a tooth can also be obtained, which shows children/young people the internal structure of teeth. This might help when discussing the anatomy and physiology of teeth, for example.

Samples and stickers

Children can have great fun with novelty samples, toys and stickers. These can be obtained from dental organisations. Examples include the following:

- Two-minute timer – for tooth brushing.
- Balloons.
- Certificates.
- Character puppets.
- Drinking bottles – for encouraging children to drink water.
- Little tooth fairy boxes.
- Packs of toothbrushes.
- Reward charts.
- Stickers (in a variety of popular well-known characters).
- T-shirts.
- Toothbrush characters, with covers.
- Wall charts.

Interactive computer items

The British Dental Health Foundation has a website with lots of interesting resources.

To coincide with their 2007 *National Smile* campaign, the foundation launched an interactive web quiz based on the theme of their campaign – *two minutes, twice a day.* Children/young people could enjoy testing their knowledge on dental health.

The website also featured a special sun timer. The idea of the timer was to help children gain a real sense of what a 2-minute tooth-brushing session felt like. The website points out that many children think that they are brushing their teeth for 2 minutes, when in fact on average evidence shows that most brush their teeth for about 45 seconds (British Dental Health Foundation, 2007). It is a helpful website presenting some interesting activities for children/young people.

Quiz

A dental health quiz can be good fun and easy to create. You could include questions on the following:

- The purpose of teeth.
- The development of children's teeth.
- Dental problems.
- How to prevent dental problems from occurring.

Put the children into teams. Members of the winning team can be treated to a prize. Obviously, the prize needs to be good for dental health.

The British Dental Foundation's website includes a variety of puzzles and games that can be downloaded. These include dot to dots, colouring and word search puzzles, for example. Your local health promotion unit may also be able to provide similar materials.

Songs and poems

Young children especially enjoy songs and poems. Include songs or poems which they might enjoy in groups. Songs about tooth fairies are often fun.

There are poems for older children too. Pam Ayres (2001) has also written a very funny poem – *Oh I wish I'd looked after me teeth*. Children love it. Also take a look at the poem *Teeth* by Spike Milligan (2001).

A range of different resources have been discussed here that could be included in activities and sessions on dental health promotion.

Assessment of learning

It is often useful to assess what children/young people have learnt. Here again you could design your own activities based on what they have been taught. Alternatively, you might find something at your local health promotion unit contained within a resource or teaching package, that could be used.

An assessment could focus on tooth brushing, for example. Send children home with a tooth brushing chart which a parent could complete with them. The chart could be ticked or a sticker given when children have cleaned their teeth each morning and evening for the required 2 minutes. Children can then bring the chart back the following week and show what they have achieved. Those children who

have achieved the target set could receive a prize. Children are receiving a reward for positive dental health behaviours.

Activity

As nurses we need to be thinking at the level of young children when planning health promotion activities with them. Example – working with children (6 years) when trying to persuade them about tooth brushing, explain in language they will understand. Make up a story about bacteria, for example. There are bugs in the mouth and they are all having a party. We need to catch them all before the party gets too big and too many of them decide to show up.

This is the kind of approach you can be taking with young children. In their minds they still believe in magical thoughts and ideas. Any factual information can always be supported with visual images. They need visual ideas to help them learn.

Importantly, remember to plan your activity carefully. Think around the following elements of the Daines et al. (1993) approach to planning:

- Aim and objectives/outcomes.
- Content.
- Methods.
- Resources.
- Evaluation and assessment.

Using the above teaching plan as a basis, design a dental health activity for a group of 6-year-olds. Remember to find out what they know already about their teeth.

Practice

Sue presents insights into community practice, whilst Helen looks at hospital practice.

Community practice

The aim of this section is to provide an overview on how dental health is promoted in the *community*. Oral health is important as it contributes to the general health of individuals. Oral health promotion aims to increase awareness of the causes and prevention of dental problems.

In practice, dental health promotion begins with the midwife at antenatal classes followed by health visitors, community nurses, community dentists, dental nurses, school nurses and community pharmacists. Dental health forms an integral part of public health. Practitioners in the community aim to advise parents/carers and their children about dental health in line with the Government's Oral Health Plan (Department of Health, 2005). The primary care trusts are required to provide oral health promotion services appropriate for the needs of local populations. The aim is to ensure that services are accessible. Parents/carers are given information, thus empowering them with the knowledge to undertake basic care related to nutrition and dental health, which impact on the oral health of their children and teenagers.

Hall and Elliman (2003) state that the most common oral diseases in children are tooth decay, gum disease and dental erosion. Nationally, many young children have problems with dental decay due to consumption of fizzy drinks. Mouatt (2003) goes on to say that dental caries are more prevalent among the lower socio-economic groups. Other factors which play an important part in the development of childhood dental problems include family stress, diet and parenting styles. These are all areas where community practitioners can help to support families with advice and care, either through individual health promotion activities or group activities. Community nurses are very effective in promoting good dental health care (Ottley, 2002).

At antenatal classes pregnant mothers are encouraged to eat healthily to help their baby's bones and teeth form. During the early years of a child's life, the health visitor provides advice about nutrition and how to take care of children's developing teeth. Powell (1998) says how important it is to stress to new parents that a healthy first set of teeth is important for general health.

Dental nurses are invited to attend community clinics to teach parents/carers how to reduce levels of sugar in the diet and promote good dental care. If needed, an interpreter can be present. When babies are 7- to 9-month olds, their parents/carers are provided with information and dental packs, which contain a soft toothbrush and toothpaste, by health visitors or community nurses.

Community dentists play a key role in detecting dental problems. Maynall (1986) maintains that some parents/carers are unaware that their children are entitled to dental treatment. Young children should attend the dentist so that early signs of decay can be detected.

The average age for permanent teeth to erupt is approximately 6/7 years; hence, this age group is an ideal target group for health promotion activities in school. Dental health messages can be introduced in a fun way. Look at cognitive theories on child development which might help in the design of activities, such as those of Piaget and Vygotsky (see Chapter 5).

Schools play a part in healthy food campaigns, whereby unhealthy foods are banned from school menus, as well as banning vending machines with fizzy drinks and unhealthy snacks. Children are encouraged to eat five pieces of fruit daily, as well as vegetables in their diet (*5 a Day* campaign, Department of Health, 2004). Scully (2001) maintains that eating a piece of cheese after meals can reduce plaque and promote mineralisation of the tooth enamel.

The Government introduced a joint initiative with Colgate several years ago, known as the Brushing for Life campaign to help all families, but particularly those in lower socio-economic areas. A purpose of this campaign was to encourage the habit of brushing children's teeth regularly with fluoride toothpaste.

In junior schools the dentist's chair is introduced so children can become familiar with sitting in it, thus helping them to feel less apprehensive on future visits to the dentist. Several games are played which include a giant floor jigsaw whereby children put different foods into food groups.

Community pharmacists play an important part in educating the public as they can advise on the use of sugar-free medicines for children, especially for prolonged medical conditions. Supermarkets can play a part too in dental health promotion. They can reinforce sweet-free zones at checkouts and shelves, so that sweets are not easily accessible to children.

The topic of dental health promotion is much debated. It is only through effective education by health practitioners in the community, working together, can changes to families' knowledge on dental health improve. Particularly important is support for families in areas where health inequalities exist. Literature or leaflets available in different languages may go someway to bridging the gap of health inequalities, as well as service accessibility.

Hospital practice

Poor dental health, as we know, is closely linked to economic deprivation, cultural differences and social exclusion. In the UK there are also differences between regions and areas within regions. These differences can be linked to poverty with social classes III, IV and V three times more likely to have lost all of their teeth in adulthood than other social classes (Department of Health, Chief Dental Officer, 2007).

Within the area that our *hospital* serves in the Midlands, there is a large proportion of the population who are economically deprived. The area has a large ethnic community and more recently a growing population of refugee and asylum seekers. Sadly, as the statistics show, these groups tend to have poorer dental health (WHO, 2005). Now that the Government has made it the responsibility of primary care trusts to provide public dental health, so there are less inequalities.

The evidence is there to see if you visit our surgical ward on Monday morning. The ward is alive with the laughter of children playing in the play area, mums and dads with them for the duration of the morning, the nurses busy rushing around the ward, preparing the children for theatre. On average 20–36 children/young people come to the ward each week for tooth extractions and conservative restoration (fillings) to their teeth.

Inequalities in dental health are not just things written about in the Government documents; they are real children. It would be reasonable to ask – Have we failed these children/young people as they have ended up at our door for treatment. It is important to recognise that although the volume of children/young people that our ward sees for dental treatment is high, that is not to say that health promotion work undertaken by other agencies has failed. Records on dental public health began over 30 years ago. The dental health of children/young people is better now than before records began; six out of ten children start school with no decay (Department of Health, Chief Dental Officer, 2007). Yet, we still lag behind other parts of Europe.

The ward treats many 2- and 3-year-olds who have rotten decayed teeth through the consumption of high levels of sugar in foods and drinks. In the primary school age group again, many children come to us for the removal or conservation of teeth that have decayed through poor diet.

Adolescents come to us for tooth extraction and conservation too, due to decay from high sugar consumption, but also tooth erosion from fizzy acidic drinks. This age group may also have oral health problems from smoking.

The ward also cares for children/young people with special needs who require dental treatment. Many of the drugs they take damage their teeth due to its sugar content. These drugs also influence the development of teeth. Some of these children suffer from dry mouths. In this situation high levels of bacteria can accumulate, increasing acid levels and decay (British Dental Health Foundation, 2007). Saliva neutralises acid from bacteria in the plaque that attacks the tooth enamel. So if a child's mouth is dry there is less saliva, thus the child will be more prone to dental problems.

The experience of coming into hospital for dental treatment is made as positive as possible for children/young people, and conducted in a safe environment. The ward's environment is designed to meet the needs of children/young people and their families and therefore is friendly and non-threatening. The dental lists are organised by dentists and dental health nurses from the community, thus providing continuity of care. A play specialist is responsible for meeting the play needs of children. The expertise of children's nurses is also available. An interpreter is provided for families who speak little or no English.

The ward area has its own playroom and dedicated recovery bay. The dental team have a purpose-built operating theatre. This allows the dental team to see many more children/young people than perhaps other hospitals. Treatments can thus be undertaken without too much waiting time.

Health promotion activities are provided in a number of different ways. The play specialist and dental nurses present poster displays on dental health and healthy eating. The play specialist also sets up games and activities that are designed to promote dental health, along with the more conventional toys and activities. There are leaflets and booklets available offering health promotion advice for families. Advice on healthy eating and how to brush effectively is also given. The ward area has toothbrushes and toothpaste that can be given out to children/young people who have been admitted to the ward unexpectedly.

Drinks and foods provided in the ward area are healthy. There are no stocks of junk food available. If parents/carers wish their children to have other foods and drinks then they are required to bring these in themselves. Children/young people are still empowered to make their own choices about what they have to eat and drink. However, the ward will only provide healthy choices (Department of Health, 2005).

The children on the dental list are followed up in the community following discharge. This is initiated by a call from the dental nursing team on the evening following the child's discharge home to check that there are no problems following dental surgery. A dental clinic appointment is also provided.

In conclusion, this section has discussed the strategies that our ward provides to promote dental health. All children/young people have the right to a good standard of dental care and I feel that our ward environment helps to contribute to this.

Conclusion

This chapter has focused on the dental health of children/young people. A variety of different ways that positive oral behaviours can be encouraged and promoted, have been considered. Although there have been improvements in dental health over the last few decades, there is still much to achieve. The health of young people's teeth does seem to be improving. There are improvements in young children's teeth too; however, these improvements seem to be slowing down. Evidence does point to geographical, ethnic and social class variations in children's/young people's dental health, as figures and reports have repeatedly highlighted.

There are a variety of dental organisations that can provide the nurse with resources and information. Using different resources for health promotion activities can really make dental health promotion a fun subject for children/young people.

The NSF (Education and Skills, Department of Health, 2004) advises that the oral health needs of children/young people are identified within local health promotion programmes. It is important that they are for children's/young people's future dental health.

References

Acheson, D. (1998) *Independent Inquiry into Inequalities in Health.* London: The Stationery Office.

Albert, D. (2005) *Understand Your Own Oral Needs.* Columbia University College of Dental Medicine. Available at: http://www.simplestepsdental.com (accessed 20 February 2007).

American Academy of Family Physicians (2000–2005) *Mouth and Teeth: How to Keep Them Healthy.* Available at: http://www.familydoctor.org (accessed 20 February 2007).

American Dental Association (2007) *Oral Health Topics – Mouth-Guards.* Available at: http://www.ada.org (accessed February 2007).

Audit Commission (2002) *Dentistry – Primary Dental Care Services in England and Wales.* London: Audit Commission.

Ayres, P. (2001) Oh, I wish I'd looked after me teeth. *Nation's Favourite Children's Poems.* London: BBC.

BDA (2002) *BDA Policy on Tackling Oral Health Inequalities.* Available at: http://www.bda.org (accessed 24 November 2006).

Blackwell's Nursing Dictionary (2005) Oxford: Blackwell Publishing.

British Dental Health Foundation (2007) *Oral Health Facts.* Available at: www.dentalhealth.org.uk (accessed 26 February 2007).

British Fluoridation Society (2007) *Fluoridation and General Health.* Available at: http://www.bfsweb.org (accessed 26 February 2007).

Brodie, I. (2006) *Mouthpiece,* 1st edn. Bingham: Bingham Dental Practice.

Daines, J., Daines, C., Graham, B. (1993) *Adult Learning, Adult Teaching,* 3rd edn. Nottingham: Department of Adult Education.

Dairy Council (2007) *Tiny Tums! Leaflet.* Available at: http://www.milk.co.uk (accessed 1 March 2007).

Department of Health (2004) *5 a Day.* Available at: http://www.dh.gov.uk (accessed 1 March 2007).

Department of Health (2005). *Choosing Better Oral Health: An Oral Health Plan for England.* London: Department of Health.

Department of Health (and Social Security) (1988) *Present Day Practice in Infant Feeding,* 3rd report. London: HMSO.

Department of Health, Chief Dental Officer (2007). *Department of Health Website.* Available at: http://www.dh.gov.uk (accessed November 2007).

Education and Skills (Department of), Department of Health (2004) *National Service Framework for Children,*

Young People and Maternity Services. London: Crown Copyright.

Hall, D., Elliman, D. (2003) *Health for All Children*, 4th edn. Oxford: Oxford University Press.

Harris, R., Nicoll, A., Adair, P., Pine, C. (2004) Risk factors for dental caries in young children: a systematic review from the literature. *Community Dental Health* 21(Suppl.): 71–85.

Marsh, B. (2002) Fears for children as millions miss out on dental care. *Daily Mail*. London: ANL Daily Mail Publishers.

Maynall, B. (1986) *Keeping Children Healthy: The Role of Mothers and Professionals*. London: Allen and Unwin (Pubs.) Ltd.

Milligan, S. (2001) Teeth. *Nation's Favourite Children's Poems*. London: BBC.

Mouatt, B. (2003) Health and fitness series 2. Dental decay and the case for fluoride. *Journal of Family Health Care* 13(2) 34–36.

National Alliance for Equity in Dental Health (2001) *Inequalities in Dental Health*. UK: National Alliance for Equity in Dental Health.

ONS (2004) *Children's Dental Health Survey 2003*. London: Office of National Statistics.

Ottley, C. (2002) Improving children's dental health. *Journal of Family Health Care* 12(5): 122–124.

Pitts, N., Evans, D., Nugent, Z. (2001) The dental caries experience of 5 year old children in Great Britain. Surveys coordinated by the British Association for the study of community dentistry in 1999/2000. *Community Dental Health* 18: 49–55.

Powell, L. (1998) Caries prediction: a review of the literature. *Community Dentistry and Oral Epidemiology* 26: 361–371.

Prodigy (2005) *Oral Hygiene*. EMIS and PIP. Available at: http://www.prodigy.nhs (accessed 26 February 2007).

Sadowsky, D. (2005) Sports safety: avoiding tooth and mouth injuries. Oral Health Made Simple. Columbia University College of Dental Medicine. Available at: http://www.simplestepsdental.com (accessed 20 February 2007).

Scully, C. (ed.) (2001) *ABC of Oral Health*. London: BMJ Books.

Secretary of State for Health (1998) *Our Healthier Nation*. London: The Stationary Office.

Seow, W. (1998) Biological mechanisms of early childhood caries. *Community Dentistry and Oral Epidemiology* 26(Suppl.): 8–27.

WHO (2005) Oral Health Country/Area Profile Programme Website. Available at: http://www.whocollab.od.mah.se/countries (accesed November 2007).

Wisdom (1999) *Keeping Your Child's Teeth Healthy. A Parent's Guide!* Wisdom.

Yaqoob, T. (2002) *Fizzy Drinks Threat to Children's Teeth*. London: ANL Daily Mail Publishers.

9 Skin Cancer Prevention

Lesley Strazds

NSF

Health promotion is about supporting families to make healthy choices for their children (Education and Skills, Department of Health, 2004).

Introduction

Action on preventing skin cancer can begin from the time children are very young. Skin protection behaviours adopted during early childhood may go on to become natural ways of living, thus help to prevent skin cancers in later life. This chapter provides details about the background to skin cancer and then goes on to discuss ways children's/young people's health can be promoted to help reduce the risks of skin cancer developing in later life.

Skin cancer can be an unfortunate consequence of too much sun, including episodes of overexposure experienced during childhood. Its importance, therefore, as a health promotion subject explored during childhood should not be underestimated, if nurses want to promote the long-term health of the next generation. NHS Direct (2007) highlights that the risk of developing skin cancer in childhood itself is relatively rare.

Too much sunlight is harmful and can damage the skin (Emis and PIP, 2006). This is the message that nurses need to promote to families, in supporting them to make healthy choices for their children and teenagers.

Incidence

Cancer Research UK (2006) reports that skin cancer is now the most common type of cancer. The year-on-year increase in the incidence of skin cancer indicates that approximately 100 000 new cases are diagnosed each year but many more may go unreported (Cancerbackup, 2006). Fortunately, most skin cancers can be successfully treated. Nonetheless, many skin cancers could be prevented if people were more careful about not exposing their skin and their children's skin to the sun. Up to 80% of skin cancers are preventable, suggests the British Association of Dermatologists (2007).

What is skin cancer?

There are three main types of skin cancer. The two most common types are basal cell carcinoma and squamous cell carcinoma. They are easily treated and rarely fatal but can become destructive, invading local tissues and resulting in scarring and disfigurement. The third and most serious type of skin cancer is malignant melanoma. Fortunately, it is the least common, but it is responsible for almost 2000 deaths each year (Statistical Information Team, Cancer Research UK).

When observing the skin for any signs of skin cancer, the British Association of Dermatologists (2007) suggests look for changes in the skin. Observe for any signs of bleeding, growing areas, changes in appearance and areas of the skin that never completely heal.

Risk factors

The most significant risk factor for skin cancer is thought to be overexposure to ultraviolet (UV) radiation in sunlight. Slight cell damage caused by UV can lead to cancerous changes occurring in the skin. Sun radiation is a contributing factor in 90% of all cases of skin cancer. It is likely that most skin damage from UV radiation occurs *before the age of 20 years*, which may be surprising fact to learn.

Information on the risks of early exposure to the sun is therefore highly significant for children/young people, as awareness of the potential damage that can be caused may influence behaviour. Children/young people may be less likely to expose their skin to the sun, and may make more effort to protect themselves from the sun's rays, if they are aware of the facts. Parents/carers need to be aware of the risks too, and how much they can do to protect their children while they are still young. A particular concern is young people, who may be keen to become sunburnt whilst on holiday.

Nurses have a key role to play in delivering messages of health promotion on sun safety. Health promotion in schools, children's centres, hospitals, and places of leisure can all help to provide important opportunities for messages on sun safety.

Health promotion

The NSF for children, young people and maternity services (Education and Skills, Department of Health, 2004) outlines a vision; all children, young people and their families are *supported*, so that they are able to make *healthy choices* in how they live their lives. The NSF goes on to stress how environmental

factors that may contribute to disease, ill health or injury, should be recognised.

Parents/carers are the main providers of health care for their children, especially in the early years. Support and information on sun safety from nurses may be beneficial. Early introduction of sun protection behaviours by parents/carers and consistent use throughout life can help to decrease a child's lifetime risk of developing skin cancer.

Sun damage

The risk of developing skin cancer is increased following episodes of sunburn. Sun damage refers to how the sun alters the look and feel of the skin. It can be acute, as in sunburn. Any episode of sunburn causes irreversible trauma within the skin's DNA possibly leading towards the development of sun damage-related conditions (http://www.dermatology.co.uk).

Malignant melanoma is most strongly linked to intermittent exposure to high-intensity sunlight (Cancer Research UK, 2006). The risk of cancer increases with the number of sunburn episodes over a lifetime (Cho et al., 2005).

Chronic sun damage, on the other hand, is seen as gradual changes in the skin caused by an accumulation of sun exposure throughout one's lifetime. This is typically associated with people who have outdoor occupations and hobbies.

It is widely known that the only beneficial effect of solar UV radiation on the skin is the synthesis of vitamin D and its role in maintaining bone health (Cancer Research, 2006). For many people it feels good to spend time outdoors, which can make it difficult to avoid excessive exposure to the sun. However, the most effective way to reduce the risk of skin cancer is to protect the skin from burning in the sun.

Sun protection

Modelling the use of sunscreen and other protection habits, such as wearing sun-protective clothing, hats and sunglasses, and seeking shade whenever possible, is an important way to teach children how to protect themselves in the sun. One way children learn is by imitation (Bandura, 1977). Through imitation, copying the behaviours of others, children can develop new skills and learn how to take care of themselves. Patterns of behaviour developed in the early years can shape attitudes and actions for the rest of children's lives.

Researchers have found that programmes promoting sun protection can be successfully implemented in childcare settings. Children as young as 4 years old are capable of learning sun-safe behaviours. Health promotion programmes, which focus on children of 8 and 12 years old, have been found to be more effective than those which focus on young people. Young people tend to be more questioning of adult advice and opinion, which may contribute to health programmes having less success with this age group, when compared with younger children.

Regular *sunscreen use* and *sun avoidance* are widely promoted by organisations and individuals interested in skin cancer prevention. Protective garments can work well. Closely woven fabrics provide good sun protection. Protection for the eyes is important too. To help avoid damage to the eyes, sunglasses that block 99–100% of UV rays should be worn.

Sunscreens have become much more effective over the years. The general consensus of experts is to select sunscreens that provide broad-spectrum protection, not only against ultraviolet B (UVB) but also against ultraviolet A (UVA). Sunscreens should offer a sun protection factor (SPF) of 15 or significantly higher, especially for young children and babies.

UVB is the part of the spectrum that causes burning and is most associated with the risk of skin cancer. UVA penetrates more deeply and is responsible for many of the common signs of premature ageing of the skin. Protection from UVA is also important as exposure can contribute to skin cancer too.

Sun avoidance is particularly encouraged between the hours of 11 am and 2 pm when the intensity of UV rays is at its greatest. It is easier to practise sun protection in an environment which supports it. Enhancing access to shade is an important aspect of many sun-safe policies.

Sunscreens

Sunscreens protect the skin by absorbing and/or reflecting UVA and UVB. Chemical absorbers within sunscreens soak up the harmful UV rays, thus reducing the amount of UV that reaches the skin, whereas physical barriers within sunscreens reflect the UV away from the skin.

Adequate solar protection is more important during childhood than at any other time during one's life (International Agency for Research on Cancer, 2001). The International Agency for Research on Cancer in their handbook *Cancer Prevention: Sunscreens* recommends the daily use of sunscreen with an SPF of greater than 15. They also advise that sunscreens are not to be used as a means of extending the duration of solar exposure or as a substitute for the appropriate clothing or shade.

Sun protection factors

SPFs found on sunscreen packaging apply mainly to UVB rays, although many manufacturers include ingredients that protect the skin from some UVA rays as well. These are known as broad-spectrum sunscreens and are highly recommended by experts.

The SPF of a sunscreen is a measure of the amount of sun protection provided and is based on the assumption that people apply 2 mg/cm^2 to the body. Studies identified by Cancer Research UK (2007) indicate that most people only apply 0.5–1.0 mg/cm^2; therefore, individuals are only getting a quarter to a half of the protection they need. This brings to prominence the importance of the correct application particularly where children are concerned. Young children love playing outdoors, but they are not aware of how the sun can damage their skin. It is, therefore, important that parents/carers take careful and necessary precautions for their children's protection. Redness of the skin, no matter how slight, is a sign that the skin has been damaged.

Calculating SPFs

A sunscreen's SPF is measured by timing – how long skin covered with the sunscreen takes to burn, when compared with unprotected skin (Health Education Authority, 1998). For example, if unprotected skin burns in 10 minutes from the sun, by using a sunscreen with a SPF2, this doubles the time spent before burning to the skin will occur. Skin will therefore take 20 minutes to burn.

Understanding skin types

An individual's skin type affects the degree to which some people burn and the time it takes them to burn. Skin types are classified on a scale of 1–6. Skin types 1 and 2 have fair skin. A low classification indicates a greater tendency for skin to burn more quickly and more severely than individuals with a high classification. The *Sun Know-how* campaign (Health Education Authority, 1998) acknowledges that although in comparison paler skinned people have an increased risk of developing sun damage, excessive exposure to intense sunlight can damage all skin types.

How to apply sunscreen

Sunscreen must be used properly to provide protection. It should be applied evenly, thickly and regularly to be effective, with attention being paid to heavily exposed areas. Experts usually recommend the initial application 30 minutes prior to exposure to the sun. This allows the sunscreen to absorb into the skin. A further application about 20 minutes after going out into the sun will help to cover any missed areas, and make sure a sufficient layer has been applied. Sunscreen applications should then be repeated at least every 2 hours during exposure to the sun. Re-application is also important especially after any activity that could remove it, such as sweating, swimming, towelling or lying on sand.

Sunscreens are important but they should not be the sole agent used for protection against the sun. Remember to use them alongside other sun protection actions outlined.

Resources

Health promotion literature

Visit your local health promotion unit, and find out details about the current sun safety campaign. The unit can provide posters and leaflets that will help to raise awareness about the dangers of overexposure to the sun for children/young people. They will also be able to provide details about where you can locate any additional health promotion materials for children on sun safety. Often activity sheets are available for children with messages of sun safety. These might include colouring activities or characters that can be cut out and dressed up ready for a sun-safe outing to the beach, which young children may enjoy.

Currently, *Sunsmart* is the United Kingdom's (UK) national skin cancer campaign. It is commissioned by the UK health department and organised by Cancer Research UK. The Sunsmart message is as follows:

- S – spend time in the shade.
- M – make sure you never burn.
- A – aim to cover up with a T-shirt, hat and sunglasses.
- R – remember to take extra care with children.
- T – then use factor 15+ sunscreen.

For more information on this campaign access their website – http://www.sunsmart.org.uk. The Sunsmart campaign produces resources, which include bookmarks with the key messages of sun safety highlighted.

Dermatology UK (2007) provides information on skin conditions, included are some useful resources for children on sun safety. They provide a number of different sun-safe stories, which children may find interesting. Dermatology UK can be accessed via their website at http://www.dermatology.co.uk.

When providing messages of sun safety in school, for example, encourage children to bring in sun hats and sunscreens for protection during the months of the year when they might be at risk of sunburn. Sun hats which cover the neck are particularly useful. More and more parents are sending their children to school with sun hats and sunscreens, so sun safety messages are beginning to take effect across the UK.

To find out the actual risks of sunburn on a particular day, access the solar UV index. The solar UV index forecast is available from the Met Office (2007) – http://www.met-office.gov.uk/weather/uv. The index is on a scale of 1–10, the higher the rate on the index, the greater the risk of sunburn on that particular day. Look out for the triangle sign.

Close

Sun protection for children/young people is really important. Nurses have a key role to play in advising children, young people and their families on how they can protect themselves. Sun safety is not necessarily a subject which receives much attention, only during periods of hot sunny weather. It needs to be an active campaign however, which receives much more attention.

References

Bandura, A. (1977) *Social Learning Theory*. Morristown, NJ: General Learning Press.

British Association of Dermatologists (2007) Available at: http://www.britishassociationdermatologists (accessed 27 November 2007).

Cancerbackup (2006) Available at: http://www.cancerbackup (accessed December 2007).

Cancer Research UK (2006) Available at: http://www.canceruk (accessed December 2007).

Cancer Research UK. (2007) *Statistical Information Team*. Available at: http://www.canceruk (accessed December 2007).

Cho, E., Rosner, B., Feskanich, D., Colditz, G. (2005) Risk factors and individual probabilities of melanoma for whites. *Journal Clinical Oncology* 23(12): 2669–2675.

Dermatology UK (2007) *Skin Cancer*. Available at: http://www.dermatology.co.uk (accessed 27 November 2007).

Education and Skills (Department of), Department of Health (2004) *The National Service Framework for Children, Young People and Maternity Services*. London: Education and Skills, Department of Health.

Emis and PIP (2006) *Sun and Health*. Available at: http://www.patient.co.uk (accessed 27 November 2007).

Health Education Authority (1998) *Sun Know How Campaign*. London: Health Education Authority.

International Agency for Research on Cancer (2001) *Cancer Prevention: Sunscreens*. Geneva: WHO publication.

Met Office (2007) *Solar UV Index*. Available at: http://www.met-office.gov.uk/weather/uv (accessed December 2007).

NHS Direct (2007) *Health Encyclopaedia*. Available at: http://www.nhsdirect (accessed 27 November 2007).

10 Accident Prevention

Karen Moyse

NSF

Heath promotion involves activities at every level – the Government policy, community strategies and individuals making healthy choices (Education and Skills, Department of Health, 2004).

Introduction

Accidents are a leading cause of death and illness in children aged 1–14 years, a recent report from the Audit Commission and Healthcare Commission (2007) has shown. The report reveals that overall child deaths have fallen. Nonetheless, there are widening gaps between the socioeconomic groups; with children from the lower socio-economic groups more likely to die from an accident than those from the higher socio-economic groups (Audit Commission and Healthcare Commission, 2007). The report urges the Government, along with local councils and primary care trusts, to take action in tackling children's accidents.

The term *accident* means an unforeseen event or mishap (Collins English Dictionary, 1998). *Safety* is described by Collins English Dictionary (1998) as being free from danger or risk. Safety is about making it less likely than mishaps, such as accidents

occur. Health promotion in the area of accident prevention is thus about promoting the safety of children/young people. Accident prevention is especially important because nurses are helping to prevent serious injuries from occurring to children, injuries that might cause death or permanent disabilities. Nurses can help in a variety of different ways. Health promotion activities can be undertaken prior to an accident occurring; educating families on how to avoid accidents happening to their children. Health promotion advice can also be given following an accident, to prevent the same incident reoccurring to a child.

This chapter focuses on health promotion advice for the prevention of accidents. Health promotion activities and campaigns, along with an examination of some of the resources available, are explored. An example from practice is presented. Further information on accident prevention campaigns can be found in Chapters 1 and 40.

What can nurses do?

Nurses have a really important role to play in preventing accidents to children/young people. This section outlines how nurses can contribute through a variety of different activities at community and individual levels. Key activities are outlined in the list below:

Community
- Policy development through the joint working of primary care trusts and local authorities.
- The development of child accident prevention courses for parents/cares.
- The development of courses for children/young people in schools.
- Community nursery nurses promoting child safety during group activities with young children and their families.
- Poster displays in the practice setting, hospital and community.
- Organising community events during Child Safety Week, such as organising fun events for children, setting up promotional stalls and distributing leaflets.
- Supporting local campaigns that are working to make the local area safer for children/young people.

Individual
- Providing child safety advice when working with individual families, so they are able to make healthy choices, thus preventing child accidents.
- Children's nurses giving safety information sensitively following an accident experienced by a child/young person, in hospital and in the community.
- Health visitors continuing their important work in relation to child accident prevention, through home visiting and family support.
- Keeping up-to-date by reading about national policy developments, national campaigns and finding out about local issues. Attending relevant study days.

This list simply provides nurses with some ideas; it is by no means exhaustive. There are undoubtedly other activities that can be undertaken. At a national level too, nurses can become involved, particularly through national campaigns.

Promoting children's safety is not only about undertaking a variety of health promotion activities, nurses can achieve much by working collaboratively with others. Nurses working *collaboratively* with other agencies, such as local councils and charities to promote children's safety, can unquestionably make an important contribution. *Partnership* working with families is essen-

tial too. This is a particularly important for health visitors when working directly with families most at risk to accidents.

Nurses can help to bring about change for children. Breen (2004) maintains that we have a key role in *advocacy*: lobbying for change, helping to make the environment safer for children. Nurses can take part and support local campaigns such as those on road safety and campaigns on safe play areas for children.

Dr Mike Hayes of Child Accident Prevention Trust (CAPT) believes that nurses are also well placed to provide local leadership on the promotion of children's safety, which is sometimes lacking. Nurses see the consequences of accidents and are thus well placed to encourage others to become involved in prevention activities.

Accident prevention

Accident prevention campaigns are vital to the prevention of accidents to children, as they raise awareness on an ongoing basis through coordinated activities. Part of these coordinated activities will involve providing families and children with health promotion information.

This section looks at accident prevention in three different areas. Initially, ways to prevent young children from experiencing accidents within the *home* will be considered. This will be followed by looking at *road safety*. Finally, a much smaller campaign will feature, which tries to promote safety in our own *gardens*.

There are many different safety campaigns, which could have been selected. However, the home, roads and gardens have been selected because they are common places where children/young people experience accidents. They have also been identified by the Accidental Injury Task Force as priority areas for intervention (Department of Health, 2002).

Sources of information

When undertaking health promotion activities which focus on accident prevention, the search for information and resources is essential. There are a number of places where the nurse might begin. The local health promotion unit is a must, a wide range of resources can be found here. These resources might include posters, leaflets, and if you are really lucky, there could be a teaching package which covers the area you particularly want to explore. Finding a teaching package will save you a great deal of work, as generally they contain a variety of different activities that can be used within a teaching session.

Another really useful place to look for resources is on the internet. Here you can log onto a variety of different websites, including those organised by charities and the Government. Note the following:

- CAPT – http://www.capt.org.uk
- Road safety (Think! 2007a) – http://www. thinkroadsafety.gov.uk/
- Royal Society for the Prevention of Accidents (ROSPA, 2007) – http://www.rospa.com
- Fire safety – http://www.firekills.gov.uk/

The charities can provide all sorts of materials, such as leaflets, posters, along with packages for specific safety events. However, be aware that some items may cost, but others will be free.

The Government too provides some useful resources. Search through the Department for Trade and Industry and Department for Children, Schools and Families websites to see what you can find. Do not forget your local library either; you might be surprised with what you find there. All these can be initial starting points in your search for information and resources.

Nurses need to have knowledge about how and where accidents occur to children, as well as up-to-date advice about prevention.

Home safety campaigns

Young children commonly experience accidents in their homes. CAPT organises many home accident prevention campaigns, as well as providing a wide range of very useful resources to go with them. CAPT plays a key role in the campaign – *Child Safety Week*.

For young children home is the place where they spend much of their time, so it is no surprise therefore that home is the place where most accidents occur. Home is where young children test out their newly acquired skills. However, in their attempts to acquire new skills, they may not always be successful, sometimes resulting in accidents occurring. Young children are not aware of the dangers that might exist around them. Children depend on others meeting their safety needs, by being aware of what they are doing and making their environments safe.

The type of accidents that happen to young children around the home include the following:

- Falls.
- Burns and scalds.
- Suspected swallowing of harmful substances.
- Inhaling or swallowing a foreign body.
- Cuts (CAPT, 2004a).

There are a number of different ways parents/ carers can make their home safe. The following provides some useful examples.

Windows, particularly those upstairs, can be quite dangerous, especially if they do not have window locks fitted. If a child falls out of an open window she/he can be left with serious injuries.

CAPT (2004b) advises the fitting of window locks or safety catches, as the best way of preventing a child from falling out of a window. Parents/carers should be encouraged to fit safety locks, thus avoiding a serious injury happening to their child.

Safety gates are another valuable safety item. They can prevent young children going into areas of the home which may be risky to them. Safety gates are particularly helpful in stopping young children falling down the stairs. CAPT (2004b) recommends placing safety gates both at the bottom as well as the top of stairs. Safety gates can be easily obtained from local children's stores or hardware shops. If parents/carers are not able to afford such items, there are often schemes available in local areas which will provide safety gates on loan.

Burns and scalds can occur to young children when at home. In severe cases such injuries can leave children with permanent disabilities. A young child's skin is thinner and more susceptible to heat than an adult's skin. Scalds contribute to 70% of thermal injuries to children, the most common being caused by hot drinks (CAPT, 2007a). Parents/carers, and anyone who interacts with young children, should always take care or even better still avoid having hot drinks in close proximity to young children.

Children can also experience burns from hot irons, open fires and cookers (CAPT, 2007a). Children should be kept away from these items. Fires and heaters, for example, should always be fitted with fireguards. It can be both surprising and concerning how frequently, as a nurse working in the community, one finds young children living in homes where fires and heaters are exposed. The dangers that these hazards present should always be highlighted.

Housefires are another concern. Children are badly injured and sometimes die through house fires. Homes should, of course, be fitted with *smoke alarms* to alert families to the danger of a fire breaking out in their home. Buying and fitting a fire alarm can be a life-saving purchase. Having a family escape plan can ensure that when the alarm does go off everyone knows what to do. Smoke alarms are especially important for children's safety and that of the whole family.

The above provides some key information on safety around the home – advice that nurses can provide to families, as well as some of the items that families may need to purchase to make the home safer for their young children.

To assist in promoting messages of home safety, use fact-sheets, leaflets and posters, which will highlight key points and reiterate ideas you want to put across. Repetition helps families remember key points, but take care not to overload them with information.

Importantly, as children become older, parents/carers can discuss with them about keeping safe around the home. When working with children on home safety yourself, try to make any activities both fun and interesting. One way to do this might be with the internet. Internet games, for example, can be useful. In relation to fire safety, access the Getfirewise website for children. It provides interactive games about staying safe at home and away from fire (Getfirewise, 2007; http://www.getfirewise.gov.uk).

Road safety

There are a number of factors that are known to reduce the severity of road traffic injuries. These include the following:

- Reduced driver speed.
- Traffic-calming systems.
- Children in car safety seats.
- Education on road safety.
- Cycle safety.

Each of these is discussed in turn.

Reduced driver speed

The faster a driver goes, the chances of a child surviving if hit by the car are lower. At 40 mph there is only a one in five chance that the child will survive. However, if the car is going at 30 mph then there is four in five chance that the child will survive (CAPT, 2007b). Drivers need to take more notice of the speed limits imposed on roads. Campaigns frequently advise about reducing driver speed, particularly at Christmas time.

Traffic-calming systems

Traffic-calming systems are designed to slow traffic down. They can be found in busy areas or spots which are known to be accident black spots. Traffic-calming systems are introduced to help make the environment safer for pedestrians and road users.

Local transport policies can help to make roads safer (Towner et al., 1996). Transport policies determine the provision of school crossing patrols and initiate changes to traffic behaviour, such as the introduction of speed restriction bumps and restricted access, for example. The evaluation of such schemes has demonstrated that they are effective in helping to reduce injuries (Towner et al., 1996). If drivers have to slow down or they are not able to access certain roads where children might be playing, this can certainly help to make the environment safer for children.

Children in car safety seats

In 2006, new laws were introduced about the wearing of child safety belts. All children should be carried in a child restraint appropriate for their size (CAPT, 2007b). This law relates to children under 12 years of age, but only if they are less than 135 cm tall (CAPT, 2007b). Above 135 cm in height, like adults, they are required to wear a seat belt.

More information on this can be found by accessing the Department for Transport website – http://www.thinkroadsafety.gov.uk/campaigns/childcarseats/childcarseats.htm. Alternatively, contact the road safety officer at your local council. When advising about car seat safety, nurses need to have a good knowledge base. Training may be of benefit in this area.

It is important that children are safe when travelling in cars. If accidents occur, the injuries are going to be less if children are wearing age-appropriate restraints.

Education on road safety

How can important messages on road safety, both for pedestrians and road users, be put across? The charities, along with the Government, through the Department for Transport have found some interesting ways. The following highlights some of what is currently available.

ROSPA is able to provide information on road safety and safety in children's playgrounds. ROSPA can be accessed via http://www.rospa.com.

ROSPA helps to support the *Stop, Look and Listen* campaign, associated with the Green Cross Code (see also http://www.thinkroadsafety.gov.uk/arrivealive/greencross.htm). You may be familiar with the hedgehog, the symbol of this campaign. The hedgehog is a cartoon character, which children find very appealing (http://www.thinkroadsafety.gov.uk/campaigns/hedgehogs/hedgehogs.htm). Access the online learning resource, where children can help the hedgehog find a safe place to cross the road (Department for Transport, 2005). The resource encourages children to think about their safety as pedestrians. Children think it is great fun.

This ROSPA resource is aimed at children of 5–10 years (Department for Transport, 2005). It might be something you would consider using when working with children, especially if you have a computer available with internet access. It can be easily downloaded during a teaching session (or before). Take points made in the resource even further through questions and discussions with children.

Another interesting way to promote pedestrian and road safety is through drama in education. The *Streetwise Road Safety Show* may be able to help. It features characters Johnnie Streetwise, the quiz host, and the not very streetwise Joe Public, the contestant. It explains six main points of the Green Cross Code. The drama is aimed at key stage 1 and 2 children (5–11 years), and can be accessed via http://www.streetwiseshow.co.uk (Larger than Life and Flash Productions, 2006).

A further example is Jugglestruck, a road safety magic show. It focuses on general road safety, the Green Cross Code, and finding a safe place to cross the road. It also features magic, puppets and juggling (Jugglestruck, 2007; http://www.jugglestruck.co.uk). Literature such as workbooks and storybooks are also available to accompany the show.

A different type of drama aimed at 16- to 17-year-olds is *Too Much Punch for Judy*. This examines a series of life events that lead to a serious road accident for a young girl. The drama looks at drink drive law, alcohol education and issues of shared responsibility (Ape Theatre Company, 2007; http://www.apetheatrecompany.co.uk).

An important resource for children is the booklet – *Arrive Alive* – a highway code for young road users (Department for Transport, 2006). This is a really useful resource providing information on walking, the Green Cross Code, rollerblading, cycling, riding in cars, travelling on buses and animals on the road. It also includes some basic road signs and traffic signals. At the end it provides children with quizzes, which might be useful for assessing their learning.

The Road Safety Unit at your local council can provide further details about different resources on road safety.

Cycle safety

Children/young people love experimenting with their bikes, not only in their own gardens but on the highways too. Safety needs to be encouraged.

A properly fitted cycle helmet is a must, as it can greatly reduce the risk of head injuries (CAPT, 2004c) (Figure 10.1). CAPT maintains that over 50% of cycle injuries involve a head injury, which clearly demonstrates the need for cycle helmets to be worn. CAPT suggests that if families link up with their local cycling shop, they can check if a child's/young person's helmet fits correctly.

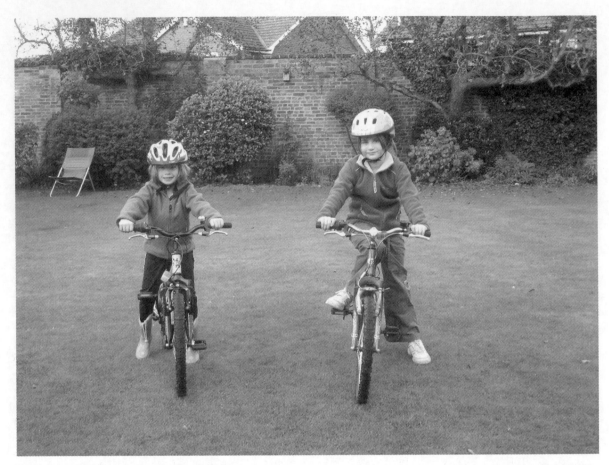

Figure 10.1 Children wearing fitted cycle helmets.

A website that might be useful for young people to access on cycle safety is http://www.cyclesense.net (Think! 2007b). The website provides information for 11- to 16-year-olds on staying safe on the road.

There are many different campaigns and resources that can be used for promoting safety on the roads for both road users and pedestrians. Carefully look around and see what fits your needs most effectively. Think carefully before choosing your resources. If aimed at children or young people, ask yourself if they will find it appealing.

Garden safety campaigns

Accidents can occur in the garden too. It is important to provide heath promotion information on garden safety so children can avoid illness and injury.

How Safe Is Your Child in the Garden? This is a really informative leaflet produced by the CAPT (2007c). The leaflet provides some good tips about making gardens safer places for children. Some general advice included in the leaflet is outlined as follows:

- Garden ponds should be filled in to reduce the risk of children drowning.
- All chemicals such as weed killers should be locked away.
- Dog and cat mess needs to be cleared away to reduce the risk of illness.
- Children need to be kept away from barbeques and bonfires, to avoid burns (CAPT, 2007c).

All the above are essential tips for children's safety in the garden.

Thought-provoking information contained within the leaflet concerns the danger of some plants. Children should avoid putting plants in their mouths. The need for supervision in the garden for young children is emphasised. As children get older, it is important to point out to them which plants may be harmful (CAPT, 2007c). In addition, the leaflet goes on to discuss the dangers of berries and also lists plants that are harmful, providing parents/carers with a really useful list to keep at hand.

Young children can so easily be attracted to the bright colours of berries, as they may remind them of sweets. Keep young children well away from berries.

The leaflet goes on to provide important advice for parents/carers on what they should do if they think their child has eaten a poisonous plant. The leaflet provides the following advice:

- Remove any remaining parts of the plant to prevent any further risks.
- Contact emergency health services for advice – accident and emergency (A + E) or general practitioner.
- Keep a sample of the plant to take to A + E or general practitioner.
- Do *not* try to make the child vomit.

NHS Direct can be quite helpful too with information related to poisonous substances.

Another interesting resource CAPT produces on garden safety is a garden quiz. The quiz is a fun and interesting way to learn information about garden safety. The garden quiz has been developed for use with parents/carers, but perhaps it could be used with older children. Ten multi-choice questions about hazards in the garden are presented.

Details of all the information on garden safety can be found by accessing the CAPT website.

This section has provided some insights into the risk of accidents occurring in the home, on the roads and in gardens. Ways to reduce the risk of accidents occurring have been discussed through the use of safety campaigns and providing families with health promotion advice.

Children's accident prevention session for parents/carers

The NSF for children/young people talks about supporting parents/cares (Education and Skills, Department of Health, 2004). Providing parents/carers with information on accident prevention is one way of supporting them to care for their children. An example from practice is presented in this section.

Outlined below is an accident prevention session recently put together for a group of first-time mothers. They had young children (under 5 years) and wanted some basic home safety advice.

Once literature had been gathered and resources selected for the session, the focus was the group itself. The starting point was helping the mothers feel relaxed with one another, so they would feel comfortable learning together. Often the group size can have an influence on this. Rogers (1993) states that small adult learning groups of about 10–25 individuals works well together. Generally, I find that groups slightly smaller than this are better, say 8–15 adults. It can be a little daunting for some people to work in a group as large as 25, resulting in low levels of group participation. Smaller groups may be more appropriate for community work, particularly where participants are not familiar with working in groups, or may be less confident in such situations.

Rogers (1993) points out the benefits of an adult learning group. The group can provide a rich source of information for each other, as well as being a good source of support.

Adults working together as a group can help to broaden each others' knowledge; all have different experiences to share. However, it is important to be aware that occasionally some individuals can be more forceful than others in sharing their ideas. The nurse, as the facilitator of such a session, needs to be sensitive to this and take action to avoid such difficulties arising. This can be achieved by drawing others in, for example, and exploring the points they raise, thus shifting the focus.

The group for the accident prevention session consisted of ten mothers. This felt quite a comfortable size for many of them to get to know each other and share their ideas. A few *ice-breaking* activities were undertaken initially to help facilitate the group getting to know each other. One activity included splitting the group into pairs and asking them to introduce their partner to the rest of the group.

It was important to find out what the group wanted to know and present it to them in a way that they would find appealing. Fortunately, I was able to meet with them individually prior to the session. In practice this is not always possible. Alternatively, a quick phone call might help, enquiring what each individual wishes to know. Then as facilitator you can be confident your health promotion session is based on the needs of your group.

Teaching plan

Below is the teaching plan for this session (Box 10.1).

Box 10.1 Accident prevention session for parents/carers of young children – teaching plan.

Group: Ten mothers with children under 5 years.

Aim

To help mothers advance their knowledge on how to prevent accidents, so they can keep their young children safe at home.

Objectives/outcomes

At the end of the course the mothers will be able to do the following:

- Discuss the potential for accidents within their own homes.
- Discuss how young children's accidents can be prevented.
- Identify local safety schemes.

Content and methods

- Introduction and ice breakers (activities).
- Group members discuss their own experiences of accidents within the home (discussion).
- Questionnaire from CAPT about children's accidents within the home (individual or pairs activity).
- Why young children are more vulnerable to accidents (discussion)?
- Consider your own home environment – where might the potential lie for accidents to occur? (Pairs activity and discussion.)
- Different ways children's accidents might be prevented within the home (Powerpoint presentation).
- Details about local safety schemes (talk).
- Questionnaire from CAPT about accidents within the home, repeated (individual or pairs activity).
- Summary.

Resources

- The groups' knowledge and experiences.
- CAPT questionnaire.
- Information on child development.
- Information about accident risks and how to prevent them (handouts).
- Information about local safety schemes (leaflet).
- Activity sheets.
- Safety information posters.
- Relevant books and leaflets on display.

Assessment of group learning

Mothers' responses to the CAPT questionnaire – the first and second time responses are compared.

Evaluation

Mothers complete an evaluation questionnaire which explores their thoughts on the session.

Reflection on the session

It is important for nurses to reflect on their health promotion sessions so that these can be improved upon. Some reflection points are noted below.

Discussing home accidents experienced might be a little daunting for some participants. If the nurse as the facilitator provides the first example then participants may feel a little less apprehensive about sharing their experiences. By going first it also shows that you as the facilitator are as vulnerable as anyone else to accidents occurring. This strategy seemed to work well as mothers were happy to share their experiences.

A quiz from CAPT was used on two occasions. This provided the opportunity to find out if the mother's knowledge and understanding had increased as a result of the session. The quiz was used at the beginning and then again at the end of the session. It demonstrated that their knowledge had indeed improved. Mothers enjoyed the activity and were also able to witness an improvement in their knowledge.

Some of the session content was delivered by Powerpoint presentation, particularly on different ways child accidents might be prevented within the home. An alternative approach could have been to use a more interactive method. Since this session I have devised room cards, where participants can work together discussing how rooms can be made safer for young children. If each pair discusses one room, by the end of the session the whole house has been covered room by room. Each pair has then provided different perspectives on preventing accidents within the home.

As well as reflection, it is useful to evaluate your health promotion sessions. A questionnaire was devised for use with participants. They were asked to make a few comments about the session as follows:

- Did the session meet their needs?
- Was the session presented appropriately?
- Should anything else have been included?

The last question can be quite useful as it can provide ideas for future work.

Presenting sessions on children's accident prevention can be a useful way to support families, so they can learn how to make their homes safer for young children. Reflection on such sessions takes practice forward, helping the nurse to more effectively meet the needs of families.

Health promotion activities for children/young people

When working with children/young people, age-appropriate resources are essential. This section examines some health promotion activity sheets on accident prevention. Activity sheets can help to make health promotion more interesting; they can help to bring a sense of reality to health promotion teaching. The charitable trusts produce a variety of activity sheets. CAPT particularly produces a wide range of these resources.

Activity sheets can be used individually with children/young people or in group situations. Another way to use them is at a community event. Children/young people can complete them at your stand, and then points raised can be used as a basis for discussion. Alternatively, you might want to include them in an accident prevention goody bag, along with other health promotion literature and freebies.

For children between the ages of 5 and 7 years, CAPT produces a variety of colouring activities. Children can colour traffic situations, for example, which depict the safest place to cross the road (CAPT, 2004d). The activity sheets also include related questions, helping to increase children's knowledge.

For children aged 7–11 years, CAPT provides safety scrambles. A series of clues are presented. For each clue a scrambled word is highlighted. Children have to unscramble the word to find the answer. For example – *this gives you time to escape if there's a fire in your home ... mealormask* (CAPT, 2005a).

The answer to the above word scramble is *smoke alarm*, but I am sure you have already worked this out.

For young people (11+ years) CAPT has produced a series of worksheets. The worksheets are designed to help increase young people's understanding about preventing accidents and promoting safety. One worksheet, for example, asks young people to consider information about a serious accident (CAPT, 2005b). They need to think about what might have caused the accident and how it could have been prevented.

Young people enjoy texting each other. Interestingly, CAPT produces an activity sheet which allows young people to actively engage in the process of designing an important safety text message. The text has to appeal to other young people so that they will actually read the message (CAPT, 2004e).

The activity sheets can be downloaded from http://www.capt.org.uk. They can also be photocopied, as long as all the correct logos are presented.

Nurses may find some of these resources useful when putting together health promotion activities for children/young people.

Conclusion

This chapter on accident prevention has examined a variety of ways safety can be promoted. Promoting safety involves working at a number of different levels; this might include individually, at a community level and in some cases nationally. Nurses can do much on all these levels to promote the safety of children/young people. Safety advice and campaigns in specific areas have been focused upon – homes, roads and gardens. There are lots of resources available to help nurses when promoting safety messages. The aim of all this work is to prevent injuries from occurring which might have long-term consequences on children's/young people's health. Think about what you might be able to achieve in your area and how you can get others involved.

References

Ape Theatre Company. (2007) *Too Much Punch for Judy*. Available at: http://www.apetheatrecompany.co.uk (accessed 3 May 2007).

Audit Commission and Healthcare Commission (2007) *Better Safe than Sorry: Preventing Unintentional Injury to Children*. London: Audit Commission.

Breen, J. (2004) Road safety advocacy. *British Medical Journal* 328: 888–890.

CAPT (2004a) *Home Accident Fact Sheet*. London: Child Accident Prevention Trust.

CAPT (2004b) *Safety Quiz*. London: Child Accident Prevention Trust.

CAPT (2004c) *Cycle Helmet Checks*. London: Child Accident Prevention Trust.

CAPT (2004d) *Activity Sheet – Check it Out, Activity for Children 5–7 Years*. London: Child Accident Prevention Trust.

CAPT (2004e) *Activity Sheet – Chancing it, Activity for 11 Plus*. London: Child Accident Prevention Trust.

CAPT (2005a) Safety scramble activity sheet. *Activity for Children Aged 7 to 11*. London: Child Accident Prevention Trust.

CAPT (2005b) Imagine. *Activity Sheet for Young People Aged 11 to 14 Years*. London: Child Accident Prevention Trust.

CAPT (2007a) *Burns and scalds*. London: Child Accident Prevention Trust.

CAPT (2007b) *Child Car Restraints – Fact Sheet*. London: Child Accident Prevention Trust.

CAPT (2007c) *How Safe Is Your Child in the Garden?* London: Child Accident Prevention Trust.

Collins English Dictionary (1998) Glasgow: Harper Collins.

Department of Health (2002) *Preventing Accidental Injury – Priorities for Action. Report to the Chief Medical Officer from the Accident Injury Task Force*. London: The Stationery Office.

Department for Transport (2005) *Hedgehogs – Stop, Look, Listen, Live*. London: Department for Transport. Available at: http://www.hedgehogs.gov.uk (accessed 12 February 2007).

Department for Transport (2006) *Arrive Alive*. London: Department for Transport.

Education and Skills (Department of), Department of Health (2004) *National Service Framework for Children, Young People and Maternity Services*. London: Crown copyright.

Getfirewise (2007) Available at: http://www.getfirewise.gov.uk (accessed 12 February 2007).

Jugglestruck. (2007) *The Road Safety Magic Show*. Available at: http://www.jugglestruck.co.uk (accessed 3 May 2007).

Larger than Life and Flash Productions (2006) *The Streetwise Road Safety Show*. Available at: http://www.streetwiseshow.co.uk (accessed 5 June 2006).

Rogers, A. (1993) *Teaching Adults*. Milton, Keynes: Open University Press.

Royal Society for the Prevention of Accidents. (2007) Available at: http://www.rospa.com (accessed 12 February 2007).

Think! (2007a) Available at: http://www.thinkroadsafety. gov.uk/ (accessed 12 February 2007).

Think! (2007b) *Cycle Sense*. Available at: http://www. cyclesense.net (accessed 12 February 2007).

Towner, E., Dowswell, T., Simpson, G., Jarvis, S. (1996). *Health Promotion in Childhood and Young Adolescence for the Prevention of Unintentional Injuries*. London: Health Education Authority.

Theme 4

Promoting Health in Minor Illness and Minor Injury

Chapter 11 Sure Start Community Children's Nursing Service – Developing a Minor Illness/
Injury Service

Chapter 12 Fever Management in Young Children (0–5 Years)

Chapter 13 Health Promotion in Young Children's Minor Illnesses

Chapter 14 Health Promotion in Minor Injuries

11 Sure Start Community Children's Nursing Service – Developing a Minor Illness/Injury Service

Karen Moyse and Zo'e Ellis

NSF

National Service Framework (NSF), standard 6 – children/young people who are ill (Education and Skills, Department of Health, 2004, pp. 4–5):

Standard

Children who are ill should receive *timely, high-quality* and *effective care*, as close to home as possible.

Marker of good practice

Parents and children should receive *information*, advice and *support* to enable them to manage minor illnesses themselves and access appropriate services when necessary.

Introduction

Parents and carers become concerned when their young children are ill (Kai, 1996). Sometimes children's illnesses are minor and can be managed at home. Much of the time parents and carers have the knowledge and skills necessary to deal with their young children's minor illnesses (Education and Skills, Department of Health, 2004). However, sometimes they may not and need to seek further advice from health practitioners.

This chapter looks at a new service that was designed to support families in caring for their young children at home, when unwell with a minor illness or minor injury. The service provides nursing care and health promotion advice. The chapter discusses how the service was developed.

Terms used frequently in this chapter include *acutely ill child* and *community children's nurse*. The acutely ill child has been defined as: *the parent who seeks help for their child on an urgent or immediate basis* (Department of Health, 2003a, p. 2).

A community children's nurse has been defined as: *a qualified nurse who provides hands on care and training in the home, and also training to carers, to become confident and competent in the care of their child in acute and chronic illness* (House of Commons Health Committee, 1997, p. xiv).

Concerns about managing children's minor illnesses

Coping with sick children

Evidence demonstrates that parents will seek help if they feel they need it when their young children are acutely ill, but can still remain concerned (Kai, 1996). Neill (2000) maintains that parents feel they are not able to spend enough time with health practitioners when their children are acutely ill.

Additional time spent with a health practitioner, when families need it, may prove to be an effective strategy in caring for acutely ill children in the community. It could ease parental concerns, as well as perhaps providing improved health outcomes for children.

Services for children need to provide good quality health care and information, appropriate to the needs of acutely ill children, as well as being easily accessible (Education and Skills, Department of Health, 2004). Parents may then feel more empowered in their child's care, with more information and support at their fingertips. Children's nurses can play an important part in making this happen, particularly for young children, as this chapter demonstrates.

Fiona Smith, Paediatric adviser to the Royal College of Nursing, highlights the value of children's nurses. Fiona maintains that they have high-quality skills in caring for children (Ganguli, 2003). Children's nurses, particularly community children's nurses (CCNs), can support families in the care of their sick children, helping them to be cared for at home.

How children's nurses could help

Parents' *knowledge and skills* are essential in the recognition and management of children's illnesses and injuries. Parents are effective at recognising when their children are ill (Kai, 1996). Interestingly, the NSF highlights that over 80% of illnesses in childhood are managed by parents without reference to any health care systems (Education and Skills, Department of Health, 2004). So it would seem that parents manage themselves most of the time when their children are acutely ill. However, when they do seek help for their children, there seems to be a need for greater levels of support (Neill, 2000) and more information (Kai, 1996).

The children's NSF suggests improving local access for acutely ill children and recommends that children's nurses could do this (Education and Skill, Department of Health, 2004). The document suggests that children's nurses based within a GP practice would be ideal. However, children's nurses could equally work from a Sure Start centre or children's centre, providing care in the community. Children's nurses would be able to spend more time

with the family when a child is sick, than potentially other health practitioners do currently. Children's nurses would be able to spend more time because the service they provide would be a dedicated service, meeting the needs of acutely ill children unwell with minor illnesses and minor injuries.

Emerging findings (Department of Health, 2003b) highlights an example of a mother who needs to attend the GP surgery with her young child who is sick. The mother has another young child, who she has to take with her to the surgery. Accessing the GP in these circumstances can be difficult and can be even more difficult, the document maintains, if the family live in a rural area due to transport difficulties.

However, some of these difficulties could be avoided with the provision of a home nursing service, delivered by a children's nurse. There may not even be a need for the child to attend the surgery at all. The children's nurse could carefully assess the child and help the mother in the provision of care and provide advice. Obviously, if following careful assessment by the nurse, the illness turns out not to be minor, the nurse would refer on appropriately to the GP or hospital services.

Community children's nursing services

There has only been a growth in CCN services since the 1980s (Whiting, 1988; Tatman and Woodroffe, 1993). Traditionally, CCNs have cared for chronically ill children (House of Commons Health Committee, 1997) and more recently *hospital at home* services have developed in some parts of the country. Few CCN services currently exist which provide purely a minor illness and minor injury focus. Although, some established CCN teams are extending their scope of practice to include minor illness and injury care for children. CCN services visiting in the home could be one way forward for the management of acute minor childhood illnesses.

Developing a minor illness/injury service for young children

Sure Start community children's nursing: a new service for sick children

Within a small rural area within Derbyshire, a CCN service has been established which helps families in the care of their acutely ill children. It is a home-visiting service that specialises in the care of young children (0–4 years), who are unwell with minor illnesses and minor injuries.

Moyse (2005) found that parents and carers who accessed this CCN service felt it helped to improve their knowledge and skills about children's minor illness and injury management. Parents and carers felt they had ready support available when their young children were ill, through provision of this service. Although, they did point out that extending the hours of the service would be of great value in making the service more accessible (Moyse, 2005).

Needs

Before the CCN service was established, the health needs of the local community were carefully assessed. The community was a deprived one, which was looking to improve children's health. The community was situated in a Sure Start area.

Deprivation and health

Deprived areas generally suffer poorer health. The association between poor health and deprivation is well documented (Townsend et al., 1988). The Acheson (1998) inquiry has further explored this issue. Acheson (1998) points out that childhood is critical, where poor socio-economic circumstances have lasting effects. Acheson (1998) recommended that if health inequalities were to be reduced, a wide range of policies needed to be implemented to achieve an improvement in health. This would be an issue for several Government departments.

The aim of the Acheson (1998) inquiry was to identify priority areas for the future Government policy – interventions that would help to reduce some of the inequalities in health that existed, including those relevant to children. By the late 1990s policies were introduced to support families. In the document *Supporting Families*, the Government provided details of its commitment to supporting families: advice for parents about their children's health and advice on parenting (Home Office, 1998). Sure Start emerged as an initiative to help children in the early years of life and to support their parents (Home Office, 1998). Sure Start has subsequently

> **Box 11.1** Objective 2.
>
> Supporting parents in caring for their children to promote healthy development.
> Reduce the number of children (0–4 years) admitted to hospital as an emergency, with gastroenteritis, respiratory infection or injury.

been an enormous development nationally. It has been a catalyst for change both in terms of health and education for young children.

Sure Start target

The aim of Sure Start was to work with families and their young children to promote child development, particularly for those children who were disadvantaged. The aim was to try to break the cycle of disadvantage for the current generation (Sure Start, 2003/4).

Sure Start had several objectives. Objective 2 (Box 11.1) was about improving the health of young children in the local community. Objective 2 related directly to preventing young children from being admitted to hospital due to acute illness, particularly gastroenteritis, respiratory illness and injury.

All Sure Starts had to meet the same objectives that were set by the Sure Start unit in London. Services were developed and implemented by local Sure Starts based on the needs of their local communities, in line with national Sure Start objectives.

Within the Sure Start area in Derbyshire objective 2, focusing on reducing hospital admissions for young children, was felt to be really important and needed careful consideration. It provided the opportunity to help improve health outcomes for local children.

A research-based needs assessment proved invaluable. The health needs of young children in the local area, current health services available for them and options for development, were carefully explored over a 6-month period by Walmsley (2003). Following Walmsley's (2003) research the local Sure Start and primary care trust (PCT) decided to address objective 2 with its own dedicated service – a

CCN service specialising in the care of acutely ill young children (0–4 years).

There were a number of health needs that existed in the local community, that were of particular concern:

- Disadvantage community – high rates of poverty were significant in this Sure Start community. Alongside this there were high rates of morbidity across the spectrum of age groups (North Eastern Derbyshire Primary Care Trust, 2003).
- Access – families living in the more rural parts of the community experienced problems accessing health services due to transportation difficulties. Many families within the area did not have their own transport; thus, accessing health services was not easy. As the Acheson (1998) inquiry points out, a lack of access to transport is likely to decrease opportunities for access to facilities and services.
- Accessing health services *out of hours* – local families, once again living in the more rural parts of the Sure Start area, expressed concern about accessing out-of-hours health services particularly at night (Moyse, 2005). They would sometimes attend accident and emergency (A + E) as this was more easily accessible.

There is an association between deprived areas and A + E use; deprived areas have higher rates of A + E attendance (Beattie et al., 2001). A + E is perceived as convenient and better; it is not subject to the same as barriers as other health care services, and some families believe they will receive better care (Sanders, 2000). There are problems associated with A + E, however. It may not be the best place for a child at night, who is unwell with a minor illness, to receive care. There is also the potential risk of exposure to other infections.

- Some parents and carers in the area highlighted a lack of knowledge and skills in the management of young children's minor illnesses and injuries, and wanted more information. Parents' and carers' knowledge and skills are key determinants in the management of minor illnesses and injuries (Education and Skills, Department of Health, 2004).

Parents/carers and practitioners felt that having a dedicated CCN service to help families could improve the quality of health care for young children in the local community. Having more information available would help to *empower* families and give them more confidence. It was important too that the new service should be easily *accessible* for them.

As previously stated the NSF (Education and Skills, Department of Health, 2004) recommends developing a change in services for acutely ill children. Sure Start in this community developed a new service for acutely ill children. Importantly, as part of this process, they considered the key issues for families with young children. Particularly significant were the health needs of the local population, as well as local geography and transport links. Parents/carers were also invited to become involved in decision-making about the new service.

The new service

A project team was created, consisting of both local practitioners and local parents and carers. The purpose of the project team was to meet on a regular basis and discuss plans for the new nursing service.

The Sure Start CCN service, as it became known, began work in November 2003, 6 months after the presentation of Walmsley's (2003) research. Funding was initially allocated for 18 months. The service operated initially Monday to Friday 9 am until 5 pm.

Aims of the service

The Sure Start CCN service needed to have clear aims from the outset. Sure Start wanted the local communities to know exactly how the service could help them when their young children were ill. The project team had to consider local health practitioners' understanding of the service too, as they were going to play a key role in recommending the service to families. Box 11.2. highlights the aims of the Sure Start CCN service.

Box 11.2 Aims of the Sure Start CCN service.

Aims of the Sure Start CCN service for young children are as follows:

- Improving parents/carers' knowledge and skills in caring for their young children when unwell with minor illnesses/minor injuries.
- Preventing children's admissions to hospital with minor illnesses.
- Reducing children's attendances at A + E departments with minor illnesses/minor injuries.
- Referring children to GP and hospital services, where appropriate, to avoid deterioration in children's health.

Box 11.3 Family-centred and child-centred care.

Family-centred

- Providing families with the opportunity to refer directly to the service.
- Appreciating families' knowledge and understanding about their child.
- Discussing with families when they felt it would be appropriate to discharge their child from the service.
- Providing families with health promotion information related to their child's care.

Child-centred

- Child-centred communications.
- Stickers, as rewards for children.
- Plasters, featuring cartoon characters.

Principles

A *family-centred* service that would meet the needs of acutely ill children and their families, providing *support* and *care*, as well as *information*, was needed. The principles of the service were developed with these concepts in mind.

To be a supportive service for parents/carers communication was going to be fundamental. The *communication* style of the service was given considerable thought, as this was felt to be really important for families in their use and relationship with the service.

Based on practice experience in the local area and research, the project team certainly felt that there was a real need for the new service to be *approachable*. The team wanted families to feel that they could approach the service about their concerns, and feel able to ask questions. Some families had pointed out to Sure Start that when using some services they had felt uncomfortable about asking questions related to their child's care. This corresponds with evidence found by Kai (1996).

It was important that families could feel that the CCN service had an empathetic understanding of their situation. Usherwood (1999) maintains empathy is needed by patients and their relatives. The project team wanted families to feel comfortable in sharing their experiences with nurses.

Fundamentally, the service needed to be competent in *nursing sick children*. The service was going to be staffed by qualified children's nurses, experi-

enced in the care of sick children both in hospital and at home.

It was essential that as the service was for children, that naturally it should be *child friendly*, young children's needs at the forefront of care. In achieving this principle of child friendliness in its care, the service needed to use child-centred methodologies, as advocated by the NSF (Education and Skills, Department of Health, 2004).

The service needed to promote the care of sick children by advancing parents'/carers' *knowledge and skills* in the management of young children's minor illness and minor injuries. The Sure Start CCN service would provide parents/carers with *health promotion information* about the care of their sick child. As research by Kai (1996) and Neill (2000) highlight, parents/carers want more information about their child's health problems and care.

Box 11.3 demonstrates how some of these principles were applied to the service.

Objectives

Objectives were set for the Sure Start CCN service, as Box 11.4 illustrates. The objectives provided specific details on exactly what the service should achieve.

Box 11.4 Sure Start CCN service objectives.

The service will:

- care for sick children;
- support parents/carers in the care of their acutely ill children;
- develop health promotion resources for parents/cares;
- develop and establish systems of communication between primary and secondary care;
- monitor the activities of the service;
- evaluate the service using research methodologies;
- explore the potential for future developments to the service.

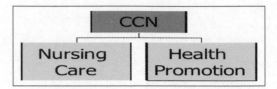

Figure 11.1   Sure Start community children's nursing model.

Action plan

An action plan was thus devised as follows:

(1) The need to design a model of care to help guide the service in its development, with its focus on support, care and information for families with young children.
(2) Marketing the service to the local community and local practitioners (hospital and community), so that families and practitioners were aware of its existence.
(3) Developing CCN policies and guidance information to ensure safe practice and good quality care for young children locally, as recommended by NSF (Education and Skills, Department of Health, 2004).
(4) The development of CCN nursing records, to help ensure safe practice. This is an essential requirement of nursing practice (Nursing and Midwifery Council, NMC, 2004).
(5) The development of health promotion resources; written information to support the verbal information given to families.
(6) To set up data monitoring systems that would enable Sure Start to have an understanding of the exact nature of referrals made to the service.
(7) The Sure Start CCNs to access appropriate training to assist in the development of the service.
(8) To set up audit/research systems to measure parents' and health practitioners' views about

the service. Toalso explore areas for future development of the service.
(9) To implement the service for young children and their families in the Sure Start area.

Elements of the action plan

A model of care was developed centred on the need for *nursing care* so children could stay in their own home when unwell. Importantly too, the model needed to include *health promotion advice* to assist parents and carers when nursing their sick children at home (Figure 11.1).

To help with marketing the service, so that the local community knew the service was in existence, materials were developed to distribute in the local community. Local community groups were visited by the Sure Start CCNs, as well as discussing the service with local health practitioners such as GPs, health visitors and community nurses. Sessions were also held at local hospitals, on the wards and in A + E departments, informing practitioners about the service. On two occasions the CCNs, along with a Sure Start parent advisor, set up a stall in the local market publicizing the service. These activities were undertaken during the early months of the project and continued periodically, just to remind families about the service.

Nursing policies for the service were developed on – *referrals, managing pyrexia (fever), respiratory infection, gastroenteritis* and *accidents in young children*, in line with the Sure Start target (2003/4).

Nursing records were developed according to standards identified by the NMC (2004). Along with Sure Start CCN policies, the nursing records were presented to the PCT clinical governance group and were approved for use.

Health promotion leaflets were devised on the management of pyrexia (fever), respiratory infections, and gastroenteritis in young children for use by parents/carers. The development of these resources was based on evidenced-based literature and discussions within the project team.

Data monitoring systems were devised and put in place for the launch of the service. These monitoring systems detailed referrals made to the service and any referrals made by CCNs to hospital services.

Access to training was important for the Sure Start CCNs. Sure Start CCNs undertook the Extended Nurse Prescribing course, so that could prescribe appropriate medications for young children when unwell. First aid courses were also undertaken, as well as study days on the management of children's eczema and asthma.

For audit/research purposes questionnaire surveys were designed and used to evaluate aspects of the service.

Home visiting for sick children

It was decided by the project team that the service would not only care for young children (0–4 years) with the illnesses identified in the Sure Start (2003/4) objective, but the service would care for young children with any minor illness or minor injury.

Referrals were received by Sure Start and forwarded on to CCNs out in the community. CCNs would assess children, provide care and health promotion advice, or refer children on to other health services, if appropriate. CCNs would visit families several times a day if necessary to provide care and advice. Visits would cease once the family felt their child was well again, or they felt confident to care without support.

Importantly for acutely ill children, CCNs were able to provide repeated observation, assessment and care. A few hours observation is an important tool in managing illness, either in hospital or primary care as the children's NSF has highlighted (Department of Health, 2003a).

CCNs were able to identify if a child's health was deteriorating and thus could refer on. If a parent/carer was really worried or the CCN herself was uncertain about the child's condition, a referral on to the child's GP or local hospital would be made.

The Department of Health (2003a) has highlighted that parents/carers have less confidence in their own judgement when their child is seri-

ously ill. Research, however, has in fact shown that parental assessment of illness and the need for hospital attendance correlates well with that of doctors (MacFarl et al., 1994). Parents/carers should always be listened to, so that an acutely ill child can be directed to the most appropriate service. The Sure Start CCNs could refer on or encourage parents/carers to do so themselves. Having the CCN service available gave parents/carers the confidence to refer on, which sometimes they do not always have themselves.

Parents' perspective

The following outlines a parent's perspective on the Sure Start CCN service. It has been written by Zo'e, who has accessed the service several times, and has worked with the service as part of the project team.

At the launch of the new service within our village, as normal, some barriers did come up from parents, but explanations were given regarding the service. The role of the CCN in the first instance was promotion of children's health, and this was gratefully received by all Sure Start parents. Our GP practice at the time was small. One problem that parents were having in our village at the time was the lack of appointments available when their children were ill. As any parent will know a child can become very ill very quickly.

When the CCN service was in its embryo stage, I felt honoured to be part of such a pioneering service, as a member of the project team. It was like a breath of fresh air, ideas to help when your child is ill.

The service needed to be approachable, available and friendly. Not only did the service need to give you peace of mind that your child had been checked by a health practitioner, but it also had to help educate families for future episodes of illness. The service fulfilled all this and more.

The CCN was such an angel at times. When I had been up 24 hours and had done all I could within my abilities for my sons, she would knock at my door. It was like a weight had been shared. The CCN is the most caring person, at a time when you need reassurance and encouragement, help is there.

The CCN readdressed all the things I had done. She would make slight alterations in the order of medication perhaps. The CCN helped to control the situation. She gave me an information sheet on temperature management, which she went through with me so I had a full understanding.

The impact of the service within my community is incredible. The service gives parents full back up with follow-up visits, until you as a parent are confident that your child is well again. It has empowered parents to understand what is needed for their sick child and what signs to look out for. This service is now part of my community. It enhances the work of Sure Start and other agencies, such as the PCT.

The CCN service is well known throughout my community. Different generations within families are aware of what this service offers. Families welcome the CCN service into their home with open arms. Personally, at times, when I just did not know what to do, I feel my sanity was saved by the CCN.

Zo'e's account describes what the service hoped it would achieve for families. Many documents have recommended this type of service for sick children, from Platt (Ministry of Health, 1959) and Court (1976), right through to contemporary documents such as the NSFs for children/young people (Education and Skills, Department of Health, 2004). Perhaps this is what Platt and Court envisaged all those years ago. Maybe now we can start to make it a reality in some communities. It is such an obvious and simple service to provide. Yet, it can help to achieve so much for some children and their families – children's nurses visiting in the home, helping parents to care for their acutely ill young children.

Challenges and achievements

Amazingly quickly parents and even grandparents picked up on what the service was able to offer. They understood why the service was there. Disappointingly, some practitioners did not see that the service was offering anything different. Yet, there was clearly a gap in service provision for the care of acutely ill children and their families locally. Walmsley (2003) had already demonstrated this in line with the Sure Start (2003/4) objective.

Other practitioners have been very supportive of the new service. One local GP practice worked really well with the service, making referrals and responding to requests for appointments for chil-

dren. This practice has also been very supportive with the training of CCNs.

The Sure Start CCN service received over 500 referrals during the first 3 years of its existence. It also received local health care awards and was shortlisted for some national awards. An article was published in *Paediatric Nursing* about developing the service (Walmsley and Moyse, 2006).

Future developments

Nationally, similar developments are beginning to take place in some parts of the country. Children's nurses are providing care and support in the home to acutely ill children with minor illnesses and minor injuries. In other places children's nurses are providing health promotion courses in the community to help parents/carers manage minor illnesses. Children's nurses and nurse practitioners/practice nurses are also holding minor illness/injury clinics for young children in children's centres and GP practices.

For this Sure Start CCN service, the scope of practice moves forward in an interesting way. There have been changes to nurse prescribing, broadening the scope of prescribing for CCN nurse prescribers (National Prescribing Centre, 2006). Additional diagnostic skills have also been acquired by some CCNs.

Concluding comments

This chapter has explored the development of an acute CCN minor illness/injury service for young children and their families, in a rurally deprived community. The purpose of this service is to address parents'/carers' concerns when their young children are acutely ill with minor illnesses and minor injuries. The service was developed in line with the Sure Start (2003/4) objective – *to improve the health of young children living in a deprived community.*

The implementation of this new service, the Sure Start CCN service, was carefully planned. The service was subsequently well supported by families. It continues to develop in line with standards and markers of good practice contained within the NSF (Education and Skills, Department of Health, 2004). Importantly for families, the service spends time with them, listens to their concerns and responds to their needs.

The service has helped families in this community, however it may not be appropriate for every community; what works in one context may not necessarily be appropriate for another. The needs of all communities will differ; local needs and current services available will be different. Importantly, the views of parents and carers are fundamental to any change in service provision for young children. Parents/carers views about the type of service they wanted in this community for their young children, helped to make the CCN service such a success. Their views influenced the way in which the service developed.

References

Acheson, D. (1998) *Independent Inquiry into Inequalities in Health*. London: The Stationary Office.

Beattie, T., Gorman, D., Walker, J. (2001) The association between deprivation level, attendance rates and triage category of children attending a children's accident and emergency department. *Emergency Medical Journal* 18: 110–111.

Court, D. (1976) Fit for the future. *The Report of the Committee of Child Health Services*, Vol. 1. London: HMSO.

Department of Health (2003a) *National Service Framework for Children, Young People and Maternity Services, Ill Child Module – Ambulatory Care Sub Group Report*. London: Department of Health.

Department of Health (2003b) *Getting the Right Start: The Children's National Service Framework, Emerging Findings*. London: Crown Copyright.

Education and Skills (Department of), Department of Health (2004) *National Service Framework for Children, Young People and Maternity Services, Standard 6 – Children/Young People Who are Ill*. London: Education and Skills, Department of Health.

Ganguli, P. (2003) Analysis, can nurse practitioners fill the gap in paediatric care. *Nursing Times* 99(31): 10–11.

Home Office (1998) *Supporting Families*. London: Stationery Office.

House of Commons Health Committee (1997) *Health Services for Children/Young People in the Community: Home and School*, 3rd report. London: Stationery Office.

Kai, J. (1996) Parents' difficulties and information needs in coping with acute illness in preschool children: a qualitative study. *British Medical Journal* 313: 987–990.

MacFarl, R., Glass, E., Jones, S. (1994) Appropriateness of paediatric admissions. *Archives of Disease in Childhood* 71: 50–58.

Ministry of Health (1959) *The Welfare of Children in Hospital. Platt Report*. London: HMSO.

Moyse, K. (2005) *Sure Start Community Nursing Service: Evaluating the Service*. Derbyshire: Sure Start Creswell, Langwith/Whaley Thorns and Shirebrook. North Eastern Derbyshire PCT.

National Prescribing Centre (2006) *Extension of Nurse Prescribing*. Available at: http://www.npc.nhs.uk (accessed 31 March 2006).

Neill, S. (2000) Acute childhood illness at home: the parents' perspective. *Journal of Advanced Nursing* 31(4): 821–832.

North Eastern Derbyshire Primary Care Trust (2003) *Health Inequalities – Local Delivery Plan*. Derbyshire: North Eastern Derbyshire Primary Care Trust.

NMC (2004) *Code of Professional Conduct*. London: Nursing and Midwifery Council.

Sanders, J. (2000) A review of health professional attitudes and patient perceptions on 'inappropriate' accident and emergency attendances. The implications for current minor injury provision in England and Wales. *Journal of Advanced Nursing* 31(5): 1057–1105.

Sure Start (2003/4) *Aim and Objectives*. London: Sure Start. Available at: http://www.surestart.gov.uk (accessed October 2004).

Tatman, M., Woodroffe, C. (1993) Paediatric home care in the UK. *Archives of Disease in Childhood* 69: 677–680.

Townsend, P., Davidson, N., Whitedhead, M. (1988) Inequalities in health: the Black report. *The Health Divide*. London: Penguin Books.

Usherwood, T. (1999) *Understanding the Consultation*. Buckingham: Open University Press.

Walmsley, C. (2003) *To Improve Children's Health (Sure Start Objective)*. Derbyshire: Sure Start: Creswell, Langwith/Whaley Thorns and Shirebrook.

Walmsley, C., Moyse, K. (2006) Sure Start community children's nursing: setting up a minor illness and injury service for children up to 5 years of age. *Paediatric Nursing* 18(3): 30–33.

Whiting, M. (1988) Community paediatric nursing in England in 1988. In: Eaton, N. (2001) Models of community children's nursing. *Paediatric Nursing* 13(1): 32–36.

12 Fever Management in Young Children (0–5 Years)

Karen Moyse

NSF

National Service Framework (NSF) for children, young people and maternity services (Education and Skills, Department of Health, 2004a, b) recommends the following:

- Parents/carers should receive information, advice and support to enable them to manage their children's minor illnesses.
- Advocates improving access to safe and effective medicines for children.
- Parents/carers should receive up-to-date and comprehensive information on the safe use of medicines for their children.

Introduction

The focus of this chapter is on health promotion advice and support in the community for the care of young children (0–4 years) who have a fever due to a minor illness. The theory presented will look at the signs and symptoms of a fever, as well as how to manage a fever. Practice examines a variety of different interventions devised by the Sure Start community children's nursing (CCN) service to help parents and carers manage young children's fevers at home.

There are different terms which can be used to describe a child who is feeling warm or hot when unwell. These terms include the following, with definitions provided:

- Fever – *an elevation in body temperature above the normal, usually as a response to infection* (Blackwell's Nursing Dictionary, 2005, p. 229).
- Pyrexia – *fever, elevation of the body temperature above the normal* (Blackwell's Nursing Dictionary, 2005, p. 498).
- Temperature – *the degree of heat or coldness of an object or substance as measured by a thermometer* (Blackwell's Nursing Dictionary, 2005, p. 596).

An additional term that may be of use to the reader is the following:

- Antipyretic – *an agent that reduces fever* (Blackwell's Nursing Dictionary, 2005, p. 43).

Why is it important for nurses to learn about fever management?

Parents can become very concerned when their young children are ill with a fever. Kai (1996) found that it was one of the symptoms that concerned parents the most when their children were ill. Fever is very common in young children. NICE (2007) states that it is the most common reason why children attend their general practitioner (GP). Moyse (2005) found that fever was one of the most common reason why young children were referred to the Sure Start CCN service, a service especially for young children with minor illnesses.

There is a perceived need to improve the *recognition*, *evaluation* and *treatment* of young children who present with feverish illness (NICE, 2007). The nurse working with young children has an important role to play in this process, as this chapter highlights.

Why might a child have a high temperature?

A fever in a young child indicates an infection of some kind (NICE, 2007). Infectious diseases remain a major cause of childhood mortality and morbidity in the UK (NICE, 2007).

Prodigy (2006) maintains that fevers are commonly associated with viral infections in children, which they usually recover from quickly. Bacterial infections can also cause a high temperature, but are not as common as viral infections (Prodigy, 2006). Bacterial infections are likely to cause quite serious illnesses.

Serious illnesses

This chapter does not explore in any depth the management of young children where the fever is due to a serious illness. However, when a nurse is first called out to see a child with a high temperature, the nurse does not know if the fever is due to a minor illness or something more serious. This section highlights briefly some of the key signs and symptoms that will alert the nurse to a situation where the fever may be due to a more serious illness.

When assessing a child with a fever, there are certain aspects of the clinical situation that the nurse should always check, not simply the temperature (NICE, 2007). These are listed below:

- Skin colour.
- Activity level – response to social cues.

- Respiratory rate.
- Hydration state – is the child feeding, what is the urine output like?
- How long has the child had a high temperature? (NICE, 2007).

Where the child has a serious illness, the nurse may find on assessment that one or more of the following clinical features are present. This list provides a summary of the clinical features highlighted by NICE (2007):

A child at high risk

- Skin colour – pale, mottled, ashen or blue.
- Activity level – unable to rouse, or if aroused does not stay awake; the child may have a weak cry or high-pitched cry or even be continually crying.
- High respiratory rate – above 60 beats per minute (bpm).
- Indrawing of chest – moderate or severe.
- Grunting.
- Bile stained vomit.
- Signs of dehydration – reduced skin turgor.
- Bulging fontanelle.
- Non-blanching rash.
- Neck stiffness.
- Focal neurological signs.
- Focal seizures.
- Swelling of a limb or child not wanting to use it (NICE, 2007).

A child at intermediate risk

- Pallor reported by parent/carer.
- Wakes only with prolonged stimulation.
- Decreased activity.
- Not responding to social cues, no smile.
- High respiratory rate >50 bpm, age 6–12 months; >40 bpm, age >12 months.
- Oxygen saturations <95% in air.
- Crepitations (sound heard with stethoscope on chest examination).
- Nasal flaring, age <12 months.
- Poor feeding.
- Reduced urine output.
- Capillary refill time ≥3 seconds.
- A new lump >2 cm.
- Fever for 5 days (NICE, 2007).

Consult the original text for more details – *Feverish Illness in Children*, NICE (2007).

Whether the illness is minor or serious, the nurse should always listen to what parents/carers have to say about their child's health. Parents/carers perceptions of their child's fever should always be taken seriously (NICE, 2007). A parent/carer will know when their child is unwell, and may well recognise when a fever is present.

Signs of a fever

What is considered to be a high temperature?

A raised temperature is one that elevates above the normal daily variation (NICE, 2007). Temperatures vary within the individual and between individuals (NICE, 2007). Many studies highlight a temperature of 38°C or above to indicate a high temperature (NICE, 2007).

NICE (2007) advises that where a baby of less than 3 months old has a temperature of 38°C or above she/he should be admitted to hospital. Where a child has a temperature of 39°C or above she/he is at risk of serious illness (NICE, 2007).

What signs and symptoms may indicate a fever?

There are a number of different signs and symptoms to look out for when a child has a fever. The child can present with some of the following:

- Flushed face.
- Warm or hot to touch.
- Irritable.
- Drowsy.
- Raised temperature on recording.

Following treatment the child may feel a little better within an hour or two, but may not if the illness is serious.

Caring for children with minor illness: what does the nurse in the community need to consider?

Careful assessment of the young child presenting with a fever is essential. The nurse should not only look at the signs and symptoms, which indicate that the child has a fever, but an overall assessment of the child needs to be undertaken. This will help to provide a more accurate assessment, allowing the nurse to recognise, advise, and evaluate on appropriate treatments.

As the NSF (Education and Skills, Department of Health, 2004a) highlights, at the onset of an illness it can sometimes be difficult to distinguish between a minor illness and a more serious one. A thorough assessment, with repeated assessments if necessary, will help determine the appropriate action to take. On repeat assessment the child's condition may have improved. However, a marked deterioration in the child's condition may develop, which will indicate a need for the child to attend hospital.

When assessing a child with a fever, as NICE (2007) indicates, assess not only the temperature, but also respiratory rate, heart rate, check how well hydrated the child is, check capillary refill time, and importantly check skin colour for anything usual such as skin rashes or cold extremities. Importantly, check the responsiveness level of the child. If any of these observations are not normal, the child should be referred on to a paediatric specialist.

In summary, the nurse will be checking the following:

- Temperature.
- Skin – colour, rash and cold extremities.
- Heart rate.
- Respiratory rate.
- Consciousness level.
- Capillary refill time.

If a child presents with a skin rash, the nurse should check the rash using the glass test.

A clear glass is pressed against the skin. If a septicaemia is present, which might be associated with meningitis, the rash will not fade on testing (Meningitis Trust, 2001) and the child will need emergency care.

Why help to reduce the child's temperature?

Simply, by reducing a child's temperature she/he is going to feel so much more comfortable. This is a very important reason for reducing a child's temperature (NICE, 2007). The difference it can make to how a child's feels is incredible.

In a minority of cases, if a child's temperature becomes too high, she/he may experience a seizure (Prodigy, 2005). There is only a very small risk of this occurring. Prodigy's (2005) guidance on febrile convulsions states that 3 in 100 children may experience a convulsion before they are 6 years old. Febrile convulsions most commonly occur between the ages of 18 months and 3 years, and are likely to be associated with a viral infection (Prodigy, 2005).

Management of a fever – non-pharmacological approaches

Initially, establish that the child has a high temperature with the use of a thermometer. If high, there are a number of different strategies that parents/carers and nurses can use to bring the temperature down. Prodigy (2006) suggests giving the child appropriate medication, give cool drinks, and perhaps take off some of the child's clothing, if the room is of *normal room temperature*.

The monitoring of a child's temperature is a very important part of the process in bringing the temperature down. This should be more than a one-off measurement. The parent/carer or nurse will want to ensure that the child's temperature is actually coming down. The impact of any treatment approaches applied need to be assessed.

When measuring a young child's temperature, there are recommended sites in the body to use. The fever guidelines produced by NICE (2007) advise that the oral and rectal sites should *not* be used. The axilla is a safe site with the use of an electronic thermometer. The ear can also be used for temperature measurement, where a tympanic thermometer is available (NICE, 2007).

Non-pharmacological approaches to temperature management will be discussed.

Fluids

The fever guidelines (NICE, 2007) recommend the importance of giving regular fluids, in an effort to help bring down a child's high temperature. This will help to keep a child cool. Small amounts of fluids given often can be useful. Where an infant is being breastfed, extra feeds can be given.

Clothing

Removing some of the child's clothing may help. Prodigy (2006) states that this depends on the temperature of the room the child is in. If the room is of normal temperature, then it is fine to remove some layers of clothing (Prodigy, 2006).

There is a risk sometimes that parents/carers will overwrap a child who is hot. As the Prodigy (2006) guidance goes on to say, it is wrong to overwrap a child with a fever, and this should not be undertaken. From observation it is not unusual for some parents/carers to overwrap a child with a fever. In the community a child may sometimes present with quite a few layers of clothing on. Reducing some of these layers can enable the child to feel more comfortable. Further, the Department of Health and the Foundation for Sudden Infant Death (2005) in the leaflet *Reduce the Risk of Cot Death* discuss the importance of a child *not* being overwrapped.

At home

Importantly, parents/carers will need to check their child overnight (NICE, 2007). This will help determine if the child's condition is worsening, and if the child needs more urgent care. Parents/carers are on hand to observe and act upon any immediate changes in their child. The nurse must provide the family with information about what to do should their child's condition deteriorate. Depending on the circumstances, this may involve NHS Direct, *out of hours* GP service or accident and emergency department.

Tests

Where a child is particularly unwell, there may be a need, depending on the clinical picture, to either undertake or refer the child for tests. Where a child (between 3 months and 5 years) has no features of a serious illness, a urine test should be performed for signs of infection (NICE, 2007). The child should also be assessed for signs and symptoms of pneumonia (NICE, 2007).

Children who are more seriously ill, depending on their signs and symptoms, will have appropriate tests performed by paediatric services. This might include, depending on the clinical picture, urine tests, blood tests, lumbar puncture and chest X-ray (NICE, 2007).

Management of a fever – pharmacological approaches and nurse prescribing

Pharmacological approaches to fever management

Antipyretic medication can be used to help reduce a child's fever. This medication should be given according to instructions outlined in the British National Formulary for Children (BNFC, 2007). Paracetamol or ibuprofen can be given (BNFC, 2007).

Young children do not always take medication readily. Tablets they often find difficult to swallow. It is helpful if medication can be given in liquid form, which allows for ease of swallowing. However, children can sometimes be reluctant to swallow medicines if the flavour is not to their liking. Antipyretics are now available in different flavours, which children find a little more acceptable. Most paracetamol preparations are strawberry flavoured and ibuprofen medicines are available in strawberry or orange flavours. If children have a preference for a particular flavour, find this out, as it may make a difference to whether they take their medication or not. It is also important to consider the use of sugar-free medicines, in an effort to reduce tooth decay.

Oral syringes are useful where a child is taking a very small dose of medicine, as the correct dose can be easily drawn up. Medicines management (Education and Skills, Department of Health, 2004b) advises the use of an oral syringe where the amount of medicine a baby/child might be taking is small – less than a 5 mL spoon.

Paracetamol

Paracetamol can be used for fever and pain in children (BNFC, 2007). It is sometimes described as the preferred medication for fever management (BNFC, 2007).

Paracetamol reduces fever by inhibiting the formation and release of prostaglandin in the central nervous system (Gillman and Rall, 1990).

This is controlled by the hypothalamus in the brain, the heat-regulating system (Skidmore, 2001). Prostaglandins have been defined as a group of several hormone-like physiologically active substances, produced by the body (Blackwell's Nursing Dictionary, 2005).

The following provides an overview of the information provided on paracetamol by the BNFC (2007). For exact details, particularly frequency and doses required by children at different ages, consult the BNFC (2007).

Cautionary labels apply to the use of many medications. In the case of paracetamol, label 30 applies; do not take with other products which contain paracetamol (BNFC, 2007). Paracetamol is not advised where there is hepatic impairment and in some cases where there is renal impairment. Parents/carers should be advised *not* to exceed the stated dose of paracetamol in any 24-hour period. Side effects are rare with paracetamol. Parents/carers should be advised that if any side effects do occur however to contact the nurse or doctor immediately.

Ibuprofen

Ibuprofen can be given for fever (BNFC, 2007). Ibuprofen is a non-steroidal anti-inflammatory drug (NSAID). There are a number of cautions associated with the use of NSAIDs in young children, which nurses need to consider. The BNFC (2007) advises caution in the following circumstances:

- Where a child has a history of hypersensitivity to any NSAID.
- Caution is also advised where coagulation defects exist.
- When a child has an allergic disorder, NSAIDs are not advised.
- Caution is also advised where a child has a cardiac, hepatic or renal problem, as NSAIDs have the potential to reduce renal function in these situations.
- It is also advised to avoid where there has been previous gastrointestinal ulceration or bleeding.

Ibuprofen has fewer side effects compared to other NSAIDs (BNFC, 2007). Side effects of ibuprofen can include gastrointestinal discomfort, nausea and diarrhoea. Interestingly, the BNFC (2007) maintains that children appear to tolerate NSAIDs better than adults, resulting in less gastrointestinal side effects.

Ibuprofen is the least likely NSAID to cause side effects and the only one licensed for sale to the public. Ibuprofen can be used successfully to bring down a child's fever. For details about dose and frequency according to child's weight and age, consult the BNFC (2007).

Combined approaches

From observation in practice, it would seem that sometimes when a child has a high fever, paracetamol and ibuprofen are used in combination to reduce the temperature. Mayoral et al.'s (2000) paper on the use of paracetamol and ibuprofen in combination states that there is not sufficient research evidence to support the combined use of these medications for managing fever in children. Guidance from NICE (2007) does not support the combined use of paracetamol and ibuprofen in practice as routine for the management of fever in young children. NICE (2007) recommends that further research needs to be undertaken in this area.

Prescribing independently

An independent prescriber assesses patients with undiagnosed conditions and makes prescribing decisions (Courtney, 2001). When prescribing for children there are a number of important factors that need to be in place before the nurse can prescribe:

- The nurse must have completed an appropriate nurse prescribing course.
- Nursing and Midwifery Council (NMC, 2004) – the nurse must of course be registered with NMC, both to nurse, and be a nurse prescriber.
- The nurse must be authorised to prescribe by her/his employer (primary care trust).
- The nurse must prescribe within her/his area of expertise.
- The nurse should use the BNF for children (BNFC, 2007). This provides essential and accurate information about prescribing for young children.
- The nurse needs to adhere to local guidelines and local formularies related to prescribing.

- The nurse must use the prescription pad she/he has been issued with by the employer.

Seven principles of good prescribing

The National Prescribing Centre (1999) has developed seven principles to good prescribing, which are available to nurses. The principles can help nurses learn how to prescribe and act as a guide when prescribing. The following provides an edited summary of these principles in relation to prescribing for a child:

- Assess the child's needs.
- Provide a strategy for managing the child's care.
- Prescribing – consider the choice of product.
- Communication and negotiation with the family.
- Review the child.
- Record keeping following prescribing.
- Reflection and evaluation (National Prescribing Centre, 1999).

Prescribing support

As a nurse, when one first starts prescribing it can be very daunting. Yet, with good peer support these initial apprehensions can soon be overcome. It can be useful to have other nurse prescribers around to consult with over prescribing issues. Community pharmacists can also be invaluable where the nurse has any queries about prescribing. Otway (2001) discusses the importance of good support from colleagues when learning how to prescribe. Hurley (2003) suggests that support from colleagues can help facilitate safe prescribing practice.

Practice interventions

The CCN service, a minor illness service for young children, put in place a number of interventions to help parents/carers manage fever with their young children. Fever is a common symptom of minor illness, and parental/carer concern (Kai, 1996). Parents/carers in the Sure Start area had expressed concern about managing fever in young children (Moyse, 2005). The Sure Start CCN service thus felt temperature management was an important subject upon which to increase parents'/carers' knowledge and skills.

Free thermometers

Parents/carers often know when their child has a fever. They may be able to tell by feeling their child's forehead, which will feel warm, or the fact that their child is miserable will alert them that something is wrong. Their child may even say that she/he does not feel well. However, there are occasions when parents/carers are uncertain if their child is ill. It can be useful for parents/carers to know exactly what their child's temperature is, as this will help in assessing their child's health. A thermometer can be essential. In practice, for example, a mother thought her child had a high temperature. Having a thermometer to hand, she found her child's temperature to be above 40°C. The mother then knew she needed to act quickly. Her child was admitted to hospital and found to have a serious infection. The simple measure of having a thermometer alerted the mother to how ill her child actually was.

The Sure Start CCN service provides each family with a free digital thermometer. This enables the family to measure their child's temperature when unwell. Families are advised to keep the thermometer in their first aid box, so it is ready when needed. They are also shown how to use the thermometer. Information is provided on normal body temperature and raised temperature, so that parents/carers know exactly what to look out for.

Leaflets/advice sheet

A fever leaflet has been devised for use by parents/carers. It has been created as an additional information source, to support the verbal information given by the CCN, when a child has a high temperature. Medicines Management standard (Education and Skills, Department of Health, 2004b) states written information can help with children accessing safe and effective medication. The Sure Start CCN service developed the leaflet, so that parents/carers would have an information source readily available to remind them about the treatments their child would need to bring down a fever. The leaflet is usually placed with the parent-held record, along with a contact telephone number for the Sure Start CCN service.

The content of the Sure Start CCN leaflet was devised in consultation with parents/carers, as well as other health practitioners. The leaflet was validated by Sure Start and the local primary care trust (PCT), and is updated every 2 years (Sure Start and North East Derbyshire PCT, 2005).

The content of the leaflet includes the following:

- What can cause a fever.
- Non-pharmacological approaches to temperature management.
- Pharmacological approaches to temperature management.
- Who to contact if parents/carers are concerned about their child.

If parents require further written information, copies of related leaflets are available from the Prodigy website – http://www.cks.library.nhs.uk/patient_information/pils. These include the following:

- Coughs and colds in young children.
- Febrile convulsions.
- Paracetamol.
- Temperature (fevers) in children.

Nurse prescribing

The Sure Start CCN service is able to prescribe medication for young children who present with fever. The CCNs are qualified independent nurse prescribers. They can prescribe paracetamol or ibuprofen for young children with fever, where appropriate, and according to the guidance presented in the BNFC (2007).

The service:

- assesses the child;
- discusses the need (or not) for medication with parents/carers;
- prescribes, if felt appropriate, consulting the BNFC (2007);
- documents;
- reassess the child to ascertain if the child's condition has improved or deteriorated.

In May 2006, regulations changed on nurse prescribing. Qualified independent nurse prescribers are now able to prescribe licensed medicines for any medical condition within their competence (Department of Health, 2006). There are restrictions associated with controlled drugs (Department of Health, 2006). Any additional training needs to be addressed through continued professional development.

For the Sure Start CCN service, this has meant that a broader range of medications can be prescribed for minor illnesses, including throat infections, ear infections and chest infections. To assist with this, additional training has been undertaken in the area of diagnosing minor illnesses.

Documentation

An important part of prescribing is to ensure that the act of prescribing has been documented appropriately. Parents/carers need to know exactly what has been prescribed for their child. Other practitioners involved in the child's care also need to know what has been prescribed.

Hall and Elliman (2003) maintain that the parent-held record was designed to encourage partnership between parents/carers and health practitioners. The Sure Start CCNs always note down in this record what has been prescribed for the child, why, and what side effects to look out for. The service discusses all this and what to do if side effects occur with parents.

Within the nursing record for the child, similar details are noted down. The NMC (2004) advises that nursing records are an important tool in protecting the patient. Nursing records should provide clear details about care of patients.

Courtney (2001) discusses how the nurse must provide details about prescribed medications within the GP records too, which must be undertaken within 48 hours of prescribing. This is essential for safe practice, avoiding errors and duplications of prescriptions.

First-dose medication for fever

The Sure Start CCN service really wanted to improve the safe access of medication for young children unwell with minor illness, as outlined in the NSF (Education and Skills, Department of Health, 2004b). Children unwell with a fever can sometimes feel better quickly if they have fast access to the appropriate medicine.

CCN nurse prescribers can administer first-dose antipyretics, as authorised by the PCT. The CCNs prescribe either paracetamol or ibuprofen for a young child with fever. The CCN, if she/he feels it is appropriate, along with the parents/carers then administers the first dose of this medicine. Hopefully, this helps the child feel better quickly. It also buys time for the parent in relation to obtaining the medicine from the pharmacy. The child can perhaps be feeling more comfortable at home, with the temperature coming down, while parent is out obtaining the medicine.

Home care for children

The Sure Start CCN service is able to provide all these interventions for young children through its home visiting service. The service provides parents/carers with information, advice and support at home, when their young children are ill with a fever. Obviously, sometimes children are seriously ill, and thus it may not be appropriate for them to be cared for at home. The service in this situation would refer on to a GP or hospital services. Home care has been shown to help reduce the stress and anxiety that might be caused for children by being admitted to hospital (Stein and Jessop, 1984).

Health promotion course

The Sure Start CCN service devised a minor illness course for parents/carers to help them manage their young children's minor illnesses. During the course a session is presented on fever management. The list below outlines the content of this session, as well as the teaching methods and resources used.

Managing a high temperature

- What is a high temperature?
- What causes a high temperature?
- What can I do to bring down my child's temperature down?

- Febrile convulsions.
- Rashes.
- Where to go for further advice.

Teaching methods

- Discussion.
- Pairs activities.
- Presentation of information.

Resources used

- Handouts.
- PowerPoint.
- Thermometers.

The health promotion course is aimed at parents/carers with young children. Extended family members are also invited to attend.

How the service links with NSF

The NSF maintains that parents/carers should receive information, advice and support to enable them to manage their children's minor illnesses. The Sure Start CCN service provides information, advice and support to families on caring for their children when they have a minor illness. This enables parents/carers to manage their children's minor illnesses at home, with less need to consult other health services (Moyse, 2005).

The NSF advocates improving children's access to safe and effective medicines. The Sure Start CCN service participates in this process by being able to prescribe young children with medication, where appropriate, when unwell. The service is also able to administer a dose of antipyretic on first contact, where a child is unwell with a high temperature and it is appropriate to do so. This allows the child to receive prompt treatment and care, so that she/he feels more comfortable.

The NSF also recommends that parents/carers should receive up-to-date and comprehensive information on the safe use of medicines. An important part of the work of the Sure Start CCN service is to provide parents/carers with up-to-date information on the safe use of medicines, particularly when prescribing.

Activity

As a community children's nurse working within a minor illness service, you have been called out by another to see her young child (2 years old) with a fever. How would you assess and manage the situation?

You are a qualified nurse prescriber; therefore, upon assessment you may feel it is appropriate to prescribe antipyretic medication and administer the first dose, involving the mother at each stage. Use the BNFC (2007) to enable you to prescribe appropriately.

What information will you provide for the mother to help her manage this situation? What further action might you take yourself to evaluate the outcome of your initial assessment and management?

Conclusion

There is a perceived need to improve the *recognition*, *evaluation* and *treatment* of young children who present with feverish illness (NICE, 2007). The nurse working with young children has an important role to play in this process, as this chapter has highlighted. The development of a home nursing service for young children with minor illness has certainly helped to improve the management of feverish illness in one Sure Start area in the East Midlands.

This chapter has presented information on the importance of assessing young children with a fever, signs and symptoms, as well as management. The section on practice interventions has highlighted how simple measures, such as providing free thermometers, providing literature, as well as a health promotion course for parents/carers, can all help in the care of young children with a fever. Having in place a home nursing service, which is able to assess and treat young children, has been an especially significant development for this Sure Start community. The Sure Start CCN service hopes that the developments it has introduced will not only help the children who come into contact with the service, but will also impact on the knowledge and skills of other families members, so the health of all children locally can be improved.

Recent resources

Hay, A., Costelloe, C., Redmond, N., Montgomery, A., Fletcher, M., Hollinghurst, S., Peters, T. (2008) Paracetamol plus ibuprofen for the treatment of fever in children (PITCH): randomized controlled trial. *British Medical Journal* 337: a1302. Available at: http://www.bmj.com (accessed September 2008).

Royal College of Nursing (2008) *Caring for Children with Fever. RCN Good Practice Guidance for Nurses Working with Infants, Children/Young People.* London: Royal College of Nursing.

References

Blackwell's Nursing Dictionary (2005) Oxford: Blackwell Publishing.

BNF for Children (BNFC) (2007) British Medical Association, Royal Pharmaceutical Society of Great Britain, Royal College of Paediatrics and Child Health, Neonatal and Paediatric Pharmacists Group. London: BMJ Publishing Group Ltd.

Courtney, M. (2001) *Current Issues in Nurse Prescribing.* London: Greenwich Medical Media Ltd.

Department of Health (2006) *Nurse Independent Prescribing.* Department of Health. Available at: http://www.dh.goc.uk/policyandguidance/ medicinespharmacyandindustry/prescription (accessed 9 Februay 2007).

Department of Health, the Foundation for Sudden Infant Death (2005) *Reduce the Risk of Cot Death.* London: Department of Health.

Education and Skills (Department of), Department of Health (2004a) *National Service Framework for Children, Young People and Maternity Services, Standard 6 – Children and Young People Who Are Ill.* London: Crown Copyright.

Education and Skills (Department of), Department of Health (2004b) *National Service Framework for Children,* Young People and Maternity Services, Standard 10 – Medicines Management. London: Crown Copyright.

Gillman, A., Rall, T. (1990) *Goodman's and Gillman's Pharmacological Basic of Therapeutics,* 8th edn. New York: Pergamon Press.

Hall, D., Elliman, D. (2003) *Health for All Children,* 4th edn. Oxford: Oxford University Press.

Hurley, G. (2003) Enhancing partnership in prescribing. *Practice Nurse* 25(7): 21–25.

Kai, J. (1996) What worries parents when their preschool children are acutely ill and why: a qualitative study. *British Medical Journal* 313(7063): 983–986.

Mayoral, C., Marino, R., Rosenfeld, W., Greensher, J. (2000) Alternating antipyretics: is this the alternative? *Pediatrics* 105(5): 1009–1012.

Meningitis Trust (2001) *Meningococcal Septicaemia.* Stroud: Meningitis Trust.

Moyse, K. (2005) *Sure Start Community Children's Nursing: Evaluating the Service.* Derbyshire: Sure Start Creswell, Langwith/Whaley Thorns and Shirebrook.

National Prescribing Centre (1999) Signposts for prescribing nurses – general principles of good prescribing. *Prescribing Nurse Bulletin* 1(1): 1–4.

NICE (2007) *Feverish Illness in Children.* London: National Institute of Clinical Excellence.

NMC (2004) *Code of Professional Conduct.* London: Nursing and Midwifery Council.

Otway, C. (2001) Informal peer support: a key to success for nurse prescribers. *British Journal of Community Nursing* 11: 586–591.

Prodigy (2005) *Febrile Convulsion* (patient information leaflet). Copyright – EMIS and PIP. Available at: http://www.cks.library.nhs.uk/patient_information/ pils (accessed 19 January 2007).

Prodigy (2006) High temperature (fever) in children (patient information leaflet). Copyright – EMIS and PIP. Available at: http://www.cks.library.nhs.uk/ patient_information/pils (accessed 19 January 2007).

Skidmore, L. (2001) *Mosby's Drug Guide for Nurses,* 5th edn. St Louis: Philadelphia.

Stein, R., Jessop, D. (1984) Does paediatric home care make a difference for children with chronic illness? *Pediatrics* 7(6): 845–853.

13 Health Promotion in Young Children's Minor Illnesses

Karen Moyse

NSF

The National Service Framework (NSF) for children/young people and maternity services asserts that parents should receive *information*, *advice* and *support* to enable them to manage their young children's *minor illnesses* (Education and Skills, Department of Health, 2004a).

Introduction

Health promotion in young children's minor illnesses discusses the development of a health promotion course aimed at parents/carers to help support and provide them with information about the management of young children's minor illnesses. (The term parents will be used throughout to indicate both parents and carers.)

Health promotion courses for parents have been available for many years, which provide them with information about how to cope during the early weeks of their child's life, traditionally called *parentcraft classes*. There have been demands from parents for more information from such courses, to help them beyond these early weeks, so they are better informed about their children's health.

In recent years, with the development of Sure Start and children's centres, a wider range of courses for parents have become available, covering a variety of different issues related to child health, both physical and emotional. These courses are commonly referred to as *parenting courses*. They may focus on such issues as children's behaviour management and children's play and development, for example.

The Government, nurses, along with other practitioners, acknowledge that parenting courses are valuable. However, there are few parenting courses that offer advice about young children's minor illness management. Yet, the management of young children's minor illnesses is something parents feel they need to know more about as Kai (1996a, b) and Neill (2000) have highlighted.

Parents want information, as well as advice and support, to enable them to manage their young children's minor illnesses successfully. This chapter examines a Sure Start health promotion course on minor illness management, developed in the East Midlands. It has been developed with the aim of increasing parents' confidence when caring for their young children when unwell with a minor illness. The chapter examines key health promotion subjects explored within the course, which includes gastroenteritis and mild upper respiratory tract infections, as well as some additional health issues that parents felt were important to know about.

The situation for parents

When a child is ill with a minor illness, parents may need extra help and support with their child's care. As any parent knows sometimes it can be pretty scary when your child is ill. Uncertainties surround what is wrong with your child. Sometimes uncertainties may also exist about where to go for help, along with not always being able to access the right help when needed.

When a young child (0–5 years) is ill, it can be even more frightening because the child is not able to say exactly how she/he feels, which may blur the picture surrounding diagnosis. Further, a young child is more vulnerable; her/his health can deteriorate more quickly than that of an older child or adult. A minor illness course is perhaps one way of helping parents to be better prepared for when their young child becomes ill.

Developing the minor illness course

A minor illness has been outlined as being in poor health, but not suffering from a major health problem (Concise Oxford Dictionary, 1982). When a child has a minor illness she/he can be acutely ill, particularly during the early stages of the illness. During an acute illness a parent may seek help for their child (Department of Health, 2003).

In the early years of life, it is not unnatural for a child to be ill frequently with minor illnesses. Evidence has shown that during a typical year a preschool child can see a general practitioner (GP) about six times. Additionally, up to one-half of infants, aged under 12 months, will attend an accident and emergency (A + E) in 1 year (Education and Skills, Department of Health, 2004b). However, over 80% of all episodes of illnesses in childhood are managed by parents without making any reference to health care services (Education and Skills, Department of Health, 2004b).

Nurses can help parents to be better informed on how to care for their young children when unwell, and provide details about what health care services are available in their local area. Doing so can be beneficial, raising parents' confidence. Research recently undertaken with the Sure Start community children's nursing service (which provides acute care for children under 5 years) demonstrated

that parents' confidence could be improved with more *information* and *support* about the management of young children's minor illnesses (Moyse, 2005). As part of this research, parents were given health promotion information on the management of minor illnesses through a health promotion course, as well as information and support when their children were ill, with the involvement of a community nursing service. Being prepared for minor illnesses helped parents cope better when their children were actually ill. The development of this minor illness course will be discussed.

The course

Parents, within the local area, wanted a health promotion course that would inform them about how to manage their young children's minor illnesses. As a result of parents' requests a minor illness course was designed and implemented.

A number of issues had to be considered in developing the course. These included the following:

- Course availability.
- Accessibility.
- Publicity.
- Exploring the content.
- The course.
- Teaching methods and resources.
- Evaluation.

Availability

Initially, it was felt that the course should simply be available to parents of young children. However, families within the local area have very strong extended family networks. Family can be a strong source of support when young children are ill. It was therefore felt that the course should be available to extended family members as well. Different members of the same family group could be provided with up-to-date information on minor illness management.

Accessibility

Nurses involved in the design of the course considered where would be the best location to hold the course in the local community, as well as the time of day that would be most suitable for families to attend. A number of families were asked for their opinion on these issues.

Publicity

Leaflets were printed and distributed in advance of the course, so that the local community were aware that it was available. Sure Start also helped to publicise the course through its various groups.

Exploring the content

The main health promotion subjects featured within the course included the management of high temperatures, gastroenteritis and mild upper respiratory tract infections, in line with the Sure Start target (Sure Start, 2003/4). Parents were also provided with the opportunity to explore particular illnesses that concerned them.

The course

The aim of the course was to advance parents' knowledge and skills in the management of their young children's minor illnesses. The course itself consisted of five sessions, held for 1 hour each week. The course ended shortly before school pick up time, so those families with older children could then travel on to school.

Teaching methods and resources

A variety of different teaching methods and resources were used. Some of the teaching methods included pairs activities, demonstrations, discussions, quizzes and sharing experiences. Resources used involved Powerpoint, books, equipment, handouts, posters and games.

Evaluation

At the end of the course parents were given an opportunity to evaluate it. They were asked if and how the course had met their needs.

The following discusses some of the course content in more detail.

Health promotion in gastroenteritis

Gastroenteritis, one of the sessions featured within the course, will be discussed. Gastroenteritis is an infection of the intestinal tract. It causes diarrhoea,

and it can also cause vomiting (Prodigy, 2006a). Children usually recover spontaneously (Prodigy, 2006a).

The session explores the *signs* and *symptoms* of gastroenteritis. Details are also provided about the *care* and *management* of babies and young children with gastroenteritis.

As part of this session it is important to highlight that vomiting and diarrhoea are not simply symptoms of gastroenteritis, but they can also be associated with other conditions in babies and children. Parents need to be aware of this, so they do not assume that their child is suffering from gastroenteritis, when it may be something else. Importantly, this issue is highlighted to parents as part of the session. For example, babies with a urinary tract infection may present with diarrhoea and vomiting (Prodigy, 2006b). It is important, therefore, that parents and practitioners alike do not make assumptions that vomiting and diarrhoea is always due to gastroenteritis. As Carter and Dearmun (1995) assert, the specific nature of gastrointestinal problems can be difficult to determine, especially in young children. Symptoms of vomiting and diarrhoea can be associated with different anatomical systems.

It is important too that parents are reminded about the external issues linked to gastroenteritis. For example, Walmsley (2003) maintains that poor hygiene is associated with inadequate sterilisation of infant feeding equipment, and can contribute to diarrhoea and vomiting. Breastfeeding is known to reduce the risks of gastroenteritis (Sure Start, 2000).

When babies and young children have gastroenteritis, they are normally nursed at home by their parents until they recover. Admission to hospital is unusual, unless as Carter and Dearmun (1995) highlight that vomiting and diarrhoea become progressive, and fluids are not being tolerated. These symptoms would suggest dehydration, and need urgent attention.

Health promotion information related to signs and symptoms

The information below outlines some of the main signs and symptoms that parents should look out for with gastroenteritis, which are explored with them during the session:

- Diarrhoea – soft, watery bowel actions, which may occur frequently.

- Sickness.
- Dehydration – more likely to occur if the baby/child is reluctant to drink.
- Lack of energy/lethargy.
- Raised temperature.
- Stomach pains (crampy pains).
- Sore bottom.

The severity of this condition can vary; some children may only experience a mild episode, whilst others can be quite ill. Prodigy (2006a) highlights how the severity of gastroenteritis can range from a mild tummy upset lasting for a couple of days, to more severe diarrhoea lasting for much longer.

If vomiting occurs it should only last for a day at most (Prodigy, 2006a). Parents should be advised to seek help from medical or nursing services, if the vomiting lasts for longer than this (Prodigy, 2006a).

It is useful to point out to parents that unlike vomiting bowel actions may take several days to return to normal. Based on practice experience, parents are frequently concerned about the diarrhoea continuing for several days from the start of the illness. Simple reassurance can ease these concerns. However, if blood appears in the bowel actions, medical help should be sought.

There is a risk of *dehydration* with gastroenteritis. The signs and symptoms of dehydration should be explored with parents during the session, so they are fully aware of what they need to look out for. Try to make the presentation of this information as interesting as possible. Interactive teaching approaches can often be used, as some parents seem to have quite good knowledge on dehydration, and are keen to demonstrate what they know.

Signs of dehydration in babies/children include (Carter and Dearmun, 1995) the following:

- Sunken fontanelle (babies).
- Poor urine output.
- Lethargy.
- Reluctance to feed or drink.
- Skin – may lack elasticity due to fluid loss.
- Behaviour – miserable and unsettled.

Health promotion information related to care and management

Care and management is discussed with parents, and information is presented.

The aim of care and management is to keep babies and children with gastroenteritis well hydrated. The most important aspect of health promotion to get across to parents therefore is *maintaining hydration*.

Carter and Dearmun (1995), along with Prodigy (2006a), highlight that aspects of care and management should include the following points.

The key health promotion messages are as follows:

- Prevent dehydration with plenty of fluids.
- Breastfed babies should continue to breastfeed.
- Bottle-fed babies should be fed with their normal strength feeds, and in addition can be given rehydration drinks.
- Children can continue with food now and then; however, they may not want to eat, wait until their appetite returns. They must continue with frequent drinks, as fluids are the most important thing.
- Monitor fluid input and urine output, so parents are promptly aware if dehydration is occurring. A low urine output or very dry nappies will indicate to parents that dehydration may be occurring. Contact should be made with medical/nursing services for further advice, if this occurs.
- If a baby or child is hot, parents should be advised to keep their baby/child cool.
- Resting will help with recuperation.
- To prevent a sore bottom, keep clean and dry and apply a barrier cream.
- To prevent the spread of infection around the family, regular hand hygiene is essential.

As the above information highlights, frequent drinks are essential. During the session nurses discuss with parents different ways they can encourage their young children to take fluids, such as offering their favourite drinks or even ice lollies. It is suggested they avoid fizzy drinks, as children may feel uncomfortable.

Health promotion in mild upper respiratory infections

Another important session featured within the course is on mild upper respiratory tract infections. Most upper respiratory tract infections involve the nose, throat and ears (Lissauer and Clayden, 2006). This session explores colds and mild sore throats only. Another session on the course looks at tonsillitis and ear infections, but will not be explored here.

The *signs and symptoms* of mild respiratory infections (colds and sore throats) as well as the *care and management* are presented. The teaching methods used in the session are outlined in the teaching plan at the end of this section.

Mild respiratory illnesses are very common in young children. Respiratory illnesses account for 50% of GP consultations for acute illness in young children (Lissauer and Clayden, 2006). It is important that parents feel equipped to manage mild respiratory illnesses, as they are managed at home, unless they become more serious.

It is important to highlight to parents that an increased risk of respiratory illnesses can be associated with environmental factors, as well as general health. Lissauer and Clayden (2006) state that these factors can include overcrowding and damp housing conditions, poor nutritional status, prematurity, smoking and congenital abnormalities of a baby's/child's heart and lungs.

Health promotion information related to signs and symptoms

Initially, during the session the signs and symptoms of mild respiratory illness are explored together with parents. In pairs parents identify the signs and symptoms (pairs activity). The nurse then discusses the results from this activity together with the group as a whole, using a flip chart to highlight specific points made by parents.

Some of the following signs and symptoms are identified and discussed:

- Coughing (not present in young babies).
- High temperature.
- Loss of appetite.
- Runny nose.
- Tiredness.
- Sneezing.
- Sore throat Prodigy (2006c).

Not all these symptoms may necessarily present with each respiratory illness, which is pointed out to parents.

Parents then explore how their baby/child might feel with these symptoms. It is particularly highlighted that some babies may experience difficulty breathing and feeding due to a blocked nose (Lissauer and Clayden, 2006). The importance of continuing to give milk feeds, small amounts and often, is highlighted as a method of preventing babies from becoming dehydrated. Coordinating breathing, feeding and swallowing can be difficult for babies when their noses are blocked; therefore, feeding small amounts frequently may make feeding a little easier.

Parents generally seem happy to talk about the signs and symptoms of mild respiratory infections. Invariably, their baby or child has been unwell with a mild respiratory illness, so they have experiences to share.

With mild respiratory illnesses, parents worry about specific symptoms. Neill (2000), in her literature review on acute childhood illness at home, highlighted that persistent cough and fever were the symptoms that families were most concerned about. Experiences with the Sure Start community children's nursing service suggest the similar; parents worried about a persistent cough and fever.

During the respiratory session parents are advised that most of the symptoms will seem to be worse during the first 2–3 days, but will gradually clear up (Prodigy, 2006c). However, it is not unusual for the cough to last several weeks.

Health promotion information related to care and management

The aim of care and management is to help ease the symptoms, particularly to make breathing as easy as possible for the baby or young child.

As part of the session parents are asked to consider what the key aspects of care might be in relation to the symptoms. Information is then presented. Key points on care and management are listed below. They include the following:

- Observations of baby's/child's condition, particularly breathing.
- Making breathing easier.
- If temperature is raised, lowering the temperature (fever).
- Ease pain, if present.
- Maintaining hydration.

- Avoidance of passive smoking.
- Information on what to do if the baby's/child's condition becomes more serious.

Observations

Parents are encouraged to be vigilant, observing their baby's/child's breathing and colour. If parents become worried they are advised to contact local medical or nursing services for help and advice. Details of these are provided, including NHS Direct. The signs and symptoms of a baby/child deteriorating with a respiratory illness are discussed during the session.

Making breathing easier

Techniques can be discussed with parents about how to make breathing easier for their baby or child.

Decongestants are one option. These can be obtained from the pharmacist. Decongestants help to provide relief for several hours (BNF for Children, 2007), making breathing easier. There are restrictions associated with age, particularly in babies under 3 months (BNF for Children, 2007). Parents are advised to check with their pharmacist for advice.

Nursing the baby/child on a gently raised tilt when resting can help with breathing. Raise the baby's/child's head and shoulders very slightly, by gently tilting the upper end of the mattress. Appropriate support and safety, while on a raised tilt, always need to be considered. A child can also play sitting up, rather than lying down, which can help to make breathing easier too (Sure Start and NED PCT, 2006).

High temperature

For details and advice about managing a high temperature, consult Chapter 12.

Easing pain from a sore throat

A young child will sometimes complain of pain from a sore throat. If the child indicates she/he has a sore throat, medication can be given to ease pain and make swallowing easier. Paracetamol or ibuprofen can be used for pain relief (BNF for Children, 2007). Advise parents to always read the instructions given with the medication. Advise parents to never give more than the stated (or prescribed) dose appropriate for their child's age.

For a child with a sore throat soft foods can also be given. Ice cream, jelly and yoghurts tend to go down well. Children may particularly enjoy having something cool and refreshing.

Maintain hydration

The importance of maintaining a baby's/child's hydration is emphasised. Parents are advised to offer plenty of drinks, small amounts and often. If there are problems drinking, advise parents to offer their child's favourite drinks, or even ice lollies.

Avoidance of passive smoking

Passive smoking can exacerbate coughing and respiratory illness (Walmsley, 2003). It is important to protect babies from passive smoke, particularly those who are vulnerable to respiratory illnesses. Encourage families to smoke away from the baby or child or even better still to stop smoking altogether. Stopping smoking is often not a popular topic with parents. However, it is an issue that needs to be raised, particularly in relation to children's respiratory illnesses. A baby/child who lives with a smoker has an increased risk of developing coughs and colds (Prodigy, 2006a).

Symptoms becoming more serious

It is important to highlight to parents what to look out for if a mild respiratory illness is developing into something more serious. Parents should seek help from health care services – GP practice, for example. If out of hours, parents should contact their GP's *out-of-hours* service or NHS Direct for advice.

If the baby's/child's health is seriously deteriorating, advise parents/carers to attend A + E. If the baby/child is having breathing difficulties, advise parents/carers to call an ambulance.

When a respiratory infection is becoming much worse, Lissauer and Clayden (2006) maintain that some of the following signs and symptoms may be present. These are discussed with parents, so they know what to look out for:

- Raised respiratory rate.
- Increased heart rate.
- Agitation.
- Tiredness.
- Change in child's colour – may be pale or grey.

- Drawing in of the chest – sternal recession and subcostal and intercostal recession may be present.

Written literature is provided to support much of the information given verbally in the session. Cards are provided with the NHS Direct telephone number on. Parents are advised to keep the card in a safe place, so they can access it when needed. The teaching plan included outlines how this respiratory session is undertaken with parents (Box 13.1).

Parents' choice – more serious illnesses

Parents are able to select a variety of health topics for discussion on the course. If there are particular child health issues they need to know about, the nurse will provide that information. In some cases, where the subject is one that the nurse feels may be more appropriate for someone else to teach, an expert can be called upon. One group wanted to know about children going into hospital for minor surgery, for example. A children's nurse from the local hospital came along to discuss the care of young children on the surgical ward. Parents found this helpful, as some of their children were due to undergo surgical procedures.

Meningitis and septicaemia (not minor illnesses)

Although meningitis and septicaemia are *not* minor illnesses, nurses teaching the minor illness course found that parents had real concerns and wanted to know more. Parents wanted to know what they should be looking out for, and what they could do. The health promotion course seemed an ideal opportunity to provide them with this important information, raising their awareness.

Meningitis and septicaemia can kill within hours (Diggle and Glennie, 2005). Meningitis is a term used to describe swelling of the meninges that surround the brain and spinal cord. Septicaemia (also known as blood poisoning) occurs when bacteria in the bloodstream multiply rapidly and cause infection (Meningitis Trust, 2006).

Meningitis and septicaemia can strike at any age, but mainly affect babies, small children/young people (Diggle and Glennie, 2005), so pertinent information for our parents. Meningitis and septicaemia can be associated with mortality and long-term morbidity problems, such as deafness and intellectual impairment (Diggle and Glennie, 2005). Children can be left with permanent disabilities, but recovery can occur too.

Importantly, some forms of meningitis can be prevented through immunisation. Parents need to be aware of this.

If meningitis is suspected the child should immediately go to hospital by the quickest means of transport available, which may be a 999 ambulance. Ambulance staff do need to know that meningitis/septicaemia is suspected (Diggle and Glennie, 2005).

If the child is attending a GP surgery, antibiotics may be given before the child goes to hospital. Pre-admission antibiotics have been known to save lives (Diggle and Glennie, 2005).

Common signs and symptoms of meningitis are as follows:

- Fever.
- Refusing food or vomiting.
- Fretful.
- Pale, blotchy skin.
- Fontanelle may be bulging.
- Spots.
- Listless/drowsy.
- Unusual cry.

Signs and symptoms of septicaemia are as follows:

- Fever, cold hands and feet.
- Refusing food or vomiting.
- Pale, blotchy skin.
- Irritable.
- Rash, red or purple spots/bruises that do not fade under pressure (glass test).
- Floppy/listless.
- Rapid breathing.
- Drowsy/difficult to wake (Meningitis Trust, 2006).

The glass test can be used to check if the rash is meningitis/septicaemia – using a clear glass, press

Box 13.1 Teaching plan for the session on mild upper respiratory infections.

Aim

Parents will have increased knowledge and skills in the management of mild upper respiratory infections in babies and young children.

Objective/outcome 1

Parents will be able to recognise the signs and symptoms of mild upper respiratory infections (colds and sore throats).

Content

The signs and symptoms of mild respiratory illness in babies and young children are discussed.

Method

Pairs activity
The groups share their thoughts on the signs and symptoms of mild upper respiratory illnesses in pairs. Their thoughts are noted on a flip chart and discussed further within the group.

Objective/outcome 2

Parents will be able to discuss the care and management of babies and young children, when they are unwell with a mild upper respiratory illness.

Content

Presentation of information on the care and management of babies and young children with mild upper respiratory illness.

Method

Talk with participation
Parents are asked questions about the care and management of babies/children with mild respiratory illness. Following parents' answers further details on care and management are provided.

Resources

Flip chart
Worksheets
Powerpoint
Handouts

Assessment of parents' learning

Game
Parents are able to test their knowledge and skills on respiratory illnesses with the use of a respiratory game that has been devised for the course (by Moyse and Surguy). They have to identify the signs and symptoms that might be associated with different respiratory illnesses and the care that babies/children may need.

Group interaction
Parents' learning can also be assessed by observing how they demonstrate their knowledge through group interactions during the session.

Activity

Plan your own teaching session on minor illness management for young children, with parents in the community. Select a minor illness, gastroenteritis, for example, and put together a teaching session using the headings outlined below (the previous teaching plan may help):

- Aim.
- Objective/outcome.
- Content.
- Methods.
- Resources.
- Assessment of parents' learning.

the side of the glass against the skin. The rash will *not* fade if the infection is present (Meningitis Trust, 2006). As the Meningitis Trust urges, do not wait until the rash appears, as it may be the last sign to appear or in some cases it may not appear at all (Meningitis Trust, 2006). Importantly too, only some of the above signs and symptoms may be present, emphasize this to parents. Remember that prompt action can save lives.

When undertaking health promotion activities on raising awareness about meningitis/septicaemia, the Meningitis Trust may be able to help. They can provide information and health promotion resources. Sometimes they can provide a representative, who will discuss meningitis and septicaemia with parent groups.

The Meningitis Trust provides a wide range of resources – leaflets, booklets, as well as an advice line for help. Particularly interesting are their resources aimed at primary school children. Children can find out about meningitis through *Monty the Duck*. This is available via an interactive website – http://www.meningitis-learning.org. There is also a book – *When Monty Had Meningitis*. The book is written to help children understand the experience of meningitis/septicaemia and attending hospital (Meningitis Trust, 2006).

Preventing infectious diseases

Nurses delivering the minor illness course not only felt that it was important to present details on the

management of minor illnesses, but to discuss with parents how they could prevent their young children from becoming ill. There are a number of different ways illnesses can be prevented, and these were discussed with parents. This includes hand washing, encouraging a healthy diet, and ensuring that children have sufficient sleep.

The NSF (Education and Skills, Department of Health, 2004a) advocates the routine immunisation of children, as a really important way of preventing infectious diseases. Immunisation has certainly had a significant impact on preventing infectious diseases. Due to immunisation certain diseases are not so much in evidence today, compared to several decades ago. However, parents' perception of the seriousness of some diseases has declined. They may not have witnessed certain diseases and thus do not realise the dangers that they present. Consequently, they may be less inclined to immunise their children. This can be evidenced currently with the measles vaccination (measles, mumps and rubella, MMR). Some parents do not realise the dangers that measles can bring, particularly its side effects. They may fail to have their children immunised. Currently, there is a rise in the incidence of measles. Recent figures produced show that there have been significant reductions in the uptake of MMR vaccine. The Government is urging parents to give their children the MMR vaccine. During 2007 the first child death from measles for some years was reported in the UK.

The NSF states that health practitioners need to boost the uptake of MMR vaccine (Education and Skills, Department of Health, 2004a). The health promotion course is an ideal opportunity to promote young children's immunisations. Details are provided on the current immunisation schedule for young children (available from http://www.immunisation.nhs.uk), as well as responding to any concerns that parents may have about particular vaccines, such as the MMR vaccine. Parents are also referred to their health visitor for further advice, if needed.

The health promotion course can really encourage parents to share information. Some parents may have already given their child the MMR vaccine, and can discuss their experiences with other members of the group. On a number of occasions this helped to ease parental concerns about the effects of MMR vaccine.

Conclusion

This chapter has explored the development of a health promotion course on the management of young children's minor illnesses. The health promotion course has been a success in the local community for which it was developed. Creating similar courses in other communities may help to reduce some of the anxieties parents experience when their young children are ill, enabling them to feel more equipped to cope with the symptoms of minor illness.

The NSF for children/young people and maternity services asserts that parents should receive *information*, *advice* and *support* to enable them to *manage young children's minor illnesses* (Education and Skills, Department of Health, 2004a). Health promotion courses can help parents achieve this by empowering them with the knowledge to manage minor illnesses, but to also help them identify when they may need to seek further advice from health care services.

Resources

http://www.immunisation.nhs.uk
http://www.meningitis-learning.org
http://www.mmrthefacts.nhs.uk
http://www.cks.library.nhs.uk/home

References

BNF for Children (2007) London: BMJ Publishing Group Ltd. Royal Pharmaceutical Society of Great Britain, RCPCH Publications Ltd.

Carter, B., Dearmun, A. (1995) *Child Health Care Nursing, Concepts, Theory and Practice*. Oxford: Blackwell Science.

Concise Oxford Dictionary (1982) London: Guild Publishing.

Department of Health (2003) *External Working Group: The Acute Module Phase 2 – The Ill Child*. London: Department of Health.

Diggle, L., Glennie, L. (2005) Recognition and prevention of meningitis and septicaemia. *Community Practitioner* 78(2): 42–45.

Education and Skills (Department of), Department of Health (2004a) *National Service Framework for Children, Young People and Maternity Services*. London: Education and Skills, Department of Health.

Education and Skills (Department of), Department of Health (2004b) *National Service Framework for Children, Young People and Maternity Services – Ill Child*. London: Education and Skills, Department of Health.

Kai, J. (1996a) What worries parents when their preschool children are acutely ill, and why: a qualitative study. *British Medical Journal* 313: 983–986.

Kai, J. (1996b) Parents' difficulties and information needs in coping with acute illness in preschool children: a qualitative study. *British Medical Journal* 313: 987–990.

Lissauer, T., Clayden, G. (2006) *Illustrated Textbook of Paediatris*, 2nd edn. Edinburgh: Mosby.

Meningitis Trust (2006) *Understanding Meningitis, a Guide for Early Years Professionals*. Gloucestershire: Meningitis Trust.

Moyse, K. (2005) *Sure Start Community Children's Nursing: Evaluating the Service*. Derbyshire: Sure Start: Creswell, Langwith/Whaley Thorns and Shirebrook.

Neill, S. (2000) Acute childhood illness at home: the parents' perspective. *Journal of Advanced Nursing* 31(4): 821–832.

Prodigy (2006a) *Prodigy Guidance – Gastroenteritis*. Available at: http://www.prodigy.nhs.uk (accessed 11 April 2004).

Prodigy (2006b) *Prodigy Guidance – Urinary Tract Infection – Children*. Available at: http://www.prodigy.nhs.uk (accessed 9 April 2006).

Prodigy (2006c) *Prodigy Guidance – Sore Throat – Acute*. Available at: http://www.prodigy.nhs.uk (accessed 10 February 2006).

Sure Start (2000) *Sure Start: A Guide for 2nd Wave Programmes*. London: Sure Start.

Sure Start (2003/4) *Sure Start: Aim and Objectives*. London: Sure Start. Available at: http://www.surestart.co.uk.

Sure Start: Creswell, Langwith/Whaley Thorns and Shirebrook/North Eastern Derbyshire (NED) PCT (2006) *Health Promotion Literature: Managing Respiratory Ilness in Young Children*. Derbyshire: Sure Start, NED PCT.

Walmsley, C. (2003) *Sure Start Objective: To Improve Health*. Creswell: Sure Start.

14 Health Promotion in Minor Injuries

Karen Moyse and Chrissie Bousfield

NSF

The National Service Framework (NSF, standard 2, Education and Skills, Department of Health, 2004) highlights how parents/carers value support and advice on key health issues. Children experience minor injuries, particularly when they are young; therefore, parents/carers may value advice and support when their children experience minor injuries.

Introduction

Children, young children especially, are at risk of sustaining *minor injuries*. Young children are more at risk because of their development; they do not have the skills to avoid danger, and are not aware of what situations expose them to danger. Parents/carers need to supervise their young children, as well as making the environments where they play and inhabit as safe as possible. Older children and teenagers are at risk of minor injuries too. Nonetheless, they are more able to understand what situations may present themselves as dangerous, and how they might avoid an accident occurring.

Minor injuries need to be managed appropriately. Parents/carers, as well as older children/young people, may value advice on what to do should a minor injury occur. Health promotion has a role to

play, both in the prevention of minor injuries (see the chapter accident prevention) and the care of minor injuries themselves. Children's nurses can provide valuable advice in both situations.

This chapter focuses on minor injury care, but specifically relating its focus to one type of minor injury – a minor burn injury. This type of minor injury has been selected because it is something experienced by children, young children especially. The chapter also discusses how parents/carers can learn about the management of their young children's minor injuries, so they are prepared should an injury occur. Importantly too, older children/young people can be taught simple principles on how to care for minor injuries.

Minor injuries

A minor injury can be defined in the following way. Collins English Dictionary (1998) describes an injury as physical damage caused to a person, and minor as something small. A minor injury therefore, in this context, is some small damage caused to a child's skin, as in the case of a minor burn.

Children are naturally adventurous and have lots of energy (Paterson, 2002). This is something that perhaps as adults we forget from time to time. Children are keen to try new things. They are learning – testing their bodies, the environment, and what they can do and achieve in that environment. It is therefore not surprising that from time to time children experience injuries as a result of trying out new things. Children may unintentionally encounter different types of minor injuries, in their attempts to live life to the full.

Minor injuries are made up of many different types. The British Red Cross (2002) outlines some of these to include minor cuts, blisters, nose bleeds, minor burns or scalds, bruises and insect bites. All have the potential to become more serious, or to be serious within themselves, which the nurse must consider. A first-aid manual will provide details on how to care for a wide range of minor injuries.

When do nurses provide health promotion advice on minor injuries?

The nurse in her/his attempts to provide care and advice on the management of children's minor injuries will do so in different circumstances. This advice may be given at the time an injury occurs. It may also be in advance of an injury occurring, teaching others the skills to be able to assist an injured child.

Opportunistic health promotion can be provided too. Opportunistic advice is given in response to questions posed by parents, for example, during a contact on another health matter. Or as Hall and Elliman (2003) describe, the contact is initiated by parents for a purpose, and the practitioner or parents use the contact for additional information. This might include a request for health promotion advice on minor injury care, for example.

A nurse can provide minor injury advice both in hospital and community settings. In the community this advice might be given in the patient's home, at clinic, in schools, or as part of parenting classes.

Minor injuries – minor burns

A burn injury has been defined as a heat injury to the skin (Prodigy, 2004). A scald is a burn caused by moist heat, either steam or hot liquid (Blackwell's Nursing Dictionary, 2005). It should be remembered that burn and scald injuries not only cause physical damage, but have the potential to cause emotional distress for children.

A minor burn injury, as discussed here, can be calculated on the basis of type, depth and percentage body surface area of the burn, as well as the part of the body that is injured (Purcell, 2003). It might appear *superficial* with red, unbroken skin. Or *partial thickness* – blisters will be evident. When the blisters burst the underlying skin is pink and tender (Purcell, 2003).

There may be a combination of the above present. Remember it depends on the actual extent of the injury, which determines whether it is a minor injury or something more serious. It is always important to consider that the proportions of a child differ from those of an adult (Purcell, 2003). Assessing burn wounds is discussed later in the chapter.

Incidence

In 2002 there were almost 37 000 children under the age of 15 years in the UK who suffered from either burn or scald injuries, and the majority of these injuries happened to children under 5 years of age (28 000) (Child Accident Prevention Trust, CAPT, 2007).

The most common age for a young child to experience a burn injury is 1–2 years of age, with a boy/girl ratio of 3:2 (Bousfield, 2002). Scalds mainly occur in the under 4-year age group with both sexes being equally affected (Bousfield, 2002).

Ten per cent of all burn injuries happen to older children and teenagers between the ages of 5 and 14 years (Hettiaratchy and Dziewulski, 2004). Older boys are more likely than girls to suffer a burn, because of their tendency to engage in risk-taking behaviours (Bousfield, 2002).

Although major injuries are not the focus of this chapter, it is a useful reminder to consider the danger that some burns can present. In 2005, 18 children under 11 years died as result of house fires (CAPT, 2007).

Significantly, in recent years burn injuries have been declining due to the use of smoke detectors and low flammability clothing (Bousfield, 2002). There is also a move away from the use of open fires as a form of heating due to central heating (Bousfield, 2002). However, in some parts of the UK, open coal fires may remain the main source of heating, particularly in some rural communities.

Like many other health issues, poverty is a related factor. There is an association between burn injuries and children living in poverty. Children in the lower social classes are more likely to experience burns than those in the higher social classes (Bousfield, 2002). Living in cramped conditions and family stress can all contribute to the risk of a burn occurring.

Health promotion campaigns

Children under 5 years, as highlighted, are at increased risk and thus form the key target group for health promotion campaigns on preventing burns and scalds (Department for Trade and Industry, 1999). Health promotion campaigns feature on an ongoing basis, as there is a continual need to remind everyone of the dangers.

Health promotion campaigns can make an important contribution. Hettiaratchy and Dziewulski (2004) highlight the success of a number of health promotion campaigns in recent years, and suggest repetition is essential in the effort to prevent burns and scalds. Although, they do point out that the success of any campaign really depends on individuals changing their behaviour, which may not always happen (Hettiaratchy and Dziewulski, 2004).

A health promotion campaign on the prevention of scald injuries is currently underway. Hot liquids cause 70% of scald injuries to children, with hot drinks being the most common offender (CAPT, 2007). Hot drinks close to young children can be hazardous, great care needs to be taken. It is very easy for a toddler, or even a baby in some cases depending on age, to reach out and pull a mug of hot tea or coffee, causing the drink to spill and a scald injury to result. It is essential that parents and carers place hot drinks well out of the reach of babies and young children. CAPT, with the support of the DTI, is organising a campaign called – *Fancy a cuppa? Preventing hot drink scalds in babies and young children*. CAPT (2002) produces a very useful leaflet, which accompanies the campaign. Video and further information can be obtained to support any work practitioners might be undertaking in association with the campaign.

Case study

Burn or scald injuries, when they occur, can be very distressing for young children. It is important that strong efforts are made to prevent them. A case study will be presented here, which will enable you to explore and reflect on caring for a young child with a minor burn injury.

Young children are at risk of burns if they are in contact with heaters, open fires, candles and cookers, for example (CAPT, 2007). Hair straightens are a more recent cause of burn injuries due to current trends in hair fashion.

The case presented here highlights the situation wherein a young child who, following close contact with an open fire, sustains a minor burn injury. Safety devices can protect children from such dangers. Where there is an open fire in the home, a fireguard is going to be an essential purchase. The Department for Trade and Industry (1999) advises using a fixed fireguard to prevent children touching or getting close to a fire. Fireguards are available on loan or at reduced cost in many local communities. Nurses can advise families about where and how to obtain fireguards.

Activity

As a community children's nurse, working in an acute care role, you are asked to see a young child who has just sustained a burn injury. Sally, a 2-year-old, has burnt a small area of her arm on an unguarded fire at home.

Think about the care she might need, first-aid management and continued care. What health promotion advice are you going to give, both in terms of caring for the burn itself and home safety? Write your thoughts in response to this case and see where they lead you.

The following two frameworks might be useful for guiding your thinking. The first introduces a framework which can be used when reflecting upon practice. The second provides a framework for care.

With the reflection framework, *reflective care*, the headings are there simply to guide your thinking. They not only allow you to consider the care provided, but also to consider that care critically. Essentially, you are reflecting upon practice. Johns (2003) believes that reflection is able to provide a valuable cognitive problem-solving approach to practice. Reflection can be really helpful in this way, so give it a go.

Reflective care:

- Practice situation.
- Care and management (care given and why).
- Reflection on care and management (critically considered).
- Recommendations for future practice (key points).

When thinking about *recommendations for future practice* – what aspects of care provided in this situation, would you consider using again? A few key points may only be needed, focusing on your new learning.

The second framework, *principles of care* (Bousfield, 2002), guides you through the different stages of care. Apply this framework as subheadings within your *care and management* section of the previous framework. Bousfield (2002) asserts that with a burn injury there are certain principles of care that need to be followed; these are outlined below:

- First-aid management.
- Pain assessment – analgesia and comfort.
- Assessment of the injury (including social factors involved).
- Wound care.
- Infection control.
- Follow-up.

Care and management (care given and why)

The following notes provide you with some pointers on caring for Sally in relation to the principles outlined above. Read these carefully before completing the activity.

First-aid management

Appropriate first-aid management needs to be undertaken. This will consist of cooling the burn immediately under gentle cold running water for 10 minutes (British Red Cross, 2002). This can be continued for up to 20 minutes, particularly as it reduces pain and swelling, as well as cleansing the wound by removing harmful substances (Hudspith and Rayatt, 2004). Cooling removes heat and prevents progression of the burn (Hudspith and Rayatt, 2004).

Cooling is effective if performed within 20 minutes of the injury (Hudspith and Rayatt, 2004). Note the use of topical creams should be avoided at this stage as they may interfere with assessment of the injury. Cooling gels may be used to relieve pain in the early stages.

The injury may be superficial, and thus can be treated by the nurse at home. However, it may be more appropriate for Sally to attend the emergency department at the local hospital depending on the seriousness of the injury and how Sally is reacting.

If Sally needs to attend hospital, cling film is an ideal first-aid cover for the burn (Hudspith and Rayatt, 2004). It acts as a temporary barrier, protecting the skin, until such time when it can be appropriately treated. Cling film is non-adherent so will minimise pain to exposed nerve endings. Further, its transparent nature allows the wound to be observed. Consider what alternatives you might use if cling film is not available.

The following provides information in relation to Sally's continued care, using Bousfield's (2002) principles of care.

Pain assessment – analgesia and comfort

To help Sally feel more comfortable she will need pain relief. Paracetamol syrup or ibuprofen suspension can be given for the management of pain in children (BNF for Children, 2007). The community children's nurse may be a nurse prescriber, and will thus be able to prescribe pain-relieving medication (analgesia). Consider how you can help Sally take her medicine, obviously with her parents' involvement. Sally may not be keen to take it, as sometimes happens (see Chapter 25).

How you communicate with Sally and her family is going to make an important difference to how they deal with the situation. A comforting cuddle from a parent is going to be especially important to Sally at this time, along with the company of her favourite toy. A calm but guiding approach from the nurse will be supportive for the whole family.

Assessment of the injury (including social factors involved)

The depth and extent of the burn injury must be assessed. Bousfield (2002) states that an estimate in terms of percentage can be calculated using a burn assessment chart developed by Wilson et al. (1987), which looks at percentage by age. Depth of the injury will be assessed using history, cause and appearance of wound, presence of blisters and sensation, which may require the expertise of hospital staff.

When assessing Sally, it is also essential to find out if she is suffering from any other injuries or illnesses (Hudspith and Rayatt, 2004). The nurse does not want to overlook anything.

Importantly too, how did the injury occur? The nurse must ask this question. Was the injury accidental, or was it perhaps a non-accidental injury? If there are any doubts about explanations provided, contact the nurse specialist for safeguarding children, for further advice.

Wound care

Wound care is obviously going to be influenced by an accurate assessment of the wound itself and what it might need. If it is a fairly superficial wound, it will obviously need less input than something that is more serious.

The aim of wound care is to protect the wound from infection and to promote a moist environment for wound healing. Hudspith and Rayatt (2004) maintain that a burn wound is essentially sterile and should be kept that way. Consider how you are going to keep it clean, and what you might need to achieve this.

There is some controversy about the management of blisters. If there are small blisters these should be left intact. Larger blisters, if present, might need to be deroofed and dead skin removed with sterile scissors (Hudspith and Rayatt, 2004). However, in this case there are no large blisters present.

A standard treatment for a minor burn might include the following:

● Application of a non/low-adherent primary dressing (which may include silicone dressings).
● Followed by an absorbent layer of gauze to soak up exudates.
● A bandage to secure.

There are many different types of dressings that can be used. In determining the type of dressing, consider where the burn injury is located on the child's body, as this will be influencing factor. Limb burns should be elevated to minimise swelling.

Infection control

The wound will need to be observed for any signs of infection. Some sources advocate the use of antibiotics in children prophylactically to prevent toxic shock syndrome (Bousfield, 2002).

Follow-up

The wound will need to be reviewed, and the dressing will need replacing. The recommended time for a dressing change is 48 hours following injury (Hudspith and Rayatt, 2004). However, the dressing should be changed immediately if the wound becomes painful, smelly or wet. Dressing changes thereafter will depend on the product used and the healing rate of the wound. Note any burn not healed within 2 weeks should be referred to the plastic surgery unit. Remember too that encouraging a young child to keep a dressing on can be quite challenging.

Healed burns become dry and scaly; to aid relief, application of a moisturizing cream is encouraged. Once the burn has healed, it is really important to emphasise that it is kept out of the sun due to a loss of pigmentation from the skin.

Additional points

Record keeping, as always, is essential aspect of care. Consider how you are going to document in Sally's nursing record. Do not forget details to include in the parent-held record as well, so parents can remind themselves about Sally's care. The Nursing and Midwifery Council (NMC, 2004) discusses the importance of accurate record keeping by all nurses.

In the future patient records will be computerised. The Department of Health is promoting electronic patient records in health care settings. In the community, for example, nurses will be able to access a summary of the child's general practitioner record (Hall and Elliman, 2003). For community nurses this will help with prescribing and keeping up to date with the child's health care.

The above principles of care (Bousfield, 2002) with related information are there to help guide your thinking, both for first management and continued care. Determine from the outset characteristics of the wound, so you are clear about the type of burn injury you are dealing with. Is it superficial or is it superficial with some partial thickness areas?

When looking through the literature to find out more information, do not be surprised to learn that there are different perspectives on the same issues, which make clarity difficult. To discover more about the management of burn injuries, discuss with your local emergency department, or if there is one close by, a burns unit.

Health promotion advice for parents/carers

Parents/carers can be prepared for their young children experiencing accidents and learn how to manage minor injuries should they occur. Obviously, preventing accidents in the first instance would be better. This section provides information that will help when teaching parents/carers about managing young children's minor injuries.

Literature sources

There are a variety of literature sources that parents/carers might consult:

- *Birth to Five* book.
- The NHS Direct self-help guide.
- Leaflets on minor injury care/accident prevention.
- *First Aid for Children Fast* (British Red Cross publication).

Birth to Five book

The *Birth to Five* book is produced by the Department of Health (2006). It is issued to first-time parents when their baby is a few weeks old, usually by health visitors. It provides practical advice on a wide range of health issues.

NHS Direct self-help guide

NHS Direct, which provides a telephone helpline service on health 24 hours a day (http://www.nhsdirect.nhs.uk), also produces a self-help guide. The guide gives advice on the management of symptoms of illness and injury in children, as well as adults (NHS Direct, 2003). It contains information on what to do if a child has experienced an accident, and how to initially manage any injuries that result.

Leaflets on minor injury care/accident prevention

When a child attends a hospital or community health service requiring an injury to be treated, written information can be given to accompany care and verbal health promotion advice given. Written information is usually available in the form of leaflets. These leaflets include information on how to care for the injury, as well as details on what complications to look out for.

First Aid for Children Fast (British Red Cross publication)

This is a great little book that provides clear injury guidance. It is very user-friendly, enabling the reader to find relevant information quickly, when needed.

Courses and advice

Courses

There are a variety of different courses that parents/carers might find useful to access. First-aid courses are available through different organisations, such as St John's Ambulance or the British Red Cross. Sometimes local children's centres are able to provide first-aid courses for parents/carers, which focus specifically on the first-aid care of young children.

Health visitors/school nurses/practice nurses

Many community nurses will be happy to provide advice on the care of children's minor injuries. Contact the local health centre or general practitioner practice for information.

Health promotion advice for older children

Older children/young people themselves may value advice on preventing minor injuries and what to do if they find themselves in a situation where a friend needs help. Here we will consider middle years children, 8–11 years.

Children in this age group are able to think and understand how accidents can be prevented, as well as what care may initially help. Due to increased cognitive growth, their thinking is more logical and they have a greater ability to remember. Cole et al. (2005) discuss how their behaviour changes to reflect this; they are becoming more independent and are able to be more responsible. When teaching this age group about minor injuries, Bousfield (2002) suggests the use of drawings, diagrams and simple explanations as useful techniques.

Healthy schools

School nurses have a really important role to play in promoting the health of children/young people in school. The Government has particularly highlighted the role of the school nurse in its strategy to encourage schools to become *healthy schools*. The Government believes schools should discuss their health priorities with their school nurses (Department of Health, 2005). Healthy schools are about helping children to develop healthy behaviours. The Government believes that by focusing on health in schools, this can promote children's health (Department of Health, 2005). Accident prevention could be an area that school nurses might like to take forward within their schools. Accident prevention is about promoting the safety of children, helping to prevent injuries. Information on the management of minor injuries could be introduced.

Literature sources

Sometimes when teaching health promotion to children, it can be difficult getting explanations just at the right level. To help support any teaching, have a look at the Usborne Pocket Scientist Series (Usborne, 2001). Featured within this series is a section on *what makes you ill?* The section includes details on what happens when children cut or burn themselves. These books are specifically written for children. They are well illustrated, contain simple explanations and have internet links (with safety warnings). Children will find them a really useful resource.

First-aid courses for children

Children's first-aid courses can be useful too. They can be put together to be used either in schools, or in leisure situations, such as Brownies (badge activities). The nurse needs to make the teaching sessions short, interactive and fun, which can help to maintain children's interest. Discuss children's own experiences of minor injuries. They are often keen to share their experiences. It also enables them to put the subject into some sort of context.

Remember to explore how to avoid accidents, removing themselves from danger, calling for help if in trouble, as well as the first-aid treatment of some minor injuries. Consider what is appropriate and safe to teach them. Children are keen to know how to help, especially girls, perhaps budding nurses of the future.

Conclusion

There are many types of minor injuries, which need to be cared for in different ways. This chapter has considered one aspect of minor injury care – the care of a minor burn injury. Health promotion advice and care on minor injury management is a wide remit, where information frequently changes. The nurse needs to work hard to keep up her/his knowledge and skills up to date. Advice about the management of minor injuries can provide valuable support for parents/carers. As children become older they may find such health promotion information useful too. Importantly, being prepared, should a minor injury occur, not only helps to advance an individual's knowledge and skills, but means that the individual is able to care for and help an injured child.

References

Blackwell's Nursing Dictionary (2005) 2nd edn. Oxford: Blackwell Publishing.

BNF for Children (BNFC) (2007) London: BMJ Publishing Group Ltd. Royal Pharmaceutical Society, RCPCH Publications.

Bousfield, B.C. (ed.) (2002) *Burn Trauma Management and Nursing Care*, 2nd edn. London: Whurr Publishing.

British Red Cross (2002) *First Aid for Children Fast. Emergency Procedures for All Parents and Carers*. London: Dorling Kindersley Book.

CAPT (2002) *Fancy a Cuppa?* London: Child Accident Prevention Trust, Department of Trade and Industry.

CAPT (2007) *Burns and Scalds*. London: Child Accident Prevention Trust.

Cole, M., Cole, S., Lightfoot, C. (2005) *The Development of Children*, 5th edn. New York: Worth Publishers.

Collins English Dictionary (1998) Glasgow: Harper Collins.

Department for Trade and Industry (1999) *Government Consumer Safety Research, Burns and Scald Accidents within the Home*. London: Department for Trade and Industry.

Department of Health (2005) *National Healthy Schools Status*. London: Crown Copyright.

Department of Health (2006) *Birth to Five*. Available at: http://www.doh.gov.uk (accessed 18 June 2007).

Education and Skills (Department of), Department of Health (2004) *National Service Framework for Children, Young People and Maternity Services. Standard 2 – Supporting Parents*. London: Education and Skills, Department of Health.

Hall, D., Elliman, D. (eds) (2003) *Health for All Children*, 4th edn. Oxford: Oxford University Press.

Hettiaratchy, S., Dziewulski, P. (2004) ABC of burns. *BMJ* 328: 1366–1368.

Hudspith, J., Rayatt, S. (2004) ABC of burns. First aid and treatment of minor burns. *BMJ* 328: 1487–1489.

Johns, C. (2003) *Becoming a Reflective Practitioner*. Oxford: Blackwell Publishing.

NHS Direct (2003) *The NHS Direct Self-Help Guide*. Leeds: NHS Direct. Available at: http://www.nhsdirect.nhs.uk (accessed 18 June 2007).

NMC (2004) *Code of Professional Conduct*. London: Nursing and Midwifery Council.

Paterson, G. (2002) In: British Red Cross (2002) *First Aid for Children Fast. Emergency Procedures for All Parents and Carers*. London: Dorling Kindersley Book.

Prodigy (2004) *Prodigy Guidance: Burns and Scalds*. Available at: http://www.prodigy.nhs.uk (accessed 9 April 2006).

Purcell, D. (2003) *Minor Injuries: A Clinical Guide for Nurses*. Edinburgh: Churchill Livingstone.

Usborne (2001) *Usborne Pocket Scientist Series – the Blue Book*. London: Usborne Publishing.

Wilson, G., Fowler, C., Housden, P. (1987) A new burn assessment chart. *Burns* 13: 401–405.

Theme 5

Children/Young People in Hospital

Chapter 15   Health Promotion for Pre- and Postoperative Care
Chapter 16   Surgical Wound Healing and Health Promotion
Chapter 17   Planning Hospital Discharge

15 Health Promotion for Pre- and Postoperative Care

Julie Spice and Annette Dearmun

NSF

The National Service Framework (NSF) outlines standards for the care of children/young people in hospital (Department of Health, 2003). Children/young people and their families receiving surgical interventions need appropriate health promotion information, so they can plan and participate in decisions about their care.

Introduction

It could be argued that on the surface, largely as a result of technological advance, children are in better physical health now than in the past. Furthermore, although there are more children with complex needs, the quality of life and health for these children is also much improved and many are surviving into adulthood. The surgical interventions available to address a wide range of medical conditions are increasingly sophisticated. The average length of stay in hospital for children has been reduced, with many surgical procedures performed as day cases.

Despite these improvements there are still reported inequalities and it was to address these that in 2004 the NSF for children/young people (Education and Skills and Department of Health, 2004)

was published. The NSF laid down consistent standards for service provision. The main aims were as follows:

- To improve services.
- To address inequalities.
- To enhance the partnerships between professionals working with children and their families.

It was envisaged that by introducing standards some of the inequalities between advantaged and disadvantaged families, different ethnic groups and geographical locations, would be reduced.

The first standard, focusing on the experience of children in hospital (Department of Health, 2003), addressed three main aspects:

- The provision of child-centred services.
- Attention to quality and safety of care.
- The importance of the quality of setting and environment.

Each of these themes has been used to provide the basis for this chapter.

It is essential that when children/young people are to undergo surgery that they are in optimal health in order to aid healing and recovery. In both elective and emergency situations particular measures can be taken to promote the health of the child. This chapter discusses the ways in which nurses, as advocates for children, young people and their families, are able to promote health in its broadest sense. Throughout this discourse the particular focus will be upon practical examples and the role that health practitioners can play in promoting the health of children/young people prior to, during and after surgery.

It is commonly recognised that a child's admission to hospital for surgery can create many stresses and anxieties, both for the child and their family. There are a number of measures which can be taken to minimise these, including organising care in order to enhance a sense of *normality*, encouraging parents to be with their child during critical events and reducing length of stay, thereby returning the child to familiar surroundings as quickly as possible. Overall, the goal of care should be to deliver services according to the child's needs. To this end it is important that the focus is upon the *whole child*, rather than just her/his medical condition. Health promotion and prevention of ill health will be an integral part of this package of care.

Child-centred services

A fundamental aspect of health promotion, before and after surgery, is providing a child-centred service, and this will mean working in partnership with the child/young person and their family within a philosophy of *family-centred care*. It is anticipated that through promoting activities which enhance family-centred care and partnership at every available opportunity, services will be improved and in turn this will optimise health. Therefore, within this section the main themes of child and family-centred care in relation to preoperative assessment and information sharing and the use of play will be explored.

Family-centred care

The philosophy of family-centred care has long been recognised as an essential part of nursing children. There are several espoused models, but in all of these the child and family are the central focus (Audit Commission, 1993; Nethercott, 1993; Coyne, 1996). The degree of involvement that the child and family have, may largely depend on their in-

dividual needs. Appropriately qualified staff, using a holistic approach, will be able to identify these needs and empower the child and family to make informed choices. This assessment can be best achieved within a child-friendly environment and rely on health practitioners having a particular understanding of children and the knowledge, skills and aptitude to work effectively with them. The following list includes factors which nurses working with children need to consider when assessing the child and family's needs:

- The child's age.
- Their stage of cognitive, moral and emotional development.
- Whether the admission is planned or as an emergency.
- The knowledge the child and family already have regarding the child's admission.
- The willingness of the child and family to engage with the staff.
- The child and family's previous experience of hospital.

Whether an admission is for a planned procedure or an emergency, the child and their family are likely to experience a degree of stress and anxiety. In addition to the strategies mentioned previously, involving them and empowering them to make choices may also reduce anxiety and promote optimal recovery. Although generally the move towards a reduction in the average length of stay in hospital is positive, it may have implications for those caring for the child – who will need to look after their child during the convalescence period at home? For this reason it is important that families are given sufficient information and support to prepare them for this. Preoperative assessment carried out as part of a pre-admission programme offers a useful opportunity not only to assess fitness for surgery, but also to explore any issues relating to aftercare.

Preoperative assessment

There is evidence that preoperative assessment is one of the most valuable ways to assess needs prior to admission, thereby reducing the risk of postoperative morbidity and mortality, addressing concerns (Janke et al., 2002) and laying down plans for discharge home. Using this opportunity to assess the child's health prior to surgery, the potential risks are identified, information is shared, plans are made to address the individual child's needs and discharge planning is commenced. These strategies will aid postoperative recovery and ensure length of stay is kept to a minimum. This will be an advantage to both the individual and organisation.

Within the framework for assessing the child's health, in addition to the focus on a child's physical needs, their social, emotional and spiritual needs are also acknowledged as being of equal importance. Pre-admission programmes which incorporate pre-assessment (including clinical assessment and history taking) have been developed to help assess and meet these individual needs prior to elective surgery. There are many different programmes available. These range from a telephone conversation to a visit to the hospital prior to surgery. When the child, young person and family are able to attend a pre-admission session, they can familiarise themselves with the environment and meet some of the staff who will be caring for them.

The overall aim is to provide an opportunity to share information relevant to the operation in advance of surgery. A member of staff will make a comprehensive assessment of the child's health and family's needs; supply relevant, written and verbal information; identify concerns the child or family may have; identify other members of the multidisciplinary team who may need to be involved prior to surgery and, where necessary, liaise with them.

Historically, these assessments were undertaken by junior doctors, but in contemporary practice this is often undertaken by experienced nurses. Evidence suggests that doctors tended to assess the child's physical fitness for surgery, whereas nurses use a more holistic approach (Rushforth et al., 2000). An example of the benefits of preoperative assessment in relation to health promotion is discussed later in this chapter.

There may be a number of reasons why the child, young person and family are unable to visit the hospital prior to surgery. Many procedures take place in specialist centres and families have a distance to travel. It may be an emergency procedure or there may be insufficient notice of the impending admission date; parents/carers may not be able to take time away from work or they may be reluctant to visit the hospital in case they cause more anxiety to their child.

In some of the specialist children's hospitals in conjunction with telephone contact, the internet is used to provide comprehensive information. The limitations of this are recognised, not least, it is seldom possible to speak with the child; thus easier to conceal anxieties. It is not possible to observe the child and therefore features such as obesity are not identified. However, parental fears and anxieties may be identified through careful phrasing of questions.

So far the focus has been on children admitted for elective procedures, but there are some strategies which can be used to prepare children in advance for an unexpected admission to hospital; for example, nurses can visit schools, playgroups and other organisations in order to give general information to groups of children. Depending on the education provision in hospital, it may be possible to organise school visits to the hospital school as part of key stage 1 skills, and therefore age-appropriate health promotion can be included in the visit. However, there will still be a need to prepare the individual child for impending surgery.

Play

Play is a natural part of a child's development. Through play, a child may be able to express their fears (even when they are unable to verbalise them), rehearse life events and debrief afterwards. Most pre-admission programmes offer children the opportunity to learn about the admission through educative and therapeutic play. Visual aids including books, pictures and videos, rehearsal by dressing up in theatre gowns and visiting the relevant departments are all examples of ways in which children may be prepared for their experience. The preoperative assessment will have identified the child's concerns, and these may include being in pain, needle phobia, disfigurement following surgery, or they may have misunderstandings from information previously attained from family members or the media. The fear of needles is a good example of a concern, which can be overcome through play, coupled with the use of topical anaesthetic creams or spray. Many hospitals have play specialists trained to work with children to help them overcome their fears through play.

When a child's emotional needs are addressed preoperatively, this will contribute to their general recovery postoperatively. All staff working with children should have knowledge of age-appropriate play and preparation techniques (Chambers and Jones, 2007).

The needs of the child, young person and their family are paramount to the care they receive. They will be better able to make choices about their treatment if they receive appropriate information and are involved at all stages. When their fears and anxieties are identified, addressed and accurate, evidence-based information has been given, this will minimise actual and potential risks, enhance recovery, facilitate early discharge planning, reduce the child's length of stay and promote health.

Information sharing

The information given to the child, young person and family should take into account their age and cognitive development. Although young children may not have sufficient level of understanding to be able to consent for the operation, they can still make choices, which will allow them to have some control. For example, whether they want medicine in liquid or tablet form, what teddy they will take to theatre or how they will travel to theatre, on the bed, walk or via other forms of transport available in the hospital. Older children may wish to have more detailed information about the operation and be more concerned about pain or altered body image. Whatever the age of the child, these differences are best addressed by appropriate staff who have the knowledge and skills to work with children/young people.

Another important aspect of information sharing is to gain information about other significant life events which may have an impact on the health and well-being of the child or other family members. Wherever possible the date of surgery should take these into account; for example, important examinations, family illness which may affect the ability of the parents to care for the child postoperatively, pregnancy, the care of other children, planned holidays. For these and many other issues, postponement of surgery may need to be considered.

Discharge planning should commence at the preoperative assessment stage, thus ensuring the child spends a minimum amount of time in hospital. Informing the parents/carers will allow them to prepare their own plan of care. They may need to arrange time away from work or enlist the help of other family members or friends to be available to care for siblings during the child's stay in hospital and on return home. As part of the process of assessment, physiotherapists or occupational therapists may be required to do a home assessment prior to surgery to determine the need for specific equipment, for example, the temporary use of a hoist.

Staff caring for children and families should have a comprehensive knowledge of consent, ensuring assent/consent has been obtained from the child and/or their legal guardian, and that all the risks have been discussed. Formal consent is usually obtained by the clinician or a member of the team performing the operation. Informed consent can be provided by any member of the multi-professional team caring for the child, and the permission of the child should be sought prior to undergoing any procedure.

Several examples of good practice which benefit children and their families have been highlighted in this section including the use of pre-assessment programmes, joint working with schools and the hospital. There is evidence that if the child and family are the central focus through individualised preoperative assessment, information sharing and play, it is more likely that the child will have a positive experience of their hospital stay. This in turn will aid recovery, enable timely discharge and ensure the child resumes their normal activities at the earliest opportunity.

Quality and safety of care provided

Hospitals have a duty to provide safe care to children, young people and families by employing appropriately qualified staff. This section discusses the association that clinical governance, pain and medicines management have in relation to promoting health in the pre- and postoperative setting.

Clinical governance

The quality of service and care children receive in hospital is audited by the Healthcare Commission

(Healthcare Commission, 2007). Auditing will highlight a hospital's performance in the deliverance of care to children undergoing surgical procedures.

The audit assesses the number of staff, including medical staff trained in basic life support, safeguarding children, the skills of the surgeons and anaesthetists, including the number of procedures performed on children in any 1 year. The aim is to establish if staff have sufficient exposure to practice to maintain their skills. Following the review, recommendations for developments or improvements to be made are fed back to individual trusts.

Such recommendations may include arranging child-specific theatre lists, networking with larger trusts to negotiate training for surgeons or referring children, particularly those under 2 years of age, to centres where there are appropriately skilled surgeons and anaesthetists. Every trust is responsible for ensuring that they respond to the recommendations in order to ensure quality in service delivery.

All staff caring for children, including doctors and anaesthetists, should produce evidence of recent training, especially in relation to safeguarding. This is important in order to minimise the adverse effects on the health of children whose maltreatment may go undetected by health practitioners. The enquiry into the death of Victoria Climbié in 2003 showed that health staff had failed to document their concerns or communicate with other agencies. Laming (2003) concluded that if staff had all been more aware of concerns, her untimely death may have been prevented.

Pain

Other training issues which emerged from the Healthcare Commission (2007) document include the need for all staff to be trained in the assessment and management of pain in children. Nurses have a responsibility to ensure a child's pain is managed effectively. The consequences of unrelieved pain can have a significant impact on the child's physical and psychological recovery postoperatively (Glasper and Richardson, 2006). There is a recognised link between pain and anxiety; preparing the child for a procedure can reduce this. A pain history should be obtained during the preoperative assessment or on admission, which will take into account the child's age and cognitive development, as well as the child's previous experiences of pain. Regular assessment of the child's pain, using appropriate age assessment tools, may enable the child to communicate the intensity of the pain more effectively. The nurse or parents/carers are thus less likely to make assumptions on the child's behalf. It would be useful to draw on the comprehensive guidelines which have been produced to help nurses recognise and assess pain in children (Royal College of Nursing, 1999).

Using the assessment as a basis, pain can be relieved using pharmacological and non-pharmacological approaches. Assessment of the type of analgesic drugs to be administered, via the appropriate route and according to the severity of pain, should be undertaken by nurses who have the skill and understanding of medicine management. Nurses administering medication should have an understanding of the side effects, contraindications and correct dose, based on the child's weight. The practitioner, usually the nurse, administering the medication is responsible for the safe and reliable administration of the medication (Nursing and Midwifery Council, 2007).

Communication within the multi-professional team will ensure this happens. Dosage of medication is usually calculated by weight; therefore, children should be weighed at pre-admission or on admission. When it is not possible to weigh the child on admission, for example, following trauma, a recognised formula can be used to estimate a child's approximate weight. This formula is age + 4 × 2.

Educating the child and family in pain management through verbal and written information and age-appropriate tools at all stages of their journey will empower them to make informed choices. This will improve their hospital experience, aid their recovery, thus promoting their health.

Equality of care

Another feature of the promotion of children's health pre- and postoperatively is related to providing a quality service to children, young people and their families, regardless of their ethnicity or area they live in. To ensure minimum standards are met, the quality and appropriateness of the service is audited annually (Department of Health, 2003; Royal College of Surgeons of England, 2007).

Quality of setting and environment

The health of children and families will be greatly enhanced if the environment is conducive to their needs. When considering the quality of the environment in relation to the promotion of health of children having surgery, attention should be paid to the emotional and physical safety of the child, young person and family. The appropriateness of the setting, nutritional requirements and specific health-related topics according to the age and developmental needs are areas for discussion within this section, all of which have an impact on the health of children.

Emotional safety

Children should only be admitted to hospital when it is absolutely necessary. Careful pre- and post-operative planning, including discharge planning at the earliest opportunity will prevent delayed discharge. This reduces potential psychological effects to the child and family. Child-friendly day care facilities should be developed wherever possible, and children undergoing elective surgery should have access to separate facilities away from adults and other children requiring emergency treatment (Royal College of Surgeons of England, 2007).

It is now unusual for children to be separated from their parents/carers for long periods. Over 50 years ago early pioneers, such as Bowlby (1951), recognised the traumatic effects that separation from their mothers had upon children. This culminated in the family-centred approaches, which are such a familiar feature of caring for children today. Facilities for families to stay are available in many hospitals. Encouraging a family member to be resident is integral in the promotion of children's health and emotional well-being.

Working within this philosophy, parental presence is a key feature and therefore it is important to address their needs throughout the hospital stay in order to enable them to contribute effectively, support their child and make informed decisions regarding care. Parental/carer presence may reduce the child's anxiety. By being present, parents/carers are able to support their child more effectively. For example, they are encouraged to accompany their

child to theatre. It is recognised that not every parent or carer feels able to do this. If, after discussion at pre-admission they wish to appoint another person to carry out this task and focus their attention on caring for their child after surgery, they should be fully supported in their decision.

Children should be nursed on wards appropriate for their age and stage of development (Department of Health, 2003); and particular attention should be paid to the needs of young people. Young people may not feel comfortable being cared for in an area decorated for babies and may prefer to be nursed with other young people of their own age. To this end many hospitals have designated areas for young people. If there is no young person's facility, they should be given the option about where they are cared for, in a children's ward or adult ward. Regardless of the setting they should have access to appropriately qualified staff with the skills and knowledge to care for their specific age-related needs.

Physical safety

Access to all children's departments should be secure and limited only to authorised personnel. In most hospitals the access to the children's department is regulated and there is closed circuit television in operation. All trusts are required to have safety and security policies and procedures in place, and these are regularly reviewed. Policies must include systems for protecting children from abduction and measures for preventing children from self-harming. On admission children and families should be made aware of the security measures. Consideration must be given to the safety of equipment and the provision of training for staff to enable them to operate it safely.

Toys and equipment should be age-appropriate and in good working order. For example, the environment where young children are nursed should not have toys with small parts, which children may swallow.

Fluids and nutrition

Assessment of a child's fluid and nutritional status should be undertaken at preoperative assessment or on admission because there is a positive link between optimal nutrition and recovery. Diet and fluids should be withheld prior to anaesthetic to prevent inhalation of stomach contents. The recommended time for fasting is 2 hours for fluids, 4 hours for milk-based products and 6 hours for food (Royal College of Nursing, 2005).

Young children are unable to understand the reason for fasting and are more likely to become fractious and are vulnerable to the effects of dehydration, so their period of fasting should be kept to minimum. This may be achieved by placing them first on the operating list.

An important part of the healing process is the resumption of diet and fluids. Fluids should be reintroduced as soon as possible postoperatively, unless there are contraindications. Small volumes of non-acidic fluid are preferable; once these are tolerated, food can be introduced. If there is to be a delay in recommencement of fluids, an intravenous infusion should be commenced prior to or during theatre. Children who have undergone tonsillectomy should be encouraged to take frequent, small amounts of diet and fluids to promote healing and prevent infection. Regular analgesia is advised to prevent poor diet and infection, which can lead to secondary bleeding several days following surgery. The dietary information and pain management is an important part of the preoperative assessment.

The diet offered to children/young people in hospital should be healthy, nutritious and appealing. Careful consideration should be given to the planning of children's menus, with children/young people included in the design of menus. Availability of *finger foods* can be as nutritionally balanced as a hot meal, particularly for toddlers who want to explore and feed themselves. Children with allergies and food intolerances should not be disadvantaged in their choice of meal. Food should be available for children at varying times of the day, especially post-surgery. Facilities should be available to ensure breastfeeding mothers are encouraged to eat regular nutritious meals whilst in hospital with their child.

Health promotion messages

A child's stay in hospital is an opportunity to discuss different health-related subjects, not necessarily associated with their reason for being there. Poster displays are one method of communicating messages. Seasonal topics such as road safety campaigns, sun safety and dangers of fireworks can be displayed in the department. Specific topics relevant to young people and parents, such as smoking cessation, drug and alcohol abuse, can also be displayed as posters or leaflets.

A particular health-related topic causing much concern across the nation currently is childhood obesity. There are increased risks associated with having surgery and an anaesthetic to children who are obese. Identifying children who are obese prior to surgery is one example of health promotion in pre- and postoperative management of children. One example of a health trust addressing this issue is described here.

All children attending preoperative assessment have their height, weight and body mass index recorded. A child's body mass index is defined as weight (kg) divided by height (m). This can be plotted against BMI charts appropriate for age and sex of the child (Cole et al., 1995). If a child's BMI is found to be outside the recommended range for their age, trained staff can use this meeting to promote a healthy lifestyle through verbal and written information and referral to the dietician. If the BMI is found to be grossly outside the normal range, in addition to the above actions, the surgeon and anaesthetist will be informed to assess the risks of surgery anaesthesia on the child.

Conclusion

This chapter has demonstrated the importance of assessment of children, young people and families before and after surgery. Whether the child is undergoing an emergency or elective procedure, the aims are the same, namely to ensure they are cared for in the appropriate setting, by staff who recognise and focus on individual needs and implement care to promote recovery which is as pain and stress free as possible, ensuring discharge occurs at the earliest opportunity. Health promotion plays a key part in all these aspects of care. Delivering a quality service is of benefit not only to the child and family but also to the healthcare organisation by increasing productivity, reducing litigation and making a contribution to maintaining a healthier population for the future.

References

Audit Commission (1993) *Children First: A Study of Hospital Services*. London: HMSO.

Bowlby, J. (1951) *Maternal Care and Mental Health*. World Health Organization Monograph. Geneva: World Health Organization.

Chambers, M., Jones, S. (2007) *Surgical Nursing of Children*. London: Elsevier.

Cole, T., Freeman, J., Preece, M. (1995) Body mass index reference curves for the UK 1990. *Archives of Diseases in Childhood* 73: 25–29.

Coyne, I. (1996) Parent participation: a concept analysis. *Journal of Advanced Nursing* 23: 733–740.

Department of Health (2003) *Getting the Right Start: The National Service Framework for Children, Young People and Maternity Services. Standard for Hospital Services*. London: Crown Copyright.

Education and Skills (Department of), Department of Health (2004) *National Service Framework for Children, Young People and Maternity Services*. London: Crown Copyright.

Glasper, E., Richardson, J. (2006) *A Textbook of Children's and Young People's Nursing*. London: Elsevier.

Healthcare Commission (2007) *Improving Services for Children in Hospital*. London: Healthcare Commission.

Janke, E., Chalk, V., Kinley, H. (2002) *Pre Operative Assessment: Setting a Standard Through Learning*. Southampton: University of Southampton.

Laming, L. (2003) *The Victoria Climbié Inquiry: Report of an Inquiry by Lord Laming*. Available at: http://www.victoria-climbie-inquiry.org.uk/ (accessed December 2007).

Nethercott, S. (1993) A concept for all the family. Family-centred care: a concept analysis. *Professional Nurse* 8(12): 794–797.

Nursing and Midwifery Council (2007) *Nursing and Midwifery Council Code of Professional Conduct*. London: NMC. Available at: http://www.nmc-uk.org (accessed December 2007).

Royal College of Nursing (1999) *Clinical Guidelines for the Recognition and Assessment of Acute Pain in Children. Recommendations*. London: Royal College of Nursing.

Royal College of Nursing (2005) *RCN Clinical Guidelines: Perioperative Fasting in Adults and Children*. London: RCN.

Royal College of Surgeons of England (2007) *Surgery for Children: Delivering a First Class Service*. London: The Royal College of Surgeons of England.

Rushforth, H., Bliss, A., Burge, D., Glasper, E. (2000) Nurse-led preoperative assessment: a study of appropriateness. *Paediatric Nursing* 12(5): 15–20.

16 Surgical Wound Healing and Health Promotion

Elaine Salmons

Introduction

In a previous chapter wound care has been discussed in relation to trauma. This chapter concentrates on wound care following surgery. At first consideration it may not be apparent that health promotion can play a role in surgical wound care. This chapter identifies how health promotion is related to wound care and how it may be implemented into hospital practice.

A model of health promotion can help to provide structure to the care nurses provide. Downie et al. (1990, p. 2) provide a model, known as the Tannahill model of health promotion, which they define in the following way: 'Health promotion comprises efforts to enhance positive health and prevent ill-health, through the overlapping spheres of health education, prevention and protection.'

Nurses generally approve of this model. It is a useful model as it identifies different areas for action. The three main areas are prevention, protection and health education. Nurses will find that there are

overlaps between these different areas. Tannahill's (Downie et al., 1990) model of health promotion will be applied to children's wound care in hospital. The three main areas of the model can relate to wound care in the following ways:

- Health prevention, preventive services – children's nurses working to reduce stress and anxiety for children/young people associated with hospital care, particularly wound care.
- Health protection – promotion of wound healing and prevention of infections through hospital policies.
- Health education – promoting techniques such as hand washing, infection control and wound care along with pain relief, through information and support for children and families.

When participating in health promotion on wound care it can be undertaken on two levels. Initially, promoting health to ensure that there is optimal wound healing. Secondly, health promotion can be about responding appropriately to a problem with wound healing, in an effort to regain optimal healing.

Children's care in hospital

Numerous studies have shown how the presence of parents in hospital can have a positive impact on a child's health (Robertson and Robertson, 1960; Bowlby, 1969, 1973). The NSF Standard for Hospital services outlines the importance of parents being very much involvement with their child's care in hospital (Department of Health, 2003). The NSF states that parents *being present* helps a child's recovery, and can even be a practical contribution to a child's care at the bedside.

Encouraging parents to be involved in care will help them to develop an understanding about their child's health needs. They can learn about wound care; what needs to be achieved to promote wound healing, and what skills will help them once their child has been discharged from hospital.

Hospital hygiene is essential in the prevention of wound infections. The Government is currently campaigning for cleaner hospitals. Nurses have a key role to play, as the chief nursing officer for England has recently highlighted (Department of Health, 2007). Sisters and charge nurses are expected to take overall responsibility for standards of cleanliness in their own ward areas (Department of Health, 2007). It is emphasised that matrons need to meet regularly with cleaning staff to ensure cleaning standards are being met, so overall rates of infection can be lowered (Department of Health, 2007).

Nurses therefore have an important role to play directly in the care of wounds with children and their families. In addition, working collaboratively with colleagues can help to prevent hospital infections, including wound infections. All hospital nurses have their part to play in helping to make hospitals a cleaner place for children.

Preoperative preparation

It is widely accepted that prior to hospital admission it is beneficial for children to be prepared for their stay and treatment. Preparation will help ensure that they cope well and make a good recovery following surgery (Sutherland, 2003).

It is increasingly common for children to receive their care in *ambulatory care* settings. Ambulatory care can be described as medical care that includes diagnosis, observation, treatment and rehabilitation. It may be provided on a day case basis, for example, as in day case surgery. Ambulatory care minimises the child's stay in hospital, thereby reducing some of the anxieties associated with being away from home and family.

Some children requiring surgery will need care for longer than simply a day; therefore, care will be provided in a ward setting. Surgery can be due to a variety of reasons. Children who are admitted for the following procedures will require wound care:

- A central venous line needs inserting (care of the exit site).
- External fixator for the treatment of a fracture (a metal framework that is attached to the bones in the leg or arm to restrict movement, and encourage healing) (pin site care).
- Gastrostomy (an artificial opening from the stomach to a stoma in the abdomen is made where a feeding tube is inserted) (stoma care). A gastrostomy tube can be in place for months or for even years in some cases. This means that a foreign body, the tube, has to remain in situ, breaking the continuity of the skin, so there is an increased likelihood of infection.

Once discharged, wound care in these situations will continue as the devices discussed will remain in situ. Glasper et al.'s (2007) text can provide an overview on the nursing management of these wounds.

Ambulatory care

Ambulatory care places more responsibility on parents/carers. This includes the psychological preparation for their child's admission, as well as undertaking some elements of postoperative care (Ellerton and Merriam, 1994).

Importantly, families need to be provided with information about their child's surgery. Nurses also need to lessen any fears the child and her/his family may have about the admission (May and Sparks, 1983). Visits to the ambulatory care unit may set straight any wrong ideas and give the child and family a greater sense of control. In addition, the use of verbal and written health promotion information for the family, as well as the child, can promote quality preparation prior to admission. Ellerton and Merriam's (1994) study evaluating the effectiveness of a pre-admission programme on day case surgery found that it did help to support families.

Longer admissions

Preparation is particularly important for children and young people who need surgery but will be in hospital for a longer duration. It is essential that stress is minimised. Hospital play specialists can have a key role here, working closely with children. Young people may also benefit from discussing their apprehensions with a play specialist (see Chapter 5).

A longer hospital stay may provide nurses with more opportunities for teaching families about wound care and preparing for discharge. Families can engage in aspects of care under supervision, which may help them to feel more confident to manage the wound site when they return home.

Preparation for admission is essential. An informed admission can help the child to feel more relaxed. This can help when any aspects of care are being undertaken, such as wound care. Preparation links with Tannahill's (Downie et al., 1990) health prevention sphere of the health promotion model.

Pain relief

Following surgery, the child may experience some pain particularly associated with the wound itself. In the past, pain in children and particularly babies was underestimated. The NSF states that there is still some evidence that the treatment of pain for children is inadequate. There is a need for better prevention, assessment and treatment (Education and Skills, Department of Health, 2004a).

Pain is documented as being the most common complication following day case surgery (Jonas, 2003). A child in hospital should receive appropriate pain relief to promote comfort.

Following discharge, pain relief needs to be continued, which is a caring role that will be taken on by parents at home. Jonas (2003) found that children's pain was best managed if parents were given information and suitable analgesia on discharge. It is central to the child's care that pain relief is discussed. This discussion should include details about when the medication needs to be administered, so the child is comfortable, particularly when wound care is being undertaken. Parents will then be able to take on the role of managing their child's pain from a more informed perspective.

If the child feels comfortable, she/he will feel less distressed by any aspect of care that needs to be undertaken, such as wound care. Distraction during wound's care is also very effective. This might include the child watching a favourite video or someone talking with the child or engaging in a fun activity, such as blowing bubbles or having a story. These activities will all help. Health promotion information on pain relief should be given on discharge, as discussed, but in addition information on distraction activities may be helpful too.

Information on pain relief links with Tannahill's (Downie et al., 1990) health education sphere of the model. Pain relief is an essential part of wound care, particularly in the early stages of wound healing.

Prevention of infection

Parents, along with young people, themselves may be aware of the risks associated with hospital-acquired infections. Nurses are working hard to prevent and combat such problems. Approximately 9% of UK hospital patients catch hospital-acquired infections, which costs around £1 billion per year. This is comparable to the running costs of eight National Health Service hospitals for a year (Department of Health, 2005).

Hand hygiene is widely acknowledged as the most effective way in preventing infection (Royal College of Nursing, 2006). It is essential that all who participate in wound care know how to wash their hands properly. A photographic step-by-step procedure along with a demonstration can be a very effective way of teaching hand washing. A *Glo and Tell machine*, if available, can be a really useful in highlighting the effectiveness of hand washing. The machine shows the hand areas that have been washed adequately, and particularly those areas which have not.

Alongside hand washing, management of the wound itself is important in promoting wound healing and preventing problems from developing. Dressings are sometimes not removed for 48 hours postoperatively to prevent infection. Wilson (2002) asserts that this prevents bacteria entering the skin from adjacent areas, until the wound surface has healed. Cleansing of the wound may be required in some situations and a new dressing applied. Depending on the nature of the wound, antibiotics may even be given prophylactically to prevent infection.

If infection does present, symptoms may include pain, heat, swelling around the wound itself and the child may have a fever (Wilson, 2002). The infection will need to be treated. The nurse will need to take appropriate action, which will involve finding out which organism is growing in the wound and discussing with the child's doctor about suitable treatments that will cure the wound of infection.

Promotion of wound healing and prevention of infections can be advocated through hospital policies, policies specifically related to wound care but also through more general hospital policies. Prevention of infection links with Tannahill's (Downie et al., 1990) health protection sphere of the health promotion model.

Teaching wound care

Prior to discharge, parents will need to be taught how to undertake wound care.

Demonstrations and discussions can be useful, along with opportunities to address any concerns that parents may have.

Teaching parents in an environment where they are able to focus on what the nurse is discussing is important. Environments where there are many distractions will make learning difficult. Find somewhere quiet to discuss care. The nurse needs to carefully demonstrate and explain the care needed, so parents can observe and listen to advice. Once the parents feel confident about taking on wound care and the nurse feels they can do so safely, then care will be handed over to them.

The family will become familiar with what is normal for their child's wound. They will need to know if the wound is healthy and healing appropriately. In addition, if there are changes such as signs of infection, how will they recognise these, and whom should they contact? These details need to be provided.

When teaching about wound care, hospital staff must consider what type of facilities the parents will have at home. Instead of a dressing trolley, for example, a tray may prove useful for undertaking wound care procedures.

Teaching can be undertaken in hospital and further reinforced in the community. For continuity, the procedure needs to be undertaken in the same way both by hospital and community nurses, so the family do not become confused by different procedures.

Teaching plan

Table 16.1 is an example of a generic teaching plan on wound care. The plan sets out content, method and resources that can be used when teaching wound care. Aim and objectives for such a plan might include the following:

Aim – to enable parents to competently promote and maintain safe wound healing of their child's wound.
Objectives – parents will be able to do the following:

- Promote their child's comfort whilst wound care is being undertaken.
- Care for their child's wound appropriately.
- Recognise signs of infection and know what actions to take should an infection develop.

The teaching plan is useful in ensuring all topics are discussed and can be utilised when assessing if parents understand all aspects of wound care. Times will vary at each stage depending on the needs of the individual child and parents (Table 16.1).

Preparation for discharge

Discharge, when parents are going to take responsibility for their child's care following surgery, needs preparation. Health promotion, as highlighted, has a part to play through appropriate preparation for discharge.

The NSF (Education and Skills, Department of Health, 2004b) states that parents need *support* and *information* to give them confidence to manage many health issues associated with their children. They need to be able to care for their child's wound appropriately and recognise potential complications.

The types of wound care that may be undertaken by parents tend to be the removal of a simple dressing postoperatively, where it is thought unlikely to be any complications. However, as highlighted earlier, there are parents who may need to take on wound care for a longer period, such as with gastrostomy care, where the tube may be in place

Table 16.1 Teaching plan.

Time	Content	Method	Resource
15 minutes	Negotiation	Discussion	
1–2 hours	Play preparation	Discussion	Video and pre-admission information
15 minutes	Hand washing and infection control	Demonstration and observation	Leaflet on hand washing. Glo and Tell lotion and ultraviolet light source
1 hour +	• Preparation • Pain management/distraction • Wound care • Signs of healing • General care/advice such as not riding a bicycle or playing contact sports, showers or baths, depending on the specific wound	Demonstration and observation	
15 minutes	• Signs of infection • What to do if infection presents	Discussion	
15 minutes	Points of contact for support/discharge information	Discussion/introduction to community team	Information leaflet with contact numbers

for many months or longer. Where long-term care is required, parental involvement in the provision of care should be negotiated in advance. It is important that they know what care their child requires on discharge from hospital.

All families should be supported at home if undertaking wound care. That care should be supported by a community children's nurse (CCN). The family may be able to meet their CCN in hospital, prior to discharge. This will provide the CCN with the opportunity to negotiate with the family the level of support they may need following discharge, which will help to reduce any anxieties the family may be feeling.

If access to a CCN service is not available then a district nurse or practice nurse should be available in the community to provide support.

Discharge information

Discharge information needs to be verbal and written so that the family have a clear idea about what they are expected to do. Some ambulatory care units will provide telephone advice following the child's discharge. Written health promotion information should answer frequently asked questions that will help parents to understand what is required of them.

Written information may include the following:

- Care of the wound.
- Signs of possible infection.
- When the child can have a bath or shower.
- When the child can go back to school.
- Any limitations to the child's activities or exercise routine.
- Who to contact for further advice.
- Contact telephone numbers for advice.

Additional advice about the child's nutritional needs should be considered (Wilson, 2002). The child will need to be eating a healthy diet so that the skin is able to heal effectively. Nurses can discuss with families about the importance of promoting a healthy diet in relation to wound care as well as more generally, if needed.

By going through all the necessary information again on actual discharge (repetition), it will ensure parents have a clear understanding about the care their child requires. Written information that accompanies the verbal information will enable families to refer back to specific points of care, if needed.

There may also be sources of written information available that provide explanations, with drawings, for children themselves. Seek these out or perhaps develop one for your practice area. Have any other practice areas around the country developed anything similar? Placing a request for information in a journal, such as *Paediatric Nursing*, may be a useful starting point.

By providing information and support, through teaching about wound care and preparing for discharge, the nurse is educating the family, which links with Tannahill's (Downie et al., 1990) health education sphere of the model.

Conclusion

Parents and carers are capable and often willing to take on the care of their child's wound, particularly where they are given the right support and information. It can sometimes be less stressful for the family and fit in more easily with family life, if they are able to manage wound care themselves. It can also save them the inconvenience of returning to the hospital, particularly if community care is available.

Skills parents/carers have learnt in hospital can be transferred to the home setting, such as correct hand washing and how to clean a wound, if this is required. It is essential that they have continued support once they are home to monitor the progress of the wound healing and continue good practice. Tannahill's (Downie et al., 1990) model of health promotion provides a useful framework for wound care following surgery. It highlights the need for prevention (services to prevent children becoming distressed), protection (policies to promote wound care), and health education (the giving of information and support to promote wound care).

References

Bowlby, J. (1969) *Attachment and Loss 1, Attachment*. Richmond: Hogarth Press.

Bowlby, J. (1973) *Attachment and Loss 2, Separation, Anxiety and Anger*. Richmond: Hogarth Press.

Department of Health (2003) *Getting the Right Start: National Service Framework for Children. Standards for Hospital Services*. London: Department of Health Publications.

Department of Health, Chief Nursing Officer and Chief Medical Officer (2005) *Saving Lives: A Delivery Programme to Reduce Health Care Associated Infection (HCAI) Including MRSA* (Dear Colleague letter 15 June 2005). London: Department of Health.

Department of Health (2007) *Improving Cleanliness and Infection Control*. London: Department of Health. PL/CNO/2007/6.

Downie, R., Fyfe, C., Tannahill, A. (1990) *Health Promotion: Models and Values*. Oxford: Oxford University Press.

Education and Skills, Department of Health (2004a) *National Service Framework for Children, Young People and Maternity Services*. London: Crown Copyright.

Education and Skills, Department of Health (2004b) *National Service Framework for Children, Young People and Maternity Services, Standard 6 – Ill Child*. London: Crown Copyright.

Ellerton, M., Merriam, C. (1994) Preparing children and families psychologically for day surgery: an evaluation. *Journal of Advanced Nursing* 19(6): 1057–1062.

Glasper, E., McEwing, G., Richardson, J. (2007) *Oxford Handbook of Children's and Young People's Nursing*. Oxford: Oxford University Press.

Jonas, D. (2003) Parents' management of their child's pain in the home following day surgery. *Journal of Child Health Care* 7(3): 150–162.

May, B., Sparks, M. (1983) School age children: are their needs recognised and met in the hospital setting. *Child Health Care* 11: 118–121.

Robertson, J., Robertson, J. (1960) *A Two Year Old Goes to Hospital*. Suffolk: Concord Video and Film Council Ltd.

Royal College of Nursing (2006) *Good Practice in Infection Prevention and Control: Guidance for Nursing Staff*. London: Royal College of Nursing.

Sutherland, T. (2003) Comparison of hospital and home base preparation for cardiac surgery. *Paediatric Nursing* 15(5): 13–16.

Wilson, J. (2002) *Infection Control in Clinical Practice*. Edinburgh: Baillière Tindall.

17 Planning Hospital Discharge

Jane Houghton

NSF

Hospital stays should be kept to a minimum through the coordinated delivery of care. Planning for discharge and the prevention of unnecessary readmission should be the norm for all children/young people (Standard for Hospital Services, National Service Framework, NSF, Department of Health, 2003, p. 19).

Introduction

The child's admission to hospital can be the result of an emergency or as a planned admission. The admission may only be a short stay of hours or simply minutes, or a much longer stay of days or even weeks. The discharge can be simple or complex, but it should be planned for, as early as possible during the child's stay. This can happen either at admission itself or even before the admission, whenever possible. Planning should include information for the child and parents/carers about the condition, medication and follow-up and how to access help or advice if needed. The primary care team (PCT) also needs timely information. The family should be provided with, or given access to, any medication and equipment that they may need.

The discharge should be planned by a coordinated, multidisciplinary team with set roles and responsibilities, and will include the child and family. An effective and well-planned discharge should aim to reduce the hospital stay to as short a time as possible. Health promotion information for the child and family should be available.

This chapter considers the issues for planning timely discharge from hospital for children/young people with minor illnesses as well as complex health or mental health needs. The issues of medication, information, communication and support will be considered.

Minor illnesses and discharge planning

Young children frequently have acute minor illnesses, with the vast majority being dealt with by their parents/carers without need of consulting a health practitioner. For those who do attend accident and emergency departments or are referred by their general practitioner (GP) to the *paediatric assessment unit*, it can be a frightening experience. The experience may undermine the parent's/carer's confidence in caring for their child. Most children who are admitted to hospital will be under the age of 3 years, with mild self-limiting illnesses. The figures show that 61% of these children will spend one night or less in hospital (Stewart et al., 1998).

The discharge process should be planned to provide seamless care between hospital and home as well as between secondary care and primary care. The majority of children, who attend either paediatric assessment units following referral, or accident and emergency departments, do not require inpatient admission. Nonetheless, parents/carers continue to need support after discharge, including adequate information about their child's condition, what to do if symptoms returned and how to get advice if needed (Ogilvie, 2005).

A good discharge plan will enable parents/carers to cope, reducing their anxieties and may prevent further admissions. Parents/carers play a major role in caring for their sick child and need to feel confident about carrying out care at home if early discharge is to be achieved.

The process of discharging patients is an important, yet often neglected aspect of health care delivery. The relative lack of care at discharge may undermine the overall effectiveness and safety of the hospital care (Forster, 2006).

Discharge planning

> **NSF**
>
> A child's discharge from hospital should be planned in good time and in liaison with other relevant agencies. Length of stay in hospital is kept to a minimum (standard 7, Executive Summary, Education and Skills, Department of Health, 2004a, p. 20).

Planning for discharge is an important aspect of care and has received increasing attention because of the implications of bed occupancy rates and to reduce readmission rates. There is an increasing use of day case and ambulatory care facilities with a high proportion of children with common acute illnesses staying for 24 hours or less (Jackson, 2000). Short-stay facilities such as assessment and observation units offer rapid stabilisation and early discharge with considerable financial saving, without critical incident and minimising disruption to the child and family.

Acute assessment units provide rapid consultation for the acutely ill child, with admission for hours, not days. At least 40% of children/young people referred as emergencies will be discharged without in-patient admission. However, up to 7%

may return either with worsening of the original problem or with an unrelated condition (Ogilvie, 2005). Only a small proportion of these will require admission. Acute assessment clinics provide emergency outpatient consultations. Only a small percentage of these referrals require in-patient admission. There is little evidence of serious clinical consequences in children discharged from these units. In fact, there is some evidence that users are satisfied with the service. Such units can also be associated with a reduction in in-patient activity levels (Ogilvie, 2005). The short stays reduce distress for the child/young person and disruption for the family.

There should be a smooth transition between hospital and home, with health promotion information for the parents/carers and speedy information for PCT practitioners. One method of reducing the delays for simple discharge is *nurse-led discharge*. The Department of Health (2004) states that there are no legal or professional reasons why nurses or allied health practitioners cannot take on more responsibility for the discharge process including the decision to discharge. They can:

- assess;
- liaise with the full team;
- plan timely discharge based on the agreed clinical management plan;
- write discharge letters;
- make follow-up calls;
- give advice to patient and carers.

This should be supported by agreed protocols, guidelines or criteria documented within the patient record. The person to whom this responsibility is delegated should be aware they are accountable for all their actions and have the necessary competencies. There must be clear lines of communication between the consultant/lead clinician and the health practitioner discharging the patient.

If nurses are to take on this responsibility, it is necessary to have a written, evidence-based policy setting out the discharge criteria. Higson and Bolland (2001) suggest that it can be in the form of a checklist for day surgery, but should be practical to use, provide uniform assessment for all children/young people and therefore would add medico-legal value to nurse-led discharge, but should be regularly audited. Table 17.1 demonstrates a checklist for day surgery.

Table 17.1 Checklist for day surgery.

	Discharge criteria	Yes	No	N/A
Clinical assessment	Alert and orientated			
	Walking safely			
	Stable vital signs			
	Bleeding from wound			
	Pain controlled			
	Tolerated oral fluids			
	Tolerated diet if child has had tonsils and adenoids removed			
	Nausea controlled at time of discharge			
	Passed urine if appropriate			
	Venflon removed			
Physiotherapy	Assessed by physiotherapist			
	Mobility aids used safely			
Safety	Responsible escort home in private transport			
	Written and verbal advice given to parents/carer regarding aftercare			
	Contact number given			
	Medication to take home given			
Follow-up care	Ward telephone number given			
	Outpatient follow-up appointment made			
	• Given to parent/carer			
	• To be sent to parent/carer			
	Dressing appointment arranged with			
	○ Practice nurse			
	○ District nurse			
	○ Outreach service			
	○ Dressing clinic			
	○ Ward			
	Date arranged			
	Referral form completed			
	Faxed/copied and filed in notes			
	Health visitor referral made			
	Discharge notification sent to GP			
Patient's satisfaction	Child/parents confirm they have been satisfied with day case experience			
Named nurse signature		Time		

Courtesy of Lancashire Teaching Hospitals NHS Foundation Trust (2006).

Information for the child and family

NSF

Clear, understandable and up-to-date information for children, young people and their parents is provided through a variety of media and formats which are appropriate to the child's development and circumstances (standard 10, Education and Skills, Department of Health, 2004b, p. 16).

Parents/carers want to understand their child's illness or condition, whether it is a mild, acute illness, a simple operation or a more complex condition. They want to know how to care for their child, how to prevent reoccurrence, what side effects to expect, when to seek help and how to access advice. The information should be verbal and written with opportunities for questions, and may need to be repeated as it is difficult to retain all the information at once. Smith and Daughtrey (2000) found that parents/carers need the following:

- Information about their child's illness and how to resume the care at home.
- Both verbal and written information.

- A second opportunity to ask questions.
- Support at home.
- Self-management plans.
- Clear instructions on follow-up visits.
- Speedy communication from the hospital to their GP.

Robinson and Miller (1996) recommend that the discharge instructions should be written in plain English to create an accessible and useful document to assist parents/carers in caring for the child at home. Often when health practitioners give verbal or written instructions, they do not realise that they are using jargon that is familiar to them but unfamiliar to others. At the same time the instructions should not be too simple or patronising. Ensure that parents/carers have all their questions answered and understand the information given.

The information may include education about medication or equipment. The child/young people with diabetes, for example, needs to understand how to use the insulin pen, whilst the child/young person with asthma, will need to know how to use inhalers. Wesseldene et al. (1999) introduced a simple form of education and support for children/young people admitted with acute asthma. The discharge package included a brief, individual, simple educational programme providing specific written management plans with instructions on the use of inhalers and peak flow devices, as well as on crisis management. The authors found the education package reduced the readmission rate as parents/carers had a better understanding of their child's condition, how to prevent attacks and what steps to take if the asthma reoccurred.

Parents/carers want health promotion information which may help prevent a reoccurrence of their child's condition (Smith and Daughtrey, 2000). This may also be an ideal opportunity for health promotion for the whole family. A range of topics may be included, depending on the child's illness. This could include prevention of cross-infection through hand washing, prevention of diarrhoea and vomiting through the appropriate storage of food and the cleansing of teats and dummies, and reduction of the risks of asthma through a smoke-free environment. If the child has been injured in an accident, for example, the health promotion information may include basic first aid, the use of cycle helmets, stair gates, car seats or the dangers of sunburn, as appropriate.

Medication

> **NSF**
>
> When prescribing, dispensing and administering medicines for children or young people at home, health care professionals alert parents or carers to the potential dangers of the medicines and advise them on appropriate storage (standard 10, Education and Skills, Department of Health, 2004b, p. 22).

The child/young person and family need to know about administering any medicines. They need to know how and when to give them, as well as details about the number of days they need to be continued. The person dispensing the discharge medication should instruct the parents/carers on use and storage.

Tomlin and Saunders (2001) found that delay in discharge is often due to a delay in the prescribing of medicines and sometimes in the dispensing. Readmission is often due to poor compliance, concordance and lack of understanding about the medication. Tomlin and Saunders (2001) introduced a system where the medication was dispensed at the beginning of the patient's stay in enough quantity to last for the duration of the child's stay in hospital and to take home. The medication is labelled appropriately for discharge from day 1. Tomlin and Saunders (2001) provide an environment for self/carer medication in order to improve patient's awareness.

The medication may be antibiotics, antipyretics, pain relief or specific to the condition such as insulin for diabetes. The parents/carers need to understand how to use the medicine. After minor day surgery, for example, the child/young person might be expected to experience some degree of pain. The parents/carers should be informed about how to recognise and prevent this. Most parents/carers have the potential to effectively manage their child's postoperative pain at home following minor surgery, provided they are equipped to do so. Bastable and Rushforth (2005) suggest considering the following:

- Prepare families with comprehensive verbal and written instructions on the recommended analgesia dose, timing and importance of giving it regularly.
- Consider most suitable time for giving discharge advice.
- Provide parents/carers with adequate amount of analgesia to take home.
- Educate parents/carers on basic pain cues.
- Give an age-appropriate pain assessment tool for use at home.
- Teach families non-pharmacological pain alleviation measures.
- Reassure parents/carers they can contact the hospital for advice at any time.
- Ensure suitable support is available such as telephone follow-up or children's community nurses (CCNs).

Information for the primary care team

The relationship between primary care services and the family continues as the child/young person moves in and out of specialist services. It is important to ensure close liaison between the GPs and community health services to facilitate continuity of care when the recovering child/young person is discharged home (Smith and Daughtrey, 2000). There should be a system in place for informing the health visitor or school nurse of a child's/young person's admission and ongoing care. This is often achieved by the role of the liaison nurse, who will form a link between the hospital services and the PCT. To enable them to provide this service effectively, they need the necessary details such as the correct name, address, date of birth and school of the child/young person, as well as the GP's name. The GP should receive a timely discharge letter whether this is written by medical staff or the nurse. Rapid communication with the PCT is achieved by letter, e-mail or fax to GPs, CCNs, health visitors, school nurses and practice nurses. Parents/carers are informed of this. This enables the team to be informed of the child's/young person's admission and need for any follow-up care.

For example, the CCN is informed of children/young people requiring advice to prevent constipation. Health visitors are advised of infants who have been admitted following accidental in-gestion. Practice nurses are informed about children with asthma. School nurses will be advised about children who have been admitted with fits (Jackson, 2000). Whichever communication system is used, especially fax, maintaining confidentiality must be considered. If there are concerns that the fax might not be picked up promptly or by the right person, it might be necessary to find another means of communication.

Follow-up and support

Ogilvie (2005) suggests that parents/carers continue to need support after discharge, and need to know what to do if symptoms return, as well as whom to phone for advice. Parents/carers play a major role in caring for their sick child and need to feel confident about carrying out care at home, if early discharge is to be achieved (Jackson, 2000). Aitken et al. (2005) describe how paediatric ambulatory care, especially emergency assessment, depends on the ability of parents/carers to shoulder the care provision at home. They suggest a system of follow-up phone calls the morning after discharge, as well as direct access to the unit for 24 hours after discharge, if parents/carers are concerned. Many units offer 24–48 hours access after discharge. This involves the first option of phone call advice, then direct access if necessary.

There should be clear guidance about whom the parents/carers can contact for advice, and if the parents/carers contact the ward, staff should be prepared to give appropriate advice. There should be written guidelines to ensure accuracy and consistency of advice given, and any contact should be documented.

Telephone follow-up should involve reviewing the child's/young person's progress, the need for medication and reinforcing any health promotion information given in hospital. This is another opportunity to cover any health promotion information that may be relevant to the child's/young person's condition.

CCN teams facilitate the early discharge of children so family life is not disrupted for longer than necessary. The hospital admission will be less stressful for the child (Gnanapragasam et al., 1995). CCN services are an organised alternative to traditional provision, enabling children/young people to receive treatment at home, which would otherwise be provided in hospital. Nurses provide continuity of care between hospital and community for children/young people with chronic or terminal illnesses and for children/young people with acute illnesses who are discharged early from hospital (Tatman and Woodroffe, 1993).

CCN services have come a long way in recent years to be able to provide a range of specialist nursing services for children/young people and their families in their own homes. Many children/young people, however, are still discharged home without such support being available (Smith and Daughtery, 2000). These families in particular need other options for follow-up, such as the phone call. It may be that they will get the support they need from the PCT, if the condition is suitable.

Complex discharges

Although most children/young people only require simple discharge, a sizeable minority need a more complex discharge for a possible range of reasons. They may have, for example, complex health needs, a complex mental health condition or there may be child protection/safeguarding concerns. The Laming (2003) report identified two particular areas of concern about children being discharged. One concern being the child/young person discharged who is not registered with a GP or school. In these circumstances the appropriate contact person in the PCT, via the *paediatric liaison nurse*, should be notified in order to arrange registration. The other concern is the child/young person where there may be child protection/safeguarding concerns.

Child protection/safeguarding children

NSF

Where there are concerns about a possible child protection issue, it is particularly important that there is a multi-agency action plan agreed and recorded before the child leaves hospital. The need to safeguard a child should always dictate the timing of their discharge so that the likelihood of ongoing harm can be assessed while the child is still in hospital (Standard for Hospital Services, Department of Health, 2003, p. 19).

Discharge planning, before the child/young person leaves hospital, should involve both the acute and community staff. In addition, other key stakeholders from health and social care, as well as other agencies if appropriate, such as police and education, may need to be involved.

Complex mental health conditions

NSF

Discharge planning should receive equal attention to admission planning. Aftercare has a crucial role in the maintenance of treatment gains made during admission. In a minority of cases admission may be a stepping stone towards longer term alternative care or residential schooling. The team will need to liaise with a range of local education, social and mental health services (standard 9, Education and Skills, Department of Health, 2004c, p. 34).

Those children/young people with complex mental health conditions require discharge planning with the multi-agency team. When they are discharged from in-patient services into the community, their continuity of care is ensured by partnership between all agencies. There should be agreements between health, education, social services and the youth justice service.

Children with complex health needs

NSF

Children/young people who are disabled or who have complex health needs should receive coordinated high-quality, child and family-centred services, which are based on assessed needs, which promote social inclusion and where possible enable them and their families to live ordinary lives (standard 8, Education and Skills, Department of Health, 2004d, p. 5).

Some groups of children/young people may have conditions which require more complex discharge packages, and therefore, discharge may be delayed. Effective planning, teamwork and expertise in these areas may reduce this delay.

Advances in medical technology have pushed the boundaries of life expectancy and resulted in many children with complex care needs, or who are technology dependent, being cared for at home. Children requiring complex care are described as those who may not be technology dependent but require jointly commissioned health, education and social services, that is, they require greater resources than those available within individual services. There should be a coordinated and reliable approach to discharge in preparing and setting up complex care packages for children/young people requiring technological and clinical care at home (Stephens, 2005).

The key principle in achieving home care for a child/young person with complex care needs is not to create the hospital in the home, but to achieve safety for the child/young person as simply as possible, with the least disruption to normal family life. It may be necessary to provide 24-hour support. For successful discharge planning, collaboration is essential between all practitioners involved. Potentially complex issues such as those of responsibility, risk management and quality management must be clarified within this process including the following (Boosfeld and O'Toole, 2000):

- Needs assessment.
- Identification of key workers.
- Discharge proposal.
- Multidisciplinary planning meetings.
- Recruitment and selection of home care teams.
- Training.
- Moving home.

Parents/carers are often required to assume 24-hour responsibility for their child's/young person's care (NHS Executive, 1998). They may need to learn complex nursing skills such as tracheostomy care, oxygen therapy and administering intravenous medications. For children/young people with complex needs, the situation is further confused by the number of different health, social and education professionals involved.

The Royal College of Nursing (2003) gives the principles for planning effective transition from hospital to home care:

- Each child/young person should have a named nurse or key worker with responsibility for coordinating discharge, beginning on admission and communicating with all professionals involved.
- Patient and carers are prepared so that they feel confident and are competent to take on agreed roles and care following discharge.
- The level of support and supervision required is assessed before discharge to estimate dependency.

Key considerations when planning discharge of children/young people who require ongoing nursing care or support are the following:

- Care planning in relation to the child's age, ability and condition.
- Appropriate resources for the family and home circumstances: respite care, equipment.
- Education and support needs of the family and other carers.
- Funding and financial issues.
- Responsibility for medical supervision.

Case study

An example of a simple discharge following emergency referral with a minor acute illness is outlined. Harry, aged 15 months, is referred by his GP to the paediatric assessment unit. He is assessed and treated there, and then spends 4 hours in the observation area before being discharged home. Harry's parents are given verbal information about his condition and treatment from the time of his admission.

Once a diagnosis is made they are also given written information and several opportunities to ask questions. The health promotion information includes details on how to prevent reoccurrence of the condition, and general advice to keep Harry healthy, such as the need for a smoke-free environment. The unit has various health promotion posters on notice boards and leaflets readily available. Harry's discharge medication is explained to his parents, including the type, function, dose and timings of the medication, with any possible side effects.

Harry's parents are also given follow-up information. This includes an outpatient appointment, with directions and what to expect at that appointment. In addition, a telephone contact number is provided in case there are any further concerns over the next 48 hours. His parents are offered a follow-up phone call the next morning. Harry is then discharged home, whilst the liaison nurse informs the PCT, including his health visitor. A discharge letter is sent to his GP. The next day the parents receive a follow-up phone call from the unit, and his health visitor contacts them to arrange a visit. Harry has made a full and speedy recovery at home.

The most appropriate place for Harry to recover from his illness was in his own home with his family surrounded by his own toys. By giving Harry's parents the information and support they needed to understand and treat his illness, their anxieties were reduced, enabling them to cope confidently with this illness and any other minor illnesses Harry might have in the future.

(In line with Nursing and Midwifery Council, 2004, recommendations, the child's real name has not been used.)

Summary

Most children/young people therefore will need a simple discharge after a short stay. Others may need a far more complex discharge, involving multi-agency planning, after a longer stay. However complex or simple the discharge process may be, the planning should start as early as possible into the child's/young person's admission, involve the family, and aim to keep the stay to a minimum. This will minimise family disruption and help to reduce distress for the child/young person. Every opportunity should be taken to help the parents/carers care for their child through health promotion information and support.

Problems often arise when parents/carers are not given enough information or support, leading to increased anxieties. Or there is a lack of prompt communication with the PCT, or there is poor multi-agency cooperation and coordination. Ensuring careful planning, teamwork and good communication with all concerned, the child/young person will be happier and healthier. The parents/carers will be more confident and less anxious.

References

Aitken, P., Glasper, A., Wiltshire, M. (2005) Parental satisfaction with a nurse-led emergency assessment unit. *Paediatric Nursing* 17(9): 31–35.

Bastable, A., Rushforth, H. (2005) Parents management of their child's postoperative pain. *Paediatric Nursing* 17(10): 14–17.

Boosfeld, B., O'Toole, M. (2000) Technology-dependent children: transition from hospital to home. *Paediatric Nursing* 12(6): 20–22.

Department of Health (2003) *Getting the Right Start: The National Service Framework for Children, Young People and Maternity Services – Standard for Hospital Services (Standard 7)*. London: Department of Health.

Department of Health (2004) *Achieving Timely Simple Discharge from Hospital – A Toolkit for the Multidisciplinary Team*. Available at: http://www.dh.gov.uk (accessed January 2008).

Education and Skills (Department of), Department of Health (2004a) *National Service Framework for Children, Young People and Maternity Services. Executive Summary*. London: Crown Copyright.

Education and Skills (Department of), Department of Health (2004b) *National Service Framework for Children, Young People and Maternity Services, Standard 10 – Medicines for Children and Young People*. London: Crown Copyright.

Education and Skills (Department of), Department of Health (2004c) *National Service Framework for Children, Young People and Maternity Services, Standard 9 – The mental and Psychological Well-Being of Children and Young People*. London: Crown Copyright.

Education and Skills (Department of), Department of Health (2004d) *National Service Framework for Children, Young People and Maternity Services, Standard 8 – Disabled Child*. London: Crown Copyright.

Forster, A. (2006) Discharging patients: moving beyond neglect to action. NPSA. Available at: http://www.saferhealthcare.org.uk/ihi (accessed 17 March 2007).

Gnanapragasam, S., Hanchet, S., Mills, J., Hill, M. (1995) Paediatric home care team. *Nursing Times* 91(9): 28–30.

Higson, J., Bolland, R. (2001) Paediatric discharge criteria leading to improved outcomes. *Nursing Times* 97(35): 30–31.

Jackson, K. (2000) Support following discharge: a service audit. *Paediatric Nursing* 12(5): 37–38.

Laming, L. (2003) *The Victoria Climbié Inquiry. Report of an Inquiry into the Death of Victoria Climbié*. London: Crown Copyright.

Lancashire Teaching Hospitals NHS Foundation Trust (2006) *Check List for Day Surgery*. Lancashire: Lancashire Teaching Hospitals NHS Foundation Trust.

NHS Executive (1998) *Evaluation of the Pilot Project Programme for Children with Life Threatening Illnesses.* London: HMSO.

Nursing and Midwifery Council (2004) *Code of Professional Conduct.* London: NMC.

Ogilvie, D. (2005) Hospital based alternatives to acute paediatric admission: a systematic review. *Archives of Disease in Childhood* 90: 138–142.

Robinson, A., Miller, M. (1996) Making information accessible: developing plain English discharge instructions. *Journal of Advanced Nursing* 24: 528–535.

Royal College of Nursing (2003) *Children's Community Nursing – Promoting Effective Team Working for Children and Their Families.* London: RCN Publications.

Smith, L., Daughtrey, H. (2000) Weaving the seamless web of care: an analysis of parents perceptions of their needs following discharge of their child from hospital. *Journal of Advanced Nursing* 31(94): 812–820.

Stephens, N. (2005) Complex care packages: supporting seamless discharge for the child and family. *Paediatric Nursing* 17(7): 42–44.

Stewart, M., Wernecke, U., MacFaul, R., Taylor-Meek, J., Smith, H., Smith, I. (1998) Medical and social factors associated with admission and discharge of acutely ill children. *Archives of Disease in Childhood* 79: 219–224.

Tatman, M., Woodroffe, C. (1993) Paediatric home care in the UK. *Archives of Disease in Childhood* 69: 677–680.

Tomlin, S., Saunders, D. (2001) Pharmaceutical care: improving practice for children in hospital. *Paediatric Nursing* 13(4): 25–29.

Wesseldene, L., McCarthy, P., Silverman, M. (1999) Structured discharge procedure for children admitted to hospital with acute asthma: a randomised controlled trial of nursing practice. *Archives of Disease in Childhood* 80: 110–114.

Theme 6

Promoting Health in Chronic Illness

Chapter 18   Asthma Management

Chapter 19   Managing Children's Skin Conditions

Chapter 20   Health Promotion for Children/Young People with Cancer

Chapter 21   Constipation

Chapter 22   Health Promotion in Childhood Diabetes

Chapter 23   Children/Young People with Disabilities and Complex Health Care Needs

18 Asthma Management

Annie Wing

NSF

The following National Service Framework (NSF) standards are relevant to this chapter: standard 1 – promoting health and well-being, identifying needs and intervening early, standard 2 – supporting parents, and standard 10 – medicines for children/young people (Education and Skills, Department of Health, 2004).

Introduction

Asthma affects approximately one in ten children in the United Kingdom (UK) and is the most common, chronic disease of childhood (Asthma UK, 2004). It is therefore really important for nurses working with children/young people to know how to recognise the symptoms of asthma and how to treat the condition. This chapter aims to help you work in partnership with children, young people and their families in order to encourage them to manage asthma appropriately, prevent problems from occurring and lead healthy, active lives.

What is asthma?

Children with asthma have difficulty breathing because their airways are inflamed and sensitive to various irritants or *triggers*. The airways respond by becoming increasingly inflamed and narrow, restricting the flow of air in and out of the lungs.

Asthma causes children to cough, especially at night-time, and become increasingly breathless or wheezy. These symptoms are commonly associated with other respiratory diseases, which makes it difficult to diagnose asthma in children, especially the very young. Children with asthma can experience anything from mild, intermittent symptoms to severe persistent symptoms, acute exacerbations and admission to hospital.

Is asthma on the increase?

The prevalence of recent wheeze and diagnosed asthma has increased considerably over the past 20 years, especially in children (British Thoracic Society, 2006). The International Study of Asthma and Allergies in Childhood (ISAAC) survey of children aged 13–14 years reported the UK as having the fifth highest prevalence of asthma out of 56 countries worldwide (ISAAC, 1998).

General practitioner consultations for asthma increased significantly in the 1980s and 1990s, particularly in the 0–4 years age group (Office for National Statistics, 2004). This may have been due to factors such as improved inhaled medications, better diagnosis or changes in the terminology used for diagnosis.

In the past decade there has been a downward trend in acute asthma episodes presenting in primary care in both preschool and school-age children/young people (Royal College of General Practitioners, 2004). The decrease in morbidity and mortality associated with asthma may indicate an improved understanding of the condition and earlier treatment with preventative medication such as inhaled corticosteroids.

There are now approximately 1.1 million children/young people with asthma in the UK, and it still accounts for a large proportion of admissions to hospital, health care visits, time off school and time off work for parents/carers. Doctor diagnosed asthma accounts for 5% of all consultations in children/young people in the UK (Asthma UK, 2004).

Asthma is a life-threatening condition if not properly managed. Death from asthma is uncommon before the age of 10 years and only 2% of all asthma deaths occur in childhood. However, each year approximately 1400 people die from asthma, 20–30 of who are children or young people (Asthma UK, 2004).

Asthma that is undiagnosed or poorly controlled can result in the following:

- Disturbed sleep for the child and family.
- Absence from school, nursery or playgroup.
- Reduced academic attainment.
- Inability to participate in social or leisure activities.
- Inability to participate in play, sports or other physical activities.
- Inability to integrate with peers, resulting in low self-esteem.
- Anxiety and family dysfunction.

Causes and symptoms of asthma

What causes asthma?

We do not know the exact cause of asthma, but there are many factors that contribute to its development. The tendency to develop allergies, including asthma, runs in families. The chances of a child developing asthma is higher if both parents have asthma, but it is important to remember that many children or young people with asthma do not have relatives with the condition.

The majority of children or young people with persistent asthma are more likely to have experienced their first acute exacerbation before the age of 2 years. They will often show signs of other allergic conditions such as rhinitis and eczema, all part of the atopic spectrum.

Atopy is an inherited tendency to produce antibodies in response to an allergen. Allergens are proteins such as pollen or animal dander, which set off a chain of reactions within the body's cells and release chemical messengers. About 25–30% of the population is atopic (Mygind et al., 1996).

It is quite normal for airways to react to inhaled irritants. For example, you may cough when walking into a smoky room or when a crumb goes down the wrong way. The airways of children/young people with asthma are more sensitive however, and when they are exposed to an allergen over a period of time, the cells in the airways become sensitive and set off a reaction in the lining of the airways, which results in inflammation. The inflammation causes the airways to become irritable, triggering a dramatic narrowing of the bronchial tubes. This tendency to overreact is called bronchial hyper-responsiveness or hyper-reactivity and is characteristic of asthma.

The common symptoms of asthma include the following:

- *Wheeze* – a high-pitched squeaky noise, which usually occurs on expiration as air is forced through the narrowed airways.
- *Cough* – children with asthma are prone to coughing, which can be particularly troublesome at night-time. The cough may be dry or productive depending on the inflammatory changes within the airways. Although many children with asthma present with cough alone, diagnosis cannot be made solely on this basis.
- *Breathlessness (dyspnoea)* – often associated with wheeze and cough but may also occur alone. Very young children cannot complain of breathlessness, but their parents/carers may notice that the child is working harder to breath, using words such as *breathing fast* or *stomach pumping in and out*, to describe symptoms. In older children or young people, speech can provide a useful tool to assess levels of breathlessness. In moderate airway obstruction, children or young people may only be able to talk in short

sentences. Increasingly severe obstruction may limit speech to the point where the child or young person is only able to say single words or may not be able to talk at all in extreme cases.

Diagnosing asthma

Establishing a diagnosis of asthma in children/young people involves a series of steps.

Taking a history

Taking a detailed history is one of the most important steps in helping to establish if a child has asthma. It is important to include details of the following:

- Current history and presenting symptoms.
- Past medical history, including previous medication taken for respiratory symptoms and its effectiveness.
- Family history of asthma, eczema or hay fever.

Physical examination

In addition to obtaining a detailed history from the parents or carers, the child should be examined by an experienced health practitioner. If the diagnosis is in doubt, referral to a paediatrician is essential, preferably a respiratory specialist (BTS/SIGN, 2005).

Breathing tests

Although the history may give a fairly clear indication that a child has asthma, it is also important to carry out objective measures of lung function. This will confirm the diagnosis and assess the severity of the condition. Peak flow meters or spirometers are commonly used to monitor and record simple lung function tests. Children need to be old enough to cooperate with breathing tests and the results are seldom accurate or reliable under the age of 6 years:

- Peak expiratory flow rate (PEFR) measures the maximum rate of air which the child can forcibly

exhale. When the airways narrow, the PEFR falls. The peak expiratory flow measures the airflow in the larger airways; it is not sensitive enough to identify small airway changes, which might be present despite a normal peak flow. PEFR is a simple technique that can be carried out at home. Measurements can be recorded two or three times a day and used to compare with previous best values.
- Spirometry is increasingly used to assess airflow obstruction. Spirometers measure the volume of air expired, for example, forced expiratory volume in 1 second and forced vital capacity. This test provides more detailed information than peak flow tests, but is rarely used at home.

Symptom monitoring

Children experience asthma symptoms for a number of different reasons. Monitoring and recording symptoms in a diary is an important step in helping to confirm a diagnosis of asthma for children, particularly in the under 5.

Symptom diaries are relatively easy for parents or carers to complete and provide a more accurate record than relying on memory alone. Parents/carers are asked to record troublesome symptoms over a period of time and note any recognisable patterns or reduction in symptoms whilst the child is taking anti-asthma medicine. The diaries should include details of the following:

- Night-time wakening and symptoms, for example, cough, wheeze, breathlessness, noisy breathing.
- Day-time symptoms.
- Day-time activity.
- How often medication is used and any response to treatment.

Asthma triggers

An increase in asthma symptoms is usually associated with a trigger. Common triggers of asthma include the following:

- Respiratory infections, colds.
- House dust mite.

- Pets, especially cats.
- Exercise.
- Cold air or sudden temperature change.
- Cigarette smoke/smoky atmospheres.
- Excitement/stress.

It is impossible to avoid all contact with allergens or environmental hazards, but exposure should be reduced wherever possible to try and reduce symptoms and the need for medication.

Respiratory infections

Viral infections, such as the common cold, are the commonest trigger of asthma in children. Many preschool children only wheeze with colds; this is called transient or episodic wheeze. It is common in children under the age of 3, and by the time these children reach the age of 6 years, around two-thirds will be asymptomatic (Martinez and Helms, 1998).

Most children are exposed to a wide range of infectious organisms as they socialise, making it almost impossible for them to avoid contact with respiratory viruses. Mixing with friends at nursery or school and older siblings at home should not be restricted in the hope of avoiding a cough or cold. This will only isolate the child, increase parental anxiety and encourage a negative approach to asthma. There is some evidence that early exposure to viral infections is protective against the risks of asthma and wheezing during childhood (Ball et al., 2002).

House dust mite

House dust mites are tiny creatures that live in beds, carpets, soft furnishings and soft toys. They thrive in warm, humid conditions and can be found in even the cleanest of homes. Their bodies, secretions and faeces trigger symptoms in 85% of children or young people with asthma (Sporik et al., 1990).

House dust mites are impossible to eliminate completely, but the following measures may help to reduce levels even though there is little evidence of significant clinical benefit in doing so:

- Use a vacuum cleaner with a high-efficiency filter that returns very low amounts of dust to the environment.
- Damp dust after vacuuming.

- Replace feather pillows and woollen blankets with synthetic ones if they aggravate asthma symptoms.
- Wash bedlinen weekly at 60°C and dry in a tumble dryer or in the sun to kill the house dust mite.
- Replace curtains with roller blinds or light washable curtains.
- Replace carpets with hard flooring.

There is currently no evidence to support the use of allergen impermeable bed covers for adults with asthma (Woodcock et al., 2003). However, young children spend considerably more time in bed than adults, and some parents/carers anecdotally report bed covers to be beneficial. They may give some protection from the harmful effects of dust mite for children with severe asthma or atopy (Custovic et al., 2002).

Pets

Furry or feathery animals are a common trigger of asthma symptoms. Allergens are found in pet hair, saliva, urine and shed skin. Cats are one of the biggest culprits, but rabbits, dogs, horses and birds can all cause problems. Small rodents, and even large insects, can also provoke asthma in some children/young people.

Children/young people are often very affectionate towards family pets. This increases allergen exposure and leads to an increase in symptoms and acute exacerbations. If it is not possible to find a new home for the pet, then preventive measures such as keeping the pet out of the child's bedroom or living space may help reduce symptoms. Bathing cats or dogs twice a week can help reduce allergen load, but this is not always a practical solution.

Exercise and excitement

Exercise, laughing and excitement can all trigger asthma. About three-quarters of children/young people with asthma suffer from exercise-induced symptoms. Their airways often narrow following increased physical activity or sudden bursts of energetic play, particularly when the weather is cold.

The term *exercise-induced asthma* is commonly used to describe the type of symptoms associated with taking exercise or playing sport. Activity is an important trigger at all stages of childhood. If a child's asthma is exacerbated by running or playing, it is impractical and undesirable to try and restrict what is a normal activity for children.

It is important that children/young people with asthma have fun and enjoy exercise. Exercise-induced symptoms are a sign that asthma control is suboptimal and treatment should be reviewed. Encouraging them to take a reliever inhaler before going out to play sport can prevent symptoms.

Although most children/young people like to feel that they can do all the things their friends do, some may use their asthma as an excuse not to join in activities. Parents and teachers need to be able to recognise when this is happening and encourage the child to feel more confident about taking part.

Swimming, in particular, is an excellent activity for children/young people with asthma. The warm, humid atmosphere of a swimming pool may be less likely to trigger symptoms of asthma.

Cigarette smoke

Maternal smoking during pregnancy has a significant impact on airway growth development (Gilliland et al., 2000). Children whose parents smoke are more likely to have wheezing episodes, increased respiratory infections and time off school than the children of non-smoking parents (Strachan and Cook, 1998; Schwartz et al., 2000; Mannino et al., 2002; Lewis et al., 2005). Parents/carers who smoke must be strongly encouraged to stop smoking in front of children and referred to the primary care team for active support if they wish to stop. It is important not to miss any opportunity to give appropriate smoking cessation advice.

Cigarette smoking is a common risk-taking activity in adolescence. Many young people start to smoke between the ages of 12 and 14 years, and the earlier they start smoking, the less likely they are to give it up. Each contact with a health practitioner should be seen as an opportunity to provide health promotion advice.

Treating children/young people with asthma

There is no cure for asthma, but with appropriate treatment and management, most children/young

people can achieve good control of their condition. When asthma is under control children can:

- avoid troublesome symptoms, night and day;
- use little or no reliever medication;
- have productive, physically active lives;
- have (near) normal lung function;
- avoid serious attacks (Global Initiative for Asthma, 2006).

The British Thoracic Society and Scottish Intercollegiate Guideline Network have developed an evidence-based asthma guideline (BTS/SIGN, 2005). The guideline aims to standardise the treatment of asthma for children and adults. Treatment is recommended depending on the severity of symptoms and response to inhaled medication. The stepped approach encourages treatment to be increased if symptoms persist, or stepped down once asthma symptoms are controlled.

There are two main types of asthma medications: relievers and preventers. They work in different ways:

- Relievers – help to relieve breathing difficulties by opening up the airways.
- Preventers – help to protect the airways by reducing inflammation and mucus production.

Relievers (bronchodilators)

Bronchodilators are used for relieving symptoms. They relax the smooth muscle in the walls of the airways to allow the air to move in and out more easily.

There are two types of relievers:

(1) Short-acting relievers, for example, salbutamol or terbutaline
(2) Long-acting relievers, for example, salmeterol or formoterol

Short-acting relievers relieve symptoms within minutes of taking them and the effects last up to 4 hours. They prevent exercise-induced symptoms and are essential in treating acute asthma attacks. They are usually blue in colour and are first-line treatment (step 1) for children/young people with asthma (BTS/SIGN, 2005).

Relievers are taken as required:

- At the first sign of symptoms or.
- Just before symptoms are likely to occur if this can be predicted, for example, just before exercise or sport.

For children/young people with mild, intermittent symptoms, a reliever inhaler may be the only treatment they will need. It is important that children, parents and carers understand how the medication works and when to use it. High doses of reliever medication are used to treat acute exacerbations of asthma.

Long-acting relievers are used in a different way from short-acting relievers. They relieve symptoms of asthma by relaxing the muscle in the airways, but they only need to be taken twice a day because the drug remains effective for up to 12 hours.

Long-acting relievers have been developed as an add-on therapy for children/young people who are already taking preventer treatment but whose asthma symptoms remain difficult to control (step 3). Salmeterol takes about 30 minutes to become effective (for this reason it should not be used for the relief of an asthma attack), whilst formoterol has a more rapid onset of action (and is licensed for short-term symptom relief).

Preventers (anti-inflammatory medication)

Preventers, or inhaled corticosteroids, help to reduce underlying inflammation in the airways and prevent bronchial hyper-responsiveness. Common examples include beclometasone, budesonide, fluticasone, ciclesonide and mometasone. They are usually brown, red or orange in colour and need to be taken every day, on a regular basis, to build up their protective effect.

Corticosteroids have no immediate effect on asthma symptoms, but if taken regularly, will prevent asthma symptoms from occurring. Once regular treatment is started, they take approximately 3–7 days before any benefit is felt.

Inhaled steroids are introduced at step 2 of the asthma guideline. They are considered for use in children/young people who report any of the following:

- Using reliever medication three times a week or more.

- Symptoms three times a week or more.
- Waking with symptoms one night a week or more.
- Had an acute exacerbation of asthma in the last 2 years.

It is not uncommon for children (or adults) with asthma to rely on their reliever inhaler to treat their asthma because it provides quick and effective relief from symptoms. Children/young people find it hard to understand why you need to take preventive drugs when you are not actually ill (Sanz, 2003). This means that many children/young people will forget to use their preventer inhaler, especially if it is doing its job, which is to prevent symptoms from occurring.

It may help some children or young people to remember to take their preventer inhaler if they leave it near their toothbrush, another preventive task that most children have to be reminded to do on a regular basis.

Corticosteroids are similar to the steroids produced by the adrenal gland and have been used safely in the treatment of asthma for many years. The asthma guideline recommends using the lowest dose necessary to control symptoms but many parents are naturally concerned about their use. It is important to reassure and inform parents about the differences between anabolic steroids that are often abused by body builders and the safety of inhaled steroids used in the treatment of asthma.

Growth suppression has been shown to occur with high doses of inhaled corticosteroids (Todd et al., 2002). Whilst this usually corrects itself once the child reaches adulthood (Pederson and Agertoft, 2000), height should be accurately measured every 3–6 months and measurements recorded on centile measurement charts (Fry, 1998). The risk associated with preventive treatment has to be weighed up against the risk associated with uncontrolled or acute asthma.

Combination therapy

Combination inhalers are now available and deliver long-acting reliever medication with an inhaled corticosteroid. These inhalers help to simplify treatment and increase adherence with treatment regimes.

Leukotriene receptor antagonists

A new class of anti-inflammatory medications, known as leukotriene receptor antagonists (LTRAs), are a more recent introduction to the list of asthma medications. They work in a different way by blocking the activity of chemicals called leukotrienes that are involved in airway inflammation. They are essentially a preventer drug, but they also have a slight reliever effect and are taken orally once a day.

LTRAs are recommended as additional therapy at step 3 of the asthma guideline. In children aged 5 and above, they should only be considered after a trial of long-acting reliever and inhaled corticosteroid. In children under 5 years, they may be considered as an alternative preventer therapy at step 2 if inhaled steroids cannot be used.

LTRAs have also been shown to reduce viral-induced asthma exacerbations in children with intermittent asthma aged between 2 and 5 years and relieve symptoms associated with exercise-induced asthma (Bisgaard et al., 2005; Robertson et al., 2007).

Delivery devices

Most asthma medications are inhaled to ensure the medication is delivered directly to the airways where their action is needed. The advantages of inhaled therapy are as follows:

- The medication is delivered directly to the lungs.
- The dose is small.
- Incidence of side effects is low.
- The action is rapid.

A variety of delivery devices have been developed for this reason. In asthma management the choice of delivery system is almost as important as the choice of drug. An inappropriate delivery device, or the right delivery device used wrongly, may be one of the reasons for poor asthma control.

Children/young people should use an inhaler device appropriate for their age. They must be taught to use the chosen device correctly because poor technique will affect the amount of medication entering the small airways and will reduce the potential effectiveness of the treatment. The National Institute of Clinical Excellence (NICE) has issued guidelines on inhaler devices for children under 5 and 5–15 years (NICE, 2000, 2002).

A spacer device or holding chamber, with or without a facemask, is likely to be the most efficient way of delivering inhaled medication in young children, but as they grow, other smaller devices may be suitable. Spacer devices should ideally be used for inhaled steroids, although not all children/young people want to use a spacer device. Dry powder inhalers are easier to teach children/young people to use than conventional aerosol-metered dose inhalers, but generally should be reserved for children/young people age 6 years and over (O'Callaghan and Barry, 2000a,b).

Activity

The Asthma UK website (http://www.asthma.org.uk/using_your.html) has a useful section on inhalers where you can find out more about how to use the different devices available for children/young people.

What are the key factors to consider when helping a child to choose an inhaler?

Self-management

Children and families can be actively involved in managing asthma, and many take responsibility for their own health needs (Wolf et al., 2002). The asthma guideline recommends regular structured review and education sessions to help children and their families understand the basic principles of disease management in order to prevent problems or manage acute episodes more effectively.

At the review it is important to focus on the child's needs as well as that of the parent or carer. Many children/young people accept and learn to live with regular symptoms and limitations, seeing it as an inevitable part of having asthma. By working in partnership with children and families, you may be able to help them change their beliefs about asthma and recognise how they can improve their quality of life.

In order to control asthma, children and their families should understand the following:

- What triggers their asthma and how to avoid risk factors where possible.
- The difference between reliever and preventer inhalers and when to use them.

- How to use their inhaler correctly.
- How to recognise signs that asthma is worsening and take appropriate action.
- When to call the doctor or seek emergency treatment.

Worsening asthma

Children/young people with poorly controlled asthma are more likely to experience an acute exacerbation. Parents and children need help to learn to recognise the early warning signs of worsening asthma in order to prevent further deterioration. Signs and symptoms vary for each child but common features include the following:

- Waking at night with a cough or wheeze.
- Wheezing and coughing first thing in the morning.
- Increased wheeze and cough after exercise or doing less exercise.
- Needing more and more reliever medication with less and less effect.

Poorly controlled asthma is one of the main reasons for children/young people not being able to attend school or nursery. In a class of 30 children, there will be approximately 3 children with asthma, so it is not unreasonable to expect every teacher to have a basic knowledge of childhood asthma and know what to do in an emergency.

Asthma UK provides helpful written advice for schools within a school asthma pack. They recommend that all schools should:

- have an asthma policy;
- ensure that all staff know what to do in an asthma attack;
- recognise that pupils with asthma need immediate access to reliever inhalers at all times;
- keep a record of all pupils with asthma and the medicines they take;
- ensure that all pupils with asthma participate fully in all aspects of school life.

Asthma action plans

Asthma action plans should form part of a structured education programme for the child and family. They encourage health practitioners to work in partnership with children/young people. Asthma action plans record important information such as the following:

- What to do if symptoms get worse.
- How long to increase treatment for (and when to step down).
- What to do in an acute episode of asthma.
- When and how to seek medical help.

Asthma action plans focus on the individual needs of the child and family, helping them to be in control of their asthma. Asthma UK produces an asthma action plan, which is reproduced as an example in the asthma guideline (BTS/SIGN, 2005). The action plan is available from Asthma UK as well as from their website: http://www.asthma.org.uk.

How to treat an asthma attack

One of the aims of an asthma action plan is to avoid acute episodes or breakthrough symptoms. Inevitably, a number of children/young people, despite following their plan, will have an acute exacerbation. Because of the variable nature of asthma, an exacerbation can occur at any time, even when symptoms are apparently controlled. Deterioration may be gradual or sudden in onset.

In an acute exacerbation of asthma you should:

- stay calm and reassure the child/young person;
- give two puffs of reliever medication immediately, preferably through a spacer;
- help the child to breath by getting them to sit up and slightly forward – do not hug them or lie them down;
- loosen tight clothing;
- if there is no immediate improvement, continue to give one puff of reliever medication every minute for 2 minutes or until symptoms improve;
- encourage the child to breath slowly and calmly.

The reliever inhaler should start to work within 5–10 minutes and the child can return to normal activities.

Call 999 urgently if the child or young person:

- is breathless at rest;

- does not respond to reliever medication after 5–10 minutes;
- is distressed or unable to talk;
- appears agitated, drowsy or exhausted;
- has blue lips or extremities.

It is safe to continue giving further doses of the reliever medication while you are waiting for help to arrive.

Health promotion

It can be an emotional experience to be told you or your child has asthma. Most people either know someone with asthma or have personal experiences or beliefs that influence what they understand about the condition.

Of the 5.2 million people with asthma in the UK, it is estimated that more than half of them have poor asthma control and reduced quality of life due to factors other than disease severity (Asthma UK, 2004). Effective health promotion is an important part of asthma management because it can produce changes in knowledge and understanding or ways of thinking (Tones, 1997). Structured education programmes help children and families to learn more about asthma and its management and gain confidence in managing their own condition more effectively. Educational interventions delivered by health practitioners trained in asthma management can improve asthma outcomes by improving symptom control and reducing school absence and exacerbation rates (Hoskins et al., 1999).

It is important to establish what children and their families already know about asthma and not give too much information at once. Remember to involve the child as much as possible and address their concerns as well as their parents. Information should be tailored according to individual need and circumstances. It is good practice to recap on information on a regular basis.

Asthma is a multifaceted disease. It presents different problems for different children. Because of this, no single intervention will be effective in improving outcomes for children/young people with asthma. Instead, health promotion activities should focus on community-based approaches as well as individual care for each child. This will help to improve health status and quality of life as well as ensuring more appropriate use of medical services.

There is a wide choice of good quality, educational literature available from a variety of sources, for example, Asthma UK or the British Lung Foundation. The internet can be a rich source of useful information; for example, the Asthma UK website (http://www.asthma.org.uk) contains accurate and up-to-date information for all ages. All their booklets and fact-sheets can be downloaded and are available in different languages. There is also an e-mail support service or telephone helpline staffed by asthma-trained nurses.

Conclusion

- Asthma is the most common, chronic disease of childhood.
- Childhood asthma presents in many different patterns of frequency and severity.
- Asthma is an inflammatory condition of the airways caused by allergens, irritants or respiratory infections.
- Poorly managed asthma is a frequent cause of absence from school.
- Correct management includes relevant allergen avoidance advice, appropriate treatment administered through an appropriate inhaler device and regular assessment.

Children/young people with asthma should aim for the following:

- Have minimal symptoms day and night.
- Use little or no reliever medication.
- Experience minimal absence from school, nursery or playgroup.
- Participate in all social or leisure activities.
- Participate in play, sports or other physical activities.

Resources

Asthma UK

Asthma UK is a charity, providing information and help for adults and children with asthma. Its website includes details for health practitioners.

Publications are available free of charge – http://www.asthma.org.uk

British Lung Foundation

This charity aims to support adults and children affected by lung disease. Publications are available free of charge – http://www.lunguk.org

Education for Health

This is an educational charity, providing training and education for health practitioners to influence best practice in respiratory and cardiovascular care. A wide variety of modules and short courses are available. Their *Simply Devices* pocketbook gives straightforward and very practical advice for health practitioners on the use of different inhaler devices, nebulisers and nasal therapies for use in patients with asthma. For further information visit http://www.educationforhealth.org.uk

References

Asthma UK (2004) *Where Do We Stand? Asthma in the UK Today*. London: Asthma UK. Available at: http://www.asthma.org.uk.

Ball, T., Castro-Rodriguez, J., Griffith, K., Holberg, C., Martinez, F., Wright, A.L. (2002) Siblings, day-care attendance and the risk of asthma and wheezing during childhood. *New England Journal of Medicine* 343: 538–543.

Bisgaard, H., Zielen, S., Garcia-Garcia, M., Johnston, S., Gilles, L., Menten, J., Tozzi, C., Polos, P. (2005) Montelukast Reduces Asthma Exacerbations in 2- to 5-year-old children with intermittent asthma. *American Journal of Respiratory and Critical Care Medicine* 171: 315–322. Available at: http://ajrccm.atsjournals.org/cgi/content/full/171/4/315.

British Thoracic Society (2006) *The Burden of Lung Disease*, 2nd edn. A statistics report from the British Thoracic Society. Available at: http://www.brit-thoracic.org.uk (accessed March 2007).

BTS/SIGN (2005) *British Guideline on the Management of Asthma*. Revised edition (SIGN publication no. 63). Edinburgh: British Thoracic Society, Scottish Intercollegiate Guidelines Network. Available at: http://www.sign.ac.uk/guidelines/fulltext/63/index.html.

Custovic, A., Fortser, L., Matthews, E., Martin, J., Letley, L., Vickers, M., Britton, J., Strachan, D., Howarth, P., Altmann, D., Frost, C., Woodcock, A. (2002) The effect of mite-allergen control by the use of allergen-impermeable covers in adult asthma: the SMAC trial. *Thorax* 57(Suppl. III): S152, iii45.

Education and Skills (Department of), Department of Health (2004) *The National Service Framework for Children, Young People and Maternity Services*. London: Crown Copyright. Available at: http://www.publications.doh.gov.uk/nsf/children.

Fry, T. (1998). Growth and asthma: regular height assessment is an important part of managing childhood asthma. *The Asthma Journal* 3(1): 74–76.

Gilliland, F., Berhane, K., McConnell, R., Gauderman, W., Vora, H., Rappaport, E., Avol, E., Peters, J. (2000) Maternal smoking during pregnancy, environmental tobacco smoke exposure and childhood lung function. *Thorax* 55: 271–276.

Global Initiative for Asthma (2006) *Global Strategy for Asthma Management and Prevention*. Available at: http://www.ginasthma.org (accessed March 2007).

Hoskins, G., Nevill, R., Smith, B., Clark, R. (1999). The link between practice nurse training and asthma outcomes. *British Journal of Community Nursing* 4(5): 222–228.

International Study of Asthma and Allergies in Childhood (ISAAC) Steering Committee (1998) Worldwide variations in prevalence of symptoms of asthma, allergic rhinoconjunctivitis, and atopic eczema: ISAAC. *Lancet* 351: 1225–1232.

Lewis, S., Antoniak, M., Venn, A., Davies, L., Goodwin, A., Salfield, N., Britton, J., Fogarty, A. (2005) Second-hand smoke, dietary fruit intake, road traffic exposures and the prevalence of asthma: a cross sectional study in young children. *American Journal Epidemiol* 161: 406–411.

Mannino, D., Homa, D., Redd, S. (2002) Involuntary smoking and asthma severity in children: data from the Third National Health and Nutrition Examination Survey. *Chest* 122: 409–415.

Martinez, F., Helms, P. (1998) Types of asthma and wheezing. *European Respiratory Journal* 12(Suppl. 27): 3s–8s.

Mygind, N., Dahl, R., Pedersen, S., Thestrup-Pedersen, K. (1996). *Essential Allergy*. Oxford: Blackwell Science.

NICE (2000) *Guidance on the Use of Inhaler Systems (Devices) in Children Under the Age of 5 Years with Chronic Asthma*. Technology Appraisal Guidance No. 10. London: National Institute for Clinical Excellence.

NICE (2002) *Inhaler Devices for Routine Treatment of Chronic Asthma in Older Children (Age 5–15 Years)*. Technology Appraisal Guidance No. 38. London: National Institute for Clinical Excellence.

O'Callaghan, C., Barry, P. (2000a). Asthma drug delivery devices for children. *British Medical Journal* 320: 664.

O'Callaghan, C., Barry, P. (2000b). How to choose delivery devices for asthma. *Archives of Disease in Childhood* 82: 185–191.

Office for National Statistics (2004) Asthma and allergic diseases. *The Health of Children and Young People*. London: Office for National Statistics.

Pederson, S., Agertoft, L. (2000) Effect of long-term treatment with inhaled budesonide on adult height in children with asthma. *NEJM* 343(15): 1064–1069.

Robertson, C., Price, D., Henry, R., Mellis, C., Glasgow, N., Fitzgerald, D., Lee, A., Turner J., Sant, M. (2007) Short-course montelukast for intermittent asthma in children. *American Journal Respiratory Critical Care Medicine* 175: 323–329

Royal College of General Practitioners (2004) *Mean Weekly Incidence of New Asthma Episodes (England and Wales)*. London: HMSO.

Sanz, E. (2003) Concordance and children's use of medicines. *BMJ* 327: 858–860.

Schwartz, J., Timonen, K., Pekkanen, J. (2000) Respiratory effects of environmental tobacco smoke in a panel study of asthmatic and symptomatic children. *American Journal of Respiratory and Critical Care Medicine* 161(3 Part 1): 802–806.

Sporik, R., Holgate, S., Platts-Mills, T., Cogswell, J. (1990) Exposure to house dust mite allergen (Der p 1) and the development of asthma in childhood. A prospective study. *New England Journal of Medicine* 323: 502–507.

Strachan, D., Cook, D. (1998). Health effects of passive smoking. 6. Parental smoking and childhood asthma: longitudinal and case control studies. *Thorax* 53(3): 204–412.

Todd, G., Alcerini, C., Ross-Russell, R., Zahra, S., Warner, J., McCance, D. (2002) Survey of adrenal crisis associated with inhaled corticosteroids in the United Kingdom. *Archives of Disease in Childhood* 2: 457–461.

Tones, K. (1997) Health education: evidence of effectiveness. *Archives of Disease in Childhood* 77: 189–191.

Wolf, F., Guevara, J., Grum, C., Clark, N., Cates, C. (2002) Educational interventions for asthma in children. *The Cochrane Database of Systematic Reviews*, Issue 1, The Cochrane Collaboration. Available at: http://www.cochrane.org/reviews/en/ab000326.html.

Woodcock, A., Forster, L., Matthews, E., Martin, J., Letley, L., Vickers, M., Britton, J., Strachan, D., Howarth, P., Altmann, D., Frost, C., Custovic, A. (2003) Control of exposure to mite allergen and allergen-impermeable bed covers for adults with asthma. *NEJM* 349(3): 225–236.

19 Managing Children's Skin Conditions

Elizabeth Barrett

NSF

The National Service Framework (NSF) for children, young people and maternity services, standard 10, highlights that in all settings families should be *active partners* in decisions about the medicines prescribed for them (Education and Skills, Department of Health, 2004).

Introduction

Skin conditions are involved in 15% of all consultations in primary care. Even common rashes can cause diagnostic difficulty. Experience takes time to develop. This chapter therefore is a guide to some of the common skin conditions nurses may come across and the health promotion advice that can be given.

Resources used to support this chapter came from a range of different sources. A useful source of information was the website for the British Association of Dermatologists (http://www.bad.org.uk). This is a resource that both families as well as practitioners will find useful. A further resource was the British National Formulary (BNF, 2007), which provides advice and prescribing details. In addition, stories that patients have told me over 25 years of working in primary care

and hospital practice, were also useful. The best way to look at a rash is with a colleague who knows more, and I acknowledge the mentorship of Dr Bruce Bittiner, Consultant Dermatologist at Bassetlaw Hospital, Worksop.

This chapter looks at general health promotion advice in relation to common skin conditions in children. It will focus particularly on childhood eczema.

General advice

It is helpful to have a limited range of treatments that you get used to advising on, or demonstrating. Ask your local pharmacist to let you have small pack sizes of some commonly used emollients. Try them out to see how they feel. Familiarise yourself with a range of steroids of different strengths.

Assessing a new patient

Not all rashes are instantly recognisable, so it is helpful to have a routine of enquiry when a child presents with a rash.

Take a proper history and have a good look at the child's skin. Listening establishes rapport and allows you to see the condition through the eyes of the child or parent. Ask open questions, such as *how does it affect you?* Use non-medical terms such as *rough* rather than *keratotic*, and *asthma and hay fever* rather than *atopy*.

History

How long has the rash been there? Have you had it before? Does it come and go? Is it itchy? Is the child well, or ill? Has the child been given any medication? What treatment have you tried so far? In the case of suspected eczema, *does the child have hay fever or asthma?*

Family history

Is anyone else itching? Is there a family history of asthma, hay fever or eczema?

Examination

In the interests of the child's autonomy, it is best to ask parents, or the child, to remove any clothes. Smaller children can sit on a parent's knee. Examine the skin in very good daylight, or use an examination light. Look at all the rash, including the nails and hair, if necessary. Feel the rash; run your fingers over it to see if it is rough or raised. Look for signs of scratching. Then stand back and look at the whole pattern. Is it symmetrical? Where is it most dense? Where are the areas that are not affected?

Tests and investigations

It is rarely necessary to do special tests. If a rash comes and goes, parents can be encouraged to take a photograph.

Giving health information

Information is best given to the parent in writing. Be specific about when treatments should be applied and how creams should be used, and for how long. Make review arrangements clear.

Other resources

The British Association of Dermatologists (2007) has an excellent website which provides a wide range of information leaflets for parents. Pictures of common skin conditions are shown. Both parents and children can be reassured by seeing their condition shown in a photograph.

Some common skin conditions in children

This section looks at the following common skin conditions in children:

- Viral rashes.
- Infestations.
- Urticaria and allergies.

Viral rashes

Rashes cause instant parental concern. This is mainly because of the fear of meningitis, but there are also fears of infectivity too. Parents need advice about school and nursery exclusion. Exclusion policy needs to be checked with the local Health Protection office. Giving a copy of this to parents may be helpful, so that they can bring it into school.

Viral rashes often appear quite suddenly and are usually blotchy, pink and are distributed over most of the body, although they tend to be more obvious on the trunk. They are often first noticed after the evening bath. Pressure with a glass tumbler causes the rash to fade. The same effect can be produced by pressing with your finger to see if you can blanch out the colour. Assess the general health of the child. Most viral rashes are non-specific and cannot be named. Most of them will fade in 2 or 3 days.

Fear of meningitis needs to be acknowledged and discussed. The sudden appearance of a rash in a child who seems very ill, or who has a very high temperature, is a medical emergency. In a very ill child, rash should be sought as it may not be obvious (Burns et al., 2004).

Chickenpox is a specific rash that is recognised by its numerous, discrete, red spots distributed over the whole body, including the scalp. In the early stages, it is helpful to find at least one fresh lesion with a tiny central blister. However, this may soon be scratched away because of itch.

Infestations

Scabies

Scabies is a common and important childhood rash that is often missed. Scabies can be wrongly treated as eczema, and eczema can be wrongly treated as

scabies. It is important to learn how to find scabies burrows because they look very insignificant.
You will not notice them if you do not look carefully. Ask a colleague to show you, if uncertain.
The places to look are between the fingers and on
the ulnar borders of the hands or wrists. In boys,
burrows or nodules on the penis are diagnostic of
scabies.

A burrow is a small, slightly wavy line, about
half a centimetre long. One or two burrows may
only be seen, so look carefully using a good light.
You many manage to see a tiny dot at the end of
a burrow, which is a mite. The absence of burrows
makes a diagnosis of scabies unlikely, and it is not a
good idea to treat an itch with anti-scabietic creams,
just in case. If the diagnosis is made, contacts need
to be identified and treated too. It is therefore important to be sure. Scabies is contagious and can
spread between family and friends, and enters into
hospitals.

Symptoms of scabies result from an allergy to the
mite *Sarcoptes scabiei* (Burns et al., 2004). The onset
of itch occurs 3–4 weeks after infection is acquired
for the first time. The itch of scabies is intense and is
worse at night, or when warm. It does not respond
to topical steroids or anti-histamines, so if a child
is not responding to good eczema treatment, the
diagnosis should be suspected afresh. Children of
any age can be affected. In any itching child, it is
important to ask whether other family members are
itching too.

Figure 19.1 shows a typical scabies burrow in a
typical site. These are subtle and need to be looked
for.

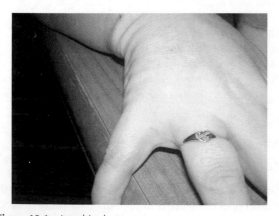

Figure 19.1   A scabies burrow.

On the rest of the body, the scabies rash can be
an unimpressive pinpoint rash, often with marked
evidence of scratching. Small blisters can be present
on the fingers. In babies, under 1 year of age, look
for burrows and blisters on the soles of the feet,
as well as on the hands. Blisters on the feet and
hands may become impetiginised (secondarily infected with *Staphylococcus*).

Treatment

Scabies spread requires close physical contact, prolonged holding of hands or sharing a bed. It is essential to identify and treat all physical contacts, even
those who are not itching, in order to break the cycle
of reinfection.

Scabies can be treated with malathion (not in children under 6 months) or permethrin (not in children under 2 months) (BNFC, 2007). Check the trade
names in the British National Formulary for Children (BNFC, 2007). A 30 g tube, or 50 mL bottle, will
be enough for two small children.

Treatment can be prescribed by the doctor or a
nurse prescriber, or bought at the chemist, if this is
more convenient. The treatment needs to be used
once, and all likely contacts should be treated at the
same time to avoid the chance of reinfection.

Help parents to draw up a list of all physical contacts in order to let them know to seek treatment.
Provide health promotion literature to support verbal health promotion advice given.

It is simplest to apply treatment last thing at night,
but not immediately after a hot bath. The lotion or
cream must be smoothed over the whole of the body,
from the neck (at the level of the ears, down) and
allowed to soak in. It may be easier to apply lotion
with a small paintbrush. Every square inch of the
skin must be covered, with particular attention paid
to the finger webs, toe webs, palms and soles.

The treatment should be left on for at least
12 hours. If this process is undertaken properly
once, it should not need to be repeated. However,
some authorities recommend a repeat application
in a week (Burns et al., 2004). Parents should be
warned about overuse of insecticides resulting from
misplaced fears of reinfection; itch may take several weeks to settle, and does not necessarily mean
the treatment has failed. Eurax or Eurax HC can be
helpful during this time.

Babies can be treated with 5% permethrin, and
the cream needs to be applied to the head, face and

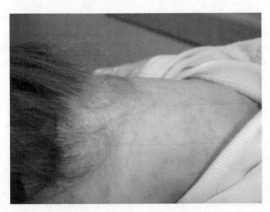

Figure 19.2   Itchy lesions at the nape of the neck (head lice).

neck as well as the body. It is advisable to seek the advice of the local dermatologist in babies under 2 months of age.

The commonest causes of treatment failure are not covering the whole body, not leaving the treatment on for 12 hours, not treating all affected people simultaneously, or reinfection from an undiagnosed, original source. It is helpful to be positive about the diagnosis, as some parents are very ashamed of scabies. Scabies is not associated with dirt. Reassure parents that scabies (unlike eczema) is curable within 24 hours, and therefore is a preferable diagnosis. Mites can survive for 24 hours in bedding or clothes, but normal washing of bedclothes is adequate, and there is no need to boil, burn or throw things out.

Head lice

Head lice are crawling insects that lay eggs (nits) that cement onto the shaft of the hair, near the base. Itch is caused by allergy to the bites of the insects. In the early stages of infestation, itch can be intense, but this can gradually lessen so that some children with chronic head lice infestation may have no itch.

The picture in Figure 19.2 shows typical lesions at the nape of the neck. These will cause discomfort; the child will find them itchy.

In severe infections, children can develop secondary staphylococcal infection (impetigo) at the back of the scalp and the hair can become stuck down and matted, usually just above the nape of the neck. Parents may need to be shown how to soak the crust away with saline soaks. The impetigo

may need to be treated with oral antibiotics (flucloxacillin or erythromycin).

Detection

Parents sometimes want a practitioner to look for live head lice. Live lice can be difficult to spot but, under a good light, you may see the grey, grain-sized insects moving. Head lice eggs (nits) are laid on the shaft of the hair, close to the scalp, and remain on the hair as it grows, giving an indication of when infestation occurred. Empty nit cases remain stuck to the hair shaft after treatment. If there is a problem of head lice at school, detection combing, once a week, is helpful, though time-consuming. Detection combing takes about 30 minutes, depending on the length of the hair. Large amounts of conditioner are needed in order to make the hair slippery and clog up the legs of live lice. The hair is divided into sections and a fine *nit comb* can be run through the whole length. Insects get caught up in the comb and can be disposed of.

Treatment

Insecticides, such as phenothrin, permethrin, carbaryl and malathion, are all effective, but concerns about resistance mean that you need to check with local guidance. The health protection nurse of your primary care trust will be able to advise. Insecticides need to be kept on the hair for 12 hours and are denatured by heat so must be left to dry, naturally. Shampoos should be avoided because the relatively low concentration may encourage incomplete treatment and, thus, the development of resistance. A further treatment in a week is logical, just in case there are any freshly hatched nits. If an alcohol-based lotion is used, be careful about open flames, as there are reported cases of burns as a result of lotions catching fire. Lotions sting if the scalp is scratched or raw, so aqueous preparations may be more comfortable in this instance. Insecticides can be purchased over the counter. Parents should be warned against regular, preventative treatment with insecticides, as this may encourage resistance.

The nurse may be called upon to show parents how to treat chronic head lice infestation effectively. *Bug busting* with repeated conditioning and combing can catch and dispose of newly hatched lice, but needs to be done regularly and properly. This requires considerable effort and commitment, and parents may need to be shown how to do it. It needs to be done at least four times a week. Large quantities of conditioner can become expensive, even if the cheapest ones are used. The success rate is only half that of malathion (Burns et al., 2004). A similar technique is used for detection combing. Siblings of a child who has head lice do not necessarily need to be treated unless head lice are detected on them.

Fungal infections

There is a tendency for parents, and often practitioners, to assume that all circular, itchy lesions are fungal. Discoid eczema is also common in children, and it often shows a pattern of central clearing, which makes parents and practitioners suspect ringworm. The *active edge* of ringworm is more florid than in discoid eczema. If in doubt take scrapings. Accurate diagnosis is important because topical steroids make fungal infection worse, and anti-fungal treatment does not work in eczema. The temptation, sometimes, is to choose a combination product such as Canesten HC or Daktacort, but it is better to make an accurate diagnosis.

Taking a good history is important, especially the speed of spread. Fungal infection can spread explosively. Enquire about a personal and family history of eczema, hay fever, or asthma. Ask whether there is a new kitten or puppy in the house, and whether parents have noticed any bald patches on any of their animals.

Taking scrapings

Most laboratories supply a fungal scraping kit, which may consist of a black piece of stiff paper which folds over and seals. A scalpel scraped gently and painlessly over the lesion will yield a fine powder of skin flakes, which are easily seen against the black. Try to get a good sprinkling to avoid the laboratory reporting that you have an insufficient sample. If the kit is not available, use an ordinary sterile sample pot but you may need a larger quantity of scrapings. Alternatively, cut a piece of coloured paper yourself, and fold it and put it into the pot.

The main sources of fungal infections in children are animals. Some forms of animal ringworm can spread rapidly, doubling and trebling in numbers every few days. This causes florid, juicy lesions with a ring of active pustules at the edge. Fungal infection in the scalp can cause circular patches of hair loss. These are rough and scaly, which distinguishes

them from another common cause of circular hair loss – alopecia areata. (The scalp in alopecia areata is very smooth and shiny and there are often stubbly hairs at the edges, known as *exclamation hairs*.) Occasionally, animal ringworm in the scalp can cause a boggy, oozy lesion called *kerion*, which is easily mistaken for impetigo. This is an acute inflammatory reaction to fungus and it needs to be treated promptly. It can cause permanent hair loss through scarring.

Treatment

If there are only one or two patches of ringworm, topical anti-fungal treatment may be effective. Rapidly spreading ringworm, or ringworm in the scalp, requires oral anti-fungals. Few oral anti-fungals are licensed in children. Fluconazole could be used, but carefully check the dosage for age and weight of the child in the BNFC (2007). Your local pharmacist, or the pharmacy advice service at the local hospital, will help.

Urticaria and allergies

Urticaria

Urticaria is generally described as an *allergy* or *nettle rash*, though the cause of the allergy is rarely identifiable. It can occur suddenly and is one of the commonest rashes that will bring patients to the doctor in an emergency. Urticaria causes short-lived swelling and redness of the skin which is well-demarcated and itchy. The surface of the skin (epidermis) is normal. It is characterised by the speed at which it comes and goes and the way it *moves around* the body. An area covered by florid urticaria at the time of leaving home may be completely clear by the time the child arrives at the surgery, only to have come up somewhere else during the journey.

Figure 19.3 shows urticaria on a baby's arm, with noticeable dermal oedema. This was gone the next day. Note the normal surface of the skin.

The most important treatment for urticaria is explanation and reassurance. It has no underlying serious cause, and no special tests need to be done. Skin contains many different types of cells, one of which is the mast cell. Mast cells contain histamine and their activation releases histamine into the tissues, causing wheal and flare. Explaining the condition in terms of the mast cells and the *instability*

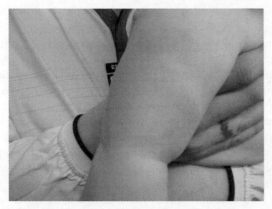

Figure 19.3   Urticaria on a baby's arm.

of the immune system is generally acceptable to parents, as long as its benign nature is emphasised. Food allergy or intolerance is rarely identifiable as a cause of urticaria. In children the commonest preceding event is an upper respiratory tract infection (Burns et al., 2004).

Parents worry more about urticaria on the face, especially if it causes deep swelling (angio-oedema). If this is a recurrent problem, parents should keep antihistamines ready, and if swelling of the throat or larynx is considered to be a risk, then a pre-filled adrenaline pen would be prescribed.

Oral non-sedating anti-histamines are the treatment of choice for urticaria. These can be given continuously or intermittently, depending on how the condition behaves. Most urticaria in children melts away within days, though it can persist for months or even longer.

Food or nut allergy

This is a difficult area for parents and for practitioners because of the worry of rapid, serious reactions, especially anaphylaxis or oedema of the throat or larynx. Parents often place great faith in food allergy as a cause of skin problems, and this faith is rarely shared by practitioners. It is an area where good listening and explanation are essential.

The suspicion of any food or nut allergy is based on history. Parents need to keep a close note of the relationship between certain foods and the development of swelling, especially if it is of the mouth and tongue. Keeping a food diary may help, noting any reactions.

It is possible to do a blood test to nuts (RAST testing). This may identify a particular type of nut, but it is still necessary to go on an accurate history. It may be necessary for children to carry a pre-filled adrenaline pen, and someone needs to have clear instructions as to how and when to use it.

How to treat childhood eczema

There are two main types of eczema that are seen in children. By far the most common is *atopic eczema*, but *seborrhoeic eczema* occurs in babies, and it is important to know the difference.

Seborrhoeic eczema (or dermatitis)

Seborrhoeic dermatitis is a distinctive and curious condition that occurs in young babies in the first few weeks of life and spontaneously resolves, often within a few weeks (Burns et al., 2004). Its relationship with atopic eczema is unclear. Typically, the baby is content, and does not scratch, but the parent is distressed about the appearance, as it can look very florid and sore. (In atopic eczema, in contrast, the baby scratches as soon as clothes are removed.) Seborrhoeic dermatitis often starts in the napkin area, but it is common on the cheeks, under the arms and under the chin. Seborrhoeic eczema has a greasy appearance, and can look very like psoriasis. In flexures, and in the nappy area, it is nearly always infected with candida, and can be bright red, sore and well demarcated. This is one of the few circumstances where the use of a product that combines an anti-fungal with a mild topical steroid (Daktacort, Canesten HC, or Trimovate), is needed. In non-occluded areas, seborrhoeic dermatitis can be treated with a mild topical steroid without an anti-fungal. This needs to be pitched to the severity of the condition. Hydrocortisone 1% or Eumovate are the steroids of choice. (Consult the BNFC for exact details.)

Atopic eczema

Atopy is a genetic condition. An atopic child can have any one, or a combination of all of the atopic conditions of asthma, hay fever or eczema.

Eczematous children have dry skin. Regular use of an emollient to moisturise is a fundamental part of good skin care, as is avoidance of bubble baths and soaps. Ointments are greasier than creams and are preferable, but it is important to go with patient preference on all products, as their acceptability determines whether they will be used. If creams or ointments sting or itch, then they should be changed to something more comfortable.

Eczema is a chronic skin condition, which flares and settles, often for no reason, and parents often blame themselves for flare-ups. It is important to be able to guide parents and children on what to expect and give them confidence in their management. Broken nights and complicated treatments can come to dominate household routines, and compliance can be difficult for busy families. Detailed instructions are essential; *use as directed* and *apply twice a day* are not adequate instructions. Apart from all the obvious reasons for poor compliance, practitioners contribute by some of the following:

- Giving inadequate or muddled instructions about how to use treatment and what to expect.
- Making it difficult for parents to obtain adequate supplies.
- Not reviewing the child to assess response to treatment and amounts needed.
- Steroid phobia.

Detailed instructions

It is not uncommon for parents to accumulate large numbers of different tubes of cream for their child's eczema. There may be several tubs of emollient, and several different strengths of steroids at home. The more there are, the more likely there is to be confusion about how to use them. A survey of parents of children with eczema in 1993 showed that 65% of parents wanted advice on how to use prescribed eczema treatments (Long et al., 1993).

Give written instructions, preferably with some idea about how much cream you expect the child to use per month. Ask parents to bring in whatever they have, and throw out the tubs and tubes that you do not want them to use. It may be best to keep things simple and use the same product for washing with, and for using as a moisturizer.

Emollients can be put on, all over, before getting into the bath or shower, and then washed off with the water. More can be put on after drying off with a towel. Emollients should be applied thinly and quickly. Many emollients are marketed as bath oils, and these are very acceptable because they are easy to use. All emollients can be used as soaps, and some can be dissolved by whisking with a tablespoon in a jug of hot water and adding it to the bath as a liquid (emulsifying ointment). (For safety reasons obviously keep the jug of hot water well away from the child.)

Baths needs to be washed out with warm water and detergent to avoid the greasier products blocking the plughole and downpipes. All emollients make the bath slippery, so there needs to be a bathmat available for the unwary. If there is a real objection, it is acceptable to bathe in water and then put emollient on after the bath, while the skin is still warm and damp.

Steroids

The word *steroid* is an emotive one, and many parents and practitioners worry about their use. The concerns are mainly around skin thinning. Parents may refuse to use topical steroids and prefer to identify a single cause, so that they can prevent their child's eczema. Many practitioners prescribe steroids fearfully and transmit this fear to patients: *'The doctor gave me this but told me not to use it.'* This fear is reinforced by information leaflets, friends, neighbours and sometimes by the pharmacist.

Unrealistically, small amounts of steroid are sometimes issued with the expectation of it lasting a month. Parents may fear or resent the disapproval of practice receptionists if they ask for more. Leaflets frequently give advice not to use steroids for more than a few days at a time. So, if you want parents to apply steroids you must say exactly how you want them used and preferably write it down as well.

One of the commonest problems with eczema is undertreatment, and many families suffer needlessly by trying to control severe eczema with emollients and oral anti-histamines. It is essential that parents have an understanding of how eczema behaves, and what constitutes *mild* eczema, what constitutes *severe* or *infected* eczema and how these different stages should be treated.

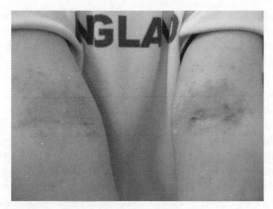

Figure 19.4 Scratched and infected atopic eczema in a typical site.

Steroid creams should be applied to active eczema only. These can be described as the *red and itchy bits*, and can be classified as mild or severe depending on how red and itchy they are.

Infected eczema is cracked and oozy. A sudden widespread flare-up of bright red eczema, especially if a child is shivery or unwell, is known as *erythrodermic* eczema (Figure 19.4). Infected or erythrodermic eczema will respond well to even 2 or 3 days of oral anti-staphylococcal antibiotics (flucloxacillin or erythromycin), and it is useful for some parents to keep a prescription in hand, rather than have to make an appointment to see a doctor.

There is little agreement as to whether steroids should be put on before or after emollients, so you need to decide on your own set of instructions and stick to them. Putting a steroid on before an emollient seems logical although evidence is lacking. Instructions should be to apply steroid cream *thinly*, rather than *sparingly* (because for some people sparingly means rarely).

The steroid should be applied to active eczema, allowed to soak in, and then emollient should be applied to the whole body, if possible. If the family is in a hurry to get ready for school, it is better to apply the emollient immediately, than not at all. It is best not to make creaming routines too cumbersome or complicated, or they may be avoided altogether.

Using brand names

It is safer to use brand names for steroids. Generic names are difficult to pronounce or remember, and some of them can sound very alike, which constitutes a clinical risk. Some steroid creams contain antibiotics, which can be very useful for infected eczema. Most creams with a letter after their name (Locoid – C, or Betnovate – N, for instance) contain an antibiotic.

Estimating correct amounts

Emollients should be prescribed in large amounts, usually in 500 g tubs. This allows you to differentiate between emollients and steroids, because steroids only come in tubes. It also reinforces the message that emollients should be used often. Nurses should advise parents to go on using emollients, even when the skin is in good condition. In very dry skin conditions, it is quite possible to use up to 500 g of emollient per week, and it is important to let the surgery know that these are the sort of quantities that may be required. Otherwise, parents may run into difficulties getting repeat prescriptions. While emollients should be used even when the skin is in good condition, children should stop using steroids once the skin is no longer red and itchy.

Requirements for steroids need to be gauged approximately. Application is sometimes quantified as *finger tip units* or FTUs (the amount of ointment that can be squeezed onto an adult finger between the tip of the finger and the first crease) (BNFC, 2007). However, it is probably more useful to work out with the parents how much is being used per month and where it is being used. If a tube of 30 g lasts 3 months, for instance, then 10 g is being used per month. The amount of steroid cream needed depends on the amount of eczema. The strength of the steroid depends on the site.

Weak steroids, such as hydrocortisone 1% can be used, though sometimes Eumovate is needed for short bursts. Stronger steroids are needed where eczema is thickened by scratching, or where the skin is naturally thicker, as on the hands, feet and knees. The strength of a steroid is increased by occlusion, including the natural occlusion of flexures, so it is not appropriate to use anything stronger than hydrocortisone or Trimovate in areas where there are deep folds of skin. For details about the potency of different steroids consult the BNFC (2007).

Alternatives to steroids, such as picrolimus or tacrolimus, are rarely necessary, and should not be routinely used as a way of circumventing steroid phobia. The long-term effect of these products is not yet established.

Although antihistamines may be helpful in reducing itch, especially at night, the priority should be to reduce itch by better management of the eczema. Avoid daytime sleepiness by using nonsedating antihistamines in the day.

Repeat prescriptions of steroids

While it could be considered wise not to have stronger steroids on repeat prescription for children, the hurdles placed in the way of obtaining them should not be so high that parents are put off using them appropriately. Single, acute, prescriptions may give a false message that the condition will be cured by the end of treatment. There needs to be a balance between the risk of overlooking review and the risk of making life difficult for parents. Unlike tablets, there is no set time for a tube to last, especially as eczema is a variable condition. Putting review instructions, or quantity suggestions, on the prescription may help to remind parents when to come for review. Bear in mind, however, that labels fall off tubes of creams, or become easily smudged.

Bandaging and wet wrapping

Wet wrapping is rarely necessary for mild or moderate eczema, but occasionally it can be useful, especially if a child cannot help scratching at night. The easiest places to wet wrap are the limbs.

Special diets and allergy testing

There is no evidence to support special diets as a way of preventing or managing atopic eczema. However, if parents notice that their child reacts badly to a particular food, they will usually have taken steps to avoid it already. As long as an extreme diet is not being imposed on a child, or they are made to feel too different from their peers, it is reasonable to support parents in things that will help their child. The problem is that eczema waxes and wanes, often for no particular reason, and it can be very difficult to make connections between foods and outbreaks of eczema.

Atopic eczema is a genetic predisposition and atopic individuals tend to have multiple positive results on allergy testing. These are not clinically useful. It may help to explain to parents that there is no external cause, and that the cause is in the chromosomes. This explanation may help to calm their search for an individual cause. For most children, eczema becomes less severe as they get older, and frequently disappears altogether, despite their genetic predisposition.

Reviewing

Formal review of skin conditions is not always easy in primary care because appointment systems do not always favour continuity of care. However, an offer to review the clinical condition gives parents confidence and it underlines that eczema is a chronic condition and that you do not expect one tube of cream to cure it. At each review it is important to clarify what emollient is being used, how often, and to gauge the amount of steroid being used per month. In addition, enquire about sleep, scratching and school. Always ask parents to bring in all creams and ointments to the review. Offer to throw out items that are finished or are not being used.

Conclusion

This chapter has explored some of the more common skin conditions of childhood. Treatment and health promotion advice have been outlined. The BNFC (2007) is an essential resource when prescribing treatment for children. To help ensure treatment is undertaken, provide families with written health promotion advice to accompany any verbal advice given. Do not forget the importance of reviewing children's skin to ascertain the impact of any treatment.

Importantly, as the NSF highlights, when prescribing for children, involve families in the prescribing decisions (Education and Skills, Department of Health, 2004). If they are involved in this process, they are going to be more likely to participate (concord) with treatment. They have taken part in the decision; therefore, they will have some confidence in that decision, more so than if their views had not been considered.

References

British Association of Dermatologists (2007) Available at: http://www.bad.org.uk (accessed July 2007).

British National Formulary (2007) London: British Medical Association, Royal Pharmaceutical Society of Great Britain, RCPCH Publications Ltd.

BNF for Children (BNFC) (2007) London: British Medical Association, Royal Pharmaceutical Society of Great Britain, Royal College of Paediatrics and Child Health, Neonatal and Paediatric Pharmacists Group.

Burns, T., Beathnach, S., Cox, N., Griffiths, C. (2004) *Rook's Textbook of Dermatology*, 7th edn. Oxford: Blackwell Publishing.

Education and Skills (Department of), Department of Health (2004) *National Service Framework for Children, Young People and Maternity Services, Standard 10: Medicines*. London: Crown Copyright.

Long, C., Funnell, C., Collard, R., Finlay, A. (1993) What do members of the National Eczema Society really want? *Clinical Experimental Dermatology* 18: 516–522.

20 Health Promotion for Children/ Young People with Cancer

Louise Soanes

NSF

Young people who have survived cancer will want to be participating in many of the same life experiences as their peers. They will want to be taking on more responsibility for their own health. The National Service Framework (NSF) for children, young people and maternity services talks about young people being provided with the opportunity to become more responsible for their own health (Education and Skills, Department of Health, 2004). Nurses working with young people recovering from cancer can be supportive, teaching them how to take care of themselves so they remain in good health.

Understanding cancer

Over the past three decades, the overall incidence of childhood cancer in Europe has risen by 1% per year for children aged 0–14 years and by 1.5% per year for young people aged 15–19 years. Nevertheless, there have been enormous advances in treatment which have improved survival rates (Steliarova-Foucher et al., 2004). In contrast to a *5-year survival rate* of 10% for children with leukaemia in the 1960s, for example, the *survival rate* has now increased to 80% (Stiller, 2007). This success is reflected in many other childhood cancers too. As a result there is now a growing population of young people and adults who have survived childhood cancer and its treatment; in 1971 there were 1400 adult survivors of childhood cancer in the United Kingdom (UK), and by the beginning of the twenty-first century, there were over 15 000 (Stiller, 2007). It is predicted by the year 2010 that approximately 1 in 250 adults will be a survivor of childhood cancer (Wallace and Green, 2004).

Guidance produced by the National Institute for Clinical Excellence (NICE, 2005), *Improving Outcomes in Children and Young People with Cancer*, recommends service provision for children and young people with cancer. Health promotion is implicit rather than explicit within this guidance. It is recognised that *supportive care* – interventions used to support children/young people through treatment – has played a major role in increasing survival rates and children's general well-being. Health promotion at this stage is often led by nurses and other practitioners.

Health promotion prior to cure from cancer is aimed at promoting optimal recovery from treatment and supporting children/young people. The need for good nutrition, protection from infection, maintenance of home and school life, psychological health and the early detection of side effects are all key elements that enable children/young people to come through their often arduous treatment. A large and collaborative multi-professional team is available to support them. Once treatment is complete, families must be reassured that care will continue (Gibson and Soanes, 2001). Success raises its own challenges. Not least of which is how to ensure that once cured, survivors will retain their health and avoid risk-taking behaviours that may be a threat to their health.

Young people surviving cancer

After treatment has ended, the emphasis of care and health promotion focuses upon the ongoing health of children/young people. Consultant follow-ups at outpatient clinics will be needed for life. For the first 5 years follow-up will be with the treating consultant. At this stage the aim of follow-up is twofold – physical and psycho-social. Physically, the aim is to monitor, detect and treat recurrence, and to detect side effects from treatment that need intervention or referral. Psycho-socially care is about monitoring social and psychological rehabilitation. After the first 5 years of survivorship, many move on to what is frequently known as the *long-term* or *late-effects clinic*. It is often during this stage that children move into adolescence. Adolescence is a time when they become more independent, moving away from some aspects of parental/carer supervision, with friends becoming especially important. It is at this time that young people may be exposed to risk-taking behaviours, such as smoking and poor diet, which can challenge their health. The continued support of nurses can help young people make positive health choices at this time. This chapter focuses its attention on *health promotion* related to the care of *survivors of childhood cancer*, during *adolescence*, when they will be presented with many challenges to their health.

The current model of care for survivors of childhood cancer

The management of survivors varies according to their individual needs to ensure the best possible future for them. The normalisation of survivors' lives and encouragement to incorporate healthy behaviours begins as soon as treatment ends. In the UK it is currently recommended that young peo-

ple treated for cancer should be followed up for life (SIGN, 2004; Skinner et al., 2005). This ensures that any adverse effects can be detected and treated early. In addition, information can be gathered to inform modification of treatment protocols (Wallace et al., 2001).

Acute and late effects commonly occur because of the non-specific nature of cancer treatment. These effects can be static or progressive, and they can appear at the time of treatment or many years later. Acute problems such as myelosuppression, mucositis and alopecia, which emerge during treatment, last for a short period and usually resolve soon after the completion of chemotherapy or radiotherapy. However, after completion of therapy longer term problems may emerge. Chemotherapy with multiple drugs, radiotherapy and surgery can cause long-term problems. The challenge is to identify and manage the delayed consequences of cancer treatment (Ganz, 2001). The risks of long-term effects are related to the treatment given, the dose of chemotherapy or radiotherapy, surgery, the young person's age at the time of treatment and gender. Long-term follow-up addresses these late issues. The aim of long-term follow-up is to optimise the quality of life for survivors. The nurses' role is becoming increasingly important in long-term follow-up and is discussed later.

Young people need to know about their past disease and treatment. They need to take responsibility for their own health as they become young adults. The Childhood Cancer Study Group has produced an *Aftercure* booklet, as well as treatment-related fact-sheets. With the use of these resources, young people should receive a treatment summary which includes total doses of chemotherapy, radiotherapy, surgery and any anticipated late effects that might develop (NICE, 2005). Nurses with expert knowledge about late effects can play an important role in providing information and completing the aftercure treatment summary card, in collaboration with young people.

Young people with busy lives need to understand the future health benefits of continuing to attend long-term follow-up clinics, long after their treatment has been completed. Compliance is a problem and innovative ways need to be developed to monitor young people. Some cancer centres are extending the length of time between clinic visits by sending an annual health questionnaire.

Health behaviours and health promotion in survivors of childhood cancer

Current treatments for childhood cancer are associated with considerable success. Although considered cured, these survivors may be affected by one or more late effects as a consequence of their cancer and/or its treatment. These include physical problems such as cardiac dysfunction, growth problems, obesity and infertility, as well as educational, emotional and behavioural issues. In addition, there is a small risk of cancer recurrence or a second cancer. For these reasons survivors need to be *knowledgeable and vigilant about their health*. Whilst the cause of childhood cancer is not known, it is assumed that those who survive are more at risk from cancer-causing agents than their healthy peers. Survivors need to understand the reasons for avoiding risk-taking health behaviours, such as smoking and poor diet, for example.

As the population of survivors grows, it will become increasingly important to normalise their lives and teach them to incorporate healthy behaviours. Gender differences in perceived health status are known to be apparent amongst survivors, girls reporting more worries about their health than boys (Smith and Bashore, 2006). Nurses working with cancer survivors need to pay particular attention to the levels of worry and anxiety in female survivors.

Health promotion provision

The long-term follow-up (LTFU) clinic is an ideal place to provide health promotion advice. Young people already attend the clinic, which focuses upon health issues. They may have built up a trusting relationship with nurses working within the clinic. The provision of health promotion advice can increase the quality of care young people receive. Health promotion advice will help to influence the health choices young people make, hopefully reducing risks of illness.

Specialist clinics too can add to the quality of care young people receive. These can include fertility, neuro-oncology, bone marrow transplant and endocrine clinics. Neuro-oncology and bone marrow transplant clinics focus on specific conditions with the benefit of specialisation and increasing knowledge. The endocrine and fertility clinics deal with the late effects of treatment.

As many survivors are young when they are diagnosed and treated for cancer, they are familiar with their parents/carers taking responsibility for interactions with health practitioners. In addition, some may have an all-powerful opinion of practitioners. The nurse, using specific communication skills, can encourage survivors to become more assertive and open with health practitioners. These communication skills can include the following:

- Speaking directly to young people during interactions.
- Asking questions about their health behaviours.
- Listening.
- Providing them with opportunities to make their own health choices.
- Providing them with health promotion information and resources to assist with those health choices.

Communicating directly with young survivors as illustrated can help foster their growing autonomy and a sense of responsibility for their own health. Nurses, working within LTFU clinics, can provide different opportunities to promote young people's health, through the use of effective communication skills.

Nurses working in LTFU clinics are often clinical nurse specialists in the field of cancer nursing. They care for and provide health promotion advice for young people. Although they have a valuable role in the UK, there are few clinical nurse specialists working with survivors of childhood cancer (Gibson and Soanes, 2001). There is a need for more clinical nurse specialists in this area of nursing. Clinical nurse specialists are vital in providing theses services to the ever-growing population of survivors.

Case study

The following case study provides an example of how health promotion can be undertaken with a young person who has survived childhood cancer. In line with recommendations from the Nursing Midwifery

Table 20.1 Drugs used to treat Deana and their potential long-term side effects.

Drug	Cardiac	Growth	Fertility	Renal	Respiratory	Neurological	Hearing	Liver	Second malignancy
Cyclophosphamide							X		
Cytarabine	X	X	X	X	X	X		X	
Doxorubicin	X		X	X					
Methotrexate			X	X	X	X			
Vincristine		X							
Dexamethasone	X								
Thioguanine								X	
Asparaginase								X	

Council (NMC, 2004) on confidentiality, names and details have been changed.

Deana is 17 years old, and lives with mother (Danielle) and young brother (David). Her parents are divorced, but Deana's father (Douglas) is in regular contact with the family and has a good relationship with the family. Deana previously suffered from *acute lymphoblastic leukaemia (ALL)*, which was diagnosed when she was 8 years old. She was treated on the United Kingdom Acute Lymphoblastic Leukaemia 97/99 protocol treatment, and finished 7 years ago. The drugs used to treat Deana and their potential long-term side effects are shown in Table 20.1.

Key health issues now for Deana to focus include the following:

- Weight – overweight.
- Smoking – smokes occasionally, if with friends who smoke.
- Drinking – alcohol consumption is 3/4 units on a Saturday night.
- Drugs – has tried cannabis once, no other drugs are used.
- Menstruation.
- Relationships – has a boyfriend but Deana is not sexually active.
- Emotional health – Deana is anxious about her health all the time.

Children/young people diagnosed with standard risk ALL often have few or no long-term side effects from treatment. However, those with high risk ALL, or those who have experienced relapses with intensive treatment, often pay a higher price. Early follow-up is advocated primarily to detect re-

lapse or recurrence. The balance changes for long-term survivors, where it becomes important to identify the late effects of therapy.

Systematic guidance for follow-up of long-term survivors of childhood cancer is published by the Childhood Cancer and Leukaemia Group – *Therapy Based Long Term Follow Up* (Skinner et al., 2005). This information allows the practitioner to anticipate late adverse effects that may need to be considered and sometimes treated. A suitable follow-up plan can then be put into place.

More recently, survivors have been provided with a record of their treatment and what it means for them in the future with the Aftercure booklet, factsheets and treatment cards, along with details of the Aftercure website – http://www.aftercure.org. These have been launched to allow survivors to have information at their fingertips. The treatment cards and fact-sheets also act as a good foundation for ongoing health promotion advice.

Assuming that Deana had standard risk ALL with no relapse, as most diagnosed with ALL do, she will be attending the primary treatment centre where she was originally treated for ALL, once a year. Deana will attend the long-term follow-up clinic held there. At this clinic Deana will see a paediatric oncologist and possibly a clinical nurse specialist. Using the United Kingdom Children's Cancer Study Group guidelines, all survivors who received chemotherapy are screened for the potential problems outlined below:

- Chemotherapy impaired quality of life.
- Secondary malignancy.
- Transfusion-associated complications.
- Dental caries.
- Pigmented skin lesions.

- Impaired immunity against vaccine-preventable infections.

Screening related to specific cytotoxic and other therapies will be given.

In reality, due to time restraints, purpose of the visit and lack of specialist staff, the visit for most offers little chance for a great deal of health promotion advice, despite the valuable nature of this advice for many young people.

Specific health issues

There are a number of specific health issues that need to be considered in relation to Deana's health. These are outlined below.

Obesity and short stature

Children/young people treated for ALL, particularly those who receive cranial irradiation, are at risk of obesity (Razzouk-Bassem et al., 2007). All survivors of childhood cancer are questioned on concerns regarding physical appearance, exercise, diet, including implications for weight and bone density. Dietary advice, such as eating a varied diet but one that is low in fat, salt and sugar and rich in fruit, vegetables and balanced in protein, will be advised. Deana's intake of calcium is important for maintaining adequate bone intensity. This is particularly important in girls who have received treatment for cancer.

This health promotion information will be given by a doctor or nurse leading the clinic. The information given is not only sound advice for maintaining health, but is also important for cancer prevention. A key issue for survivors of childhood cancer is how to avoid developing a second cancer. These risks can be minimised by preventing the development of obesity, avoiding smoking, unprotected sex and sunbathing.

But if, as in Deana's case, being overweight becomes a problem, then referral to a dietician will be needed for more in-depth advice on safe weight loss. Being overweight following childhood cancer is often seen as an acceptable price to pay for survival. However, being overweight and its link to survivors' self-image, esteem and levels of anxi-

ety is worthy of proactive intervention and support (Zebrack and Chesler, 2001; Cantrell, 2007).

Physical activity can bring about many physiological and psycho-social benefits and should be advocated. These can include the following:

- lower blood pressure.
- increased lung function.
- lower blood sugar.
- lower blood cholesterol.
- decreased mineral bone loss.
- decreased body fat and weight.
- improved flexibility.
- increased stamina.
- improved sleep quality.
- decreased stress levels.
- improved mood and self-esteem (Bomar, 1996).

It is therefore important to help control Deana's weight, particularly if she becomes overweight.

However, Deana may find exercise difficult to achieve, due to ongoing fatigue and muscle weakness as side effects of her treatment. Ongoing cardiac problems, though rare, may also occur as she would have received an anthracycline (doxorubicin) as part of her treatment. Health promotion on the signs of this, such as shortness of breath, fatigue, wheeze, rapid/irregular heat beat and poor tolerance of exercise, should be reported straightaway. To monitor cardiac function Deana will have an echocardiogram every 5 years.

Smoking, alcohol and drugs

Risk behaviour is a normal part of adolescence (Pasternak et al., 2006), and childhood cancer survivors will often want to do the same as their healthy peers. In fact, they are encouraged to go and lead a normal life. For young people they may choose to undertake behaviours that carry risks. Acknowledging that experimentation with smoking, alcohol, drugs and sex is part of life maintains a pathway for *open communication* between practitioners and long-term survivor. Good communication can allow the increased risks associated with such behaviours to be explained. These risks will include second cancers, cardiac problems, premature emphysema and lung fibrous. The key message for survivors is – *if you don't smoke, don't start, and if you do, try to stop.*

Explaining these risks to Deana will give her the health promotion information she needs to understand more fully the consequences of the risks she is taking. Giving information on quitting smoking programmes, for example, which there are many (Department of Health, 2004), will provide her with further options.

Similarly with alcohol, Deana is not legally old enough to drink alcohol, but like many of her peers she does. There is an increased risk from drinking alcohol due to the potential hepatotoxic side effects of cyclophosphamide. Once again the health promotion approach should be about counselling and information on responsible drinking. Written information should be given to support any verbal details provided.

The approach for health promotion will be dependent on the recreational drug being used. However, most of the recreational drugs have neuropsychological effects (Health Education Authority, 1996; Department of Health, 2002). Recreational drugs can increase problems in those who have been treated for brain tumours, radiotherapy to the central nervous system or chemotherapy treatment with intrathecal methotrexate or cytarabine (Horne, 2008), the last two of which Deana would have received in her treatment.

Sex and fertility

Female fertility is not normally affected by treatment for ALL, unless cranial spinal irradiation that included the ovaries or high doses, >10–15 g of cyclophosphamide. For the majority of girls treated therefore, normal sexual development, fertility and the chances of having a normal pregnancy and birth are the same as the general population. It cannot be assumed that Deana is aware of this. Adult and teenage survivors of childhood cancer may have only a vague understanding of their previous illness, its treatment and consequences. They are often too young to remember or be involved in such discussions at the time. They are too embarrassed to ask their parents/carers or prevented from doing so, because their family may feel uncomfortable in discussing the past. Gaps in their knowledge may therefore exist. There remains a misconception in the public that all chemotherapy causes infertility. This is not the case. But Deana needs to be made

aware of this; therefore, discussions about safe sex with someone who she can trust are essential.

Emotional health – anxiety

Many survivors of childhood cancer and their families are anxious. This may be related to fear of relapse or side effects. The most vulnerable among them include females, people in poor financial conditions, the unemployed and those with low education (Massimo and Caprino, 2007). If the anxiety becomes too much, it may compromise their quality of life and ability to seek appropriate health care. Fundamentally, survivors become afraid of knowing. Practitioners can provide essential information and support to help lessen any fears that may exist. Most importantly, listening to their concerns is paramount.

Activity

Imagine that you are a clinical nurse specialist working in an LTFU clinic. Make some notes on what health promotion advice you might provide to Deana, in relation to the health issues outlined above. Consider how you could provide this advice, using your communication skills and health promotion resources. If this task seems too great, select only two health issues and explore these further.

Conclusion

This chapter has provided some background information on childhood cancers. It has considered the current model of care in relation to survivors of childhood cancer, and it has focused upon the importance of health promotion for their future health. Although health promotion activities are being undertaken by clinical nurse specialists, there is scope for a greater development of this role with young survivors of childhood cancers.

Nurses, clinical nurse specialists particularly, working with young people recovering from childhood cancer, have an important contribution to make in relation to promoting their health. They can be supportive by listening to their concerns. In addition, they can provide health promotion information, which will help these young people to become more independent, and thus take on more responsibility for their own health. Essentially, clinical nurse specialists can contribute to advancing young survivors' health through health promotion activities in LTFU clinics.

References

Bomar, P. (1996) *Nurses and Family Health Promotion.* Philadelphia: W.B. Sanders Company.

Cantrell, M. (2007) Health-related quality of life in childhood cancer: state of the science. *Oncology Nursing Forum* 34(1): 103–111.

Department of Health (2002) *The Score – Facts about Drugs.* London: Department of Health.

Department of Health (2004) *Choosing Health.* London: Department of Health.

Education and Skills (Department of), Department of Health (2004) *The National Service Framework for Children, Young People and Maternity Services.* London: Crown Copyright.

Ganz, P.A. (2001) Late effects of cancer and its treatment. *Seminars in Oncology Nursing* 17(4): 241–248.

Gibson, F., Soanes, L. (2001) Long-term follow-up following childhood cancer: maximizing the contribution from nursing. *European Journal of Cancer* 37: 1859–1868.

Health Education Authority (1996) *A Parent's Guide to Drugs and Alcohol.* London: Health Education Authority.

Horne, B. (2008) Health promotion in long term survivors. In: Gibson, F., Soanes, L. (eds) *Cancer in Children and Young People – Acute Nursing Care.* Chichester: Whiley.

Massimo, L., Caprino, D. (2007) The truly healthy adult survivor of childhood cancer: inside feelings and behaviours. *Minerva Pediatrica* 59(1): 43–47.

NICE (2005) *Improving Outcomes in Children and Young People with Cancer.* London: National Institute for Clinical Excellence.

NMC (2004) *The Code of Professional Conduct.* London: Nursing Midwifery Council.

Pasternak, R., Geller, G., Parrish, C., Cheng, T. (2006) Adolescent and parent perceptions on youth participation in risk behaviour research. *Archives of Pediatrics and Adolescent Medicine* 160(11): 1159–1166.

Razzouk-Bassem, I., Rose, S., Hong-eng, S., Wallace, D., Smeltzer, M., Zacher, M., Pui-Ching, H., Hudson, M. (2007) Obesity in survivors of childhood acute lymphoblastic leukaemia and lymphoma. *Journal of Clinical Oncology* 25(10): 1183–1189.

SIGN (2004) *Long Term Follow Up of Survivors of Childhood Cancer.* Scottish Intercollegiate Guideline Network. Available at: http://www.sign.ac.uk (accessed 23 January 2008).

Skinner, R., Wallace, H., Levitt, G. (2005) *Therapy Based Long Term Follow Up.* Childhood Cancer and Leukaemia Group (CCLG). Available at: http://www.ccig.org.uk (accessed 23 January 2008).

Smith, A., Bashore, L. (2006) The effect of clinic-based health promotion education on perceived health status and health promotion behaviours of adolescents and young adult cancer survivors. *Journal of Pediatric Oncology Nursing* 23(6): 326–334.

Steliarova-Foucher, E., Stiller, C., Kaatsch, P., Berrino, F., Coebergh, J., Lacour, B., Parkin, M. (2004) Geographical patterns and time trends of cancer incidence and survival among children and adolescents in Europe since the 1970s (the ACCIS project): an epidemiological study. *Lancet* 364(9451): 2097–105.

Stiller, C. (2007) *Childhood Cancer in Britain, Incidence, Survival and Mortality.* Oxford: Oxford University Press.

Wallace, H., Green, D. (2004) *Late Effects of Childhood Cancer.* London: Hodder Arnold.

Wallace, W., Blacklay, A., Eiser, C., Davies, H., Hawkins, M., Levitt, G., Jenney, M. (2001) Developing strategies for long term follow up of survivors of childhood cancer. *British Medical Journal* 323(7307): 271–274.

Zebrack, B., Chesler, M. (2001) Health-related worries, self-image, and life outlooks of long-term survivors of childhood cancer. *Health and Social Work* 26(4): 245–256.

21 Constipation

Ali Wright

NSF

The National Service Framework (NSF) for children, young people and maternity services (Education and Skills, Department of Health, 2004) discusses children/young people with long-term conditions. Children with constipation, in some cases, can experience problems over a long period, which may give rise to emotional issues.

Introduction

This chapter aims to give practical health promotion ideas and information to children's nurses, both hospital and community based, to use with families which may be experiencing problems of constipation with their child. Health visitors, school nurses, and community children's nurses are in an ideal position to support families whose children may be suffering from constipation in the community. If a child is referred on for hospital care, children's nurses can continue to provide support and information. Nurses will be building a continuing relationship with the child and her/his family and will see the outcome of any interventions they have advised. As Muir and Burnett (1999) state, in order to achieve successful management of childhood constipation, families require a consistent and supportive approach.

It is hoped that information contained within this chapter will enable practitioners to become more confident about their knowledge in the management of children with constipation.

The information will enable the practitioner to:

(1) develop an understanding about children's constipation and its management, both in hospital and the community;
(2) recognise the signs and symptoms of constipation and factors that can lead to its development;
(3) identify normal milestones for children in relation to bowel habits and to recognise changes from the norm;
(4) recognise the importance of assessing the child's history in relation to her/his toileting needs;
(5) recognise, through health promotion strategies, how healthy eating and drinking, as well as being active, can help children to overcome constipation;
(6) develop an understanding about how medicines can help constipation, and how to support families who are using a medicine management plan;

(7) support families in the longer term manage-
    ment of their child's health;
(8) explore the case history of a young girl attend-
    ing a nurse-led clinic for childhood constipa-
    tion and see how health promotion messages
    are introduced.

Facts about constipation

What is constipation in children?

Constipation is a disorder of the gastrointestinal
tract. Constipation has been described as painful
and difficult defecation (Clayden, 1996). The medical words used for constipation include bowel actions, faeces and stools. However, many children
and families understand the word *poo* better. In
practice, it is always helpful to use words children
understand; therefore, the word poo will be used
here.

Signs and symptoms of constipation

The Rome III classification system is based on the
premise that for each disorder there are symptom clusters that remain consistent across clinical and population groups. This type of organised framework provides a means for identification of patients, which can then be modified as
new scientific data emerge (Drossman, 2006). The
decision-making process to define Rome III criteria for children aged 4 to 18 years old consists
of arriving at a consensus based on clinical experience and review of literature (Rasquin et al.,
2006).

The term *functional constipation* describes all children in whom constipation is not caused by organ
problems.

Diagnostic criteria for functional constipation
in infants up to 4 years of age are outlined
below:

- Two or fewer poos per week.
- At least one episode per week of incontinence
  (after the acquisition of toileting skills).
- History of excessive poo retention.

- History of painful or hard bowel movements.
- Presence of a large mass in the rectum.
- History of large-diameter poos that may ob-
  struct the toilet.

Accompanying symptoms may include irritabil-
ity and decreased appetite. The accompanying
symptoms disappear immediately following passage of a large bowel action (Hyman et al.,
2006).

Diagnostic criteria* for functional constipation in the child or adolescent

Diagnosis must include two or more of the following in a child with a developmental age of at least 4
years, with insufficient criteria for diagnosis of irritable bowel syndrome:

- Two or fewer bowel actions in the toilet each
  week.
- At least one episode of bowel incontinence each
  week.
- History of retentive posturing.
- History of painful and hard bowel actions.
- Presence of a large poo in the rectum.
- History of large-diameter stools that may ob-
  struct the toilet.

*Criteria fulfilled at least once per week for at
least 2 months before diagnosis (Rasquin et al.,
2006).

Soiling

Soiling is the involuntary passage of a bowel action
into the underwear as a direct result of chronic constipation (Clayden, 1992). It is also known as *overflow soiling*. Soiling happens over a period of time,
because as the child becomes constipated, the poo
becomes harder and large, so much so that the child
cannot pass it. If the child associates pain with going to the toilet, the child will stop pushing. Liquid
or soft poo pass around the hard large poo in the
rectum and leak out of the bottom, causing stain-
ing of poo on the child's underwear. It is important to note that children have no control over this
soiling.

Withholding

Constipation often develops when the child begins to associate pain with pooing. Once this association is made, the child starts to withhold poo to avoid discomfort (Rogers, 2004).

Factors that can lead to constipation

Social

- Poor diet.
- Overfeeding in infancy.
- Insufficient fluid intake.
- Excessive milk intake.
- Faddy eating.
- Potty training difficulties.
- Problems with school toilets.
- Changes in lifestyle and routine.
- Lack of exercise.
- Lack of privacy.

Psychological

- Perceptions and beliefs about normal bowel habits.
- Poor bowel habits – ignoring the urge to go, withholding.
- Eating disorders.

Physical

- Anal fissure.
- Mild pyrexia, dehydration and immobility.
- Position for defecation.
- Weight – under or over.
- Children who have been sexually abused may present with pain on pooing or rectal bleeding (Gordon, 2005).

Constipation develops because the poo becomes harder, and as more poo is made it is held in the rectum, stretching the rectum. As the rectum becomes larger the poo is more difficult to push out. The feeling of needing to go the toilet is not felt by the child or simply ignored. The child continues to hold onto the poo as she/he knows it will hurt to pass it. More and more poo is stored in the rectum. Soiling will begin because the new liquid poo is pushed down around the large mass of poo, and leaks onto the child's underwear.

Facts about constipation

Some of the following facts illustrate how common constipation in children can be. Nurses may find this information useful when talking to parents/carers who have concerns about their child's toileting needs:

- In about 25% of all cases, constipation starts when the child is still a baby (Nelson et al., 1994).
- Constipation is most common in children between the ages of 2 and 4 when they are potty training (Nelson et al., 1994).
- About one-third of 4- to 7-year-olds are constipated at any one time (Farrell et al., 2003).
- Five per cent primary school children become constipated for more than 6 months (Young and Beattie, 1998).
- Majority (over 95%) of children, who experience constipation, have functional constipation, which is not caused by organ difficulties (Staiano and Tozzi, 1998).

Hirschsprung's disease

Hirschsprung's disease may need to be considered as a cause of illness, if a child with a history of constipation fails to respond to medical management over a period of time. Hirschsprung's disease is a functional intestinal obstruction, which results from the congenital absence of parasympathetic ganglion cells in the mesenteric plexus of the distal bowel. These cells are responsible for the peristaltic movement of the bowel, and when they are absent, constipation results (Sinfield, 2007).

A rectal biopsy will be needed to establish if the child has Hirschsprung's disease. If the disease is confirmed, surgical interventions may be necessary. If rectal biopsy excludes Hirschsprung's disease, the child will be managed using a medicines management plan.

History and assessment

Working with children the nurse may begin to identify that a child is having problems with constipation. Parents/carers may be mentioning issues that fit into the diagnostic criteria previously mentioned. The child's eating pattern may be changing, the amount of drinks may be altered, the nappy/toileting pattern may be altered and there may be issues around going to the toilet at school.

When taking this history, the nurse can begin to build up a rapport with the child and family. The nurse can help them to look at health promotion strategies, using preventative approaches, educational and information-giving techniques or client-centred approaches. However, the nurse needs to recognise when the child needs more help, and should encourage the family to see their general practitioner (GP), as a medical approach using medicines may be needed. If the problem cannot be solved in the community, a referral to hospital will be needed.

Key health promotion messages

Eating, drinking and going to the toilet are part of day-to-day life. The child and family need to see how constipation links with everyday activities, eating habits and exercise, for example. Health promotion information can be given verbally, as well as in writing (Figure 21.1).

An important part of health promotion, where a child has constipation, is to help the child and her/his family understand how the body works, and what is happening when the child is constipated. The nurse needs to explain these issues to the child and family. The nurse should offer possible solutions in a positive way and use health promotion messages that are age appropriate, so the child is able to understand.

Normal activities of living

Eating

An explanation suitable for a child might be:
As we eat and drink, water and food goes into the stomach, where it is mixed up and digestion begins. The nutri-

ents are absorbed into the blood and are circulated around the body, giving us our energy source each time. We all need to eat a balanced diet, giving us proteins, carbohydrates, sugars, fibre and vitamins. If enough foods containing fibre are not eaten this can cause constipation – not being able to poo.

Practical ideas to encourage healthy eating might include some of the following:

- Pureed fruit and vegetables can be introduced into a baby's diet when weaning begins.
- For some children just eating more fibre may help soften the poo.
- Children should be encouraged to eat as much fruit and vegetables as they can, not strictly five per day.
- Encourage children to have breakfast. Breakfast foods such as brown bread and cereals are a good source of fibre.
- Fibre is found in the following:
  - the skins of fruit and vegetables such as apples, grapes, jacket potatoes and potato wedges.
  - brown, wholemeal and granary bread.
  - wholemeal pasta and brown rice.
  - wholegrain cereals.
  - baked beans.
- Encourage children to eat meals rather than eating snack foods, as these tend to be low in fibre, unless they are portions of fruit or vegetables.
- Encourage all of the family to eat healthily, rather than just the children.
- Praise children when they eat something different; using a star or reward chart with stickers may help (Figure 21.2).
- Encourage the child and family to keep a food diary to show to health care practitioners what has been eaten.

Approximately 30 minutes after eating many people get the urge to go the toilet. Ask the parents/carers to encourage children to sit on the toilet after meals.

Drinking

We all need to drink to keep our bodies hydrated. Drinks are a source of energy too, especially for

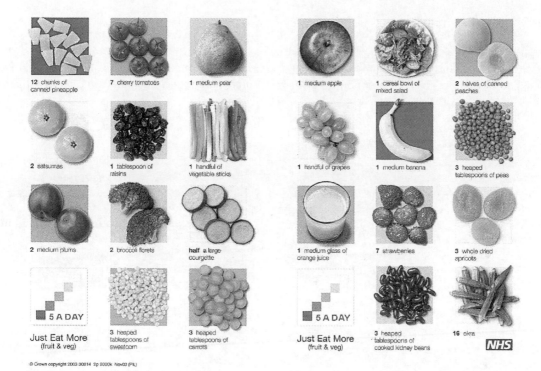

(a)

(b)

Figure 21.1 a and b 5 a day leaflet.

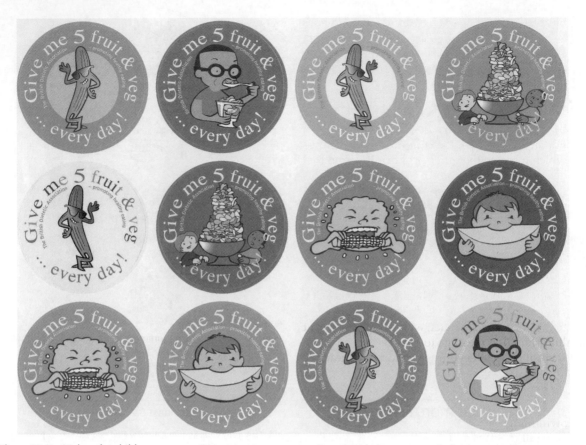

Figure 21.2   Stickers for children.

babies. If children do not drink enough then this can lead to constipation. For some children simply drinking more may help. Practical ideas to encourage drinking can include the following:

- If parents/carers notice their baby straining to do a poo, try offering cooled boiled water or diluted fruit juices between breast or formula feeds.
- Add extra milk to a child's cereal, as this all counts as fluid.
- Encouraging a child to drink will help to keep the poo soft, which means it may be easier to pass (six to eight drinks per day will help). Use the child's usual drinking cup.
- Families may need advice on how to fit in the number of drinks required per day. During

school time ask school staff to help, as many schools now encourage drinks to be taken into school. ERIC (Education and Resources for Improving Continence) is promoting a *Water Is Cool in School* campaign.
- More drinks are needed for hot days, and if the child is very active or sweaty.
- Too much milk can fill a child, which will reduce the amount of food the child can eat, which can lead to constipation. A balance diet is needed.
- To prevent tooth decay, water-based drinks are best rather than sugary drinks.
- Encourage the child to drink her/his favourite drink, as long as it is a healthy option.
- Vary drinks offered.
- Choose cups with colourful designs which may be appealing to the child.

- Simple explanations of how much a child needs to drink may be easier for all to understand, such as how the drinks can be spaced out during the day – two cups before lunch, for example.
- Praise the child when they drink certain amounts. Using a star/reward chart may help, if drinking is an issue for the child.
- Fun activities – ask the child to colour pictures which indicate the number of drinks taken that day, using a colour code for different drinks (orange = orange juice, red = fruit juices, green = apple juice, blue = water).

Exercise

Children should be encouraged to be active each day. Exercise keeps the body healthy, and this helps to maintain bowel activity too. Being active can help children go to the toilet, which is an important health promotion message to get across.

Practical ideas to encourage children to be active can include the following:

- Team games and races.
- Swimming.
- Football for boys and girls.
- Walking/cycling to school and with the family.
- Exercise awards and stickers.
- Encourage family exercise activities together.

Going to the toilet

An explanation suitable for a child might be:

Food passes through the tummy into the bowel and the good stuff is absorbed into the body. What is left over is not needed and passes through into the large bowel where it becomes poo. Then the poo travels all the way along the large bowel to the back passage where it is stored. When the back passage is full, nerves within the bowel wall send a message to the brain telling us we need to go the toilet. When we sit on the toilet, we have the urge to push down, and this opens the muscles in our bottom and poo is pushed out of the body into the toilet. This pushing continues until our bottom is empty. When the poo has been pushed out, the muscles in the bottom tighten until

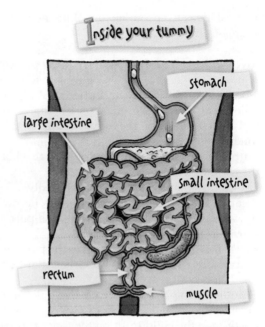

Figure 21.3   Inside your tummy (illustration by Bruce Waite).

we need to poo again and the poo cycle starts all over again (Figure 21.3).

Potty training and toilet training

Potty training is the time when a child is ready and understands that they can use the potty or toilet to have a wee or poo. Each child is an individual and the age at which she/he becomes potty trained will vary, from 18 months to 3 years is usual.

The time to start potty training may be when the child can say or shows an adult they want to have a wee or poo and/or the child understands simple commands. Parents/carers should encourage their child to:

- sit on the potty a couple of times each day;
- regularly ask the child if she/he needs the potty;
- praise the child when she/he uses the potty appropriately;
- sit the child on the potty/toilet (for a short time) after meals;
- do not rush the child to the potty/toilet.

Practical ideas to encourage use of the potty and toilet are outlined below:

- Involve the child when buying a potty or toilet seat.
- Does the child feel safe on the toilet? A child's toilet seat may be useful to help the child feel secure, and not at risk of falling into the toilet.
- Putting a stool at the child's feet may also help the child to feel secure.
- Use clothes that a child can take off easily.
- Wearing pants will help the child to feel grown up. Accidents will happen, but that is part of learning.
- Praise the child when she/he uses the potty appropriately. Using a star/reward chart may help.
- Read storybooks.
- Encourage the child to sit on the toilet after meals.
- Encourage the child to sit on the toilet and use their tummy muscles to push may help.
- Praise the child when she/he sits on the toilet.
- Is the child confident to use school toilets? Families may need to negotiate with school staff about any issues the child might have. ERIC is running a scheme called *Bog Standard*, promoting better toilets for pupils at school.

Eating, drinking and going to the toilet are part of day-to-day life, the child and family need to see how constipation links with everyday activities. Some of the key health promotion messages in helping children to develop toileting skills, as well as avoiding constipation, have been outlined.

Medicine management

Some children who become constipated will need medicines to help overcome their constipation. These medicines are called *laxatives* and are taken by mouth. The aim of treatment with medication is to help the child have a regular poo and to experience no discomfort when passing it. Medicines may be needed for many months or even longer to ensure the child can poo regularly without problems. The bowel is then likely to return to its normal size.

There are several sorts of laxatives. The following information outlines different types.

Stimulant

A stimulant increases intestinal motility (BNF for Children, 2007). It is usually taken in the evening and works in about 8–12 hours. This group of laxatives can cause colicky tummy aches. Stimulant laxatives are best used after softener laxatives have softened the poo.

Osmotic

These medicines increase the amount of water in the large bowel, either by drawing fluid from the body into the bowel or retaining the fluid administered at the time the medication is taken (BNF for Children, 2007).

A combination of laxatives may be used, as many hospitals have guidelines for the use of laxatives, and doctors may have a preference for certain types. The way in which a child presents to a health care practitioner may impact on treatment. If a child is constipated and has impaction of the rectum, the first treatment will be to empty the bowel. The child may need to be admitted as an in-patient. A maintenance medicine plan should then be formulated. The medicines used should ensure a regular bowel habit for the child.

Children are normally managed by their GP, using mild laxatives. If the child continues to be constipated on medicines, the GP may refer the child to a community paediatrician or paediatric gastroenterologist, who will manage the child's treatment or offer an opinion on treatment options.

The role of nurse is to understand which medicine is being used and why, and support the family in giving the medicines to their child. Families may need help in finding ways of giving medicines in a way that their child will tolerate. Nurses take a lead role in supporting children and families with problems of constipation, as families perceive nurses offer a sensitive and holistic approach (Farrell et al., 2003).

Medicines for Children (RCPCH, 2003) and the BNF for Children (2007) are useful sources of up-to-date prescribing information. To monitor progress it is helpful if families keep a diary, which includes the following:

- Medicine dose and time taken.
- Description of the poo (using stool charts).
- Any accidents/soiling episodes.
- Tummy aches.

Looking at the diary can help to see which medicines are working, and see what has helped the most. Doses of medicines can be altered in response to the number of times the child is going to the toilet and the consistency of the poo. Medicines should not be stopped abruptly, as the problem may return. It is better to gradually reduce the dose, ensuring the child continues to poo according to her/his established routine.

It is important that a child who is taking medicines is seen by a doctor or nurse regularly to assess progress. In order to achieve successful management of childhood constipation, families need a consistent and supportive approach (Muir and Burnett, 1999).

The long-term treatment of a constipated child should be focus on a strategy in which the need for stimulants and laxatives is cautiously eliminated, with a gradual increase in fibre and fluid intake over a period of time (Rogers, 2005).

Behaviour

Incontinence is distressing for children and can be indicative of not only physical problems, but emotional problems too (Education and Skills, Department of Health, 2004).

If constipation continues over several months with no improvement, the child may:

- develop low self-esteem.
- suffer bullying from other children.
- have low school attendance.

Where a child is not making progress, a referral may be needed to a child and family mental health team. They will be able to explore the child's concerns and put in place some support strategies. The aspects of management that can be invaluable when supporting a child with constipation are encouraging concordance with the management plan and

behaviour management techniques with rewards. Putting in place rewards will help to keep the child interested and motivated.

Government policy

In relation to the Government policy on this area of practice, the nurse may want to seek information from the following documents:

- *National Service Framework for children, young people and maternity services, standard 6 – children/young people who are ill:*

  Point 10 – Children with long-term conditions
  Point 10.17 – Children with incontinence
  (Education and Skills, Department of Health, 2004)

- *Good Practice in Continence Services* (Department of Health, 2000).
- *National Institute for Clinical Excellence*, clinical guidelines 14th wave (April 2007). The Department of Health Ministers has referred the following topic to the National Institute for Clinical Excellence for the production of clinical guidelines: diagnosis and treatment of childhood constipation. Remit: To prepare a clinical guideline on the diagnosis and treatment of idiopathic childhood constipation, focusing on:

  initial presentation;
  diagnosis;
  management;
  referral.

Case study

Olivia was $2\frac{1}{2}$ years old when she was referred to a paediatric gastroenterologist by her GP. Olivia had a history of struggling to have her bowels open from about 1 year of age, with constipation for the last 6 months. The GP managed her care for 3 months, initially using appropriate medication. Parents and the GP were concerned about her lack of progress and whether to start potty training, and jointly decided to seek further advice.

Olivia was referred to a paediatric gastroenterologist. He assessed her health. Olivia usually ate well, but now she was having a poor appetite. She was also reluctant to drink and had experienced changes in mood. Olivia was having large painful poos. When Olivia needed to poo in her nappy she would hide from her parents. Olivia attended nursery.

Olivia was diagnosed with constipation due to a previous and continuing anal fissure. This is a crack in the mucous membrane at the anal margin (Blackwell's Nursing Dictionary, 2005). Her management plan consisted of the following:

Medicines to soften the stools even more than previous treatments.
Olivia needed to unlearn the *holding on* reflex associated with having a poo. The pain would then stop, as the stool would be smaller, softer and easier to pass.
Referral to the nurse-led constipation clinic.

Over several years Olivia overcame her constipation. By using medicines to soften the poo, Olivia learnt how to go to the toilet normally. She progressed from nappies to pants, probably at a slower pace than her peer group, but in a way that matched her needs at the time.

At each contact with the children's nurse, health promotion messages were used relating to eating, drinking, toileting, and her parents were supported in the giving of medicines. Olivia herself was encouraged with lots of praise and support from her parents, nursery staff and the children's nurse at the nurse-led clinic. Once normal bowel habits were established without the need for medicines, Olivia was discharged from the nurse-led constipation clinic service.

Name and details have been changed as required by Nursing Midwifery Council (NMC, 2004).

Conclusion

Supporting children with constipation and their families is an important role for the nurse. Careful assessment of what the issues might be that are causing constipation need to be explored. Health promotion information can help guide a family to find solutions. The value of an appropriate diet, along with drinks and exercise, should not be underestimated. Children can be encouraged with praise and support. In some cases medication may be needed, but where this is not successful or there are other concerns, referral to a hospital specialist will be needed.

References

Blackwell's Nursing Dictionary (2005) Oxford: Blackwell Publishing.

BNF for Children (2007) Royal Pharmaceutical Society of Great Britain, RCPH. London: BMJ Publishing Group Ltd. British Medical Association, Royal Pharmaceutical Society of Great Britain, Royal College of Paediatrics and Child Health.

Clayden, G. (1992) Management of chronic constipation. *Archives of Disease in Childhood* 67: 340–344.

Clayden, G. (1996) A guide for good paediatric practice: childhood constipation. *Ambulatory Child Health* 1: 250–255.

Department of Health (2000) *Good Practice in Continence Services*. Department of Health. London: Crown Copyright.

Drossman D. (2006) The functional gastrointestinal disorders and the Rome III Process. *Gastroenterology* 130: 1377–1390.

Education and Skills (Department of), Department of Health (2004) *National Services Framework for Children, Young People and Maternity Services, Standard 6 – Children and Young People Who Are Ill*. London: Crown Copyright.

Farrell, M., Holmes, G., Coldicutt, P., Peak, M. (2003) Management of childhood constipation: parents' experiences. *Journal of Advanced Nursing* 44: 479–489.

Gordon, J. (2005) Childhood idiopathic constipation. *Gastrointestinal Nursing* 3(9): 25–30.

Hyman, P., Milla, P., Benninga, M., Davidson, G., Fleisher, D., Taminiau, J. (2006) Childhood functional gastrointestinal disorders: neonate/toddler. *Gastroenterology* 130: 1519–1526.

Muir, J., Burnett, C. (1999) Setting up a nurse led clinic for intractable childhood constipation. *British Journal of Community Nursing* 4(8): 395–399.

Nelson, R., Wagget, J., Leonard Jones, J. (1994) Constipation and megacolon in children and adults. *Diseases of the Gut and Pancreas*. Blackwell Scientific.

NMC (2004) *Code of Professional Conduct*. London: Nursing and Midwifery Council.

Rasquin, A., Di Lorenzo, C., Forbes, D., Guiraldes, E., Hyams, J., Staiano, A., Walker, L. (2006) Childhood functional gastrointestinal disorders: child/adolescent. *Gastroenterology* 130: 1527–1537.

RCPCH (2003) *Medicines for Children*. Royal College of Paediatrics and Child Health. London: RCPCH Publications Limited.

Rogers, J. (2004) Paediatric bowel problems. *Gastrointestinal Nursing* 2(4): 33–39.

Rogers, J. (2005) Reducing the misery of constipation in children. *Practice Nursing* 16(1): 12–16.

Sinfield, M. (2007) In: Glasper, E., McEwing, G., Richardson, J. (eds). Ulcerative Colitis. *Oxford Handbook of Children's and Young People's Nursing*. Oxford: Oxford University Press.

Staiano, A., Tozzi, A. (1998) Diagnosis and treatment of constipation in children. *Current Opinions in Paediatrics* 10: 512–515.

Young, D., Beattie, R. (1998) Normal bowel habit and prevalence of constipation in primary school children. *Ambulatory Child Health* 4: 277–282.

22 Health Promotion in Childhood Diabetes

Helen Thornton

NSF

The National Service Framework (NSF) for children, young people and maternity services: standard for hospital services suggests that other NSFs apply to children/young people (Department of Health, 2003a). For example, with this chapter strong links can be made with the NSF for diabetes (Department of Health, 2001).

Introduction

With over 246 million people in the world with diabetes, the United Nations General Assembly passed a landmark resolution in December 2006 recognising diabetes as a chronic, debilitating and costly disease associated with complications. Governments have acknowledged, for the first time, that a non-infectious condition poses as serious a threat to world health as infectious diseases such as HIV/AIDS, tuberculosis and malaria (United Nations Resolution, 2006). Diabetes is the most common metabolic condition of childhood which children's nurses will encounter (Royal College of Nursing, RCN, 2006).

The National Collaborating Centre for Women's and Children's Health (NCC-WCH) reported in 2004 that around 16 000 children/young people aged 0–16 years had attended paediatric diabetes centres in England. Ninety-five per cent of these children had type 1 diabetes (NCC-WCH, 2004). In the past, children's nurses would only encounter type 1 diabetes, but now they will see other types of diabetes. They must therefore develop an understanding of the underlying physiology, treatment and health promotion requirements of these different types of diabetes.

As children/young people with other conditions such as childhood cancers and cystic fibrosis live longer, they develop their own type of diabetes with treatment challenges (Spence, 2005). The rise in childhood obesity and lack of exercise is blamed for the appearance of type 2 diabetes in white British adolescents, as well as in the known high-risk groups of children/young people from Asian and African origins. Furthermore, as we develop a greater understanding of genetics we have discovered types of diabetes which arise from inherited gene mutations. Another type of diabetes described as maturity onset diabetes of the young has been discovered.

Children/young people have particular needs which differ from those of adults with diabetes, whichever form of diabetes they are living with. This chapter discusses key documents and what they recommend in relation to diabetes care for children/young people. How to promote the health of these children/young people will be explored using health promotion principles and case discussion.

Key documents and recommendations

The overall goal of managing diabetes is to enable the children/young people to lead a normal life, as free as possible from the clinical and psycho-social complications of the disease (RCN, 2006). This section looks at different documents which provide recommendations for the care of children/young people with diabetes.

Every Child Matters

Children/young people living with a long-term condition, such as diabetes, need additional support to enable them to achieve the main outcomes of *Every Child Matters* (Education and Skills, 2003), outlined below:

- Being healthy – enjoying good physical and mental health.
- Staying safe – being protected from harm and neglect.
- Enjoying and achieving – getting the most out of life.
- Making a positive contribution – being involved with the community and society.
- Economic well-being – not being prevented from achieving potential due to disadvantage.

Nurses need to consider these outcomes when working with children/young people with diabetes.

National Collaborating Centre for Women's and Children's Health (NCC-WCH)

Children/young people with type 1 diabetes should be offered an ongoing integrated package of care by a multidisciplinary paediatric diabetes care team. The diabetes care team should include members with appropriate training in clinical, educational, dietetic, lifestyle, mental health and foot care aspects of diabetes for children/young people. This will help to optimise the effectiveness of care and reduce the risk of complications (NCC-WCH, 2004). The team should consist of the following members:

- Designated consultant paediatrician with a specialist interest in diabetes.
- Paediatric diabetes specialist nurse.
- Senior paediatric ward nurse with experience in diabetes.
- Paediatric dietitian with a special expertise in childhood diabetes.
- Access to appropriate psychological support from experts in child mental health.
- Specialist services in podiatry and ophthalmology should also be easily available.

The specific needs of these children/young people can be met by a nurse who is a qualified children's nurse, with extended skills in paediatric diabetes care (RCN, 2006). The children's nurse should be an effective educator, counsellor, manager, researcher, communicator and innovator, and therefore accountable for her/his own actions (RCN, 2006).

Diabetes is a condition which requires 24-hour care and attention. Many children/young people with diabetes, especially those with type 1, will need to learn how to inject insulin regularly. This can be quite a challenge for families to take on board. Education, support and encouragement with this task are essential. Certainly, in the early stages when diagnosis has just been confirmed and everyone is familiarising themselves with what needs to be achieved, support will be invaluable.

Diabetes affects all aspects of children's/young people's lives and requires an in-depth understanding of the complex interactions between lifestyle, diet, insulin, exercise and growth. Children/young people and their families need to acquire the necessary knowledge and skills in diabetes itself, as well as becoming empowered to develop self-management skills (Sengbusch et al., 2006).

As the child's/young person's progresses through childhood and adolescence, different health promotion topics will need to be delivered in age-appropriate ways. These include the following:

- What is diabetes?
- Principles of treatment.

- Support groups both, local and national.
- All aspects of insulin management including storage, preparation, obtaining supplies, administration, injection sites, sharps disposal and adjustments in treatment.
- Dietary management in diabetes, including carbohydrate counting, as required.
- Managing special occasions such as Christmas, Easter and parties.
- Lifestyle issues/emotional well-being.
- Management of hypoglycaemia (low blood sugar).
- Illness management including ketone testing.
- Management of exercise.
- Blood sugar monitoring, including blood sugar targets, recording and interpretation of results.
- Diabetic control and how it is assessed.
- Complication screening.
- School/nursery.
- Holidays, including crossing time zones.
- Dental care.
- Immunisations.
- Foot care.
- Growth and puberty.
- Insulin pump therapy (if appropriate).
- Alcohol.
- Smoking.
- Benefits.
- Tattooing and body piercing.
- Pregnancy/sexual health.
- Exams.
- Career advice (some professions are not open to people with diabetes).
- Transitional care.
- Leaving home/university.
- Helpline numbers for paediatric diabetes care team.
- Driving.
- Self-care skills.
- Current and future research.

At a young people's consultation day, which was organised in collaboration with the National Children's Bureau for the development of guidelines for type 1 diabetes, it was found that young people wanted consistent, accessible, up-to-date information on all aspects of living with diabetes. Young people were found to be positive about accessing information through leaflets, CD-ROMs, videos and websites. However, parents/carers felt that health information should be delivered through one-to-one or group sessions with a specialist nurse (NCC-WCH, 2004).

The NCC-WCH commissioned by the National Institute for Clinical Excellence (NICE, 2004) published comprehensive guidelines on the management of type 1 diabetes in children/young people. This information is also contained within type 1 diabetes: diagnosis and management of type 1 diabetes in children, young people and adults clinical guideline number 15 (NICE, 2004).

Competency-based frameworks have now been developed to support staff in managing a child or young person with diabetes and what information they require. These can be accessed from the *Skills for Health* website – http://www.skillsforhealth.org

National Service Framework for diabetes

In 2001 the National Service Framework for Diabetes (Department of Health, 2001) was published. It outlined 12 standards of care to be delivered over the next 10 years. This was the first NSF that dealt specifically with a chronic disease. But when it was developed there was an awareness, by its authors, of certainly some interdependency with other NSFs, which were about to be produced, particularly those for children/young people and long-term conditions.

Children/young people feature in 11 of its 12 standards:

- Prevention of type 2 diabetes.
- Identification of people with diabetes.
- Empowering children, young people and adults with diabetes.
- Clinical care of adults with diabetes.
- Clinical care of children/young people with diabetes, including the transition from specialist paediatric diabetes services to specialist adult diabetes services.
- Management of diabetic emergencies.
- Care of people with diabetes during admission to hospital.
- Diabetes and pregnancy.
- Detection and management of long-term complications of diabetes and the provision of integrated health and social care.

National Service Framework for children/young people and maternity services

The publication of NSF for children produced core standards, which could universally apply to all children/young people, including those with a long-term condition such as diabetes (Education and Skills, Department of Health, 2004a). Standard 10, medicines for children/young people, is particularly relevant to paediatric diabetes care teams (Education and Skills, Department of Health, 2004b). This is because the prescription of any medication should be in the relevant formulation, by appropriately trained personnel, providing the child/young person and their family with up-to-date evidence-based treatments and information to support concordance (Education and Skills, Department of Health, 2004b).

Many paediatric diabetes specialist nurses have completed their nurse prescribing course to enhance their service delivery to children/young people. This enables the children's nurse to prescribe relevant treatments for diabetes and other conditions. From 2006 qualified nurse prescribers were able to prescribe from the current British National Formulary, a full range of medicines within their area of competence (Department of Health, 2006a).

Children/young people in school

Another area of diabetes care which links into standard 10 (medicines management) is the management of diabetes in the school setting. In 1996, a good practice guide for supporting pupils with medical needs was introduced (Department for Education and Employment, Department of Health, 1996). This was later replaced by managing medicine in school and early years setting guidelines (Education and Skills, 2005).

Children/young people who have diabetes may need to administer extra glucose or snacks, monitor blood sugar levels or inject insulin within the school environment. Tang and Ariyawansa (2007) maintain that there are difficulties facing children/young people in their day-to-day management of diabetes in school. Children/young people with diabetes are covered by the Special Educational Needs (SEN) and Disability Act 2001 (Act of Parliament, 2001), and schools should be aware of this when dealing with pupils with diabetes. Schools are required to ensure reasonable adjustment so that the school does not discriminate against the child/young person in reasons relating to the disability. Within the school someone will have responsibility for overseeing this. It is important that all staff know who the pupils with diabetes are and know how to treat a hypoglycaemic episode as a lack of knowledge is not acceptable under this Act.

Children/young people with diabetes can also not be discriminated against in extra-curricular activities, such as school trips or after-school activities. Reasonable adjustment may be required to accommodate their needs.

If children/young people with diabetes have been losing time from school, then there may be a need to discuss with family and the special needs co-coordinator to see if there is a requirement for an individualised education plan. Regular severe hypoglycaemic episodes may impair cognitive function. If this is suspected then assessment may be required via the SEN code of practice (Thornton, 2007). The paediatric diabetes specialist nurse, working in partnership with the family, can provide education to school staff, concerning the management of diabetes in school. The possible topics covered are outlined below. Providing such information is not only health promotional but also contributes to the outcomes of *Every Child Matters* (Education and Skills, 2003).

Topics to be discussed with schools (Thornton, 2007) are as follows:

- What is diabetes, recognition of symptoms and how to refer a child/young person.
- Outline treatment principles of diabetes.
- Dietary requirements.
- Blood sugar monitoring, including detailed training if staff require.
- Insulin injections, including safe storage and sharps disposal.
- Exercise.
- Management of hypoglycaemia.
- Management of illness.
- Treats and parties.
- School trips including individualised care planning, as required for residential trips.

- Exams.
- Career advice.
- Specialised equipment.

Support for the family and the school can be provided by the paediatric diabetes specialist nurse, enabling the child/young person to have a happier and more successful time at school.

Health promotion

Health promotion principles in diabetes management

Health promotion is not only about individual lifestyle choices but it is also about a more environmental approach to health as outlined in the Ottawa Charter for Health Promotion (1986). Within the analytical models of health promotion, there is a realisation that health promotion has a broad sociocultural framework (Jones and Naidoo, 2002). This is true of children/young people with diabetes, as the environment they grow up in and the support services they are offered have a direct result on their health.

Health promotion should promote self-esteem and autonomy (Jones and Cribb, 2002). It should recognise the developmental stages of childhood and support a young person to independence, from paediatric through to adult services.

Many health promoters use counselling techniques. Some hold a formal qualification in counselling; certainly training in counselling is advised. There are many different approaches in counselling; directive and a non-directive approaches are often used. These differ; a directive approach gives guidance to enable behavioural change to take place, whereas the non-directive approach gives the individual time and space to reach a decision. Individuals will be more successful in health-related behavioural change if a combination of these two styles is used, as Sidell (2002) suggests. Change will only occur if the individual has readiness and motivation to make change happen.

Prochaska and Di Clemente (1984) describe a motivation to change model. Within this model there are four distinct phases: pre-contemplation, contemplation, action and maintenance (Prochaska and Di Clemente, 1984). In helping children/young peo-

ple to change their behaviour, the health promoter must recognise that health-related behaviours are influenced by social and cultural attitudes and belief systems (Sidell, 2002). If the health promoter effectively accesses the child's/young person's readiness and motivation to change, then more positive health behaviours may begin to emerge.

There are three areas of health promotion which are focused upon by paediatric diabetes care teams:

- Diabetes-specific health promotion.
- General health promotion, which is then made diabetes specific.
- Age-specific health promotion.

Each of these areas of health promotion will be explored.

Diabetes-specific health promotion

The care process experienced within paediatric diabetes care can influence the outcomes in adulthood, especially in the development of micro- and macro-vascular complications. The Diabetes Control and Complication Trials (DCCT, 1993) confirmed what had always been suspected; good diabetic control prevents long-term complications. Children/young people with type 1 diabetes and their families are informed that the target for long-term glycaemic control is an HbA1c level (diabetes control test) of less than 7.5% without frequent disabling hypoglycaemia. Their care packages are designed to attempt to achieve this (NCC-WCH, 2004). All children/young people with diabetes receive screening for diabetes complications and associated conditions annually. Some screening does not commence until the age of 12 years, while other screening commences earlier (see Box 22.1). Dines (2003) suggests that screening is an important part of health promotion.

Diabetic retinopathy is the commonest form of blindness in the working age group. It is important that screening takes place, because the early stages of diabetic retinopathy can be treated effectively with laser therapy, but by the time there are sight changes it could be too late (National Retinopathy Screening Programme, 2006). In 2006 digital retinal screening programmes for the detection of diabetic retinopathy were rolled out across the United

Box 22.1 Screening recommendations.

Type 1 diabetes: diagnosis and management of type 1 diabetes in children/young people
National Collaborating Centre for Women's and Children's Health
Commissioned by the National Institute for Clinical Excellence (September 2004)

Children/young people with type 1 diabetes should be offered screening for coeliac disease and thyroid disease as these are both autoimmune conditions which are associated with diabetes. They also require screening for micro-vascular complications such as retinopathy (eye disease), renal disease associated with diabetes and macro-vascular disease by blood pressure checks.

Kingdom (UK) to fulfil the diabetes NSF requirement that 80% of patients with diabetes will have been offered retinal screening by April 2006 and 100% by the end of 2007 (Department of Health, 2003b). Retinal screening is recommended from the age of 12 years (NCC-WCH, 2004), but some children/young people with diabetes, due to the duration of diagnosis, may require screening prior to the age of 12 years. The provision of such a service would be determined locally.

Screening programmes are public health services that need to be managed at the level of a large population to monitor quality effectively. In the UK, this is carried out by the National Screening Committee. The criteria for appraising the viability, effectiveness and appropriateness of a screening programme should always be applied. The National Diabetes Retinopathy programme has strict quality assurance standards to ensure its effectiveness (http://www.nscretinopathy.org.uk).

General health promotion, which is then made diabetes specific

There are a wide range of issues; some are outlined here.

Immunisation

Paediatric diabetes teams work in collaboration with health visitors and school nurses to ensure routine immunisation schedules are met. Blood sugars need to be monitored more closely in the post-vaccination period, especially if a live vaccination has been given. There is also a requirement to avoid the vaccinated limb for 1 month post-vaccine for administration of subcutaneous insulin injections, due to erratic absorption of insulin that could occur if there was any localised swelling (Thornton, 2000). In addition, children/young people with diabetes are offered an annual influenza vaccination, and if not previously vaccinated a pneumococcal vaccination. All people with diabetes including children/young people are classified as a high-risk group and are given priority in these vaccinations programmes each year (Department of Health, 2006b).

Dental health

All children/young people should receive routine dental screening every 6 months. Individuals with diabetes are more prone to periodontal disease, which in itself can contribute to poor diabetic control. Other studies have suggested that high HbA1c test result, which indicates poor diabetes control, is associated with increased dental carries (NCC-WCH, 2004). Children/young people with diabetes eat more frequently than is recommended by dental practitioners; their diet has three meals and three snacks per day. The last meal is at bedtime which increases the acid within the mouth prior to sleep. They also consume pure sugar in the form of sugary drinks in the treatment of hypoglycaemia, often in night-time hours, sometimes without attention to their dental hygiene. Dental hygiene is therefore very important.

The following case study provides details of what would happen if a dental extraction was required by a child/young person with diabetes. Special attention is required if dental extractions are to be performed.

Age-specific health promotion

Sexual health

The NSF for children, young people and maternity services requires primary care trusts and local authorities to ensure interventions to improve young people's sexual health and reduce teenage

Case study

An 11-year-old boy, Tom, with type 1 diabetes attended his dental practitioner, along with his mother. Tom required dental extraction due to overcrowding of his teeth prior to orthodontic treatment. The dental practitioner wanted to refer Tom to the local sedation clinic. The mother was aware from education that she had received from the diabetes care team, that her son required specialised support for any surgery, and asked the dental practitioner to liaise with the diabetes care team. The dental practitioner made contact and arrangements were made for an in-patient stay in hospital, which carries out dental procedures on children/young people with complex needs. Tom was admitted to hospital, starved appropriately, receiving insulin therapy and monitoring before, during and after the dental procedure. He also had antibiotic cover to prevent infection.

(Tom's name and details have been changed as required by Nursing Midwifery Council guidelines (NMC, 2004).)

pregnancy (Education and Skills, Department of Health, 2004a). There are plans for every school to provide comprehensive personal, social and health education, including education on sex and relationships (Department of Health, 2003c).

Pregnancy in women with type 1 and Type 2 diabetes in 2002–2003 (Confidential Enquiry into Maternal and Child Health, CEMACH, 2005) was the largest ever enquiry into diabetes and pregnancy undertaken in the UK. It examined the outcomes of 3733 women accounting for 3808 pregnancies between 1 March 2002 and 28 February 2003. It found that women with diabetes are much more likely to have difficulties compared with the general population:

- Deliver early.
- Require an induction in labour.
- Be delivered by a caesarean section.
- Their babies may have complications.

The management of pregnancy in a young woman with diabetes is a highly intensive and interventional process, with the requirement of multiple injections and blood tests each day to maintain near normal blood sugars. Other medications have to be reviewed as they can cause fetal abnormalities, and high-dose folic acid has to be taken to help prevent

neural tube defects (CEMACH, 2005). With planning and specialist support services, young women with diabetes can reduce these risks and have a normal birth (St Vincent's Declaration, 1989; Department of Health, 2001).

For the male with diabetes there is the possibility of impotence resulting from poor diabetic control. Both groups can also contract sexually transmitted diseases, similar to the general population. These infections can impact on their overall diabetic control.

There are four guiding ethical principles in health promotion: respect for autonomy, beneficence, nonmaleficence and justice (Jones and Cribb, 2002). Providing a sexual health service within an adolescent diabetes clinic involves the promotion of self-esteem and autonomy in young people, by empowering them to make informed choices about their sexual health. It is also important to sign post them to specialist services, if needed.

In my own area a sexual health advisor, with additional training in diabetes, attends the adolescent diabetes clinic to provide an integrated, confidential sexual health service for young people. The advisor can facilitate referral onto a wider network of sexual health services as and when required.

Conclusions

The management of diabetes in children/young people is an example of health promotion on many dimensions. This chapter has demonstrated that health promotion activities are not only diabetes specific, but can also be age specific. Health promotion can be adapted to meet the needs of children/young people with diabetes and their family. As diabetes is now so common, all children's nurses must ensure they develop an understanding of the management principles of diabetes and how to access specialist services to enable appropriate advice and guidance to be given.

References

Act of Parliament (2001) *Special Educational Needs and Disability Act 2001*. Available at: http://www.opsi.gov.uk/acts/acts/2001/20010010 (accessed 10 December 2006).

Confidential Enquiry into Maternal and Child Health (CEMACH) (2005) *Pregnancy in Women with Type 1 and Type 2 Diabetes in 2002–2003, England, Wales and Northern Ireland*. London: RCOG Press.

Department for Education and Employment, Department of Health (1996) *A Good Practice Guide for Supporting Pupils with Medical Needs*. London: Crown Copyright.

Department of Health (2001) *National Service Framework for Diabetes: Standards*. London: Crown Copyright.

Department of Health (2003a) *The National Service Framework for Children, Young People and Maternity Services – Standard for Hospital Services*. London: Crown Copyright.

Department of Health (2003b) *National Service Framework for Diabetes: Delivery Strategy*. London: Crown Copyright.

Department of Health (2003c) *Effective Sexual Health Promotion, a Toolkit for Primary Care Trusts and Others Working in the Field of Promoting Good Sexual Health and HIV Prevention*. London: Department of Health.

Department of Health (2006a) *Medicines Matter a Guide to Mechanisms for the Prescribing, Supply and Administration of Medicines*. London: Department of Health.

Department of Health (2006b) *The Influenza Immunisation Programme 2006/2007*. London: Crown Copyright.

Diabetes Control and Complication Trials (DCCT) (1993). The effect of intensive treatment of diabetes on the development and progression of long term complications in insulin-dependent diabetes mellitus. *New England Journal of Medicine* 329(14): 977–986.

Dines, A. (2003) A case study of ethical issues in health promotion – mammography screening: the nurses' position. In: Sidell, M., Jones, L., Katz, J., Peberdy, A., Douglas, J. (eds) *Debates and Dilemmas in Promoting Health. A Reader*, 2nd edn. Basingstoke: The Open University in association with Palgrave.

Education and Skills (Department of) (2003) *Every Child Matters*. London: Crown Copyright.

Education and Skills (Department of) (2005) *Managing Medicines in Schools and Early Years Settings*. London: Crown Copyright.

Education and Skills (Department of), Department of Health (2004a) *National Service Framework for Children, Young People, and Maternity Services*. London: Crown Copyright.

Education and Skills (Department of), Department of Health (2004b) *Medicines Standard: National Service Framework for Children, Young People and Maternity Services*. London: Crown Copyright.

Jones, L., Cribb, A. (2002) Ethical Issues in health promotion. In: Katz, J., Peberdy, A., Douglas, J. (eds) *Promoting Health: Knowledge and Practice*, 2nd edn. Oxford: The Open University in association with Palgrave.

Jones, L., Naidoo, J. (2002) Theories and models in health promotion. In: Katz, J., Peberdy, A., Douglas, J. (eds) *Promoting Health: Knowledge and Practice*, 2nd edn. Oxford: The Open University in association with Palgrave.

National Collaborating Centre for Women's and Children's Health (NCC-WCH) (2004) *Type 1 Diabetes: Diagnosis and Management of Type 1 Diabetes in Children and Young People*. National Institute for Clinical Excellence. London: RCOG Press at the Royal College of Obstetricians and Gynaecologists.

National Retinopathy Screening Programme (2006) *Eye Screening for People with Diabetes – the Facts*. Available at: http://www.nscretinopathy.org.uk/ (accessed 10 December 2006).

NICE (2004) Type 1 diabetes: diagnosis and management of type 1 diabetes in children, young people and adults. *Clinical Guideline 15*. London: National Institute for Clinical Excellence.

NMC (2004) *Code of Professional Conduct*. London: Nursing and Midwifery Council.

Ottawa Charter for Health Promotion (1986) In Katz, J., Peberdy, A., Douglas, J. (eds) (2002) *Promoting Health: Knowledge and Practice*, 2nd edn. Oxford: The Open University in association with Palgrave.

Prochaska, J.O., Di Clemente, C.C. (1984) In: Katz, J., Peberdy, A., Douglas, J. (eds) (2002) *Promoting Health: Knowledge and Practice*, 2nd edn. Oxford: The Open University in association with Palgrave.

Royal College of Nursing (RCN) (2006) *Specialist Nursing Services for Children and Young People with Diabetes*. London: RCN Publishing.

Sengbusch, S., Muller-Godeffroy, E., Hager, S., Riintje, R., Hiort, O., Wagner, V. (2006) Mobile diabetes education and care: interventions for children and young people with type 1 diabetes in rural areas of northern Germany. *Diabetes Medicine* 23(2): 122–127.

Sidell, M. (2002) Supporting individuals & facilitating change: the role of counselling skills. In: Katz, J., Peberdy, A., Douglas, J. (eds) *Promoting Health: Knowledge and Practice*, 2nd edn. Oxford: The Open University in association with Palgrave. 140–160

Spence, C. (2005) Cystic fibrosis-related diabetes practice challenges. *Paediatric Nursing* 17(2): 23–27.

St Vincent's Declaration (1989) International Diabetes Federation. Available at: http://www.idf.org/home/index (accessed 10 December 2006).

Tang, W., Ariyawansa, I. (2007) Difficulties facing young people with diabetes at school. *Journal of Diabetes Nursing* 11(1): 27–31.

Thornton, H. (2000) A simple influenza campaign for young people with diabetes. *Journal of Diabetes Nursing* 4(1): 8–11.

Thornton, H. (2007) New year, new challenges in diabetes care. *Journal of Diabetes Nursing* 11(1): 20–21.

United Nations Resolution (2006) *Caps Momentous Year for Diabetes World*. Available at: http://www.unitefordiabetes.org/news/campaign. International Diabetes Federation (accessed 27 December 2006).

23 Children/Young People with Disabilities and Complex Health Care Needs

Sarah V. Wilcock

NSF

The National Service Framework (NSF) (Education and Skills, Department of Health, 2004) talks about promoting the health of disabled children, whose health needs may be great.

Introduction

Children/young people who are disabled and/or have complex health needs, just like any other group, will benefit from health promotion. However, sometimes their needs may be great simply because of the complexity of their needs.

This chapter focuses on health promotion with children/young people who have disabilities and/or complex health needs. How health can be promoted with this group, so they can develop their potential, will be discussed. The chapter explores how a community team of children's nurses and support workers promote the health of children/young people with disabilities and/or complex health needs, in the East Midlands.

Here the nurse is promoting health in a slightly different way to that discussed within other themes in the book. Health promotion work is focusing on tertiary prevention, limiting the impact of an individual's disease once it is present (Hall and Elliman,

2003) and promoting the individual's potential. Working in partnership with children/young people and their families, along with other practitioners, nurses can help to achieve much for them.

Needs

Children/young people with disabilities and/or complex health care needs include a broad spectrum of individuals. Around 770 000 children/young people in the UK are disabled and 100 000 have complex health care needs (Education and Skills, 2007).

There does not appear to be any agreed definition for *children with complex health care needs* (Price and Thomas, 2007). However, this chapter considers children/young people with complex health care needs and disabilities as those who are dependent on some kind of technology or medical equipment to sustain, maintain and improve their lives. Sadly, some of these children/young people may not survive into adulthood.

Currently, this group is high on the Government's agenda. The aim is to ensure they receive *services of a high quality*, which meet their diverse needs. It is important that they are helped to live *ordinary lives* (Education and Skills, Department of Health, 2004; Education and Skills, 2006, 2007). Indeed, it is paramount that they are seen as children/young people first and foremost, thus given opportunities to develop and achieve their potential (Education and Skills, 2003; Education and Skills, Department of Health, 2004). Accomplishing this can sometimes be challenging, particularly where there may be restraints placed upon service provision (Audit Commission, 2003; Education and Skills, 2006).

Practice

As team leader for a continuing care and respite team, in the East Midlands, the care of these children/young people and their families is really important to me. The team itself consists of qualified children's nurses, as well as support workers, who have a nursery nurse qualification. They are all trained to care for a range of children/young people on a named child basis, each responsible for the care of particular children/young people.

A wide range of services are provided for those cared for by the team. This includes meeting their health care needs along with play and development needs. The aim of care is to provide opportunities for promotion and improvement in health, so children/young people are encouraged and supported to develop their potential.

Care is provided in a number of environments, predominately in the child's or young person's home, also in hospital, school, nursery and other community settings. The team works closely with different practitioners, and families themselves, to ensure an appropriate service is given.

The children/young people in our care have a variety of different medical conditions; cerebral palsy, chronic lung disease, muscular dystrophy are some of the conditions they may present with. In some cases, depending on the condition, they may need a range of equipment to help sustain life. This might include home ventilation equipment, tracheostomy devices or oxygen to support breathing. To help meet nutritional needs, gastrostomy feeding may be a priority of care.

During a visit the children's nurse or support worker will take over the care from parents/carers or simply assist them. Parents/carers are looking after their child on a continual basis, and may, as in many cases, need a break from the repeated demands of caring. Our team is able to provide that relief.

The team implement a *play and development programme*. This programme is tailor-made to meet the child's/young person's needs, with the involvement of the whole family and other practitioners. It is paramount that the team links with other practitioners, in particular physiotherapists and occupational therapists. Essentially, this is to ensure the programme will assist the child/young person to achieve her/his potential and promote health.

The therapists usually have specific areas of care that the child/young person will need to be working on. For example, physiotherapists may be working on breathing. By working with therapists closely, the team can compliment the therapist's programme. The therapist may only see the child/young person each month. However, members of out team may be involved weekly or even daily in some cases. This more frequent contact provides the opportunity to further practise aspects of care or skills, which will help to enhance or promote the child's/young person's health.

The team aims to support the family in the care of their child. The family may, with all the other demands of caring, find it difficult to undertake specific aspects of care or the play programme itself. Team members provide them with a break and undertake the programme with their child. The team are facilitating the family with a period of respite, care and promoting the child's health simultaneously.

Another aspect of the team's role is liaison; this includes liaison with other practitioners on behalf of the family. The team can liaise with practitioners to resolve any issues over equipment, for example. Difficulties may be experienced in getting hold of equipment or replacing items, which may be urgently needed. The family will be busy taking care of their child and do not have the time to repeatedly chase items.

Case study

To highlight how the play and development programme is implemented, this case study demonstrates how a simple programme can promote the health and development of a child with complex health care needs.

Jack, 2 years old, has learning and physical difficulties. He requires a range of health interventions daily to maintain and promote his health and development. This involves gastrostomy feeding, a range of medicines and a daily physiotherapy programme. (Jack's real name has been changed in line with guidance from Nursing Midwifery Council, 2004.)

Jack's main carer is his mother who has health problems herself. She finds it difficult to carry out Jack's physiotherapy daily, as it is too physically demanding for her. Jack's father works full time and there are other children in the family. To undertake Jack's physiotherapy each day is difficult for the family. As health practitioners we have to be very aware of what realistically can be expected of parents in caring for their child's complex health care needs. The extra care that a child such as Jack requires can be immense, and it is paramount that practitioners provide services to assist families.

To help Jack and his family, the team provides daily assistance with his physiotherapy programme. This involves a member of the team undertaking various physical exercises and movements which incorporate play.

Prior to starting this programme with Jack, a support worker from the team undertook a play and development assessment. This assessment would have been carried out in conjunction with his nursing assessment. Both assessments are combined to minimise the number of in-depth contacts with the child and family. The future aim is to have a multi-agency assessment, where different practitioners who are going to be involved in the child's care assess the child together.

For Jack the play and development assessment was undertaken with him and his mother. Close liaison with the physiotherapist and occupational therapist was involved. Liaison with other practitioners is essential to ensure that the play and development programme is written for Jack and meets all his development needs.

Jack's play and development programme focused on five areas of development:

- Cognitive.
- Communication.
- Emotional.
- Physical.
- Social.

All these areas of Jack's development are addressed during his visits from members of the team. This may happen at each visit or over a period of visits, depending on Jack's needs at the time.

Visits with Jack are always documented in his family-held record on what activities have been carried out and how Jack has responded to them. Documenting in this way helps to monitor Jack's progress. It clearly highlights what areas of development have been worked on, how Jack has responded and what areas need further input. The family-held record is often used as evidence with his physiotherapist when updating her on Jack's programme, as it clearly demonstrates how he is progressing.

Jack's play and development programme is maintained by his support worker from the team. His support worker ensures that it is reviewed every 3–6 months. The support worker also liaises regularly with Jack's mother and his named nurse from the team to make any changes to the programme.

Every 6 months his support worker carries out an updated assessment with Jack's mother and his named nurse, also liaising with his physiotherapist and occupational therapist. At a team meeting all team members, who provide care for Jack, discuss his progress and offer opinions on what has worked and further ideas on what might help Jack. The purpose of this is to ensure Jack's health is being promoted in a way that will best meet his needs.

The team is also able to quickly identify if Jack is outgrowing a piece of equipment. His named nurse can liaise with the occupational therapist for reassessment of his equipment needs. Barriers to long waiting times for vital pieces of equipment needed by Jack can be reduced. Help from the team can take away pressure for his parents and reduce the number of practitioners that need to make contact with the family. Many families often report that they are constantly on the phone to one practitioner or another, trying to sort out different issues for their child. Having the programme in place, with the involvement of the team, can reduce these pressures for families.

In conclusion, the play and development programme has benefits for the child and family. Importantly, for the child the programme can offer play opportunities, which aim to be a fun experience. The team will work very closely with the family. Issues such as equipment, which are essential for promoting the child's health, can be resolved more readily when using the programme.

Evaluations have demonstrated that the play and development programme is valued highly by families. The team's regular input and reviews with the family provide a valuable source of support for them. Jack's case highlights how a simple play and development programme can have an important influence on promoting the health of a child with complex health care needs.

Conclusion

The NSF describes the importance of supporting children/young people with disabilities and/or continuing health needs and their families (Education and Skill, Department of Health, 2004). It maintains that their needs should be identified early. The earlier their needs are identified, the sooner interventions can be put into place to meet those needs. Partnership working with families and other practitioners is absolutely essential. The community nursing teams discussed in this chapter are working hard to effectively identify and meet the needs of this group of children/young people, support their families, as well as liaising with other practitioners involved.

Children/young people with disabilities and/or continuing health care needs can have a great many health needs. Health promotion activities with them and their families may involve not only information giving as with other groups, but the teaching of skills, developing and implementing programmes of care and child development to help them reach their potential and support their families.

The play and development programme outlined here is simple to implement and has many benefits. It can assist parents/carers and practitioners to help children/young people achieve their potential and promote health in a fun way.

References

Audit Commission (2003) *Services for Disabled Children: A Review of Services for Disabled Children and their Families*. London: Audit Commission.

Education and Skills (Department of) (2003) *Every Child Matters*. London: Crown Copyright.

Education and Skills (Department of) (2006) *Every Disabled Child Matters*. About Every Disabled Child Matters. Available at: http://www.edcm.org.uk (accessed 9 September 2007).

Education and Skills (Department of) (2007) *Aiming High for Disabled Children. Better Support for Families*. London: HM Treasury.

Education and Skills (Department of), Department of Health (2004) *National Service Framework for Children, Young People and Maternity Services. Standard 8 – Disabled Children and Young People and those with Complex Health Needs*. London: Crown Copyright.

Hall, D., Elliman, D. (2003) *Health for All Children*, 4th edn. Oxford: Oxford University Press.

Nursing and Midwifery Council (2004) *The Code of Professional Conduct*. London: NMC.

Price, M., Thomas, S. (2007) Continuing care needs. In: Lowes, L., Valentine, F. (eds) *Nursing Care of Children and Young People with Chronic Illness*. Oxford: Blackwell Publishing.

Theme 7

Medicines Management

Chapter 24   Medicines Management

24 Medicines Management

Roger Kirkbride

NSF

The National Service Framework (NSF) for children, young people and maternity services, standard 10, focuses on medicines management. Standard 10: children, young people, their parents or carers, and health care professionals in all settings make decisions about medicines based on sound information about risk and benefit. They have access to safe and effective medicines that are prescribed on the basis of the best available evidence (standard 10, Education and Skills, Department of Health, 2004, p. 4).

Introduction

The range of medicines available to the prescriber continuously increases; new drugs may have new indications or provide better or adjunctive treatments; new formulations make medicines easier to take or mitigate side effects. In order to improve access to effective treatment, prescribing rights have been extended and more non-medical health care practitioners are prescribing medicines in a variety of situations. The cost of medication to the National Health Service (NHS) rises substantially every year and accounts for a significant percentage of the NHS budget. But children/young people often do not benefit from their medication as well as they could or should. Medicines may not be optimally prescribed; they may not be dispensed, taken or administered correctly; or children/young people may experience adverse effects or unwanted side effects. Some children/young people experience harm through their medication regime and a significant proportion of hospital admissions can be attributed to medication. The process by which the safety, efficacy and cost-effectiveness of drug therapies are improved is termed *medicines management*.

Definition of medicines management

There is no one clear and agreed definition of medicines management – it is a complex process; Simpson Prentiss et al. (2003) found that the understanding of what it means depends on the perspective of health care practitioners involved. The Audit Commission (2001, p. 5) defined medicines management in hospitals as: 'the entire way that medicines are selected, procured, delivered, prescribed, administered and reviewed to optimise the contribution that medicines make to producing informed and desired outcomes of patient care'. The National Prescribing Centre (2002, p. 5) defines medicines management as: 'a system of processes and behaviours that determines how medicines are used by patients and by the NHS'.

Many of the definitions come from those involved in the profession of pharmacy; the definition proposed by Tweedie and Jones (2001, p. 248) attempts to encompass all health care practitioners together with involvement of the patient: 'The systematic provision of medicines therapy through a partnership of effort between children/young people and practitioners to deliver best patient outcome at minimised cost'.

Although definitions vary in terms of scope and emphasis, they all share a number of common themes:

- Optimising a medication regime – ensuring that the child/young person is prescribed the right drug at the right dose and the right frequency.
- Facilitating compliance with the medication regime – engaging the child/young person or their parent/carer in the treatment plan and helping them to stick to it.
- Organising supply and administration – ensuring that the child/young person can gain access to the medication and that it is given/taken appropriately.
- Monitoring and reviewing the medication regime – ensuring that the child/young person obtains the intended benefit from the medication regime.

Underpinning all of the above is cost-effectiveness: the NHS has limited resources and needs to use them most effectively to the benefit of all children/young people.

Why do we need medicines management?

Medicines are a major cost to the NHS; according to figures quoted in parliament (Daily Hansard, 2005) the NHS in England spent almost £9.3 billion on drugs in 2003/2004, which amounted to about 15% of total NHS expenditure. In the community this proportion rises to about 20% of expenditure – a sum of approximately £7.9 million in 2003/2004. However, these medicines are not necessarily used effectively; according to figures given in *Pharmacy in the Future* (Department of Health, 2000) almost half of medicines are not used correctly and that, each year, over £100 million of unused medicines are returned to pharmacies.

More importantly, there is evidence that children/young people fail to gain the optimum benefit from their medicines and some suffer actual harm. The Audit Commission (2001) estimates that up to 50% of people with long-term conditions do not take their medicines as prescribed, and medicine-related problems are responsible for 5–17% of hospital admissions. Although much of the data on compliance and the rate of medicine-related problems relates to older people, a similar picture emerges for children/young people, as the NSF demonstrates (Education and Skills, Department of Health, 2004). But the potential to cause harm is three times higher. A study of admissions to neonatal and paediatric intensive care units suggested that almost 15% of admissions were due to errors in prescribing or administration of medicines. Standard 10 of the NSF, the Medicines Standard (Education and Skills, Department of Health, 2004), recognises the additional complexity and sensitivity of the use of medicines in children.

Medicines management principles

The complexity of achieving good practice for children in the four themes of medicines management – optimising a medication, facilitating compliance with the medication regime, organising supply and administration, monitoring and reviewing the medication regime – are greater than for most adult groups. The age, weight and developmental stage of children need to be taken into account; information for the health care practitioner, the parent/carer and child/young person may not be easily available or appropriate, and communication problems may arise from the number of people involved in the care process.

Optimising a medication regime

The NSF, standard 10

Vision: We want to see all children/young people receiving medicines that are safe and effective, in formulations that can easily be administered and are appropriate to their age, having minimum impact on their education and lifestyle (Education and Skills, Department of Health, 2004, p. 4).

As children/young people progress from neonate to infant to child to adolescent, their ability to absorb drugs, distribute them around the body, metabolise and excrete them changes and is often very different from that of an adult. The differences are summarised by the National Prescribing Centre (2000) and include the following:

- Oral absorption may be delayed or speeded up (due to variable intestinal transit time; higher gastric pH; different gastrointestinal content; posture).
- Distribution through the body may be increased or decreased (due to a higher proportion of total body water and decreased plasma protein binding).
- Metabolism of drugs may be slowed down because enzyme systems may be absent or immature. Metabolism of drugs may be increased because children have a higher metabolic rate than adults.
- Excretion is slowed down in neonates and infants as renal function is not mature until 6–8 months of age.

Any or all of these factors may influence the choice of drug that may be used. Similarly, any or all of these factors may influence the route and formulation for administration and the dose that may be needed.

Drugs that are effective in adults may be inappropriate in children/young people; they may have a higher rate of adverse drug reactions or they have other effects that do not occur in adults. For many drugs the information available on safe and effective use in children/young people is not available. Establishing a safety profile is difficult; ethical constraints limit studies in paediatric populations and such studies that are undertaken often include only small numbers of children/young people, reducing the likelihood that the full range and severity of adverse reactions will be correctly identified. As a result, up to 50% of medicines used in children may not have been studied on the age group for which they are prescribed. Such drugs may be:

- *off label* – not licensed for use in children/young people or used outside the terms of their product licence.

- or unlicensed – not licensed at all for any indication or age group; these drugs may be undergoing clinical trials, be imported from another country, or have been made specially.

Since these medicines do not have product licences, the information on them and their use in children is generally scarce. The British National Formulary for Children (BNFC) was launched in September 2005 in order to collate and disseminate the best available information on the use of medicines in children/young people and provide advice to prescribers and other health care practitioners. The BNFC also provides advice on the formulation of medicines for children/young people and their dose.

The particular preparation of medicine selected needs to take into account the intended route of administration, age of the child/young person and the availability of suitable formulations. Moules and Ramsey (1998) state that the oral route of administration is the preferred option for administering medicines to children and is generally regarded as being the most convenient method. However, solid dose formulations may not necessarily be suitable or appropriate for children; although some children are capable of swallowing tablets, infants and many small children are not. Many drugs are available as liquid medicines; sugar-free formulations are now common and are particularly favoured for long-term therapies. But liquid medicines often still contain alcohol, dyes or other excipients that make them unsuitable for children. The formulation of liquid medicines often makes dilution inadvisable and they should never be mixed with infant feeds.

Research by Seth et al. (2000) suggests that the rectal route of administration is not popular in the United Kingdom, unlike other countries. However, it can be an effective route avoiding problems of swallowing or the taste of the medicine; for drugs suitable for administration in this way suppositories are available.

The appropriate dose will need to be calculated by reference to the age, body weight, body surface area (or a combination of these) of the child/young person. The BNFC (2007) clearly indicates which methodology should be used and provides guidance on the appropriate dose by age, per kilogram of body weight or per square metre of surface area. Where surface area is to be used the BNFC (2007) provides tables from which the body surface area can be estimated if the height and weight of the child are known. Where the BNFC does not give adequate guidance, the advice of a Medicines Information Centre (MIC) should be obtained; MICs are available in most NHS trusts; a national directory of MICs is available through an NHS site – UK Medicines Information at http://www.ukmi.nhs.uk

Facilitating compliance with the medication regime

The NSF, standard 10, wants to see children, young people, their parents or carers, and health care professionals in all settings make decisions about medicines based on sound information about risk and benefit. They have access to safe and effective medicines that are prescribed on the basis of the best available evidence (Education and Skills, Department of Health, 2004, p. 4).

According to the Health Survey for England (Information Centre, 2005), over 20% of children/young people of school age reported long-standing illness. Although the rate of long-standing illness appears to be stable, the number of children receiving active treatment for conditions such as asthma, hay fever, eczema, severe allergy, epilepsy, attention deficit hyperactivity disorder and diabetes (now including type 2 diabetes – formerly only seen in older adults) continues to increase. A smaller, but significant, percentage of children also receive treatment for an acute condition. However, compliance with, or adherence to, medication regimes is often poor, particularly where children/young people are taking medication regularly for long-term conditions. Compliance is difficult to measure accurately, but the NSF estimates that compliance with children/young people's medication regimes ranges from as low as 25% to up to 82% (Education and Skills, Department of Health, 2004). There is evidence of resulting adverse consequences in children/young people with, amongst other conditions, prophylactic antibiotic treatment, asthma and epilepsy. In smaller children compliance with diabetes medication regimes is often good, but as they grow in to adolescence compliance falls as societal pressures and a switch in the accountability for decision-making takes effect. While the child is young the parent/carer takes responsibility for administering medicines; it switches to the young person as she/he takes more responsibility for their own actions and the parent/carer has less responsibility. This process can be difficult for both parties and can have an adverse impact on compliance.

Non-compliance may be involuntary due to forgetfulness or misunderstanding of instructions; for children this may be compounded by the intervention of a parent or carer and the policy of the school that they attend. All schools should have a policy for how they manage medicines, which encompasses long- and short-term prescription medicines; the administration of invasive medicines (for example, adrenaline injections for severe allergy, or rectal diazepam for status epilepticus); over-the-counter medication; storage; and record keeping. The policy should also include a statement on the responsibilities of staff; however, teaching unions, such as the National Union of Teachers (NUT), advise their members that participation in any medicines policy is entirely voluntary and urge members to ensure that they have proper training (NUT, 2005). A survey of primary schools in London (Wong et al., 2004) showed that 86% of schools had a policy in place and that the majority of staff with responsibilities for medicines tended to be support staff; approximately 50% of schools used written care plans for pupils with diabetes, asthma or epilepsy.

Compliance or concordance?

Carter et al. (2003) found that intentional non-compliance is much more common than involuntary non-compliance and has a much more profound effect on the way that people take their medicines – particularly where medicines are taken in a preventative context. Intentional non-compliance is a response to a medication regime based on the patient's understanding of the condition, the benefits and adverse effects of medication and their beliefs about their condition and its treatment. The word *compliance* suggests that the patient is acting on the directions of the prescriber – the patient is not involved in the process of making decisions about their treatment. There is evidence that a patient-centred approach promotes better, more effective medicine taking; such an approach is termed *concordance.* Weiss and Britten (2004) assert that concordance is based on a sharing of power between the patient and the health care practitioner. It acknowledges that the patient has knowledge and experience of her/his condition and response to treatment. This experience is different from the knowledge of a health care practitioner but is equally valid; this may cause tension where the health care practitioner's use of evidence-based medicine is in conflict with strongly held beliefs of the patient. Nevertheless, it is likely that a two-way discussion exploring beliefs and checking understanding will lead to improved satisfaction with care and better knowledge of the condition and its treatment; adherence to medication is more likely, which then results in better health outcomes and fewer medication-related problems.

Children/young people should be involved in the discussions about their condition and its treatment as soon as it is feasible. Children/young people develop at different rates and will be able to participate to an increasing extent as they grow. Older children with long-term conditions should be encouraged to take responsibility for their treatment, wherever possible. However, they need support through this process; there is considerable evidence that compliance with a medication regime falls away as children reach adolescence and that the support of nurses and other health care practitioners can be crucial: such independent support and advice is valued and can be effective in promoting compliance and avoiding the complications of non-compliance.

Organising supply and administration

The NSF, standard 10, wants to see medicines being prescribed, dispensed and administered by professionals who are well trained, informed and competent to work with children to improve health outcomes and minimise harm and any side effects of medicines (Education and Skills, Department of Health, 2004).

Although the majority of supply of medicines occurs through pharmacies (hospital or community) and the majority of administration of medicines is under the control of parents, carers or children/young people themselves, there are a number of considerations for the nurse in the supply and administration of medicines for children. Figure 24.1 illustrates the medicines management cycle and how the hospital and community cycles intersect. If we use an example of a child admitted to hospital with unexplained symptoms, we can use the cycles to illustrate where the nurse needs to be

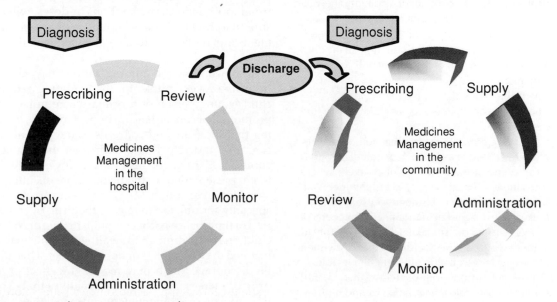

Figure 24.1 Medicines management cycle.

aware of the potential to be involved with supply and administration.

In the hospital a diagnosis may lead to the prescription of a medicine; as we have already discussed, many medicines used in children do not have product licences and some may need to be specially manufactured; the supply of such medicines will be organised through the hospital pharmacy. However, the administration of the medicine is, most often, the responsibility of the nurse and there are a number of principles, set out by the Nursing and Midwifery Council (NMC, 2006), that nurses should follow. Box 24.1 summarises these responsibilities. For full details consult the reference provided.

Box 24.1 Principles for administration of medicines (extracted from *A-Z Advice Sheet – Medicines Management*, NMC, 2006).

Registrants in exercising their professional accountability in the best interests of their patients must:

- Know the therapeutic uses of the medicine to be administered.
- Know its normal dosage, side effects, precautions and contraindications.
- Be certain of the identity of the patient to whom the medicine is to be administered.
- Check that the prescription, or medicine label dispensed by pharmacist, is clearly written.
- Consider the dosage, administration method, route and timing of the administration, in the context of the condition of the patient and coexisting therapies.
- Check the expiry date of the medicine.
- Check that the patient is not allergic to the medicine.
- Contact the prescriber or another authorised prescriber without delay, where contraindications to the prescribed medicine are discovered, where the patient develops a reaction to the medicine or where the medicine is no longer suitable.
- Make a clear, accurate and immediate record of all medicine administered, intentionally withheld or refused by the patient, ensuring that any written entries and the signature are clear and legible.
- It is also your responsibility to ensure that a record is made when delegating the task of administering medicine; clearly countersign the signature of any student who is being supervised in the administration of medicines.

Administration of medicines can take up to 40% of a nurse's time and she/he should be fully aware of their responsibilities in this respect.

It is on discharge that the role of the nurse in supply and administration becomes more diverse. The diagnosis and treatment regime needs to be communicated fully and accurately to the primary care team; while this would be carried out by the hospital medical team, the receiving general practitioner (GP) practice may well involve its nursing team in assuming effective responsibility for care. In these circumstances considerations of supply, as well as administration, come into play, particularly where the medicine is specially prepared and/or the dose regime unusual. For children/young people who have long-term conditions and are to continue with a course of treatment for some time, a repeat prescription regime may be established; this may be controlled by the practice or, increasingly, mediated through a pharmacy. It is essential that the correct information is provided to the pharmacy. This ensures that the correct medicine is provided in time so the medication regime continues uninterrupted. Dialogue with the child's/young person's preferred pharmacy, particularly about unusual formulations, preparations or doses, will ensure that the medicine is kept in stock or arrangements are in place for it to be obtained in sufficient time.

Responsibility for administration may change from the ward nurse to the parent/carer, the child/young person or a primary care nurse. The promotion of concordance is important here, ensuring that the fears and concerns of the patient and carer are understood and addressed. In some circumstances it may be necessary to investigate different presentations of medicine before deciding on a regular prescription. Many tablets or capsules are specially formulated to release the drug over a period of time, or at a particular point in the gut. Where children find it difficult to swallow, parents may be inclined to crush tablets or open capsules. This must be discouraged as it may reduce the effect of the drug or increase its toxicity; alternatives that avoid the problem of swallowing may be available.

Important in the process of allaying fears and concerns and promoting concordance is the provision of information; often the product information leaflet accompanying the medicine may not be available or may not include indications or doses for children/young people. The primary care nurse may wish to provide education and support in these circumstances or arrange for that to be provided by another member of the primary care team.

Certain medicines or preparations may require a greater degree of support in administration:

- Small children may not be able to use inhalers properly and may require the appropriately sized device to make them effective.
- Medicines to be given by injection may require continued involvement of the nurse to help ensure appropriate administration and to respond to any queries or issues raised in the treatment; the administration of growth hormone is one such example.
- Alternatively, education of the parent/carer to enable them to administer medicine by injection may be required. This may include the administration of adrenaline for anaphylactic shock; insulin for young children with diabetes; or parenteral nutrition.
- Children with diabetes who have been issued with insulin pumps may require additional support and for any therapy requiring multiple injections these sites must be examined regularly.

In the hospital the nurse is less involved in supply but is directly and intimately involved in administration; at this point she/he may be providing advice on using the medication and, particularly as the child/young person approaches discharge, health promotion advice. In the community the nurse may be more involved in the organisation of continuity of supply and more involved in providing information, education and support for administration taking place in the patient's home.

In either situation the nurse must continue to observe the impact of the medicine on the child/young person and be prepared to review its continued need. Increasingly, nurses are prescribing medicines for children/young people either as supplementary or independent prescribers, and monitoring and review of medication regimes is essential.

Monitoring and reviewing

The NSF, standard 10, primary care trusts and NHS trusts ensure that:

- All children with epilepsy have regular medication reviews (in line with the SuDEp recommendation);
- Mechanisms are in place for regular review of medicines used to treat children/young people with complex, long-term conditions;
- There is equitable access to medication reviews, where appropriate, for children in all settings including children's homes and young offenders' institutions (Education and Skills, Department of Health, 2004, p. 21).

Monitoring of a medication regime is fundamental in establishing the progress of the patient's condition; the effectiveness of the medicine(s) being prescribed and taken; and in ensuring that any adverse effects are identified. In an acute setting, monitoring is a frequent process; the patient's condition and response to medication is checked regularly and this monitoring affects ongoing treatment and duration of stay. In the community, monitoring is no less important but may be less frequent. On discharge from hospital, or after an acute episode dealt with in the community, monitoring by a health care practitioner may include daily or weekly checks on progress.

For certain long-term conditions, the NSF, standard 10, identifies the frequency with which children/young people should be formally monitored, and these standards are partially reflected in the GPs general medical services (GMS) contract quality and outcome framework (QOF). The child's/young person's or parent's/carer's contribution to continuous monitoring should not be ignored; a history of results of peak flow measurements or blood glucose tests for those with asthma and diabetes, respectively, provides all involved with important information on progress. Monitoring data may be used to trigger a medication review or as part of the information set used in a scheduled medication review.

A definition of medication review is given in *Room for Review* (Medicines Partnership, 2002, p. 12); it proposes that a medication review is 'a structured, critical examination of a patient's medicines with the objective of reaching an agreement with the patient about treatment, optimising the impact of medicines, minimising the number of medication-related problems and reducing waste'.

Four levels of medication review are identified: unstructured or opportunistic in response to a question; prescription review looking at dose rationalisation; treatment review to identify systematic issues with medication; clinical medication review carried out in the presence of the patient looking at the effectiveness of medication.

The QOF framework in the GMS contract requires all patients taking medication for long-term conditions to have a medication review every year, and the need for children taking medicines for long-term condition is important. The NSF (Education and Skills, Department of Health, 2004) states that a study of sudden unexpected death in epilepsy identified that inadequate medicines management was responsible for 47% of deaths in children; the NSFs for asthma, diabetes, long-term conditions and the NSF for children all identify the need for regular review. As they grow and develop, children's/young people's response to medication changes as does their ability to metabolise drugs and use different dose forms. Their ability to participate in discussion about their condition and follow different management strategies changes, and they may need support from health care practitioners (or people outside the home) as they face the social and emotional challenges of adolescence. *Room for Review* (Medicines Partnership, 2002) sets out a framework for a clinical medication review; good consultation skills are essential – particularly where children or adolescents are involved; obtaining the views of the patient as well as carer may require some tact and carefully constructed discussion.

Nurses working with children/young people, whether in hospital or the community, have a greater responsibility to become involved in medicines management. Children are not mini-adults and require special consideration; information on children's medicines may be inadequate and as they develop their needs and issues change. The NHS intent to use the skills of nurses and other health care practitioners has been clearly set out by the Department of Health. New options for nurses to become more involved in medicines management continue to develop.

Increasing access

Following the first Crown report in 1989, nurse prescribing was first enabled by legislation in 1992 and was rolled out across England in 1998 following successful trials between 1994 and 1998. Initially, nurses with particular district nursing and health visitor qualifications who were employed by an NHS trust or a GP practice were allowed to prescribe from a limited formulary; subsequently an extended formulary was introduced for nurses who had gained additional qualifications. Nurses able to prescribe from the Nurse Prescribers' Formulary for District Nurses/Health Visitors or the Nurse Prescribers' Extended Formulary were able to act without reference to a GP or another health care practitioner.

In 1999 the Review of Prescribing, Supply and Administration of Medicines chaired by Dr June Crown, recognising the need for patients to have greater access to medicines, introduced a broader concept of non-medical prescribing – prescribing by nurses, pharmacists and other health care practitioners (Crown, 1999). The report identified two new classes of prescriber – independent prescribers and dependent prescribers – and set out conditions for the context of their practice and establishing their competence to practice.

Subsequently, the Department of Health introduced in 2003 legislation to introduce supplementary prescribing (dependent prescribing) and in 2006 to extend the scope of independent prescribing.

The introduction of supplementary prescribing and independent prescribing now offers nurses five ways in which they can supply or prescribe medicines to children/young people in their capacity as practitioners, as described in *Medicines Matters: A Guide to Mechanisms for the Prescribing, Supply and Administration of Medicines* (National Practitioner Programme, Core Prescribing Group, 2006).

Patient-specific directions

A patient-specific direction is a written instruction from a prescriber, for medicines to be supplied or administered to a named patient. This encompasses traditional prescriptions, instruction in the patient's notes or on a patient's ward drug chart.

Patient group directions

A patient group direction (PGD) is a written instruction for the supply or administration of a licensed medicine in a particular clinical situation. The patient may or may not be identified before presenting for treatment, but the person authorised to supply or administer the medicine must be named. A PGD must be signed by a doctor (or dentist), a pharmacist and be approved by the organisation in which it will be used (generally a primary care trust (PCT) or NHS trust).

A PGD may be used where there are large groups of children/young people who need the same medication – for example, vaccination programmes; primary care nurses and school nurse are particularly involved in these.

Nurse prescribers' formulary for community practitioners

The nurse prescribers' formulary for community practitioners is the formulary used by community practitioner prescribers and certain school nurses. The formulary contains a limited list of medicines and dressings and appliances relevant to community nursing and health visiting practice. In March 2006, there were approximately 33 000 community practitioner nurse prescribers in the UK registered with the NMC (NMC, 2007).

Supplementary prescribing

Supplementary prescribing is an arrangement between an independent prescriber – a doctor – and the supplementary prescriber, to implement a clinical management plan (CMP). The CMP is a plan written for a specific patient with the agreement of that patient. The supplementary prescriber can prescribe any medicine that is specified in the plan and there are no restrictions on the medicines that can be listed in the plan. Supplementary prescribing is most suitable for managing children/young people with long-term conditions where the supplementary prescriber is working closely with the doctor. In March 2006, there were just over 7000 nurse supplementary prescribers registered with the NMC.

Independent prescribing

Independent prescribing allows nurses to prescribe any licensed medicine for any medical condition that the nurse is competent to treat, with the exception of controlled drugs where restrictions apply. The Nurse Prescribers' Extended Formulary limited nurses to 240 medicines for 110 conditions but that limitation was lifted in 2006. The nurse must be competent to assess, diagnose and make treatment decisions for the patient; this will normally be in the context of a particular area of specialism, where it is appropriate for the nurse to be operating remotely from a doctor. It is not expected that independent prescribing will be suitable for complex medical conditions or where children/young people have a number of co-morbidities.

Substantial additional training is required to qualify as an independent prescriber; at least 26 days training at a higher education institute and 12 days learning in practice spread over a period of 6 months is required; a designated medical practitioner must supervise the student and provide support. Entry requirements for training are exacting and are detailed in *Improving Patients' Access to Medicines: A Guide to Implementing Nurse and Pharmacist Independent Prescribing within the NHS in England* (Department of Health, 2006).

Many nurses who have taken up new roles as independent prescribers are working in specialist areas; these include asthma, epilepsy and diabetes. Childhood onset is a feature of these conditions and the additional complexity of prescribing for children/young people has to be taken into account. In addition, nurses are also providing specialist services for adolescents. In the community, some nurse prescribers run minor illness clinics (usually in GP practices, but sometimes in other community settings) to which babies and young children are referred by their GP colleagues or are brought directly by their parents/carers.

Collaboration

The role of the nurse in medicines management for children is changing and increasing in range, depth and complexity. It is essential that, through the medicine management process, the child/young person or their parent/carer:

- is involved in the decision-making process and that they understand what medicines are being prescribed and for what purpose they are intended;
- understand the information that is given to them – with written information being used to confirm and supplement verbal information;
- understand how and when to take/use the medication;
- understand what side effects may be experienced and how to identify them;
- knows who to contact if there is any query or problem.

For independent prescribers a framework for support and maintenance of competence is outlined in *Improving Patients' Access to Medicines: A Guide to Implementing Nurse and Pharmacist Independent Prescribing within the NHS in England* (Department of Health, 2006). In addition, each PCT provides an analysis of prescribing that allows each nurse prescriber to benchmark their prescribing against other nurse prescribers; advice and prescribing support is also available from the PCT, and clinical supervision should be provided through the GP practice to which the nurse is attached. Such formal support is supplemented by informal support; peer groups provide support through sharing information and experiences with other nurse prescribers. Nurse prescribers thus improve their practice through collaboration with their peers, medical prescribers and pharmacists acting in prescribing support roles.

Prescribing brings additional dimensions to the nurse's practice, but even without it (at the end of March 2006 only 6.2% of nurses registered in the UK had prescribing rights) the nurse has a significant role to play in all aspects of medicines management. All members of the team involved in patient care have their part to play, but medicines management may mean different things to each member of the team depending on individual perspective. It is important that each member of the team has a good understanding about the role and expertise of others. Good communication processes need to exist between practitioners; helping to ensure that children/young people derive maximum benefit from these processes. In this context nurses may take on roles that may not be considered traditional. A number of NHS trusts employ specialist medicine management nurses. For example, in Calderdale and Huddersfield NHS Foundation Trust (Guy, 2006), the medicine management nurse is employed by the pharmacy department to work across the trust to promote a multidisciplinary approach to medicines management. She leads the production of education and training on medicines management; audits policies and procedures; and educates student nurses in medicines management. The role also encompasses working across primary and secondary care boundaries to improve medicines management communication systems.

In primary care GPs, practice nurses and pharmacists may all be involved in checking children's/young person's medication. Regular checks by a specialist nurse may identify issues that need attention. An annual medication review by the GP may indicate that the regime needs to be reconsidered. A medicines use review by the pharmacist may identify concordance issues or suggest changes to the dosage scheme, which may help to make adherence easier. These inputs need to be coordinated to avoid confusing the child/young person or their parent/carer and to ensure that all members of the team are properly informed.

Conclusion

The scope of medicines management is broad and encompasses all elements that involve the prescribing, supply and administration of medicines. All nurses are involved in some aspect of medicines management to a greater or lesser extent depending on their role. Prescribing rights for nurses extend the ability of nurses to provide care for children/young people and increase their involvement in medicines management at all levels. Whether acting as supplementary or independent prescribers, nurses increasingly act with other health care practitioners as part of a team – and that team may be drawn from a greater range of professions.

For all nurses working with children/young people, the additional complexity arising from children's/young people's rapidly changing physiological and psychological development makes medicines management crucial. Nurses must act as an advocate for children/young people, considering their needs and attitudes alongside those of parents/carers, to ensure safe and effective treatment. Effective communication with families is essential; but further, the nurse needs to be aware of, and able to communicate with, other health care practitioners who may be involved in children's/young people's care.

References

Audit Commission (2001) *A Spoonful of Sugar: Medicines Management in NHS Hospitals*. London: The Audit Commission for Local Authorities and the National Health Service in England and Wales.

British National Formulary for Children (BNFC) (2007) London: British Medical Association, Royal Pharmaceutical Society of Great Britain, Royal College of Paediatrics and Child Health, Neonatal and Paediatric Pharmacists Group.

Carter, S., Levenson, R., Taylor, D. (2003) *A Question of Choice – Compliance in Medicines Taking*, 2nd edn. London: Medicines Partnership.

Crown, J. (1999) *Review of Prescribing, Supply and Administration of Medicines*. London: Department of Health.

Daily Hansard (2005) *NHS Drug Costs*. Written Answers: 15 November 2005. Available at: http://www.publications.parliament.uk/pa/cm200506/cmhansrd/cm051115/text/51115w34.htm (accessed 6 November 2006).

Department of Health (2000) *Pharmacy in the Future – Implementing the NHS Plan – A Programme for Pharmacy in the National Health Service*. London: Department of Health.

Department of Health (2006) *Improving Patients' Access to Medicines: A Guide to Implementing Nurse and Pharmacist Independent Prescribing within the NHS in England*. Leeds: Department of Health.

Education and Skills (Department of), Department of Health (2004) *National Service Framework for Children, Young People and Maternity Services, Standard 10 – Medicines for Children and Young People*. London: Department of Health.

Guy, K. (2006) *The Self-Administration of Medicines Patient involvement Participants in HMMC Wave 2*. Available at: http://www.npc.co.uk/mms/events/Calderdale Huddersfield.pdf (accessed 6 November 2006).

Information Centre (2005) *Health Survey for England 2004 – Updating of Trend Tables to Include 2004 Data*. London: NHS Health and Social Care Information Centre.

Medicines Partnership (2002) *Room for Review. A Guide to Medication Review: The Agenda for Patients, Practitioners and Managers*. London: Medicines Partnership.

Moules, T., Ramsey, J. (1998) *The Textbook of Children's Nursing*. Cheltenham: Stanley Thornes.

National Practitioner Programme, Core Prescribing Group (2006) *Medicines Matters: A Guide to Mechanisms for the Prescribing, Supply and Administration of Medicines*. London: Department of Health.

National Prescribing Centre (2000) Prescribing for children. *MeReC Bulletin* 11 (2): 5–8.

National Prescribing Centre (2002) *Modernising Medicines Management: A Guide to Achieving Benefits for Patients, Practitioners and the NHS (Book 1)*. London: National, Prescribing Centre and National Primary Care Research and Development Centre.

National Union of Teachers (NUT) (2005) *Administration of Medicines: NUT Health and Safety Briefing*. Available at: http://www.nut.org.uk/story.php?id=1580 (accessed 31 May 2007).

Nursing and Midwifery Council (NMC) (2006) *A-Z Advice Sheet – Medicines Management*. Available at: http://www.nmc-uk.org (accessed 15 November 2006).

Nursing and Midwifery Council (NMC) (2007) *Statistical Analysis of the Register 1 April 2005 to 31 March 2006*. Available at: http://www.nmc-uk.org (accessed 29 May 2007).

Seth, N., Llewellyn, N.E., Howard, R. (2000) Parental opinions regarding the route of administration of analgesic medication in children. *Paediatric Anaesthesia* 10(5): 537–544.

Simpson Prentiss, S., Atkins, K., Raynor, D., Closs, S. (2003) Managing medicines: a social worlds perspective of professional involvement. *The International Journal of Pharmacy Practice* 11 (Suppl. R92): 92.

Tweedie, A., Jones, I. (2001) What is medicines management? *The Pharmaceutical Journal* 266(7136): 248.

Weiss, M., Britten, N. (2004) What is concordance? *The Pharmaceutical Journal* 271(7270): 493.

Wong, I. Awolowo, T. Gordon, K. Mo, Y. (2004) Survey of administration of medicines to pupils in primary schools within the London area. *Archives of Disease in Childhood* 89: 998–1001.

Theme 8

Pain Management

Chapter 25   Pain Management

25 Pain Management

Elizabeth Bruce

Introduction

Recognising and treating children's pain in hospital is an important role for the nurse. Health promotion, providing information to children/young people and their families, is part of this process, thus enabling them to understand how pain can be successfully treated.

Advice on pain management in this chapter includes the use of prescribed medications, as well as other interventions. Guidelines are also provided on how to care for children/young people who need to undergo potentially painful procedures. In addition, at the very end of the chapter, an example from community practice is included – how community children's nurses (CCNs), working in an acute service, might treat young children when experiencing pain.

Importance of pain management for children/young people

It is the ethical and professional responsibility of all nurses to ensure that a child's stay in hospital is as pain free as possible. Pain has an important function in our lives, yet if it is poorly managed, ongoing pain can have damaging short- and long-term effects. It affects sleep, increases the risk of complications such as chest infections, pressure sores and blood clots, increases length of hospital stay and can also have long-term psychological effects, including behavioural problems and nightmares.

Policy

The English National Service Framework for children, young people and maternity services (Department of Health, 2003) provides several standards related to the management of pain for children in hospital (Box 25.1).

Box 25.1 Pain management (NSF standard).

Hospital policies for managing children's pain should apply to all children in every hospital department, including newborns in neonatal units. Special focus should be given to children in A + E departments, postoperative pain, pain related to procedures and long-term pain as in cancer. They should be founded on the following principles:

- Children have a right to appropriate prevention, assessment and control of their pain.
- Clinical staff should receive training in the prevention, assessment and control of children's pain.
- Children can expect the management of pain to be a routine part of any treatment or procedure.
- They can also expect to be involved as active partners in pain management.
- Protocols and procedures should support the safe use of pain-controlling medicines.
- Children's pain management should be demonstrated by regular audit.

Adapted from the Standard for Hospital Services (Department of Health, 2003)

Key messages and how to promote them

What is pain?

It is very important for children/young people and families to understand pain, as knowledge about what is happening to our bodies can help to reduce fear and uncertainty. Pain plays an important role in our lives. Its purpose is to protect our bodies from injury and serve as a warning system, alerting us to areas of damage and prompting us to protect our bodies from further harm. A person born with the inability to feel pain (a rare condition) will not move away from a hot or sharp object or think to protect a broken limb, unless she/he can actually see the damage being caused. The person will not seek medical help for a painful condition such as appendicitis, unless a symptom other than pain prompts them to visit the doctor.

The type of pain discussed above is called *acute pain* because it is usually short-lived and has an obvious cause. It is usually easy to treat and disappears once the cause has gone. *Chronic pain* is very different to acute pain. It is longer lasting (usually 3 months or longer) and may be related to a specific disease or condition, but can also occur after an illness or injury or have no obvious cause. It can be difficult to treat, and referral to a paediatric chronic pain clinic is often needed (Eccleston et al., 2006).

How do we feel pain?

Usually, when we feel pain, our body has experienced some sort of damage or injury (like stepping on a nail). The damage triggers the release of chemicals, which stimulate our nerves to send a message (electrical impulses) to the brain, where the message is processed and we feel pain. In chronic pain, the nerves are sending messages to the brain, but often there has been no damage to trigger these messages (or the original source of injury has healed).

Pain assessment

Pain is an individual and personal experience that can be difficult to describe to others. Self-report (the child's account) is the gold standard. Wherever possible, ask the child to describe it using her/his own words (*where it is, what it is like*). This is the most accurate method of assessment. It is essential that children and their parents/carers inform practitioners about the pain. Many children think that adults know when they have pain and so will not tell unless they are asked. Children may also be reluctant to tell others about their pain for fear of the consequences, such as further tests, a longer stay in hospital or foul-tasting medicine.

A number of tools can be used to assess pain in children. The most commonly used are behavioural and self-report tools. Many of these can be downloaded from the internet and used clinically without permission (see the list of Resources). Children can use self-report tools from 3 to 4 years of age, if given proper instruction. For younger children, a faces scale can be used, while for children over the age of about 8 years a numeric rating scale is helpful.

Basic principles for good pain assessment practices (RCNI, 1999; RCPCH, 2001) are as follows:

- Wherever possible, teach children to use a pain assessment tool well in advance of any potentially painful episode.

- Use previous experiences to practise using the tool to score pain.
- Always use age-appropriate words – younger children will not understand the word *pain*, so make sure you use words that they are familiar with.
- Always believe children when they tell you they have pain.
- For children who are unwilling or unable to tell you about their pain, use behavioural tools. (Physiological signs are also useful, but less accurate, so should not be used alone where possible. Behavioural and physiological signs only measure the degree of stress/distress and need to be considered in context, for example, consider any likely causes of pain, fear and distress.)

Non-drug management of pain

Information, preparation and planning

Pain is both an *emotional* and a *sensory* experience, so if a child is frightened or is expecting something to hurt, the likelihood for pain is increased. Providing information, preparing children through play and ensuring parents/carers are informed and involved are all essential to minimise fear.

Good practice points for the management of painful procedures are as follows:

- Explain the procedure well in advance, allowing children/young people to ask questions and discuss their fears. Children/young people usually want to know how the procedure is done, why it is needed and what it will feel like (Doorbar and McClarey, 1999).
- Plan techniques that children/young people can use during any painful or frightening procedures to distract and engage them.
- Encourage parents/carers to be present, but do not make them feel guilty if they feel unable to stay. Children identify parental presence as the most important factor that helps them cope with procedures (Doorbar and McClarey, 1999).
- Parents/carers will also need information about the procedure and help to plan their role. They should be encouraged to engage the child in conversation or play, rather than to

console or comfort their child, as the latter appears to increase distress (Chambers et al., 2002).
- Plan each stage of the procedure to ensure that everything is done to minimise the likelihood of pain and distress (see Box 25.2).

Distraction

There are a wide range of techniques that can help children to focus away from negative thoughts and feelings and on to positive thoughts and actions. The most commonly used is distraction. This has been shown to be effective in reducing anxiety and distress behaviour during repair of lacerations (Sinha et al., 2006). If parents are taught to use distraction with their child, then parental anxiety is also reduced (Kazak et al., 1998). Distraction techniques should be age-appropriate and chosen with the child. For younger children, interactive stories or rhymes and games that involve controlled breathing, blowing, counting or singing are effective. For older children, reciting things backwards, films and computer games are more appropriate. Older children can also use other techniques such as biofeedback and hypnosis, but these require a greater degree of training and expertise.

Box 25.2 Environmental methods of reducing procedural pain and distress.

Provide information and prepare the parent and child

- Give step-by-step information of what will happen during the procedure, including what the child will see, hear and feel.
- Use age-appropriate language and terminology and avoid medical jargon.
- Avoid high-anxiety words such as *pain*, *hurt* and *cut*. Use words such as *poking*, *freezing* and *squeezing* instead.
- Do not suggest that the procedure will definitely hurt.
- Be aware of possible misinterpretations of words and phrases such as *dye* or *put to sleep*.
- Address children's concerns (for example, *taking all my blood*).
- Consider using books describing the procedure that the child can read with the parent.

- Give information before and during the procedure, and be honest.

Parental involvement

- Ask the parents how much distress they expect from their child.
- Instruct the parent not to threaten the child (for example, *if you don't keep still they'll have to do it again*).
- Instruct the parent on coping-promoting behaviours (for example, distraction) and avoid distress-promoting behaviours (for example, reassurance and sympathy).

Practitioners' behaviour

- Be calm, confident and in control.
- Avoid reassurance, apology, sympathy and criticism.
- Avoid conversation with other practitioners and parents that may be distressing (for example, describing possible complications) in front of the child.
- Teach students how to do the procedure outside the room to minimise discussion in front of the child.

Health care setting

- Maintain a quiet, calm environment.
- Avoid stressors such as beeping monitors.
- Avoid long delays between explaining the procedure to the child and performing it.
- Avoid situations in which children can see or hear procedures being performed on other children.

Procedural details

- Allow comfort items such as favourite stuffed animals or blankets.
- For venepuncture or cannulation in thumb-sucking children, avoid the arm of the preferred thumb.
- Do not force the child to lie down if they do not want to, unless this is completely necessary.
- Consider giving the child a job, such as holding a dressing or plaster.
- Give the child choices where possible to increase their sense of control.

- For long procedures, allow *time out* if needed at set times that have been agreed in advance.
- Allow the child to *count down* from ten to one before a brief procedure.
- Use automatic lancets for finger pricks and venepuncture in preference to heel lance wherever possible.

Hospitalised children

- Use a treatment room and keep the child's room or bed area as a *safe place*.
- Give hospitalised children a predictable *safe time* when procedures will not be done.
- Plan ahead to avoid repeated procedures whenever possible.
- Avoid painful routes, such as intramuscular injections.

Adapted from Young (2005).

Sucrose

Neonates are particularly vulnerable to procedural pain. Research has shown that a small dose of sucrose (usually coated on a dummy) is effective to manage procedure-related pain and distresses up to the age of about 3 months. The use of a dummy, swaddling and breastfeeding can also reduce distress behaviours in this age group (Cignacco et al., 2007).

Drugs used to manage pain

There are a limited range of medicines that are used to manage pain in children/young people. All medicine doses are worked out by weight or age. Always advise parents/carers to follow the instructions on the label and check the drug name on the packet, as some cough and flu remedies contain a mixture of different drugs.

Simple analgesics

Paracetamol (for example, Calpol®, Disprol® and Panadol®)

Paracetamol is an effective analgesic (pain-relieving medicine). It is used to relieve mild-to-moderate pain (British National Formulary for Children, BNFC, 2007).

Ibuprofen (for example, Neurofen®)

Ibuprofen is for mild-to-moderate pain (BNFC, 2007) too. It is one of the most commonly used of a group of drugs called *non-steroidal anti-inflammatory drugs* (NSAIDs).

Other drugs in this group include diclofenac (Voltarol®), piroxicam and naproxen. The BNFC (2007) outlines that this group of drugs should be avoided in children less than 3 months of age and those with poor kidney function, clotting disorders or a history of gastric bleeding or ulceration. Caution in use is also required where children have cardiac and hepatic problems.

Ibuprofen may be given to children with mild asthma unless they develop an increase in symptoms with its use. (The BNFC, 2007, maintains that in some cases NSAIDs have the potential to worsen asthma.)

Aspirin is another drug in this group, but should not be used to manage pain in children under 16 years of age, as it is associated with an increased risk of Reyes syndrome (RCPCH, 1997; BNFC, 2007).

As well as providing effective pain relief, both paracetamol and ibuprofen are also *antipyretics* and hence are useful for reducing a high temperature.

Other forms of pain relief

Local anaesthetics

These block nerve impulses or pain messages travelling to the brain. The simplest form is a cream applied to back of hand before cannulation or blood tests. Local anaesthetics can also be injected before suturing or during an operation or can be given via an *epidural*. This is a thin catheter inserted near the spinal cord to give pain relief during and after an operation.

Opioids

The most commonly used opioids are morphine and codeine. Codeine is a moderate analgesic, and morphine a strong analgesic. Many parents worry about morphine, its potential side effects and whether their child will become addicted. Side effects such as nausea, itching and an increased level of sedation are not uncommon, and nurses should be trained to observe for and treat these. Any person who is taking an opioid for any length of time (several weeks or months) will become *tolerant* to the drug – in effect, their body becomes used to it, and the dose has

to be gradually increased to have the same effect. The individual develops a *physiological dependence* on the drug, which means that if the drug is stopped abruptly, she/he will experience unpleasant withdrawal symptoms, which include disturbed sleep, agitation and hallucinations. To prevent this, the drug is reduced or *weaned* slowly. *Addiction* is a psychological dependence or craving for a drug. This is extremely rare in children and not something for concern, even with long-term use (ANZCA, 2005).

Adjuvants

There are a wide range of other drugs that can be used to manage pain. These include clonidine and ketamine, which can be used to manage pain after surgery and also to manage some types of chronic pain. Gabapentin, amitriptyline and carbamazepine have also been found to be helpful in managing *neuropathic* or nerve pain, which is a common type of chronic pain. All of these drugs were originally introduced to manage other symptoms or conditions, but have since become useful in pain management.

There are certain restrictions as to their use, so consult the BNFC (2007).

Activity

As a staff nurse on a surgical ward, you are looking after Sarah, a 9-year-old girl who is having an appendicectomy tomorrow. Sarah is due to have a cannula inserted later today, which will be left in until after her operation. What will you tell her about the type of pain she might experience and how it can be managed:

(i) during cannulation
(ii) during her operation
(iii) and after her operation?

Which pain assessment tool would you choose for Sarah?

What drug and non-drug interventions might you plan to use to manage her pain (i) during cannulation and (ii) following surgery?

Twenty-four hours after surgery, Sarah is now able to take her analgesia orally. She has required one dose of oral morphine, but her mother is reluctant for her to have any more in case she becomes addicted to morphine. What might you tell Sarah's mother about morphine and addiction?

Sarah weighs 21 kg. Use the BNFC (2007) to work out the correct 6 hourly dose of oral paracetamol for her weight.

Conclusion

Health promotion advice can help manage children's/young people's pain in hospital. The chapter has discussed the use of non-drug and drug interventions, and advice that may be given. Importantly, the nurse needs to provide children, young people and their families with explanations that are understandable. Age-appropriate advice and care are particularly important and needs careful consideration, so that pain can be successfully managed.

A community perspective

In the community, children's pain is treated frequently by general practitioners. However, nurses and health visitors have a role too. The following outlines the management of young children's pain in the community, as undertaken by the Sure Start CCN service.

With the Sure Start CCN service, the CCNs can prescribe medication for young children where they are suffering from mild-to-moderate pain. As nurse prescribers they are able to do this. Children are obviously fully assessed, and prescribing decisions are undertaken in consultation with parents/carers. Either paracetamol or ibuprofen might be prescribed, depending on the circumstances for the individual child. The BNFC (2007) would be used as the basis for any prescribing decisions. The CCNs are also able to administer first-dose paracetamol or ibuprofen to help relieve the child's pain. Non-drug interventions for the management of young children's pain are always discussed.

Paracetamol and ibuprofen can be purchased as over-the-counter medicines. However, some families do not have the funds available to purchase them, or may have difficulty accessing their local pharmacy when their child is in pain.

Resources

Leaflets

Let's Talk About ... Helping to Manage Your Child's Pain – Intermountain Primary Children's Medical Care Centre – http:// intermountainhealthcare. org/xp/public/documents/pcmc/painmanage. pdf

Pain, Pain, Go Away: Helping Children with Pain (McGrath, P., Finley, G., Ritchie, J., 1994) – http:// pediatric-pain.ca/ppga/ppga.html

Making Cancer Less Painful: A Handbook for Parents (McGrath, P., Finley, G., Turner, C., 1992) – http:// pediatric-pain.ca/mclp/mclp.html

Helping Your Child Cope With Painful Procedures – WellChild Pain Research Centre – http:// ps1.psy.soton.ac.uk/psyweb/staff/myprofile/ mypublications/publications/cliossi/pain_leaflet-procedure3.pdf

Helping Your Child Cope with Everyday Pain – WellChild Pain Research Centre – http://ps1.psy. soton.ac.uk/psyweb/staff/myprofile/ mypublications/publications/cliossi/pain_leaflet-everyday3.pdf

Helping Your Baby Cope with Painful Procedures – WellChild Pain Research Centre – http://ps1.psy. soton.ac.uk/psyweb/staff/myprofile/ mypublications/publications/cliossi/pain_leaflet-babies3.pdf

Websites

Children's Pain Assessment Project – http://www. ich.ucl.ac.uk/cpap/

Complex Regional Pain Syndrome – http:// www.cafamily.org.uk/Direct/r17.html

Great Ormond Street Hospital for Children – http://www.ich.ucl.ac.uk/gosh/clinicalservices/ Pain_control_service/Homepage

Royal Children's Hospital Melbourne – http:// www.rch.org.au/anaes/index.cfm?doc_id=778

Toronto Sick Children's Hospital – http:// www.aboutkidshealth.ca/Pain/Pain-Home

Pain assessment tools

FLACC Behavioural Tool – http://www.wisc.edu/ trc/projects/pop/FLACCSCALE.pdf

Wong-Baker FACES pain rating scale – http://www.mosbysdrugconsult.com/WOW/faces.html

Faces Pain Scale – Revised (FPS-R) – www.painsourcebook.ca/docs/pps92.html

18 Multi-language Numeric Rating Scales – http://www.partnersagainstpain.com/index-mp.aspx?sid=3&aid=7692

References

Australian and New Zealand College of Anaesthetists and Faculty of Pain Medicine (ANZCA) (2005) Specific patient groups. In: *Acute Pain Management: Scientific Evidence*, 2nd edn. Australia: ANZCA.

BNF for Children (BNFC) (2007) London: BMJ Publishing. Available at: http://bnfc.org/bnfc/ (accessed 30 December 2007).

Chambers, C., Craig, K., Bennett, S. (2002). The impact of maternal behavior on children's pain experiences: an experimental analysis. *Journal of Pediatric Psychology* 27: 293–301.

Cignacco, E., Hamers, J., Stoffel, L., van Lingen, R., Gessler, P., McDougall, J., Nelle, M. (2007) The efficacy of non-pharmacological interventions in the management of procedural pain in preterm and term neonates. A systematic literature review. *European Journal of Pain* 11: 139–152.

Department of Health (2003) *Getting the Right Start: The National Service Framework for Children, Young People and Maternity Services – Standards for Hospital Services*. London: Crown Copyright.

Doorbar, P., McClarey, M. (1999) Ouch! Sort it out: children's experiences of pain. *Report of a Qualitative Study of Children's Experiences of Pain*. London: Royal College of Nursing Institute.

Eccleston, C., Bruce, E., Carter, B. (2006) Chronic pain in children and adolescents. *Paediatric Nursing* 18: 30–33.

Kazak, A., Penati, B., Brophy, P., Himelstein, B. (1998) Pharmacologic and psychological interventions for procedural pain. *Pediatrics* 102(1): 59–66.

Royal College of Nursing Institute (RCNI) (1999) *The Recognition and Assessment of Acute Pain in Children: Recommendations*. London: RCNI.

Royal College of Paediatrics and Child Health (RCPCH) (1997) *Prevention and Control of Pain in Children: A Manual for Health Care Professionals*. London: BMJ Publishing.

Royal College of Paediatrics and Child Health (RCPCH) (2001) *Guidelines for Good Practice: Recognition and Assessment of Acute Pain in Children*. London: RCPCH.

Sinha, M., Christopher, N., Fenn, R., Reeves, L. (2006) Evaluation of nonpharmacologic methods of pain and anxiety management for laceration repair in the paediatric emergency department. *Pediatrics* 117: 1162–1168.

Young, K. (2005) Pediatric procedural pain. *Annals of Emergency Medicine* 45: 160–171.

Theme 9

Promoting Emotional Health

Chapter 26   Baby Massage and Baby Yoga

Chapter 27   Health Promotion Course: Living with Babies

Chapter 28   Baby Play

Chapter 29   Baby Club

Chapter 30   Positive Parenting

Chapter 31   Promoting Children's Mental Health – Focus Bullying

Chapter 32   Safeguarding Children (Health Promotion)

Chapter 33   The Health of Children/Young People in Care

26 Baby Massage and Baby Yoga

Karen Moyse, Helen Surguy and Liz Whelan

NSF

Promoting the emotional health of children is essential. The National Service Framework (NSF) talks about the need for children/young people to feel secure and supported if they are to achieve their full potential (Education and Skills, Department of Health, 2004).

Introduction

Baby massage and baby yoga are discussed within this chapter. Both are complementary therapies aimed at promoting babies' *emotional health*. In recent years there has been a growing interest within nursing and health visitor practice about how these therapies can support families. Parents are becoming very interested, as an article on baby massage recently highlighted in *The Times* (Baggott, 2007).

Baby massage and baby yoga may well be beneficial for babies' emotional health, especially through the positive interactions they can experience with their parents and carers. Parents and carers are so fundamental to creating a nurturing environment, particularly in the early years (Education and Skills, Department of Health 2004). This chapter looks at some of the benefits attributed to baby massage through the work of community practitioners:

health visitor, children's nurse and nursery nurse within a Sure Start centre. Importantly too, the benefits of baby yoga will be considered through the work of Liz, a qualified yoga teacher. Both these therapies can be used as a forum for promoting positive messages about babies' health.

Positive touch and bonding

Some of the terms frequently used within this chapter are outlined. When a baby experiences massage or yoga, it is usually undertaken by the baby's mother, so the term *mother* will be used here. The term mother can also be applied to any carer in this context, as it is not always the baby's mother who undertakes massage or yoga, but another carer, normally a member of the baby's family. We must not forget that fathers too can be involved in these therapies.

The term *positive touch* will be used. This refers to a mother interacting positively with her baby, touching her baby sensitively, gently and caringly. During a massage or yoga session, for example, a baby gives out cues, which the mother respects and responds to. This could be the baby showing enjoyment in the massage/yoga taking place, which may encourage the mother to continue. Conversely, the baby may not be happy, cries, the mother stops. She is responding sensitively to her baby by observing her baby's cues.

Murray and Andrews (2000) talk about these cues or signals given out by the baby, which demonstrate how the baby feels. Examples of these cues include the baby's facial expressions and body language. Babies are giving out cues all the time, in whatever they do, not just during massage or yoga sessions. Mothers need to learn to understand their baby's cues and respond appropriately. Klaus and Klaus (1998) even propose that mothers almost have to become detectives to learn how to unravel these cues.

It is really important for the relationship between mother and baby, if the mother learns to be sensitive to her baby (Murray and Andrews, 2000). Baby massage and baby yoga can be used as strategies to help mothers develop sensitivity towards their babies. Most mothers are naturally sensitive to their babies' needs; sometimes others need a little extra help, which yoga or massage can provide. Many mothers undertake yoga and massage with their babies simply for the enjoyment that it brings to their relationship.

Bonding

Bonding is the process whereby individuals become emotionally attached to one another (Collins English Dictionary, 1998). Bonding as a concept within nursing is commonly discussed in relation to the mother/infant bond. This bond is believed to be strong and emotional (L'Abate et al., 1993). Sutcliffe's (1994) book on *baby bonding* stresses values such as secure attachments and loving relationships as fundamental for bonding to occur. A strong bond between mother and infant would seem to support and protect the infant, which is essential for its survival.

Part of Sure Start's (2000) philosophy centres on the promotion of early bonding between mothers and their babies, helping them to build warm and affectionate relationships with each other. Baby massage was implemented within our Sure Start area (Creswell, Langwith/Whaley Thorns and Shirebrook, CLWTS) to encourage and support early bonding between parents and their children (Lorenz et al., 2005).

Concern had existed within this Sure Start area for some years about the number of young children with developmental delay, particularly in the area of language development (Kirk, 2005). One way to help address this, certainly in the early months of life, Sure Start felt, was to help the attachment or bond between mothers and their babies. It was important for practitioners to encourage mothers and babies to interact together, thus supporting children's development at an early point in their lives. As psychology has shown over many years, the interactions between children and their mothers are important, particularly for language development, as Vygotsky (1962) has demonstrated, for example.

Sure Start, an initiative introduced by the Government following the publication of *Supporting Families* (Home Office, 1998), offers a supportive approach to parenting in deprived areas for families with children under 5 years of age. Currently, at the time of writing, in many areas the work of Sure Start is being encompassed within the role of children's centres, which are developing in different locations around the country.

Baby massage

Baby massage is not a new concept; it has been around for hundreds of years (Touch Learn, 2002). The use of baby massage is ancient. Its roots can be traced back to ancient Indian medicine dating from 1800 BC, and continues energetically in India today (Freedman, 2000). The following outlines some of the suggested benefits of baby massage.

Baby massage has a number of benefits. As discussed, baby massage can promote bonding, by helping mothers to become more aware of their baby's non-verbal cues. It enhances bonding as touch conveys nurturing and love, essential ingredients for emotional and physical growth (Weisberg and Day, 1998). It can also relax the baby by using these loving or positive touches to help lessen the baby's tensions. Baby massage is also a wonderful way to lessen stress for mothers.

Baby massage involves positive touch. Positive touch, as highlighted, is built upon the use of positive interactions and communications between mother and baby, with the mother learning and respecting her baby's non-verbal cues or signals. Through massage, the baby may give out positive cues, which in return build the mother's confidence in what she is doing. The mother may feel that she is doing something really positive for her baby.

Robotham and Sheldrake (2000) state that if baby massage is carried out with love, the end result is to create not only a feeling of security for the baby, but it can also relax the mind and body of the person giving the massage. Worwood (1990) believes that the baby's well-being depends on the mother's own well-being too. So anything the mother does to make life easier and happier is all to the common good.

Contemporary life is hectic, and even more so after a mother has given birth. In Western societies mothers are expected to give birth one day and then return to normal duties of keeping house, cooking, cleaning and child rearing, the next. Heller (1997) questions the high incidence of post-natal depression amongst Western mothers, with many feeling overwhelmed by the experience of caring for a new baby.

Interestingly, Brazelton (1992) believes that new mothers will be in the midst of some degree of post-natal depression following birth. Such a depression can affect physical recovery and rebalancing of hormones. Brazelton (1992) found that mothers who are depressed are usually working hard at becoming a mother. Due to the nature of the illness, mothers with post-natal depression can often feel less able to meet the emotional needs of their babies. Heller (1997) found that Western societies have a higher incidence of post-natal depression when compared to other more child-oriented cultures, which provide new mothers with the opportunity to rest during the early weeks following birth.

Baby massage may be able to help mothers suffering from post-natal depression to bond with their baby. It allows them to communicate with their baby through touch, helping to build their relationship. Mothers actively listening and responding to their babies go on to develop a mutually trusting relationship with them, through baby massage. As a result these mothers can gain confidence in the care they are providing for their baby. Pelaez-Noguerus et al. (1996) found that depressed mothers who massaged their babies could increase their babies' positive affect and attention.

Baby massage may also help to improve mood. Work has been undertaken in Florida which shows that mothers massaging their preterm babies, as well as observing their preterm babies being massaged, can help to reduce their feelings of anxiety and lift mood (Feijó et al., 2006).

It is not uncommon in Western societies for mothers to experience sleepless nights and feel shattered when caring for a young baby. Heller (1997) believes this lack of sleep contributes to the high incidence of post-natal depression amongst new mothers. This is because they are feeding during the night, which reduces both the quantity, as well as the quality of sleep they are able to get. As a result of becoming sleep deprived, mothers can begin to feel low, cry and disorganised. The baby's cries become more grating, affecting the mother's parenting capacity.

The baby's cries may be caused by separation anxiety from the mother and can be relieved by the positive touch of baby massage, resulting in the baby feeling secure, safe and loved. It can also help to regulate the baby's breathing. Feeling the mother's heartbeat and respirations helps to soothe the baby. The smooth baby massage strokes influence breathing, helping the baby to become more relaxed (Touch Learn, 2002).

Once the baby is feeling more relaxed, she/he will fall asleep. Conversely, the baby who cries itself to sleep is going to become stressed and exhausted. Adamson (1996) states that massage produces endorphins and serotonin, which when released relieve discomfort and aid sleep. Weisberg and Day (1998) agree that massage helps the baby to learn to relax, with a sounder and longer sleep resulting.

Importantly however, always remember when caring for babies that they cry for a variety of different reasons, frequently because they are hungry. Crying can also be due to discomfort, tiredness or even boredom. Illness too is another really significant reason why babies cry, and should never be far from one's thoughts.

A mother will learn to recognise her baby's different cries; what the cry means and how best she should respond. Where comfort and companionship are what the baby is looking for, massage may help.

Some of the benefits of baby massage have been outlined. Through massage mothers and their babies can become close, setting in place important foundations for their future relationship and helping babies to feel secure within that relationship.

In Chapter 27, Helen discusses a course designed for mothers and their babies, which promotes positive health messages, while at the same time providing mothers with the opportunity to participate in baby massage.

Baby yoga

Baby yoga may be beneficial for babies' health and development. This section explores some of the benefits of baby yoga. Mothers and babies engage in baby yoga, which helps to bring them closer together. Liz is a qualified yoga teacher. She teaches baby yoga to mothers, and has taught it for some years, both on an individual level and group basis. Here, Liz discusses the benefits of baby yoga as she has observed through her teaching. The evidence presented is not based on research but through a wealth of experience.

What is baby yoga?

Yoga is able to offer babies physical stimulation and can help strengthen their bodies. Yoga postures also involve the senses, mind and psyche (Freedman, 2000). Baby yoga can give babies a sense of well-being. It is a mutual process between mothers and their babies, with a great deal of non-verbal communication taking place between the two (Freedman, 2000).

Baby yoga is a gentle exercise with relaxation for both mother and child. For those that are familiar with yoga, it is based on *hatha yoga*. Baby yoga is a playful stimulation with moves to rhymes and songs, which help to make it fun and easy to remember. Baby yoga should take place in a calm relaxing environment, where mother and baby can concentrate on what they are experiencing together.

Baby yoga provides exercise to stimulate the baby, which helps with relaxation, the letting go of tensions, thus promoting sleep. By getting enough rest during the day, babies can experience a deeper sleep at night. A gentle yoga sequence in the early evening, followed by relaxation, can help the baby drift off to sleep.

For the overtired baby gentle rocking and swinging movements or a hand and foot massage with joint relaxation may be beneficial. Relaxed holding with the mother walking can help to soothe a crying baby. If the baby is overstimulated, holding the baby with her/his face turned away from any stimulating activity may help.

Feeding creates a strong bond between mother and baby, especially breastfeeding. When feeding, the baby is in the best position to see the mother's face, her smile and hear her voice. Difficulties in feeding can cause fretfulness in the baby and tension/anxiety in the mother, thus creating a vicious circle. Relaxation is the key for both, and baby yoga can help to provide that, thus helping with the development of a successful feeding pattern and bonding.

Emotional benefits

The emotional benefits of baby yoga are related to *bonding* and the *positive interactions* that take place between mother and baby. Baby yoga provides positive interactions between the two, which enhance the baby's sense of well-being and confidence.

With baby yoga the mother and baby get to know each other at a deeper level, and the baby's sense of trust and security is heightened by the touch, smell and voice of its mother. Baby yoga encourages the feeling of calm and relaxation in both (Freedman, 2000).

A mother can let her baby know that she has a sense of what the baby is feeling through imitation. For example, when a baby squeals with delight the mother uses the same pitch in her voice when responding. If the mother fails to demonstrate this empathy, the baby may either stop expressing these feelings or show an increase in a different behaviour to gain attention. Baby yoga helps the mother to be more aware of her baby's emotions and needs, and as a result the baby gains confidence that her/his needs will be met.

Baby yoga has benefits for mothers too. Mothers can find handling their new baby a little anxiety provoking, at least initially. Baby yoga can help to improve mothers' confidence in handling their new babies.

Although there are no studies at this time to support any claims that baby yoga helps mothers with post-natal depression, it would be interesting to research its impact. From experience with mothers who have post-natal depression, baby yoga seems to offer them something different. By undertaking baby yoga in a class or alone, mothers and babies learn to handle their emotional relationships. In a class environment, for example, mothers interact with each other, so positive emotions are shared. Babies interact with each other too.

By undertaking baby yoga alone, the mother and baby are sharing quality time together, enjoying each other's company and enjoying what they are doing together. When first undertaking baby yoga, it is important to choose a time when both mother and baby are more likely to be relaxed. As the techniques and exercises become more familiar, calming a distressed baby will become more effective and will take less time. However, as Freedman (2000) states, it can take considerable skill before a distressed baby can be calmed quickly.

Physical benefits

There are a number of physical benefits associated with baby yoga. Baby yoga can help to strengthen the baby's muscles (Freedman, 2000). Strengthening the muscles can help with the baby's physical development. Baby yoga helps babies explore by discovering ways of moving and using their muscles. Some examples are provided.

A baby's muscle control starts to develop gradually. One of the first noticeable developmental changes in a newborn baby is head control. After a week or so the baby will begin to lift its head for a second before flopping it back down again (Sheridan, 1997). A baby will practise head control by repeatedly lifting and flopping its head down, almost head butting its mother's shoulder in the process. The head needs support to prevent flopping.

Babies have physical actions that come from the primitive brain. Sheridan (1997) has outlined some of these. Newborn babies appear to attempt crawling movements when laid on their tummies or even walk when held upright with their feet just touching a firm surface. The handgrip of a baby is incredibly strong. A baby can grasp with its fingers when the palm of its hand is touched at 1 month of age (Sheridan, 1997). This strength of grip passes over time, but some degree of it still remains. Baby yoga aims to encourage the baby to hold onto its mother with this strong handgrip.

The primitive action of a handgrip appears to have survival value for the baby, which can be understood by looking at the behaviour of other cultures. In some Eastern countries babies are carried on their mother's back or front, wherever they go.

Babies within these cultures continue to have the ability to hold onto their mothers. In Western countries mothers do not do this. (Mothers might be accused of spoiling their babies if they were to carry them everywhere.) Babies in Western cultures therefore lose the ability to hold onto their mothers.

Other physical benefits of baby yoga are associated with the skin and touch. Baby yoga can stimulate the receptors in the skin, which in turn increases blood flow around the body, making the body system more efficient. The touch and moves of baby yoga can help babies feel relaxed. Relaxation helps with breathing and the release of tension.

Conclusion

The bond between baby and mother can be strengthened by the closeness, experienced through baby yoga. The baby will develop trust in her/his mother and can enjoy the activity they are both participating in together. The mother can also experience increased confidence and satisfaction in her own parenting role.

The emotional and physical benefits of baby yoga described in this chapter can create a sound basis for the development of a well-rounded individual. It may help the child's growing sense of who they are and sensitivity towards others. It may also eventually influence the child's own role as a parent.

As Liz describes baby yoga may have benefits for babies' health and development. Many mothers really enjoy the experience.

Cautions

Baby massage and baby yoga should only be undertaken by a person trained to do so. With baby massage, mothers are trained by a qualified baby massage teacher. The same with baby yoga, mothers are trained by a qualified baby yoga teacher. Mothers undertake these techniques on their own baby. As a nurse, do not undertake these techniques yourself, unless qualified to do so.

As qualified baby massage or baby yoga teachers ourselves, having learnt with recognised organisations for the training of baby massage and baby yoga, we would only be permitted to massage on a doll. We would not be able to undertake massage on a child, unless it was our own child. Nurses therefore need to be clear about what they are permitted to do, within the realms of their qualification. If undertaking such a course, check with your training body about the regulations that apply to you.

Before introducing baby massage or baby yoga, always make sure the baby is well enough to participate in such a session. If a baby has a health problem or specific condition, seek medical advice. Sometimes it may simply not be the right time for massage or yoga; the baby may simply be too tired. Respond to the cues given by the baby; never undertake if the baby is not interested.

Guidelines on the use of complementary therapies in nursing have been produced by the Royal College of Nursing (RCN, 2003). The RCN (2003) advises that the use of complementary therapies in nursing should only be introduced if it is in the *best interests* of the patient/client and *safety* guidelines are followed. Relevance to practice is indeed an essential consideration and is strongly advocated by the NMC (2004). Baby massage was relevant to our practice, as the promotion of bonding between mothers and babies was a high priority for practitioners within Sure Start.

Safety about baby massage and baby yoga must always be an essential consideration. The NMC (2004) has highlighted that nurses must be satisfied about the safety of any new therapy before introducing it. For example, before we introduced baby massage into our practice, the subject was examined carefully. We attended a recognised training course, as well as undertaking a period of supervised practice. Together with some of our colleagues within the primary care trust (PCT), we developed guidelines for practice and designed written resources for use by parents.

Associated chapter

Baby yoga is a recent advent into practice. Not only is it growing in the care of babies, but children are being provided with the opportunity to experience yoga too. See Chapter 7 for more information.

Conclusion

This chapter has looked at baby massage and baby yoga, particularly focusing on some of the benefits that might be associated with these complementary therapies in relation to children's health and development, particularly emotional health. Both complementary therapies may help mothers and babies to become closer to one another. Hart et al. (2003) found in their evaluation of health visitor run baby massage classes, that mothers did feel that it strengthened the bond between themselves and their babies. Although Sure Start's work on baby massage has not been formally evaluated in this area, practitioners felt that that it did help to support mother/infant bonding (Moyse, 2005). Liz, from her observations in practice, undoubtedly has similar thoughts about baby yoga and how it can impact on the bonding process.

Resources

Further information can be found about our work on baby massage in two articles published by Paediatric Nursing during 2005. They are as follows:

- *The Benefits of Baby Massage* by Lydia Lorenz, Karen Moyse and Helen Surguy.
- *Baby Massage and Baby Play* by Karen Moyse.

For baby yoga Liz suggests the following texts:

- *Baby Yoga* by Freedman (2000).
- *Baby Om* by Staton and Perron (2003), primarily for the parents and carers.

References

Adamson, S. (1996) Teaching baby massage to new parents. *Complementary Therapies in Nursing and Midwifery* 2: 151–159.

Baggott, K. (2007) The hands-on mums. *The Times* 7 July.

Brazelton, T.B. (1992) *Touch Points Birth to 3*. United States: Perseus Publishing.

Collins English Dictionary (1998) 4th edn. Glasgow: Harper Collins.

Education and Skills (Department of), Department of Health (2004) *National Service Framework (NSF) for Children/Young People and Maternity Services*. London: Education and Skills, Department of Health.

Feijó, L., Hernandez-Reif, M., Field, T., Burns, W., Valley-Gray, S., Simco, E. (2006) Mothers' depressed mood and anxiety levels are reduced after massaging their preterm infants. *Infant Behaviour and Development* 29(3): 476–480.

Freedman, F. (2000) *Baby Yoga*. London: Gaia Books Ltd.

Hart, J., Davidson, A., Clarke, C., Gibb, C. (2003) Health visitor run baby massage classes: investigating the effects. *Health Visitor* 76(4): 138–142.

Heller, S. (1997) *The Vital Touch*. New York: Henry Holt and Company.

Home Office (1998) *Supporting Families*. London: Crown Copyright.

Kirk, J. (2005) *Sure Start Creswell, Langwith/Whaley Thorns and Shirebrook (CLWTS) – Monitoring and Evaluation Report*. Derbyshire: Sure Start CLWTS.

Klaus, M., Klaus, P. (1998) *Your Amazing Newborn*. Cambridge: Perseus Books.

L'Abate, L., Weeks, G., Buchanan, W.L. (1993) *The Dictionary of Family Psychology and Family Therapy*. London: Sage.

Lorenz, L., Moyse, K., Surguy, H. (2005) The benefits of baby massage. *Paediatric Nursing* 17(2): 15–18.

Moyse, K. (2005) Baby massage and baby play. *Paediatric Nursing* 17(5): 30–32.

Murray, L., Andrews, L. (2000) *The Social Baby*. Surrey: CP Publishing.

Nursing and Midwifery Council (NMC) (2004) *Code of Professional Conduct*. London: Nursing and Midwifery Council.

Pelaez-Noguerus, M., Field, T., Hossain, Z., Pickens, J. (1996) Depressed mothers touching increases positive affect and attention. *Child Development* 67: 1780–1792.

Robotham, A., Sheldrake, D. (2000) *Health Visiting Specialist and Higher Level Practice*. London: Churchill Livingstone.

Royal College of Nursing (2003) *Complementary Therapies in Nursing, Midwifery, and Health Visiting Practice*. London: Royal College of Nursing.

Sheridan, M. (1997) *From Birth to Five Years. Children's Developmental Progress* (revised and updated by Frost, M., Sharma, A.). London: Routledge.

Staton, P., Perron, S. (2003) *Baby Om*. Ireland: Newleaf.

Sure Start (2000) *Sure Start: A Guide for 2nd Wave Programmes*. London: Sure Start.

Sutcliffe, J. (1994) *Baby Bonding, Giving Your Child a Secure Start to Life*. London: Virgin Publishing Company.

Touch Learn (2002) *Infant and Child Massage Teacher Training Course Manual*. Staffordshire: United Kingdom.

Vygotsky, L. (1962) *Thought and Language*. Cambridge, MA: MIT Press.

Weisberg, E., Day, R. (1998) *What Is Infant Massage?* Available at: http://www.childbirth.org/articles (accessed August 2007).

Worwood, V. (1990) *The Fragrant Pharmacy*. London: Macmillan London Ltd.

27 Health Promotion Course: Living with Babies

Helen Surguy and Karen Moyse

NSF

Promoting the emotional health of children is essential. The National Service Framework (NSF) talks about the need for children to feel secure and supported if they are to achieve their full potential in life (Education and Skills, Department of Health, 2004). Parents/carers have an important role to play in helping children to feel secure. Some parents/carers may need support from practitioners to achieve this.

Introduction

Living with Babies (LWB) is a health promotion course for mothers and their babies. This chapter looks at the development of the LWB course within a deprived area, a Sure Start area. The course was developed to support parenting and promote children's health.

Practitioners introduced the course as a new initiative in the community. They particularly wanted to promote emotional attachment between mothers and their babies, as well as supporting mothers with improvements in their children's health. The NSF states that mothers are central to giving their babies a healthy start. The health of children from disadvantaged communities is known to be poorer than other communities (Education and Skills, Department of Health, 2004). Practitioners hoped the course would lead to improvements in children's health locally.

Babies and children have strong feelings of affection for their parents/carers. Babies thrive on the abundance of love they receive from them. Children's health is so important, as it can provide foundations for future health. Emotional health is an integral part of feeling good and being healthy. Children need to feel safe, secure and protected (Touch Learn, 2002). Feeling secure can influence children's emotional health in a very positive way. The course aimed to help mothers influence their children's emotional health positively from an early age.

After completing a Touch Learn baby massage course, a group of practitioners (Health Visitor, Nursery Nurse, and Community Children's Nurse) realised some of the health benefits baby massage could offer. It could provide children with emotional health benefits, as well as the possibility of physical health improvements too. Baby massage also appeared to have benefits for mothers.

The practitioners thus proposed a parenting course – the LWB course. Following the recruitment of fellow community practitioners, the course was designed and implemented. The course featured baby massage at its core. It was designed specifically for mothers with babies under 1 year of age.

LWB later became part of an established parenting programme *Living with Children*, within the local primary care trust (PCT). The *Living with Children* service is a recognised parenting skills project which has successfully been supporting parents/carers in Derbyshire for over 12 years. The element of the course that is considered vital to its success is creating a relaxed environment where parents/carers and their children can relax and learn together.

Health promotion

Health promotion for disadvantaged groups is not a new concept. From evidence stated in the Black report (Black et al., 1980), almost three decades ago, health promotion for deprived families was being encouraged. This report found that although health was improving amongst the population as a whole, health inequalities were widespread. Variations in health existed between the social classes, with the lower social classes experiencing much poorer health than other social classes. Children in the lower social classes needed help. By improving children's health while they were young, it was felt that this would have health benefits in later life. Townsend et al. (1987) proposed that by increasing child benefit, and the maternity grant, as well as ensuring local authority day care for the under 5, along with nutritionally adequate school meals, and mounting a child accident preventing programme, children's health would improve, particularly in the lower social classes.

Unfortunately, evidence from the Black report (Black et al., 1980) was clearly not acted upon at the time (Townsend et al., 1988; Acheson, 1998). However, it did stimulate debate on a much wider scale (Townsend et al., 1988).

Today, the NSF for children and young people and maternity services (Education and Skills, Department of Health, 2004) and *Every Child Matters* (Education and Skills, 2003) are important strategies for promoting the welfare of children. The Government wants practitioners to address children's health promotion needs. By giving each and every child a good start in life, the aim is to reduce health problems in later life.

The emotional health of children in the early years is an important element of these strategies. The Government is encouraging parenting education which focuses on enhancing sensitivity towards children

(Education and Skills, Department of health, 2004). Children from the most disadvantaged communities are more likely to experience mental health problems than those in the higher social classes (Meltzer et al., 2000). Better parenting in the early years may help prevent such problems emerging. Developing the LWB course, a parenting course, would perhaps support parents with the emotional care of their children in the early years.

Models of health promotion

Models and concepts of health were incorporated into the LWB parenting course. To address the health promotion issues stated within the Government agenda, health needed to be the focus. Minkler (1994) argues that health-orientated programmes rather than disease-orientated programmes are more effective.

Health promotion, prevention of health problems and the protection of children are integral to their health. Promotion, prevention and protection have been included in Tannahill's (1985) model of health promotion. His interpretation is that health promotion seeks to empower by providing necessary information and helping people to develop skills, as well as a healthy level of self-esteem. Lord and Farlow (1990) argue that health practitioners should view themselves as facilitators rather than teachers of health, which helps to empower participants when promoting their health.

Empowerment is supported by the World Health Organization (WHO). The WHO (1984) believes that health promotion is a process of enabling participants to increase control over their own lives, so they can improve their health. An empowerment approach to health was certainly appropriate for the LWB, supporting mothers to improve the health of their children themselves.

Practice – setting up the course

The LWB course was written, delivered and evaluated with a group of young mothers who all had babies under 1 year of age. The LWB course encouraged mothers to understand their babies' emotional and physical needs and how to respond to them. The end result was hopefully to increase positive parenting styles especially where some mothers had experienced poor parenting themselves. It is recognised that parenting is a complex function, involving relationships, communication, social skills and the acquisition of understanding (Hall, 2000). The course was there to provide families with some different and more positive insights into how parenting might work for them.

Involvement and partnership

The Living with Children service was invited to work in partnership with Sure Start on this venture. Course materials would then be accessible to a wider range of practitioners within the PCT. More parents might then benefit from what the LWB course could offer.

The baby massage component of the course was felt to be a fundamental element. Any health practitioners who were interested and qualified in baby massage within the Sure Start team were invited to contribute to the course content. The LWB practitioners became a team comprising of a midwife, community psychiatric nurse, nursery nurses, heath visitors and a community children's nurse. This larger team enabled mothers to benefit from a wealth of knowledge and experience.

Working in collaboration with a team can enable practitioners to work closely and coordinate their efforts (Headrick et al., 1998). West (1997) described the characteristics of inter-professional collaboration as a good teamwork with a clear shared vision, effective participation and task orientation. Headrick et al. (1998) also state it is important to select a team with the right balance of skills. Importantly, however, collaboration has to be sort from the group of people who are there working together.

Practitioners worked collaboratively, and were able to recognise their colleagues' talents. The LWB team did learn effectively from working together. Having this important shared goal in the LWB course brought them closer together.

Headrick et al. (1998) conclude that real improvements are likely to occur if the range of practitioners are responsible for providing a service, share their different knowledge and experiences, as well as agreeing with the improvements they are intro-

ducing. They test practice and jointly learn from their results. LWB practitioners very much wanted to improve the health of the local community by advancing practice together.

Teaching styles

As the LWB course was designed to encourage learning in a supportive way, the team had to think about which teaching methods would be appropriate. It was recognised that a formal teaching style, where the facilitator stands at the front of a group talking, would not fit well. Within some areas of deprivation and poverty sometimes the educational level reached by individuals is not high, and there are still those who are unable to read and write (Home Office, 1998).

Rudduck (1978) suggests that group work unlike lectures maximises opportunities for learning, through a capacity to respond to developing situations. The team felt that an informal teaching style would work best for the course. Practical sessions, small group work and discussions were included to enable everyone to contribute to the learning experience.

Jacques (1984) found that groups larger than ten people will divide into subgroups, which can influence group cohesiveness. A small group was thus favoured by the team, who wanted to create a safe, trusting environment that would promote a sense of belonging for participants. Informal teaching methods, and a small group size, were felt by most practitioners as the best ways to enhance learning for participants.

Course content

The course was composed of many different health issues that practitioners considered would be of value to mothers in their parenting role. Mothers were also asked what they felt would be of value to include within the course itself. First-time mothers especially worry about common health issues with their babies. Giving mothers the understanding to deal with these situations in a positive way, practitioners felt would help them to feel more confident.

Practical elements of the course were included, such as baby massage and baby play. The benefits of baby massage to mothers can be many, but one in particular that practitioners wanted to get across was helping mothers to become *sensitive to their babies* by touching them in a positive way and observing their babies' cues and responses. Positive touch and observing babies' cues are so important to mothers in developing sensitivity towards their babies.

Baby play is an activity which babies undertake with their parents/carers within Sure Start (Moyse, 2005). It helps parents/carers learn how to play and stimulate their babies. The LWB course included baby play to demonstrate play skills to new mothers. Nursery nurses teach mothers how to interact with their babies playfully, as well as how to use and make toys. It demonstrates to mothers that they do not need to buy expensive toys to stimulate their babies.

Another practical part of the LWB course was the introduction of relaxation for mothers. Parenting can be stressful (Langley, 1998). The team therefore did not want to make the course all work for the mothers attending. It was important that mothers had time to relax away from their babies.

Discussing problems is important with mothers, particularly with those mothers who are feeling low or depressed. The mental health NSF (Department of Health, 1999) encourages health practitioners to openly discuss mental health issues and break down any barriers that exist. The course included a session on post-natal depression for this very reason, so mothers could gain insights into post-natal depression and would also be aware of the support services available locally. Mothers would then know what to do, if a problem was developing.

The team devised a 6- to 9-week course, covering the subjects listed below:

- Session 1: Introduction
  - Introduction to the course.
  - Practical – Baby massage.
- Session 2: Crying babies
  - Crying – The aim was to give mothers more insight into why babies cry. Information was included on babies' different cries and how mothers could comfort their babies.
  - Practical – Baby massage, leg and foot massage.
- Session 3: Feeding and growth
  - Information on weaning, feeding and growth was provided. Comparisons were made between home-cooked foods and bought baby foods.
  - Practical – Baby massage, chest and abdomen massage.
- Session 4: Sleeping
  - The session looked at normal sleep patterns during the first few years of life. The health benefits of sleep were discussed.
  - Practical – Baby massage, back massage.
- Session 5: Minor illnesses
  - Symptoms, along with management of some of the more common minor illnesses that babies present with, were discussed. This included information on when a baby should see a doctor.
  - Practical – Baby play, stimulation.
- Session 6: Children's safety
  - Information on child safety in the home was discussed.
  - Practical – baby play, rhymes.
- Session 7: Promoting mothers' mental health
  - Promoting mental health and preventing post-natal depression is a subject that some mothers have little knowledge of and often do not know how to recognise. This session aimed to bring mental health into the open, discuss treatments and support available for mothers.
  - Practical – baby play, making a toy.
- Session 8: Relax
  - Relaxation – Being a mother is a full-time job and at times can be stressful. Discussing with mothers how to relax was essential. A session on relaxation and yoga for mothers was provided by a qualified yoga teacher.
  - Practical – Relaxation and yoga for mums.
- Session 9: Graduation
  - Graduation, fuddle and pamper session – A beauty therapist was invited to offer treatments to mothers, such as facials, massage and nail art.
  - Graduation – For those mothers who had attended for a minimum of 6 sessions, they were awarded a certificate.

Implementation

Over a 4-month period the team had met to discuss and write the course. Plans for the first course were put into action. Decisions regarding the venue, crèche facilities and funding were made. No Sure Start buildings had been completed at this time, so a number of local venues were explored.

A group of young mothers who attended a Sure Start group had the benefit of using a counsel-owned property (rent free). This group also had a crèche, which was funded by Sure Start. The team asked the mothers if they would be prepared to be the pilot group for the course. They agreed and the pilot course took place on a weekly basis over a 2-month period.

Evaluation

The pilot group consisted of eight mothers, who had a reputation for giving frank feedback. Group members participated really well. Following the sessions, practitioners gained excellent feedback from them which was surprisingly, as sometimes their body language gave a very different impression. Brookfield and Preskill (1999) identify that egos stand in groups and can shut down meaningful discussions. The presence of peers within the young mothers group may have been overwhelming for some of the mothers but from individuals positive feedback was received.

Here are just a few of the comments received from the mothers:

- We really enjoyed the course.
- I missed some of the sessions. But the sessions I did attend, I thought, were very helpful for young mums with children under 1 year.
- I thought it was very useful; it helped me look after my child in a different way. Love and comfort especially when poorly. I am not as stressed as I used to be because of the helpful information and activities we have done together.

One aspect of the course that was felt to be essential by all practitioners was baby massage. Knowledge and skills in baby massage helped practitioners to deliver a course that was sensitive to both the needs of babies and their mothers. Baby massage was delivered only by those practitioners who were qualified to do so. Mothers and babies seemed to gain much from the experience.

The challenges

There were a variety of challenges along the way. When it came to delivering the course, there were reduced staffing levels due to staff sickness and maternity leave. Two members of staff were needed to deliver each session. But to take two members of staff away from practice for one afternoon per week for an 8- to 9-week period would put considerable strain on delivering community services for children and families. To avoid this, a total of ten Sure Start practitioners were asked to facilitate the course at different times, which worked well.

Only a small number of practitioners were able to teach baby massage. However, other members of staff underwent their training and completed this just in time to be involved in the course. All the practitioners involved gained a great deal of satisfaction from participating in the LWB course.

Future developments

What are your plans for the future development of this work?

The Living with Children service has now taken this course forward into other parts of the PCT. A resource pack has been compiled for use by practitioners when delivering the course. There have been expressions of interest about the course from different practitioners, generally within the PCT itself.

Conclusion

From humble beginnings the course has been a remarkable success and demand for it continues.

Some practitioners use the course as it has been devised, whilst others have incorporated it into their own post-natal groups and clinics.

The original idea was to help support mothers with new babies living in a deprived area, helping them to become more sensitive to their babies' needs and thus more able to promote their babies' emotional and physical needs. Hopefully, the course was able to positively influence the long-term health of these babies/children. Only time will tell if the course has influenced families in this way. Practitioners took on board recommendations contained within the NSF and made them a reality in an effort to promote the emotional health of children in a deprived community.

References

Acheson, D. (1998) *Independent Inquiry into Inequalities in Health Report*. London: The Stationery Office.

Black, D., Morris, J., Smith, C., Townsend, P. (1980) *Inequalities in Health: Report of the Research Working Group*. London: Department of Health and Social Security.

Brookfield, S., Preskill, S. (1999) *Discussion as a Way of Teaching, Tools and Techniques for University Teachers*. Buckingham: The Society for Research into Higher Education and Open University Press.

Department of Health (1999) *National Service Framework for Mental Health*. London: Department of Health.

Education and Skills (Department of) (2003) *Every Child Matters*. London: Education and Skills.

Education and Skills (Department of), Department of Health (2004) *National Service Framework for Children, Young People and Maternity Services*. London: Department of Health.

Hall, D. (2000) Promoting the health of children. *The Practitioner* 246: 614–618.

Headrick, L., Wilcock, P.M., Batalden, P. (1998) Interprofessional working and continuing medical education. *British Medical Journal* 316: 771–774.

Home Office (1998) *Supporting Families*. London: Crown Copyright.

Jacques, D. (1984) *Learning in Groups*. London: Croom Helm Ltd.

Langley, J. (1998) Successful parenting: how to live with children. *Community Practitioner* 71(9): 289–291.

Lord, J., Farlow, D. (1990) A study of personal empowerment implications for health promotion. *Health Promotion* 10: 2–8.

Meltzer, H., Gatward, R., Goodman, R., Ford, T. (2000) *Mental Health of Children and Adolescents in Great Britain*. London: TSO.

Minkler, M. (1994) Challenges for health promotion in the 1990s: social inequalities, empowerment, negative consequences and the common good. *American Journal of Health Promotion* 8(6): 403–413.

Moyse, K. (2005) Baby massage and baby play. *Paediatric Nursing* 17(5): 30–32.

Rudduck, J. (1978) Learning through small group discussion. *SRHE Monograph 33*. Guilford: University of Surrey.

Tannahill, A. (1985) What is health promotion: planning for the 1990s. *Health Education Journal* 44: 167–168.

Touch Learn (2002) *Infant and Child Massage Teacher Training Course Manual*. Staffordshire: Touch Learn.

Townsend, P., Davidson, N., Whitehead, M. (1988) *Inequalities in Health: The Black Report. The Health Divide*. London: Penguin Books.

Townsend, P., Phillimore, P., Beatie, A. (1987) *Health and Deprivation: Inequality and the North*. London: Croom Helm.

West, M. (1997) Promoting interprofessional collaboration. *Newsletter of the European Network for the Development of Multiprofessional Education in Health Studies*. February 12.

World Health Organization (WHO) (1984) *Health Promotion: A Discussion Document on the Concept and Principles*. Geneva: WHO.

28 Baby Play

Jane Blenkinsop

NSF

The National Service Framework (NSF) for children/young people and maternity services, discusses the importance of promoting children's development (Education and Skills, Department of Health, 2004).

Introduction

Baby play is the name of a health promotion initiative that helps babies to learn through play in their first year of life. This chapter looks at the benefits of early play and interaction for the promotion of infant's mental health. The chapter is divided into two sections. The first section looks at the theory behind the baby play initiative and how this links with NSF standard 2 – *Supporting Parenting*, and standard 9 – *The Mental Health and Psychological Wellbeing of Children/Young People* (Education and Skills, Department of Health, 2004). The second section provides an example of how theory has been put into practice.

Section 1 – theory

The importance of play, stimulation and positive interaction between a baby and its primary carer has been well researched and documented. The impact this positive early interaction has on the relationship, and the child's subsequent health and development is remarkable. A child who has a secure attachment has a greater chance of being healthy (Education and Skills, Department of Health, 2004). Positive interactions during an infant's first year of life provide the foundation on which future relationships are built. If a child has a secure attachment with their primary carer, a mutually trusting, loving and healthy relationship can be formed. This experience will help the growing child to develop positive relationships with others as they become more socially active (Bowlby, 1965). Children who do not have a secure attachment are more likely to exhibit aggressive behaviour, have significant social problems and experience mental health problems too (Education and Skills, Department of Health, 2004).

In encouraging a secure attachment between parent/carer and baby from an early age, practitioners are assisting in promoting both infant and parental/carer mental health. Further, this may prevent future mental health difficulties for the child in later life. Studies show that in areas of high deprivation children are more likely to be affected by mental health problems, and that a high proportion of children who present with significant psychiatric disturbance at the age of 3 years still have difficulties at the age of 8 or 12 years (Sure Start, 2004).

Evidence shows that 10% of 5- to 15-year-olds have a diagnosable mental health disorder (Sure Start, 2004). Without intervention and appropriate treatment, these problems may continue into adulthood. The prevention of mental health problems through early intervention understandably is the best way forward (Sure Start, 2004).

The NSF standard 9 (Education and Skills, Department of Health, 2004) outlines the importance of emotional well-being in children/young people for their health and development. It also states that there is now increasing evidence on the effectiveness of interventions to improve children's/young people's resilience and treat disorders. In 2003 the Government paper *Every Child Matters* was published. This document states that all children should have the right to receive the opportunity and support to:

- be healthy;
- stay safe;
- enjoy and achieve;
- make a positive contribution;
- achieve economic well-being (Education and Skills, 2003).

A child who has a secure attachment with parents/carers is better equipped to develop confidence and is therefore more likely to have greater self-esteem. Learning and achieving are likely to be enjoyed as efforts are recognised and praised. The child is going to feel able to fully participate and gain from the opportunities made available. This is even more important in disadvantaged families, where a child is likely to be less able to engage in activities due to the additional problems and constraints faced in daily life.

Many parents/carers are aware of the importance of ensuring that play and social opportunities are available for their young children. However, the need to provide play and social opportunities for babies is not generally so well recognised, and this is where baby play can make an important contribution.

How baby play began

Baby play was developed in a deprived area within rural Derbyshire during 1996. It was developed in response to growing concerns raised by local health and education practitioners, regarding the significant number of children who were entering nursery with poorly developed play skills and a lack of readiness to learn at school. Children, who start school with adequately developed skills and the ability to cope with frustration, are able to take advantage of the opportunities offered by school (Hall and Elliman, 2003).

A local health visitor developed the idea of a group for parents/carers and babies (under 1 year), with support from the local primary care trust health promotion unit. The health visitor facilitated the group on a fortnightly basis initially. Following the appointment of a community nursery nurse to the area, the group was held weekly and replicated in nearby villages. Following the development of the local Sure Start programme, baby play became a mainstream Sure Start activity. Due to its success baby play was later rolled out to many other areas within the primary care trust.

The aim of the baby play group

The aim of baby play is to provide an effective means of practically demonstrating to parents/carers the benefits of play and interaction from birth. It also aims to empower parents/carers as their child's first educator, helping development, health and learning. As Sheridan (1997) maintains, a baby's main carer has a crucial role to play not only in ensuring that a child's basic needs are met, but also in providing stimulation.

In formulating baby play it was envisaged that parents/carers would become more aware of their child's development and more confident in their role as parents/carers. For example, parents/carers would be able to deal with behavioural issues, such as temper tantrums confidently. They would simply recognise temper tantrums as another stage of normal development.

If parents/carers are helped to become empowered, and are recognised as experts in their own child's development by practitioners, it can assist their confidence. They may then go on to support their child's learning throughout the child's education. As Hall and Elliman (2003) state, parents/carers who are confident and consistent in their handling are likely to have a confident child. If a child feels supported in her/his learning, the child is likely to develop confidence and coping mechanisms, which are essential in facing the challenges of everyday life.

In providing an opportunity for interaction through play, practitioners are also encouraging cognitive development from birth. Shore (1997) has shown that early stimulation and interaction can impact on the development of the human brain. Baby play goes some way to raise parental/carer awareness of the extent to which they can contribute to their child's development now and in the future through interaction.

Section 2 – practice

The ethos of the baby play group is that it promotes play without the need for expensive toys and equipment. It is a simple, low cost and effective way of encouraging parents/carers to play and interact with their children from birth. Although toys are used in the group, many of the play resources are items which most families would have at home. Of course when using items other than toys, it is essential that the items are safe for babies to use. Importantly too, babies need to be closely supervised during the play session. This is discussed with parents/carers at all sessions.

Parents/carers are made to feel welcome. We want them to feel that the group is fun and non-threatening. It can be daunting for some parents/carers to join a group for the first time.

The group is also a good opportunity for parents/carers to have quality time, to join in play with their baby, and to enjoy each other away from the home environment and its distractions. The activities are all appropriate for babies aged from 1 to 12 months old. From 1 year of age parents/carers are encouraged to access toddler play with their child. Toddler play offers similar opportunities to baby play, but is available especially for toddlers.

List of equipment needed for baby play

Below is a list of equipment which is useful to have before starting a baby play group. It is not exhaus-

tive but outlines the basic items, and can be added to as the group develops.

Balls – a selection of various colours, sizes and textures

Use to encourage:

- Awareness of hands by stroking baby's hand with a ball.
- Bringing two hands together to reach for a ball. Start with a football-sized ball and then work down in size as skill develops.
- Sitting – use a V-shaped pillow to support the baby's head and body. Place a football-sized ball between the baby's feet to provide support and encourage head control whilst sitting.
- Turn taking by rolling the ball to an older baby and encourage her/him to push it back again.
- Posting a ball, which fits in one hand, into a container or tube.
- Encourage physical (gross motor) skills-rolling, crawling, and baby pulling up to standing, to reach towards the ball.

Safety advice

It is essential to avoid using balls which are small enough to fit in a baby's mouth. Parents/carers need to be strongly advised that such balls should not be used.

Safety mirror

Use to encourage:

- Baby to focus on self and parent/carer.
- Baby to follow her/his reflection from one side to the other.
- Helps with pre-verbal skills, such as eye contact, imitating faces and sounds, and showing anticipation.
- When baby is on her/his tummy, ask the parent/carer to hold the mirror in a position where the baby can see her/his own reflection. Parents/carers can also see the baby's reflection. This enables eye contact and verbal interaction to continue during the activity.
- Place a piece of material over the mirror the baby can remove it to reveal her/his own reflection.

- Dress up. How does baby respond to seeing herself/himself wearing a hat?

Safety advice
The use of a plastic safety mirror rather than a glass one is recommended.

Home-made rattles

Put pasta, rice, beads, water and sequins inside a small plastic drinks bottle to produce different sounds.

Use to encourage:

- Auditory stimulation, observe baby's reaction to a variety of sounds.
- Tracking sounds; does baby turn to find the noise?
- Rolling
- Banging two objects together.
- Shaking the rattle with control. Give parent/carer a rattle so they can take it in turns to make a noise.

Safety advice
Ensure that lids are fastened securely. Check regularly to ensure safety.

Margarine tubs

Use to encourage:

- Reaching to knock a tower of tubs down.
- Emptying and filling.
- Piaget's (1954) concept of object permanence, by hiding an object under a container. Does the baby know that it is still there even though it is out of view?
- Place a tower of tubs between a baby's feet while they are in a sitting position. As baby's balance in the sitting position improves, vary the distance and position of the tubs.

Safety advice
Check for sharp edges and splits in the tubs; discard if present.

Books

Home-made books of black and white images or bold patterns and colours can easily be produced

with drawings, clip art or pictures cut from suitable magazines or catalogues. Laminating these will make them more hard-wearing.

Use to encourage:

- Visual stimulation.
- Sensory stimulation if using textured or noisy books.
- A cosy, safe activity between baby and parent/carer. Baby will either be excited or soothed depending on tone of voice and expression used by parent/carer.
- Older baby's will enjoy handling books and may turn a partially opened page on a cardboard book.
- Books are a gentle activity and are good to use when a baby is sleepy or has just woken up.

Safety advice
When producing home-made books, care must be taken to avoid any sharp edges.

Stacking cups

Use to encourage:

- Banging objects together.
- Finding hidden objects.
- Hand (fine motor) skills by placing a small ball in the largest cup for the baby to remove and then work down to the smaller sizes to increase the challenge.
- Build a tower at baby's eye level to encourage balance when sitting.
- Physical skills such as rolling, reaching and crawling.

Safety advice
Purchased toy – follow any relevant safety advice on packaging.

Pans and spoons

Use to encourage:

- Banging.
- Posting, encourage baby to release objects into the pan.
- Making sounds.

- Turn taking (parent/carer and baby have a spoon each).

Safety advice
Ensure that the screws, which hold the panhandle on, are safe and secure. Reinforce the importance of close supervision to parents/carers.

Bubble blowing

This can be calm and relaxing or exciting and noisy activity depending on how the parents/carers communicate with the baby during the activity. For the added benefits of pre-verbal skills, it is helpful if parents/carers face their baby and blow the bubbles themselves, rather than using a bubble machine. Pre-verbal skills form part of the foundation for speech and language development.

Use to encourage:

- Reaching to pop bubbles.
- Early communication skills. Babies may indicate that they want more bubbles by facial expressions, physical movement or vocalising.
- Eye contact, copying faces and sounds.
- To encourage communication, for example, gesture to indicate *more* and *all gone*.

Safety advice
Avoid blowing bubbles near the baby's face, especially near the eyes. Ensure that parents/carers hold the container or wand to ensure that the mixture is not swallowed, or that the baby does not put the wand into her/his mouth.

Hats

Use to encourage:

- Observe the baby's response in seeing parents/carers appear different, whilst wearing the hat.
- Eye contact.
- A response to seeing her/his own reflection in the mirror, whilst wearing a variety of hats, once the baby is able to sit steadily.
- Development of physical skills, for example, co-ordinating arms and hands to remove the hat.

Safety advice
Check for any loose threads and that any decorations are securely attached.

Pull along toy

Use to encourage:

- Hand skills, such as the baby using pincer grasp to hold string.
- Problem solving/cause and effect – pull the string and the toy moves.
- Reaching for string and returning to sitting position without losing balance.
- Mobility, crawling and pulling to stand.

Safety advice
Supervise during the activity to prevent baby putting the string into her/his mouth or around neck. Check for fraying of the string.

Treasure basket

Provide a variety of items for babies to explore and manipulate. Include safe items in various shapes, sizes, colours and textures. You may also want to include items that produce smells and sounds.

Safety advice
Again, the strict supervision needs to be communicated with the parents/carers. Items which could fit into the baby's mouth should *not* be included. Check contents for wear and tear regularly. Particularly avoid giving this activity to a baby who is constantly mouthing objects.

Health and safety issues

It is important to ensure that all toys and play equipment are checked regularly for damage or potential danger. All items used should be easy to keep clean (we tend not to use wooden toys in the group for this reason). All toys which have been used are cleaned at the end of each session and in between use by different babies.

Parents/carers are encouraged to take babies over the age of 12 months to toddler play, as it may be hazardous for children who are toddling to be in the same small area as very young babies.

Venue

The group needs to be held in a child safe environment. Washable blankets are used to cover the floor and parents/carers and practitioners remove shoes before walking on the blankets. V-pillows are used for providing support for babies until they are sitting steadily. This allows parents/carers to have both hands free for play, and helps to encourage parents/carers to face their baby, instead of baby facing away from them.

Additional equipment

As practitioners gain experience in facilitating the group, it will become evident which additional equipment would be useful. Through engaging in play with a baby and parents/carers, practitioners will observe which new skills are emerging and can then identify any equipment that might be useful in encouraging these skills. The type of equipment needed will depend on the age and stage of the babies attending at that time. It is useful to try and select toys which can be used in more than one way. This will ensure cost-effectiveness and will make storing the toys more manageable.

Preparing for the group

- In order to facilitate the group successfully, practitioners must have a good knowledge and understanding of child development and appropriate play and activity ideas.
- Two practitioners are needed for a group of eight babies and their parents/carers. This will allow sufficient time to be spent with each baby and parent/carer. It also enhances the smooth running of the group and ensures that it is a quality experience for all participants.
- The floor should be cleared of any potential hazards, and covered with washable blankets.
- Put toys to one side rather than putting them out on the floor. Practitioners are then able to access an appropriate toy for a baby's stage of development. Parents/carers are also able to see what toys are available and which they think would be of interest to their child.

- The number of babies able to attend each session will depend on available space within the room. I would suggest setting up a second group rather than having one large group if the number exceeds eight, as this will ensure that the structure of the group is maintained.
- If the same practitioners can facilitate the group each week, this helps to build a positive relationship with parents/carers. It can also provide a good insight into each baby's development, rather than various practitioners asking parents/carers the same questions each week about their baby's development.

Starting the session

- On arrival parents/carers are welcomed into the group and a practitioner will spend time with each of them, discussing the previous week's activities. Parents/carers will often report back if their baby has started doing something new.
- A practitioner will demonstrate an activity and discuss the benefits of that activity in relation to the child's development. This is undertaken individually. Parents/carers are then given time and support if needed to try out the activity with their baby.
- Practitioners then work their way around the group, changing activities and introducing new play ideas where necessary, until all babies are engaged in an activity with their parents/carers. A baby's responses to the activity are highlighted to encourage parents/carers to read their baby's cues and respond accordingly.
- If the baby or parents/carers have lost interest, a different activity will be given. Any safety information that is relevant to the new activity is shared with them.
- Several different activity, ideas will be given for each baby within a session. As parents/carers become more aware of their baby's likes and dislikes, they will often request a certain toy.
- Practitioners emphasise the fact that all babies develop at their own rate. Practitioners therefore look at development as a series of skills all emerging consecutively, rather than focusing too much on developmental milestones which must be reached by a certain age.

- If concerns arise regarding a baby's development, this needs to be dealt with sensitively as parents/carers do inevitably compare their baby to others of a similar age. Parents/carers would be supported and encouraged to discuss concerns with their health visitor, who can make any necessary referrals. Play ideas that help to incorporate any advice given by other practitioners could then be implemented within the session.
- Breaks for feeding, sleeping or just a cuddle are important. Parents/carers are welcome to stay if they arrive with a sleeping baby. A practitioner will take time to discuss play and development with them.
- Health promotion issues do arise frequently within the group. Parents/carers will often chat to each other in between activities about weaning and sleep problems. They will often share ideas and compare notes. This is a good opportunity for practitioners within the group to provide relevant health promotion information.
- Once a baby becomes mobile, all parents/carers are asked if they need any home safety equipment, as we are able to order this at a low cost from the local home safety scheme.
- Each session is ended with a group activity. This helps to ensure that the group comes to an end positively and on time. It is also a good opportunity to encourage the use of songs and rhymes. Parents/carers can learn new rhymes to enjoy with their baby at home. Activities at the end of each session depend on the age of babies present, but by being imaginative and flexible we find a way for all of the babies to join in. Ideas for the end of group activities include singing, action rhymes, blowing bubbles, ball pool, textures and paper, musical instruments or messy play with cooked spaghetti, for example.

Baby play activities are offered to all babies in the community. The community nursery nurse visits each family with a new baby, about the time the baby is 6 to 8 weeks of age. The aim of this visit is to introduce appropriate play ideas and to discuss the benefits of play and stimulation in relation to their baby's development. It is also an opportunity to promote the baby play group. Families who are unable to attend the group may be offered baby play home visits and are then supported in attending a group at a later date.

Practitioners within the team have produced a series of leaflets, which give practical ideas for play and information about development. There are four different leaflets, each focusing on different age groups (Figure 28.1).

These include the following:

- 0–3 months.
- 3–6 months.
- 6–9 months.
- 9–12 months.

Each one gives practical tips on encouraging baby's development and relevant safety information for the age group (Coombes and Kirk, 1999). A series of activity packs has also been produced which provides age-appropriate nursery rhymes and tips on how to make them fun for babies (Blenkinsop and Winson, 2003).

A health promotion baby play course has been developed, and here parents/carers learn some of the theory behind the group. It is also quite practical with lots of play ideas and information about the developing child. Each session ends by parents/carers joining their children in the crèche to try out some new rhymes and memorise traditional ones.

Case study

The following demonstrates how baby play was used to help one family. In line with Nursing Midwifery Council guidance (NMC, 2004) names have been changed.

Samantha (18 years) and Tom (20 years) moved into the area when Samantha was pregnant. They had no relatives living nearby. Tom worked during the day. Once Mathew was born, Samantha spent much of her time at home alone with him. With encouragement from the health visitor, Samantha began attending baby play with Mathew.

Samantha was quite apprehensive in the beginning about caring for Mathew. Practitioners observed her anxiety, but they were able to recognise her strengths too. They encouraged and reassured Samantha. She attended regularly and her confidence in handling Mathew grew. Samantha now interacts positively with Mathew and is far less anxious. Samantha has also made friendships with other mums in the group, which have led to further opportunities for socialisation.

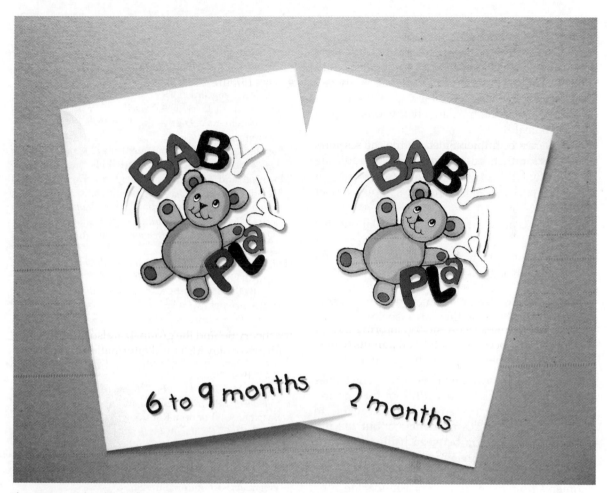

Figure 28.1   Baby play leaflets.

Sure Start provides a variety of different health promotion courses. Samantha has now attended two of these. She is enthusiastic about Mathew moving on to join toddler play in the near future. The experience has been a positive one for both Samantha and Mathew. His emotional health certainly appears to have benefited from attending baby play; he is a happy baby. Samantha's emotional health too appears to have benefited from attending the group.

Evaluation and conclusion

Feedback from parents/carers has been positively received about baby play activities. This work has evaluated favourably in the Sure Start local programme evaluation, where parents/carers comments included:

- Friendly staff.
- Feel very comfortable about attending.
- Time to play uninterrupted by other things.
- Felt isolated before but now I don't.
- Good interaction with the children (Kirk, 2005).

A large number of parents/carers who attend the group go on to attend toddler play and the local preschool. Many parents/carers have also gone on to attend some of the Sure Start health promotion courses and parent learning courses.

Early years services, especially Sure Start local programmes and children's centres, provide opportunities to recognise and address the emotional health needs of infants (Education and Skills, Department of Health, 2004). I certainly feel from my experiences with baby play that such experiences contribute positively towards infants' emotional health.

The guidance in the NSF states that all services for mothers, fathers and caregivers:

- focus on the relationship between the parent and infant;
- are offered at an early stage when relationships are forming;
- provide support to parents/carers, based on building their confidence and skills in caring for children;
- address the wider environmental circumstances of the family including their socio-economic needs (Education and Skills, Department of Health, 2004).

In facilitating baby play I have seen many babies and their parents/carers benefit from this service. I would like to see the group made available to all families, as it raises awareness about the importance of interaction between babies and their parents/carers. I feel that such initiatives go some way to establishing positive relationships and attachments from the beginning of a child's life.

References

Blenkinsop, J., Winson, S. (2003) *Baby Play Activity Packages*. Derbyshire: North Eastern Derbyshire PCT.

Bowlby, J. (1965) *Child Care and the Growth of Love*, 2nd edn. London: Penguin books.

Coombes, C., Kirk, J. (1999) *Guidelines for Establishing Baby Play in Your Area*. Derbyshire: Chesterfield Health Promotion Unit.

Education and Skills (Department of) (2003) *Every Child Matters*. London: Education and Skills.

Education and Skills (Department of), Department of Health (2004) *National Service Framework for Children, Young People and Maternity Services. Standard 2 – Supporting Parenting. Standard 9 – The Mental and Psychological Wellbeing of Children and Young Adults*. London: Crown Copyright.

Hall, D., Elliman, D. (2003) *Health for All Children*, 4th edn. Oxford: Oxford University Press.

Kirk, J. (2005) *Sure Start Creswell, Langwith/Whaley Thorns and Shirebrook (CLWTS) – Monitoring and Evaluation Report*. Derbyshire: Sure Start CLWTS.

Nursing and Midwifery Council (NMC) (2004) *Code of Professional Conduct*. London: NMC.

Piaget, J. (1954) *The Construction of Reality in the Child*. New York: Basic Books.

Sheridan, M. (1997) *From Birth to Five Years. Children's Developmental Progress* (revised and updated by Frost, M., Sharma, A.). London: Routledge.

Shore, R. (1997) *Rethinking the Brain: New Insights into Early Development*. New York: Families and Work Institute.

Sure Start (2004) *What Works in Promoting Children's Mental Health, the Evidence and Implications for Sure Start Local Programmes?* London: Sure Start.

29 Baby Club

Kate Hawksworth

NSF

The National Service Framework (NSF) for children/young people and maternity services discusses the importance of promoting children's health and development (Education and Skills, Department of Health, 2004). Community practitioners can support parents/carers in improving their young children's health and development through group activities.

Aims of baby club

A vision of the NSF standard 2, *Supporting Parenting*, is for parents/carers to be confident and able to bring up their children in a way that promotes their health, development and emotional well-being (Education and Skills, Department of Health, 2004). At the time this document was published, a health visitor and community nursery nurse team in a small rural community in the East Midlands were planning to set up a *baby club* to help support parents and their babies in the local community. Meeting the vision of NSF standard 2 with particular reference to promoting infants' emotional well-being thus became one of the main aims of baby club. A further aim included reducing social exclusion by helping parents and carers to develop a social support network, and emotional support, through attending baby club.

Planning baby club

Careful planning is essential when developing a new health promotion initiative. Working within Sure Start the health visitor had a reduced caseload and a community nursery nurse who worked $2\frac{1}{2}$ days a week, which all helped to enhance the planning and facilitation of baby club. The intention of baby club was to build on the existing success of baby play, the benefits of which have been discussed by Jane in Chapter 28. Baby play helps to promote the development of a secure attachment between infant and parent/carer by promoting positive interaction.

In the early stages of planning, the health visitor and community nursery nurse encountered significant logistical difficulties in finding a venue. This was due to the existing Sure Start centre undergoing major refurbishment. Several local venues were considered; however, none were suitable due to funding, lack of storage or rooms not being available at suitable times. The resulting delay was very frustrating for the team. However, within weeks of the new Sure Start centre opening in 2005, the hard work and planning came to fruition with the first baby club session taking place in April 2005. Poor attendance at baby club was always a concern as historically group attendance had been poor in the area. However, the team were quietly confident that the group would be well attended, as baby club was developed in response to local demand.

The health visitor invited guest speakers from other agencies who had relevant knowledge and skills in supporting parenting and health promotion topics. The visiting speakers were arranged following discussion with parents attending the group, in the club's early weeks. The health visitor recognised the importance of involving parents in planning the content of group activities for the ongoing success of baby club.

A final consideration in planning baby club was how to fund refreshments. As Sure Start funding was not infinite, the group had to be self-sufficient. With parents involvement a decision was made to charge 50p per family. Flyers were sent out with a brief description of baby club, including details of these charges. The flyers helped to ensure that parents were aware of any costs before they came.

The health visitor was strongly aware of the need to promote positive emotional health in parents, so they in turn, would be able to promote positive emotional health of their infants. It is widely accepted that children's mental health is about the ability to enter into and sustain mutually satisfying personal relationships, as well as to play and learn in line with age and intellectual ability (Kurtz, 2004). Baby play was already successful in meeting the emotional health needs of infants, with a strong focus on secure attachment. It was hoped that baby club might be able to achieve similar success.

The importance of supporting parenting in order to promote parents' emotional health was felt to be a priority by the team. All health visitors locally had been trained in the *Solihull Approach* (Solihull NHS Primary Care Trust, 2004). The Solihull Approach is based on three key concepts:

- Containment.
- Reciprocity.
- Behaviour management.

It is the concept of *containment* that the health visitor particularly felt was essential for parents'

emotional health. Parents can sometimes feel overwhelmed by very powerful emotions within their role. For example, if they have an infant who is not sleeping, they may feel strongly about this. By responding to these strong emotions, the health visitor is able to contain them and help parents to move forward. Parents in turn are then emotionally available to contain and respond to their infant's needs and emotions.

Once all emotions are contained, parents and their infants are then able to enter into a reciprocal interaction. *Reciprocity* being the second key concept of the Solihull Approach. Schore (2001) spoke about reciprocity as part of the mechanism of attachment. He believed that if parents are in tune with their infants, they are then able to promote their infants' development in so many ways.

Mental health is central to Sure Start programmes, which aim to promote the physical, intellectual and social development of babies and young children, with a particular focus on those who are disadvantaged. The Government acknowledges that a lack of appropriate stimulation in the early years may result in language delay, which in turn may lead to emotional or behavioural disorders later (Education and Skills, Department of Health, 2004). *Behavioural management* can help support behavioural difficulties. Behavioural management is the third key concept in the Solihull Approach.

Stimulating babies

If babies' and young children's development in the early years is supported and encouraged by parents, they may not develop behavioural problems. Children grow up feeling loved, and supported, with their development encouraged. Delays in areas of development, such as language, may not occur.

In the health visitor's experience, some parents do not appreciate the importance of stimulating their babies in the early months. There is biological evidence to support babies' need for stimulation. Stimulating babies' development is necessary in order that biologically synapse connections extend in the brain, which are essential for social and emotional development, as Shore (1997) has highlighted.

By 18 weeks gestation, the fetus has developed between 1 and 2 million basic brain cells (Solihull,

2004). These brain cells have some predetermined basic survival functions. However, it is not until after a baby is born that the vast majority of synapse connections (between brain cells) are formed (Begley, 1996). The first year of development is very rapid – any parent will tell you that. Phenomenal changes take place, behaviour, understanding and in the way the baby interacts with the world.

During a baby's first year of life, the brain grows and synapses make connections according to the stimulation they receive. For example, visual stimuli will wire the visual cortex of the brain. The majority of connections made in the infant's cortex are as a direct result of post-natal experience. Le Doux (1993) recognised that events in early life can and do remain an influence throughout life, particularly when experienced with strong emotions. He believed that early-experienced precognitive emotions continue to play out in later life, despite the individual having no conscious memory of the event.

Considering all these theories, the responsibilities of being a parent can be very daunting. Through baby club the team intended to support parents in achieving positive emotional health for their babies. The health visitor acknowledges the tremendous value of baby play in promoting babies' emotional health. This could be improved further still by supporting parents' emotional health, so they in turn could support their babies.

About baby club

Baby club is a 2-hour session, which runs on a weekly basis starting at 9:15 AM, post school drop-off time. This time was chosen with consideration to parents who also had school-age children. The health visitor and community nursery nurse are present each week. On alternate weeks there is a midwife available. The midwife sees her antenatal contacts and is available to offer advice and support to mums in the post-natal period.

The first hour is devoted to baby play. The community nursery nurse is invaluable in helping parents meet their babies' developmental needs. The last hour is when other team members and guest speakers are invited to join the group. To date this has included a wide variety of multi-agency workers:

- Welfare rights.
- Housing officers.
- Citizens advice.
- Local police.
- Fire officers.
- Representatives from the local home safety scheme.

During the second hour, drinks and healthy snacks are served for parents and their babies. Obviously, parents are reminded about the safety of food and drinks in relation to the care of their baby.

During snack time the health visitor can offer advice on age-appropriate foods for weaning. Snack time provides an ideal opportunity to promote the Department of Health's (2004) ongoing *5 a Day* (fruit and vegetable) campaign. The Department of Health (2004) recognises that one of the barriers to families achieving 5 a Day is awareness. At baby club the team are able to provide knowledge on buying, preparing and eating fresh fruit and vegetables. The team have seen an increase in parents' motivation to maintain 5 a Day intake for their children.

Parents are asked at the beginning of each term if they have any particular interests or requests for guest speakers. Some parents have significant input into the content of this programme. They prefer not to have a guest speaker each week as some weeks the group like time to share their thoughts and ideas. There are always frequent questions for the health visitor and midwife.

Baby massage is always a popular request. The health visitor and community nursery nurse are both trained in baby massage, so this can easily be included. A subject which causes high levels of anxiety for parents is the management of minor injuries and minor illnesses. The health visitor has accessed training on the teaching of first aid to parents and there is an acute community children's nursing service on site. So the team are able to allay parents' anxieties.

The team would like to stress at this stage the importance of being flexible to meet demand and parental requirements. Picking up on the cues of parents may well lead one away from planned activities. For example, if a parent has experienced a very bad night as her/his baby has not slept, then the health promotion topic is likely to be steered towards sleep and bedtime routines.

A further example could be a parent who is concerned that the baby/older child is refusing food. Flexibility is crucial to successful group facilitation and the team need to ensure that all concerns raised are addressed within the group. If not, arrangements are made to follow up at a later stage. Parents gain a great deal of support from each other; knowing that they have helped someone to solve a problem is an effective way of building individual self-esteem.

The team see baby club as an ideal opportunity for health promotion activities. The following health promotion topics have been presented:

- Mental health in the post-natal period
  - The Sure Start community psychiatric nurse joined the group to discuss post-natal depression.
- Antenatal and post-natal support
  - Support and advice are available from the health visitor and the midwife.
- Speech and language in babies
  - The importance of talking to your baby from birth is discussed by the community nursery nurse during baby play activities.
- The importance of books for babies
  - The Sure Start librarian joins the group on a regular basis; she encourages parents to join the library. Parents are able to borrow books for their babies through Sure Start. This service has been invaluable as the nearest library is 3 miles away.
- Behaviour management
  - Ongoing advice and support are available from the health visitor and community nursery nurse within the group, and concerns are followed up at home as necessary.
- Child development
  - Baby play facilitates a greater understanding of child development.
- Healthy weaning
  - Every week snack time provides the ideal opportunity for discussion on infant's diet and the Government's 5 a Day campaign for infants and parents/carers.
- Minor injuries and minor illness in babies and children
  - The Sure Start community children's nurse attends the group. She offers excellent advice

for parents on managing minor injuries and illnesses.
- Dental health promotion
  - The primary care trust has its own oral health promotion unit. Staff from the unit visit every 6 months. They discuss how harmful fruit drinks and juices can be, particularly if given in a bottle. Parents are always surprised about the high sugar content in baby yoghurts and cereals.
- Further education
  - A lecturer from the local college visits to discuss courses on offer for parents and carers.

The parenting role is influenced by many factors. The Solihull Approach (2004) believes that a parent's own experiences of being parented play an important part. So too, do pre-birth expectations, family structure and external factors. External factors could include poor housing or a lack of social support. Hall and Elliman (2003) recognise the need to assist parents with personal support, information, advice and material resources. Housing and benefits are known to cause great concern for many new families. At baby club the team have been able to introduce parents to practitioners working locally to support families with housing and benefits issues. The housing and benefits officers have joined the group as guest speakers. This has encouraged open discussion and an opportunity for questions and answers.

Case study

The following highlights one mum's experience of attending baby club. The case study shows how one family has benefited from baby club. In maintaining anonymity, as the Nursing and Midwifery Council (2004) advises names have been changed.

Mum was anxious during her pregnancy and following the birth of baby Rory. Due to her anxiety she felt unable to leave the house alone. This left mum and baby Rory at significant risk of social exclusion.

Working within a Sure Start area and having the advantage of a reduced caseload, the health visitor was able to visit mum very intensely during the postnatal period. During these visits the health visitor gained mum's trust. After a few months mum agreed to visit baby club, her confidence and self-esteem were still quite low. Initially, the health visitor organised for someone to collect mum and baby Rory to take them to the group. Mum enjoyed the group and was pleased to meet old friends and make new ones. Within a few weeks mum was walking to the group with other parents.

Now Rory is a happy, sociable and inquisitive toddler. Mum is visibly more relaxed. Her relationship with Rory is a warm and positive one. This supports the opinion of the Child Psychotherapy Trust (1999) who believes that parents/caregivers who feel emotionally supported themselves are more emotionally available for their babies.

The mum in this case study has benefited through support from other parents and has in turn been a great support to other mums. Rory has now outgrown baby club and has graduated to toddler play.

Conclusion

Supporting parenting, as the NSF advocates (Education and Skills, Department of Health, 2004), seems to be something that baby club is achieving for families locally. The team have witnessed an increase in confidence and self-esteem amongst parents/carers locally since starting baby club. Knowledge and skills gained by them is clearly evident in discussions within the group. With increased confidence and self-esteem, along with knowledge of child development, parents/carers are in a better position to promote the emotional health and development of their infants. Baby club appears to be achieving its aims.

Prior to baby club commencing at the newly refurbished Sure Start centre, baby play could only be delivered on an individual basis in family homes. Although very beneficial in encouraging positive attachment, there was no opportunity for new and isolated parents/carers to build their social support networks. As Hall and Elliman (2003) highlight, forming social support networks is crucial for parents/carers, as it can influence the health outcomes for families and their children. Baby club has helped to strengthen community networking. Some families have even been able to rekindle relationships that they first made at school many years ago. Baby

club gives mums-to-be, new mums and carers the opportunity to mix socially and therefore minimise the risk of social exclusion.

Baby club has been well attended from day 1 with an average of six parents/carers attending regularly. The team believe the reason for baby club's success is its ability to respond to local need. The service was originally requested by the local community itself. Parents/carers play a key role in developing baby club's activities. Further, practitioners organising the service were already known and trusted by the local community, which has thus helped to encourage attendance.

There have been unexpected positive outcomes from baby club, including an improvement in multidisciplinary team working. Through close liaison with midwifery services, antenatal contacts are now a regular occurrence at baby club. Working in partnership with the midwife in this way allows practitioners to recognise and support any mums-to-be with emotional health concerns. Mums-to-be are able to mix with new mums and share worries and concerns. Sharing concerns encourages a problem-solving approach with the added security of professional knowledge and advice from the team.

The area is one of high unemployment. The team have been delighted that many parents/carers who attend baby club have gone on to further their education. Perhaps baby club has helped to encourage this.

Baby club has demonstrated itself to be financially sustainable. Parents/carers have been happy to pay 50 p each session, which has more than covered the cost of refreshments. Using excess funds, the group were able to finance transport for an outing to a local farm park just a few months after baby club started.

Without Sure Start backing, in particular the management and administration teams, baby club would not have been the tremendous success that it has been. Access to the children's room at the Sure Start centre has been invaluable, and being part of a Sure Start team has also made it easier to link with other Sure Start practitioners. Baby club has been an ideal opportunity to introduce other Sure Start services. Parents/carers who attend baby club go on to access the Sure Start library, toy library and adult education services.

As baby club is intended to promote positive emotional health for parents/carers and their babies, it is very difficult to formally evaluate. However, baby club is now in its fourth year. The children who first attended baby club now attend nursery. Interestingly, teaching staff say they can tell which children have attended baby club, as they are more sociable and confident when entering into relationships with other children. Baby club may be a way forward for other areas where practitioners wish to support parents/carers in their parenting role, helping to improving health outcomes for children.

References

Begley, S. (1996) Your child's brain. *Newsweek*, 19 February, 55–61.

Child Psychotherapy Trust (CPT) (1999) *Promoting Infant Mental Health: A Framework for Developing Policies and Services to Ensure the Healthy Development of Young Children*. London: CPT.

Department of Health (2004) *5 a Day*. London: Department of Health.

Education and Skills (Department of), Department of Health (2004) *National Service Framework for Children, Young People and Maternity Services*. London: Crown Copyright.

Hall, D., Elliman, D. (eds) (2003) *Health for All Children*, 4th edn. Oxford: Oxford University Press.

Kurtz, Z. (2004) In: Sure Start. *What Works in Promoting Children's Mental Health: The Evidence and the Implications for Sure Start Settings*. London: Sure Start.

Le Doux, J.E. (1993) Emotional memory systems in the brain. *Behavioural and Brain Research* 58: 69–79.

Nursing and Midwifery Council (NMC) (2004) *Code of Professional Conduct*. London: NMC.

Schore, A. (2001) Effects of a secure attachment relationship on right brain development, affect regulation, and infant mental health. *Infant Mental Health Journal* 22: 201–269.

Shore, R. (1997) *Rethinking the Brain: New Insights into Early Development*. New York: Families and Work Institute.

Solihull NHS Primary Care Trust (2004) *Solihull Approach Resource Pack – The First Five Years*. Cambridge: Jill Rodgers Associates Ltd.

30 Positive Parenting

Karen Moyse

NSF

The National Service Framework (NSF) for children, young people and maternity services advocates supporting parents, in helping children to feel emotionally secure (Education and Skills, Department of Health, 2004).

Introduction

A child's relationship with her/his parents can provide a significant foundation for relationships in later life. This chapter on positive parenting looks at some of the techniques that parents can use to help them parent positively. Using positive parenting techniques may help to strengthen the relationship that parents have with their child.

What is positive parenting?

Positive parenting is a term that is now frequently talked about in Britain, through books, magazines and especially television (TV) programmes. The TV programmes are particularly interesting, and examples of these include *Supernanny* and the *House of Tiny Tearaways*. They frequently portray an expert explaining to usually exasperated parents why their current approach to parenting is not working, and how this can be changed into a more positive one. Over a period of time behavioural changes can clearly be observed in the children, with parents seeming much more confident in their parenting skills.

Positive parenting essentially is about parents developing a close relationship with their children and particularly being positive with them. The approach attempts to turn parents away from some of the more negative approaches to bringing up children, such as undermining children's confidence, and smacking. These are replaced with a much more positive approach. Positive parenting techniques include praise for children's good behaviour and time out for negative behaviour. Importantly too, parents must *not* always comment on each and every negative behaviour exhibited by their child. Positive parenting is about helping children to grow into confident, happy adults. It is also about treasuring our children for what they are themselves, so they too can recognise their own abilities.

Parenting

Having described positive parenting, it is important to consider what parenting itself actually means and involves. The Oxford Concise Dictionary of Current English (1982) defines a parent as someone who has a child, either born to them or adopted. The problem with this definition is that it fails to tell us what parenting actually involves. Once you have this child, what do you do with it? You love, care and help your child grow into a happy confident adult – the process of parenting. Sounds easy, doesn't it?

Parenting in contemporary Britain throws up a number of issues which impact on the parenting role and the relationship that a parent has with her/his child. Some of these are outlined below:

- As a parent do you have enough money to care for your child?
- Do you have somewhere suitable to live?
- Is your child healthy and developing normally?
- What do you do when your child is sick, where do you go for help?
- How will you educate your child?
- Teaching your child to have good manners and have moral values is important too.

Each of these may present different dilemmas for families.

Activity

Think about what these different dilemmas and what they might mean for some families.

Parents often have to juggle the role of parenting with other demands in their lives. This might include running the home, going to work, caring for relatives who may be sick and even studying. In addition, there may be pressures from extended family, suggesting that you are failing to fulfil the demands of your parenting role. This is before you have even considered how you are going to manage your child's behaviour – both the good and not so good. A complexity of issues it would seem, with no easy answers. At the end of the day, all parents want is to have a loving, caring relationship with their child. However, different issues seem to impact upon this.

The relationship

Parenting is an important process which should help and guide the child so that she/he develops into a happy and well-adjusted adult. Central to this process is the child and parent developing a strong loving relationship. Researchers have studied the relationship between parent and child for many years. Historically, two of the most famous theorists in this area have been John Bowlby and Michael Rutter. Bowlby (1979) believed that there was a strong causal relationship between a child's experiences with her/his parents and the later capacity to make affectional bonds. Both Bowlby (1979) and Rutter (1981) agreed that a child needed a stable loving relationship to develop normally. Rutter (1981), however, also believed that harmony within the family was as important a factor.

More recently, there has been further research on the relationship between parents and their children. Studies include work by Kurtz (2004) and Barlow et al. (2007). These studies have examined the Government's parenting programmes offered through Sure Start. Sure Start parenting programmes aim to enhance the relationship that parents have with their young children. Barlow et al. (2007) have shown that Sure Start parenting programmes can help the relationship between parents and their young children living in deprived communities.

Positive parenting in practice

It is important to consider what positive parenting can actually achieve for some families. Positive parenting can mean more fun, and less stress for all the family, with the child developing a greater sense of self-esteem (Moyse, 1999). It can provide parents with the knowledge and skills necessary to be confident and successful in their parenting role (Moyse, 1999). Hall and Elliman (2003) interestingly state that parents who are more confident in the handling of their child are likely to have a more confident and secure child.

From applying positive parenting techniques myself in practice for many years, the benefits have been clearly apparent. As a practitioner, one can see relationships between parents and their children improving, where positive parenting techniques have been adopted.

Hall (1996) comments that parents tend to replicate the style of parenting that their own parents used. However, the problem with repeating parenting styles is that there is a risk that the same mistakes may be repeated. Parents-to-be need to give some thought to how they will approach the role of parenting, before simply repeating what has gone before. Questions parents-to-be may want to ask themselves:

- How do they feel about the way they were parented?
- What do they feel worked in the relationship?
- What do they feel did not work in the relationship?
- What type of parents do they want to be?
- What kind of relationship do they want with their child?

Hall and Elliman (2003) assert that children's chances of success in life can be greatly improved with good family support and behavioural guidance. This is fundamentally what positive parenting is trying to encourage, good family support and providing families with behavioural techniques that will help guide their children.

Sure Start adopts a positive approach to parenting in its work with families living in deprived areas. It offers families advice and support on parenting their young children, as well as providing group activities in the form of parenting programmes. Importantly, Sure Start works in partnership with individual families.

Parenting programmes offered through Sure Start can impact on parenting in quite a positive way. In Barlow et al.'s (2007) research parenting programmes that started early and continued through childhood could produce good outcomes for children. The Government does view supporting parents and their children as essential for helping children out of poverty (Sure Start, 2007).

Positive parenting techniques

There are different approaches to positive parenting that can be used, such as *Triple P* (Triple P, 2003) and Webster-Stratton and Herbert (2000), for example. Having used Sutton's (2000) work myself for several years, we will discuss this approach.

Carole Sutton, a psychologist, has worked in practice and undertaken research on parenting for many years. Sutton's (2000) work has its foundations in cognitive behavioural psychology. The be-

havioural approach within psychology is concerned with learning in the social context. The cognitive approach involves the individual's thoughts, perceptions and judgements (Sutton, 2000). The cognitive behavioural approach brings all these together in its efforts to help parents and their children.

The foundations of Sutton's (2000) work are associated with helping children feel secure in the relationship with their parents. Sutton (2000) is keen to provide parents with guidance on how to cope with difficulties they might experience in the parenting role.

The techniques

Positive parenting provides different techniques that can be used. Some of these techniques are outlined:

- Positive reinforcement, which is about providing the child with praise and positive feedback for doing something well.
- Rewards – giving the chid a reward for doing something really well. (However, the child needs to find the reward actually rewarding. Each child will find different things rewarding.)
- Time out can be given for negative behaviour. Each child loves attention. The child is removed from the social situation, and not given attention for a short period. The child is then able to reflect upon her/his behaviour before returning to the social situation again (Sutton, 2000).

These are just some of the techniques Sutton (2000) advocates in her approach towards positive parenting.

There are obviously a couple of safety points to be considered in relation to using these techniques. Before undertaking these techniques, parents need to be sure that their child is old enough to be able to understand what is trying to be achieved.

When removing a young child from the social situation and into another room, for example, obviously the room has to be free from danger. The parent still needs to be close by, and ensure her/his child is safe. The child is only removed from the social situation for a few minutes.

These are techniques that can help with parenting. They do not simply focus on the child's negative

behaviour, but promote and reward positive behaviour.

Supporting families

When families are trying to resolve problems with
their child's behaviour, they may have limited support. Sometimes they are facing criticism from family, friends or school, which can make things more
difficult, rather than improving matters. There certainly needs to be much more support available in
local communities for families who are experiencing behavioural difficulties with their children.

When children are young there is quite a lot of
support available through health visitors, nursery
nurses, children's centres and Sure Start centres, for
example. However, as children become older, there
appears to be less support available. Some schools
with their accompanying school nurses can be quite
helpful. Nonetheless, there is a need to increase the
support available.

With the advent of the Government's policy
on extended schools, the situation is beginning
to change. Extended schools aim to support children and their families (Education and Skills, 2007;
http://www. everychildmatters.gov.uk). The Government views schools as being at the heart of local
communities, and thus well placed to offer support.
Extended schools are about enhancing children's
confidence, improving relationships and helping them achieve (http://www.everychildmatters.
gov.uk). In addition, children's centres are also developing services for children over 5 years.

As a nurse (with the appropriate training) you
may be able to provide families with much needed
support in helping their children to feel emotionally
supported, so they are able to go on and achieve
in school. To be able to support families the nurse
needs an in-depth understanding about child development. Sometimes parents perceive that there may
be a problem with their child's behaviour, when in
fact it may not be a problem, but a misunderstanding. Discussing with parents about what is normal development for their child may help to clarify any misunderstandings. Hall and Elliman (2003)
believe giving information on child development is
useful.

So far the issue of behaviour has been considered
from the parents' perspective, but what about the

child? What issues might be concerning the child
that seems to be affecting her/his behaviour? There
could be all sorts of reasons – school, friends, family, tiredness, ill health, or even bullying. Exploring how the child is feeling is essential. It is important that parents sit down and talk with their child,
listen, find out what might be wrong. Working together will help to resolve any problems. Importantly, children need to feel they can talk with their
parents.

Teaching parents

This section looks briefly at what nurses can do
when working with families in group situations.

There is a view that there should be more parenting groups, where parents can learn the techniques
of parenting. An independent commission recommended that the Government should provide training workshops for parents at every stage of bringing up their children. Families should not be left on
their own to cope with any problems in bringing up
their children (Carvel, 2005). This commission was
set up in 2004 by the National Family and Parenting
Institute.

Different practitioners within this book have presented information on parenting courses which
they organise in their area. The aim of these courses
is to support and provide information to parents,
usually when children are young. Perhaps in time,
as the benefits of these courses are recognised, there
may be more opportunities to develop parenting
courses to help support parents with older children.
Parenting courses not only help parents to learn new
information and skills, but also provide the opportunity to share experiences with other parents. Parents are not only helping themselves, but also supporting other parents too.

As parents we get the best of our children, but we
also get the worst of them. The important thing is
not to become obsessed with behavioural issues. It
may just simply be a transient episode, which resolves itself in time, or possibly something that is
genuinely upsetting the child and needs to be discussed. As the nurse involved with families, take
care not to label children's behaviour, so that it does
not turn into something that it is not. Putting across
the child's perspective in the group situation is really important.

Teaching session

A course on positive parenting might include some of the following information:

- Positive parenting – discussing what positive parenting is and how it can help children and parents.
- Discussing with the group about their own experiences of being parented.
- How do they feel about being a parent?
- Issues that impact on modern day parenting.
- Child development.
- How different experiences can influence children's development in the long-term.
- Introduce positive parenting techniques.
- Parents can be invited to undertake a little homework. They are invited to use positive parenting approaches at home with their child, and then if they wish these experiences can be brought back to the group for discussion. (Some parents may wish to share these experiences with the nurse individually.)

The above points might provide you with some ideas about where to start when putting together a course yourself on positive parenting. Do not forget to find out what parents themselves feel they need to know.

Evaluation

The parenting work that Sure Start does is continually being evaluated. In some cases the national evaluations have produced mixed views. One Sure Start evaluation compared families from Sure Start areas, with those from non-Sure Start areas. Evidence was very much in favour of the Sure Start families when comparisons were made on styles of parenting. Toynbee (2005) in *The Guardian* (13 September 2005) reports that the evaluation found Sure Start mothers to be warmer parents than the other group. The Sure Start mothers also demonstrated less hostility and *less negative criticism* of their children. Sure Start mothers also displayed *more affection* towards their children than the other mothers.

This is indeed an encouraging result for Sure Start, and demonstrates that its positive approach

to parenting is beginning to have an impact with some families. Details of Sure Start evaluations can be found on the Sure Start website – http://www.surestart.co.uk

Having worked within Sure Start, I have observed the impact that a positive approach to parenting can have on families. The aim is to steer parents away from some of the more negative approaches to parenting and replace these with a more positive approach. Closer bonds between parents and their children were indeed evident.

Conclusion

This chapter has explored positive parenting. It has outlined what positive parenting is, and how it can be used with families to help them parent their children in a positive way. Some of the techniques of positive parenting have been outlined, such as those used by Sutton (2000). The chapter has also provided insights into how Sure Start is helping families to be more positive in the parenting of their children.

Parenting programmes designed to help parents bring up their children are developing around the country. However, there is a need for more such programmes, especially for families who have children over the age of 5 years, where there is sometimes less obvious support available. The Government is becoming more aware of the need to support parents with older children. Parenting programmes can help to spread the word of positive parenting, helping children to feel emotionally secure through the close relationship they develop with their parents, as the NSF advocates (Education and Skills, Department of Health, 2004).

References

Barlow, J., Kirkpatrick, S., Wood, D., Ball, M., Brown, S. (2007). *Family and Parenting Support in Sure Start Local Programmes*. London: Sure Start.

Bowlby, J. (1979) *The Making and Breaking of Affectional Bonds*. London: Tavistock.

Carvel, J. (2005) *Commission Urges Workshops for Parents on Raising Children*. London/Manchester: The Guardian.

Education and Skills (Department of) (2007) *Extended Schools*. Available at: http://www.everychildmatters.gov.uk (accessed 28 September 2007).

Education and Skills (Department of), Department of Health (2004) *National Service Framework for Children/Young People and Maternity Services*. London: Education and Skills, Department of Health.

Hall, D. (1996) (ed.) *Health for All Children*, 3rd edn. Oxford: Oxford University Press.

Hall, D., Elliman, D. (2003) (ed.) *Health for All Children*, 4th edn. Oxford: Oxford University Press.

Kurtz, Z. (2004) *What Works in Promoting Children's Mental Health: The Evidence and the Implications for Sure Start Settings*. London: Sure Start.

Moyse, K. (1999) Positive parenting: the role of the children's nurse. *Paediatric Nursing* 11(4): 9–10.

Oxford Concise Dictionary of Current English (1982). London: Guild Publishing.

Rutter, M. (1981) *Maternal Deprivation Reassessed*. Middlesex: Penguin.

Sure Start (2007) *Sure Start Evaluations*. Available at: http://www.surestart.gov.uk (accessed 28 September 2007).

Sutton, C. (2000) *Helping Families with Troubled Children, A Preventive Approach*. Chichester: John Wiley & Sons.

Toynbee, P. (2005) *We Must Hold Our Nerve and Support Deprived Children*. The Guardian. London/Manchester: The Guardian Unlimited.

Triple P (Positive Parenting Program) (2003) *Triple P News*. Milton: Triple P.

Webster-Stratton, C., Herbert, M. (2000) *Troubled Families, Problem Children*. Chichester: John Wiley & Sons.

31 Promoting Children's Mental Health – Focus Bullying

Karen Moyse

Introduction

Middle-years children (children from 5/6 years, through to 10/11 years) can be delightful, happy children. Unfortunately, sometimes there are events that can spoil their childhood for them. Bullying, the focus of this chapter, sadly is one of them.

Childhood should be a time of being creative, a sense of being loved by the family, having fun with friends. One would be naïve to think that this is the way for all children. For some this is a very different picture to the life they experience on a daily basis. Friends are so important to children (Cole et al., 2005). Yet, so-called friends can sometimes be the cause of much pain, especially if they are bullies.

This chapter provides a snapshot inside one mental health promotion issue for children – *bullying*. There are many mental health promotion issues that the chapter could have focused on, but bullying appeared to be the issue that was of real concern for many children and their parents/carers, particularly in the 6- to 11-year age group. Undoubtedly for adolescents (11+ years) too, bullying can cause difficulties. Some of the issues discussed here may have relevance for adolescents, particularly *cyberbullying*.

The chapter examines the issue of bullying; looking at the unhappiness that it can cause for some children, current health promotion campaigns, and particularly how nurses can help to support children. In addition, this chapter considers the issue of bulling in relation to e-communications, better known as cyberbullying. E-communications have become so much part of our lives, particularly with the younger generation. Often we see them on their mobile phones, chatting to each other or communicating via the internet. A very contemporary way of communicating, but it can leave them vulnerable to receiving undesirable communications. Protecting children/young people from these undesirable communications is an issue that nurses need to consider.

Bullying – some facts

What is bullying?

Being ridiculed, name-calling, are all part of being bullied (Tassoni, 2007). Bullying can also include social exclusion (Elkin, 1998), being left out of group activities. These actions are bound to cause unhappiness for those children who experience them.

Bullying can start out as a simple chance comment which may then become more frequent, steadily escalating into repeated verbal attacks. Tassoni (2007) explains that it may be one or two children who initiate the bullying, but then other members of the group join in. The bullying may develop into a group activity, something that unites the group.

Being bullied can have a significant impact on children's emotional health, affecting how they feel about themselves. The Government's anti-bullying pack states that bullying can lead to depression, anxiety, loneliness and a lack of trust in adult life (http://www.dfes.gov.uk/bullying/pack/02.pdf). However, there are some children who might be able to ignore it, especially if the bullying is not persistent. Nonetheless, children should *not* have to tolerate being bullied. Parents/carers and nurses can help by providing children with coping strategies. For the victims of bullying, reporting it is the first important step in making events change. Girls are more likely than boys to take that first step (Tassoni, 2007).

Interestingly, a high level of bullying is reported amongst the 6- to 11-year age group (Tassoni, 2007). Bullying can start from as young as 6 years of age (Tassoni, 2007). As nurses we might find it hard to imagine that children aged 6 might be capable of bullying their peers, but sadly it does happen.

Insights into bullying

Evidence presented here looks at who might be a victim of bullying. It is also important to be conscious of where bullying is likely to occur, and who might be doing the bullying.

What makes someone a victim? It seems that any child can be vulnerable. Elkin (1998) considers anything that might make a child slightly different from the others; size, shape, culture, ability can make a child vulnerable. It can even be something as trivial as hair colour (Elkin, 1998).

There are children with certain *personality types* which make them more vulnerable to bullying. Tassoni (2007) says these are children who may be anxious, passive, and already have a low opinion of themselves. The mental health of these children takes a further battering, due to the bullying they receive.

There are a number of other children who may find themselves at risk. Bullies apparently target children who are frequently *alone* (Tassoni, 2007). The lone child is outnumbered and therefore easy prey for the bully. Children from different *cultures* may find themselves at risk too. As Braganza (2001) discusses, Asian girls in some communities feel quite susceptible to being bullied.

Children from the most disadvantaged communities are apparently more likely to experience mental health problems than other social classes (http://www.ons.gov.uk). Bullying might be one issue which contributes to the mental health of these children.

Where does bullying commonly occur? School is obviously a very common location. Elkin (1998) believes that it occurs on the way to and from school, in the classroom and even in the school toilets. Not forgetting, as the Government's anti-bullying pack highlights, it commonly happens in the playground too (http://www.dfes.gov.uk/bullying/pack/02.pdf). Children would probably say that these are the places where they feel most vulnerable.

Who bullies? Most of the evidence so far presented has pointed to other children being the instigators of bullying. However, it is important to remember that it is not only children who cause the problem; adults are capable of bullying children too. *ChildLine*, a confidential helpline for children, provides accounts of children who have experienced bullying by adults, such as teachers and even family members. Unfortunately, in some cases, the behaviour of these adults has gone on to influence the behaviour of other children, who start to bully the victim as well (http://www.childline.org.uk).

Psychological factors

As parents/carers it pains us to see or to be aware of bullying when it happens to children, particularly our own children. When they are young, children will happily share information about what is happening to them at school and other places. However, Tassoni (2007) states, as children become older they are less willing to share information about what is happening in their lives. This may be the time when disturbing events such as bullying are likely to occur. Yet sadly, parents/carers may be completely unaware that it is happening to their child.

Children may decide not to communicate information about being bullied to their parents/carers for a variety of reasons. One theory put forward is that children might blame themselves; the bullying is my own fault. Offler (2000) maintains that the victims of bullying sometimes believe this, which only serves to lower their self-esteem still further. Low self-esteem consists of dissatisfied and negative feelings about oneself (Cole et al., 2005).

Bullying can often have short-lived consequences. However, in some cases as research has established, it can have long-term consequences; severely impacting upon the lives of children, affecting their mental health. The family can have an important influence on how children react to it. Cole et al. (2005) point out that family life can provide an important foundation, which acts as a kind of buffer to the trials that children experience. Perhaps family life equips some children with the ability to fend off events which cause emotional stress.

How to pick up the signs of bullying

Signs of bullying can be observed. Parents/carers, as well as teachers and nurses, need to observe for changes in appearance and behaviour which may highlight that a child is being bullied. This is important especially if we consider that some children are unlikely to indicate themselves that bullying is an issue.

The signs to look out for, which help identify if a child is being bullied, may include some of the following:

- Unkempt appearance.
- Marked changes in behaviour.
- The child not wanting to attend school or a particular activity.
- Bed wetting, nightmares, difficulty going to bed.
- Cuts, bruises, minor injuries, which the child is unwilling to talk about.
- Items belonging to the child go missing.

Once bullying has been recognised or the child tells someone about it, discussions should be undertaken with care. Tassoni (2007) recommends that it should be talked about extremely sensitively. Three important steps to follow, certainly for parents/cares, include the following:

- Listening to the child.
- Telling the child that you care about them.
- Talking about where the child might be able to get help.

It is essential to provide the child with information on what to do when the bullying is actually happening. The anti-bullying pack (http://www.dfes.gov.uk/bullying/pack/02.pdf) advises that a child should do the following:

- Try to stay calm, and look confident.
- Be firm and clear, look the bullies in the eye and tell them to stop.
- Get away from the situation as quickly as possible.
- Tell an adult what has happened straightaway.

After the bullying incident has occurred, the pack recommends that a child should do the following (http://www.dfes.gov.uk/bullying/pack/02.pdf):

- Tell a teacher or another adult.
- Tell parents/carers.
- Keep speaking until someone listens.
- Use the school peer support service.
- Don't let the child blame herself/himself for what has happened.

Children need to know that they are loved and cared about. Children sometimes blame themselves, but they have no need to feel they are at fault. The psychological approach taken by loved ones and nurses can make a significant difference to how children feel about the bullying experiences they have been through.

Campaigns and strategies

There are a variety of places where further information can be sought on how to deal with bullying, as well as education that can help to prevent it. This section outlines some of these sources. Details on Government strategies are included.

Government strategies

The NSF advises strengthening children's awareness of emotional health, including tackling bullying (Education and Skills, Department of Health, 2004). School is viewed as a place where anti-bullying education can be addressed. School nurses can become involved, supporting children and the school.

Schools are aware that bullying is an issue that they need to tackle. In recent years some schools have made considerable efforts to put in place initiatives to help tackle bullying. The Government too has taken significant steps, supporting schools in their efforts. The NSF outlines how schools should approach mental health issues, with bullying highlighted as a priority area for action (Education and Skills, Department of Health, 2004).

The NSF states that children's mental health needs to be promoted in a structured way, using guidance – *DfES Guidance Promoting Children's Mental Health in Early Years and School Settings* (http://www.dfes.gov.uk/mentalhealth/pdfs/childrens-mentalhealth.pdf).

The Government's anti-bullying pack for use by practitioners – *Bullying, Don't Suffer in Silence* (http://www.dfes.gov.uk/bullying/pack/02.pdf) – is an essential resource. The pack has been complied from a wide body of recent research evidence.

The following list outlines some of the details contained in this very useful pack:

- It discusses issues such as the importance of school policy. Raising awareness and the need for consultation in the development of policy is recommended. The policy needs to be monitored to ensure that it is effective. It should be reviewed at least once every school year.
- Strategies should be in place to deal with incidents of bulling. Schools need to have effective recording systems, which include an incident book containing the name of the bully. Schools also need to listen carefully and provide opportunities for children to express their views. A multi-agency approach should be taken by schools. They also need to involve parents/carers.
- Working with parents/carers is essential. In most cases they will simply want the bullying to stop, but others may want the bully punished.
- Peer mediation can be used to resolve conflicts between children. Mediation by peers is in a structured way – a neutral person to help resolve disputes.
- The pack also recommends theatre-in-education groups to raise awareness and find solutions. Role-play in dealing with taunts can be enlightening to all.
- Raising awareness through use of a range of resources such as books, videos, DVDs can help too.

- Making classroom activities sensitive to the needs of others, as well as peer mentoring for children with disabilities who may be more vulnerable, can help raise children's awareness about the needs of their peers.
- Encouraging children to say positive things about one another, and particularly promoting this from an early age in school, for example, from the age of 5.
- Developing a playground policy – this will help children beyond the classroom. Training supervisors to recognise and help those children at risk of being bullying.
- The pack also provides details about a range of different resources that can be used.

The pack is a really helpful resource in itself, as evidenced from the summary provided.

Health promotion unit

Health promotion literature is also available through local health promotion resource centres. They will be able to provide teaching packs, books, as well as relevant leaflets. Teaching packs relevant to the school curriculum may also be obtained, which include information on bullying.

ChildLine

ChildLine is a confidential helpline for children/young people. Provide children with this number if they are finding it difficult to talk to people about being bullied.

Freephone 0800 1111

Children can also write to -

Freepost 1111
London, N1 OBR

ChildLine produces leaflets for children and parents/carers on bullying. ChildLine is a service provided by the NSPCC.

Kidscape

Kidscape is a charity organisation which aims to prevent bullying and child abuse. Kidscape has a wide range of publications available, particularly for children. Resources can be accessed via their website – http://www.kidscape.com/. It provides a telephone helpline service too.

Parentline Plus

Parentline Plus is a national helpline for parents/carers – 0808 800 2222. It produces resources too, and can be accessed via http://www.parentlineplus.org.uk

Anti-bullying alliance

The alliance is funded by the Government's Education and Skills department. The alliance organises anti-bullying week, which is held in November each year. Look out for special programmes on CBBC (Children's BBC) during anti-bullying week. The alliance can be reached via http://www.anti-bullyingalliance.org.uk.

Reading

Reading may also be a useful resource for children. Elkin (1998) highlights that if children read stories about fictional characters who have been bullied, this may help them. They can sit reflect upon their own feelings, and perhaps realise that other children have felt the same. Children can learn that bullying is not uncommon, and that they can develop strengths to deal with it, as others have done. Reading helps children reflect upon their own coping skills. Ask your local bookshop and see what they can suggest.

There are books and resources that are recommended for parents/carers too:

- *Preventing Bullying! A Parents' Guide* by Kidscape (2001).

Reading helps promote cognitive strategies and more positive feelings about what is possible.

What can nurses do to help in practice?

Nurses have an important role in the promotion of children's health and safeguarding their interests. The Nursing and Midwifery Council (NMC, 2004) believes that nurses should protect and promote the health of those in their care – children. Health promotion on protecting children from bullying falls within this remit.

Similar to any area of practice that affects children, nurses working with them need to educate themselves, find out what the literature says. Nurses need to be aware of the signs of bullying and what they can do to support children and their families.

Offler (2000) discusses two important areas to consider, *communication* and *liaison* in relation to practice. Nurses are good communicators and can sensitively support children who have been bullied. *Every Child Matters* highlights that there are many different sorts of mental health problems, but it often takes sensitivity and skill to even notice that a problem exists (Education and Skills, 2003). Nurses have that sensitivity.

Do not assume that as the nurse involved you are responsible for everything. There are other appropriate personnel who you need to liaise with about the situation. Offler (2000) discusses the importance of liaising with other members of the team. In the community this might include school nurses and teachers. In hospital youth workers and family therapists may be able to help. Parents/carers are obviously part of that team and should be involved. In more serious cases, CAMHS (Child and Adolescent Mental Health Services) may need to be contacted.

Nurses working with children in schools will not be the only nurses that come across bullying. Nurses working with sick and disabled children, both in hospital and community settings, may find that bullying is an issue for those in their care. Children, because of their health problem or disability, may be seen as different, thus making them more vulnerable to being bullied. Besag (1989) has highlighted that children with chronic health issues or disabilities may be more at risk to bullying. Be aware, as previously highlighted, that those children in our care may try to hide their difficulties, in an effort to disguise themselves as being different (Cross, 1998).

Importantly, consider their siblings too; they may find themselves vulnerable to bullying. Siblings may try to hide the fact they are being bullied. They may feel that the family have enough to do caring for their disabled brother or sister. Siblings may not want to add to family concerns.

Whatever context a nurse is working in with children, she/he may come across bullying. Be prepared, as the problem may not be identified by the others.

There are a number of different things that nurses can do to help the victims of bullying. The list below may help:

- Listen to children.
- Observe for signs of bullying.
- Supporting children and guide them in the right direction for help.
- Help children to build their confidence back up again, through praise and encouragement.
- Ensure that those who need to know are made aware of the bullying.
- Help the school develop its policies on anti-bulling.
- Raise awareness of anti-bullying through group teaching sessions and individual work with children. Discuss rights and wrongs, and respecting others.

Nurses have a range of skills that they can use to help a child who is being bullied. As Offler (2000) highlights communication and liaison are essential skills. Nurses may have that special know-how to actually identify that a child is the victim of bullying.

A critical point to consider

Nurses are not always that familiar with the issue of bullying. Nurses need to be aware that bullying is a health promotion issue that is relevant to their practice when working with children. Educating oneself is the first important step to making things better for children.

Cyberbullying

In recent years e-communications have taken off in a big way. I expect many of us could not imagine getting through the day without the use of the mobile phone or internet to communicate with colleagues, clients and the search for information.

In discussion with Emily (12 years old) and her friends recently, mobile phones and computers were highlighted as some of the most impor-

tant things they owned. Young people are especially keen on the use of their mobile phones. Texting has become a really crucial way for them to communicate with one another. Young people have developed their own text language, which some of us might have difficulty deciphering that language.

Bullying through the use of text messages and e-mails can involve the sending messages and images which are unwelcome and can cause young people much distress. This comes under the heading of cyberbullying, which involves the sending of texts and images via phones, e-mails and the internet (http://www.teachernet.gov.uk).

Safe use

It is crucial that young people, if they are going to use mobiles and the internet, they do so safely – http://www.teachernet.gov.uk (Be aware that there are some health concerns about children using mobile phones.)

As nurses when undertaking health promotion activities, we may encourage young people to use the internet, for example, to search out information. In doing so it is essential that we encourage safe use. There are dangers as the *Teachernet* website highlights; children need to be vigilant to forms of bullying, and not to misuse these forms of communication themselves (http://www.teachernet.gov.uk). Misuse can have serious consequences, not only for the victims but for the instigators of bullying too.

Stoptextbullying is a website which children and their parents/carers, along with teachers, can access for advice on how to deal with text bullying (http://www.stoptextbullying.com). The importance of keeping records of bullying incidents is stressed.

The Government has recently launched a campaign on raising the awareness of cyberbullying – September 2007. Details of this campaign can be found on the Teachernet website (http://www.teachernet.gov.uk). The website provides some very useful information for families and schools, some of which is outlined below:

- Provide advice to children/young people on cyberbullying.

- Provide advice to parents/carers on cyberbullying.
- Support for the person being bullied.
- Reporting cyberbullying.
- Investigation.
- Working with the bully and applying sanctions.
- School policies.

A very useful leaflet is also produced – *Cyberbullying, a Whole School Approach* (Department for Children, Schools, and Families, 2007).

Some essential advice for young people is given on what to do if they are the victim of cyberbullying:

- Never reply.
- Save the messages.
- Let someone else know about it.

For parents it might be useful to consider keeping home computers in a place where they can see if there is something wrong.

The Government advises that when young people are using mobile phones and the internet themselves, they need to carefully consider what they are sending to others. Importantly, respecting others is essential (http://www.teachernet.gov.uk).

Interestingly, the bullies think they are anonymous, but apparently not so. There is software available that will enable the bullies to be identified.

Cyberbullying is much more common than we might think. Nurse can do much to raise awareness about what children young people can do if they experience cyberbullying.

Safe use in practice

Having considered the negative side of e-communications, it is useful to consider its positive side too, in relation to promoting health. The Royal College of Nursing (RCN, 2006) has produced some very useful guidelines on the use of text messaging for nurses. The RCN (2006) believes that text messages can help signpost young people to health services. This might include a nurse reminding a young person about a health appointment at school, for example.

The RCN (2006) stresses that in using this form of communication, nurses must always remember client's confidentiality, as highlighted in the Nursing Midwifery Council (NMC, 2004) code of conduct. Messages need to be deleted from the mobile phone to maintain high standards of confidentiality, thus protecting clients. All messages should also be documented, in line with NMC guidelines on record keeping. Essentially, before introducing a text messaging service for young people, like any new service, potential users need to be made aware of its existence.

The NMC (2007) guidelines on record keeping have recently been updated and can be accessed via the website – http://www.nmc-uk.org

Conclusion

This chapter has provided details on how nurses can help support children that are being bullied. Details have been provided on health promotion campaigns, as well as Government strategies. How bullying can make a child feel has importantly been discussed. Recent information on the latest form of bullying, cyberbullying, has been presented.

Supporting children's and young people's mental health, so they can continue to enjoy their lives and feel good about themselves, is something positive we can do for those in our care. There are a range of resources that nurses can access, as this chapter has outlined. As a nurse be prepared; children/young people being bullied is an issue that you are likely to meet in practice. Nurses have sensitive communication skills, use those skills to support children's/young people's emotional health; allow them to discuss their concerns. Nurses can support parents/carers too, by guiding them on what they can do to support children/young people.

Resources

Anti-Bullying Week 2006 – National Strategies Update – http://www.anti-bullyingalliance.org.uk (accessed November 2006).

Working Towards a Bully-free zone – http://www.childline.org.uk (accessed 14 August 2007).

Anti-bullying Pack – Bullying, Don't Suffer in Silence. London: Education and Skills – http://www.dfes.gov.uk/bullying/pack/02.pdf (accessed 14 August 2007).

Promoting Children's Mental Health within Early Years and School Settings. London: TeacherNet, Department for Children, Schools and Families – http://www.dfes.gov.uk/mentalhealth/pdfs/childrensmentalhealth.pdf (accessed 14 August 2007).

Kidscape – Resources – http://www.kidscape.com/ (accessed 14 August 2007).

Surveys between 1999 and 2004 on Children's Health – http://www.ons.gov.uk (accessed July 2007).

Bullying – http://www.parentlineplus.org.uk (accessed 28 September 2007).

What Is Cyberbullying? – http://www.teachernet.gov.uk (accessed 20 August 2007).

Parenting Resources – http://www.stoptextbullying.com (accessed October 2007).

Cyberbullying – http://www.teachnet.gov.uk (accessed 28 September 2007).

References

Besag, V. (1989) *Bullies and Victims in School*. Milton Keynes: Open University Press.

Braganza, J. (2001) Attempted suicide by Bangladeshi adolescent girls. *Paediatric Nursing* 13(2): 26–29.

Cole, M., Cole, S., Lightfoot, C. (2005) *The Development of Children*, 5th edn. New York: Worth Publishers.

Cross, S. (1998) Sick children risk bullying by classmates. *Community Practitioner* 71(7/8): 235.

Department for Children, Schools, and Families (2007) *Cyberbullying, a Whole School Approach*. London: Crown Copyright.

Education and Skills (Department of) (2003) *Every Child Matters*. London: Crown Copyright.

Education and Skills (Department of), Department of Health (2004) *National Service Framework for Children, Young People and Maternity Services*. London: Crown Copyright.

Elkin, S. (1998) How to grab the bully by the book. *The Times*, 30 October.

Kidscape (2001) *Preventing Bullying! A Parents' Guide*. London: Kidscape.

Nursing and Midwifery Council (NMC) (2004) *The Code of Conduct, Professional Standards for Nurses and Midwives*. London: NMC.

Nursing and Midwifery Council (NMC) (2007) *Record Keeping*. London: NMC. Available at: http://www.nmc-uk.org (accessed September 2007).

Offler, E. (2000) Bullying: everybody's problem. *Paediatric Nursing* 12(9): 22–26.

Royal College of Nursing (RCN) (2006) *Use of Text Messaging Services*. London: Royal College of Nursing.

Tassoni, P. (2007) *Child Development 6–16 Years*. Oxford: Heinemann.

32 Safeguarding Children (Health Promotion)

Karen Moyse

NSF

The National Service Framework (NSF) for children, young people and maternity services, standard 5 (Education and Skills, Department of Health, 2004), sets the standard for health and social care practitioners to help prevent children suffering harm and to promote their well-being.

Introduction

Health promotion campaigns can focus on the protection or safeguarding of children, as well as the more usual health promotion issues nurses would expect. Safeguarding children has been high on the Government agenda in recent years, particularly since the publication of the Laming (2003) Inquiry, *Every Child Matters* (Education and Skills, 2003), the new Children Act (2004), and more recently with the publication of *Working Together to Safeguard Children* (Education and Skills, 2006a). There are also a number of other documents that the Government has produced, which focus on safeguarding children. (A summary of these documents can be found on the internet at various sites by using keywords such as *safeguarding children*.)

Changes in practice have occurred since the publication of these documents and with the advent of the new Children Act (2004). Some of the key changes include the creation of Children's Trusts, the setting up of local Safeguarding Boards for children, and the duty on all agencies to make arrangements to safeguard as well as promote the welfare of children (Education and Skills, 2006a). The importance of joint working between agencies has been particularly stressed. In line with joint working, information sharing between agencies is fundamental. Guidance has been produced on the appropriate sharing of information between agencies – *Information Sharing: Practitioners' Guide* (Education and Skills, 2006b).

Lots of new information and guidelines, however campaigns for change continue. With this in mind the chapter looks at two issues:

- Corporal punishment as a form of discipline.
- A campaign to bring about change – change in how we discipline our children.

This chapter is looking at the issue of *reasonable punishment* (the physical punishment of a child by a parent/carer). Positive parenting has become very important in recent years, being positive with children, yet setting clear guidelines. The idea of reasonable punishment does not fit well with all practitioners. The Government is looking at this issue again.

Corporal punishment

Positive parenting is about being positive with our children, and also avoiding negative approaches to parenting. The United Kingdom (UK) has a long history of corporal punishment. Positive parenting tries to steer families away from corporal punishment. Corporal punishment can be the deliberate infliction of pain by an adult upon a child (Leach, 1993). In addition to the physical consequences, there are the emotional consequences; a child living with the fear of being physically punished.

Hitting and smacking are disapproved of in the relationship between one adult and another, but not in the relationship between parents/carers and their children. Children are usually much more vulnerable than adults, smaller in size and younger in age, yet it is permissible to give them a smack.

The history of corporal punishment in the UK, in part, stems from the class issue which was so dominant in centuries past. As outlined in *The Observer* (2003), Britain's class system was used to legitimise corporal punishment; masters were allowed to hit their servants.

In the past, corporal punishment was acceptable within schools. It was not outlawed until 1987 (Hollingshead, 2005). Independent schools did not fall into line until more recently – 1999 (Hollingshead, 2005).

Smacking in the home was not questioned until quite recently. Newson and Newson's (1989) research, undertaken in the East Midlands, demonstrated that during the 1980s many parents/carers used corporal punishment to reprimand their children at home. In some cases children as young as 1 year of age were being smacked. Seven hundred families were included in the Newson and Newson's (1989) research. At 1 year of age, two-thirds of a 1985 sample of babies had already been smacked. A 1-year-old cannot clearly tell right from wrong, so what purpose would a smack have?

In addition, the Newsons found that as children grew older smacking became more severe, particularly where families found that their initial light smacks were no longer effective. Implements also started to be used.

The way the UK has approached childcare over the generations is interesting to explore, and provides some insights into the attitude changes to parenting that are emerging. The Victorians did not approach childcare in the way that we do today. In comparison to Victorian times, we seem to treasure our children much more, as positive approaches to parenting prove more favourable and rewarding.

The Victorians were quite different. Many children were exploited as child labourers (de Mauser, 1974). Corporal punishment was also the norm. Forms of punishment at the time included prolonged isolation, beatings and whippings (de Mauser, 1974), which would horrify us today. Children would not always survive due to the appalling conditions in which they lived and worked.

However, the Victorian era was significant; the beginnings of change for children started to emerge. Concern started to mount for the welfare of children. Legislation was introduced to protect children from cruelty (de Mauser, 1974).

Brooks (2006) states that during the 1920/1930s the approach to childcare was different again; behaviourist approaches were adopted. One significant name to emerge at this time was the behaviourist – John B. Watson. He believed that behaviours needed to be habit forming; feeding and sleeping should all be regimented routines for the young (Brooks, 2006). Disappointingly, Watson also believed that parents should not be encouraged to cuddle their children (Shipman, 1972).

Child-centric care however started to come to the fore during the 1940s, through the work of Benjamin Spock. Spock felt that it was appropriate for mothers to enjoy their children (Shipman, 1972). During the 1950s the work of Bowlby came to prominence. Bowlby (1953) stressed the importance of mothers spending time with their children during the early years. More recently there has been the work of Penelope Leach (Brooks, 2006). Leach (1993) has strongly advocated positive parenting, with no corporal punishment.

A real landmark in the UK for examining the needs of children can be witnessed through the advent of the Children Act (1989). This was recently updated with the Children Act (2004).

Today we live in an era where positive approaches to parenting are advocated, and there is much more understanding about the needs of children. Importantly, there are the NSFs for children/young people (Education and Skills, Department of Health, 2004), along with *Every Child*

Matters (Education and Skills, 2003), promoting the physical and emotional welfare of children. The Children Act (2004) providing the legal framework for *Every Child Matters* (Education and Skills, 2003). The welfare of children is considered paramount. However, the debate over corporal punishment still continues.

Sweden, along with a number of other European countries, banned smacking (Leach, 1993). Other countries are considering placing limits on parents/carers physically correcting their children.

Currently, here in the UK mixed views exist about how we should progress – whether or not to introduce a ban on children being smacked by parents/carers. Some people feel that parents/carers should be allowed to smack their children, whilst others advocate an outright ban, and actively campaign for its rapid introduction.

With the advent of the new Children Act (2004), however, there have been some legislative changes. Legislation has been introduced which places restrictions on parents/carers smacking their children. Rather than implementing an outright ban on smacking, the Government has taken the middle ground, considering the different perspectives that exist on both sides of the debate.

The legislation states that parents/carers who smack their children so hard that it leaves a mark will face imprisonment. The imprisonment could be for a maximum of 5 years. Parents/carers are allowed to give their children a mild smack as a reprimand. However, any punishment which causes bruising, grazes, scratches, minor swelling or cuts will face action (http://www.news.bbc.co.uk; British Broadcasting Corporation, 2005). These legislative changes were introduced at different stages within the four countries of the UK.

So it would seem that parents/carers continue to have the right to administer a light smack. Hollingshead (2005) writes in *The Guardian* that apparently this caused outrage during a debate on the matter in parliament. Traditionalists, he outlines, resent increasing Government interference in family life. However, organisations such as the National Society for the Prevention of Cruelty to Children would welcome an outright ban on smacking.

An article by Rosemary Bennett, Social Affairs Correspondent in *The Times* (Bennett, 2006), revealed in a recent survey that an outright ban on smacking is still not what the majority of parents/carers want in the UK. Bennett (2006) found that seven out of ten parents smacked their children. The same parents would also strongly resist any move to ban smacking in the home. Further, the parents believed that a ban on smacking would lead to a sharp deterioration in their children's behaviour (Bennett, 2006).

It would be interesting to know more about the basis on which these parents formed their views. What impact, I wonder would it have, if these same parents actually no longer smacked their children? Would their children's behaviour deteriorate or actually improve? Would the relationship between children and parents be different? It would be interesting to observe.

There are many practitioners and children's organisations who feel that an outright ban would be appropriate. Sir Al Aynsley-Green, the Children's Commissioner for England, has said that he intends as a priority of his post to ban smacking (Brooks, 2006). Sir Michael Rutter has also called for a ban on smacking children (Carvel, 2005). Along with children's organisations such as the NSPPCC, Barnardos, and Save the Children, who are all calling for a ban on smacking.

Children are at the centre of these discussions about corporal punishment. I wonder what their views are. They are the ones that are receiving the smacks. How do they feel about it? As Brooks (2006) states, children have the right to be consulted about matters affecting their lives. Surely, smacking should be one of these issues.

It would seem that British legislation is moving on, albeit in a slow but somewhat more promising direction. Perhaps, when there is a greater body of opinion which supports a ban on smacking, the law may then follow in supporting a ban. However, perhaps if the converse were true; the law actually changed, public opinion may then follow. In Sweden, the change in law actually seemed to be influential in altering public opinion that smacking children was not appropriate. Durrant (2000), in a report which discusses the Swedish experience on banning smacking, maintains that the ban along with ongoing educational campaigns appeared to be very effective in altering the social climate on corporal punishment. Maybe this is the approach the UK should take.

Changes on how we discipline our children

Nurses know that it is important to be positive with children. Many nurses work hard to spread the message of positive parenting. There is still much to be achieved, particularly in relation to the way children are disciplined.

Children can develop well with encouragement and support from their parents/carers. It is also essential that parents/carers are fair and consistent with their children, setting clear boundaries and maintaining them. Children should be encouraged to learn what behaviours are acceptable, and those that are not. The Government maintains that failing to set clear boundaries can be neglectful of children's needs (Department of Health, 2000a).

Anyone who is a parent/carer will know that it can be difficult to be consistent with children all of the time. A little advice can sometimes be useful. For some parents/carers trying to be fair with their children can be very challenging, setting clear boundaries while *not* being too harsh. Help and support may well be needed. Community nurses, such as health visitors and school nurses, are certainly well placed to provide initial guidance. They can advise on behaviour management strategies, for example. Community nurses will also know what services exist in the local area, such as the details of parenting classes, which may help.

The Department of Health (2000a) asserts that discipline which is harsh can be damaging both physically and emotionally to children (Department of Health, 2000a). The issue of physical punishment to children by parents/carers is one that has caused much debate, particularly in recent years. It is something that many practitioners working with children feel is *not* appropriate.

The Government reviewed the position on parents/carers physically punishing their children in 2000. A consultation was launched (Department of Health, 2000a). The document, *Protecting Children, Supporting Parents*, wanted to know the views of parents/carers, as well as professional organisations involved in the care of children.

The consultation came about due to a change in the law arising from the European Court of Human Rights ruling on *reasonable chastisement* – the physical punishment of a child by a parent (http://www.intute.ac.uk/socialsciences).

Many responses were received through the consultation process in England and Wales, over 900 in fact (http://www.dh.gov.uk).

The consultation at that time (Department of Health, 2000b) revealed that the majority of people who responded felt reasonable chastisement should continue. However, all the children's organisations that responded were in favour of a ban (http://www.dh.gov.uk/en/Publicationsandstatistics). The results highlighted that attitudes were beginning to change, although not the dramatic change in opinion that some practitioners wanted.

Following the consultation process, the Human Rights Act (1989) came into force in 2000. The courts have to consider several factors when deciding whether punishment amounts to reasonable chastisement, which include its emotional and physical affects on the child (http://www.dh.gov.uk/en/Publicationsandstatistics).

The new Children Act (2004) came into effect in 2005, bringing about change. Section 58 of the Children Act (2004) maintained that it was essential to strengthen the system for safeguarding children. The Act said it would be unacceptable to criminalise all physical punishment of a child by a parent. However, Section 58 removed the defence of reasonable chastisement for acts that caused children actual bodily harm, grievous bodily harm and cruelty (Education and Skills 2007; section58.consultation@dfes.gsi.gov.uk).

At the time the Government said it would review Section 58 two years hence, to find out the practical consequences of reasonable chastisement/punishment. In parliament there were concerns about the practical implications of these changes to the law, and how they would operate. The Government particularly wanted to know if the actual changes in law had helped to improve the legal protection of children. It was also felt that parents/carers attitudes towards smacking could be looked at again, at the same time (section58.consultation@dfes.gsi.gov.uk).

In June 2007 the Government commenced its review. The Department for Education and Skills invited responses once more on both the impact of the law, along with attitudes towards smacking. The Government is due to report over the coming months (at the time of writing).

A new campaign was recently launched responding to the view of reasonable punishment – The

Children Are Unbeatable Alliance. The Alliance (2007) believes that it is unjust to try to define acceptable ways of hitting children. They believe that smacking, slapping or any physical punishment is violent behaviour towards children. Adults would not find it acceptable for another adult to hit them (it is against the law anyway). Why is it acceptable for children? The Alliance (2007) is not trying to recommend a change in law but is trying to recommend a change in practice.

The Alliance (2007) makes the point that reasonable punishment sends out a dangerous message about the acceptability of violence. Importantly, the Alliance (2007) maintains in their view that Section 58 undermines child protection, and the promotion of positive discipline.

Although an outright ban was not put in place when the law changed in 2005, some changes to the law however did take place, something that might not have happened a few decades earlier, when views were very much in favour of physical punishment. Progress is moving forward, albeit slowly. It will be interesting to see what the results of this consultation process yield, and if in years to come there are further changes with regard to the law and practice on physical punishment.

The consultation process is now closed. The results from the consultation process are due to report shortly (at the time of writing). Look on the Education and Skills website for the results of this consultation.

Activities

- Look into the debate about introducing a ban on smacking. See what you can find out, and observe its progress.
- Promoting the safety of children is part of the role of every nurse who works with children. There are local procedures that all nurses *must* follow. Search these out, read what they say, ask colleagues questions on issues you do not fully understand. Your local Safeguarding Children department will also be able to help with advice. The Royal College of Nursing (RCN, 2004) also provides guidance on protecting children.

Conclusion

The campaign by the Alliance (2007) provides an example of a health promotion campaign which is trying to protect children and encourage parents/carers to be positive in their parenting. The campaign is trying to protect both the physical and emotional health of children.

The chapter has looked at a health promotion campaign aimed at safeguarding children. Key documents on the issue of safeguarding children/young people have been highlighted. The issue of reasonable punishment/chastisement has been discussed, as well as providing some details on the background to corporal punishment in the UK. It will be interesting to see in the years to come if practice and the law do change in relation to reasonable punishment/chastisement – a ban may one day happen. Observe the debate, as it will undoubtedly continue.

Resources

http://www.dh.gov.uk/en/Publicationsandstatistics/Pressreleases/DH_4011482 (accessed 20 August 2007).
http://www.direct.gov.uk/ (accessed January 2008).
http://www.intute.ac.uk/socialsciences – Note on protecting children, supporting parents (accessed 20 August 2007).

References

Alliance (2007) *Responding to the Review of Reasonable Punishment*. London: The Children Are Unbeatable Alliance.

Bennett, R. (2006) Majority of parents admit to smacking children. *The Times*. London: Times Newspaper Ltd.

Bowlby, J. (1953) *Child Care and the Growth of Love*. Harmondsworth: Penguin.

British Broadcasting Corporation (2005) *New Smacking Law Comes into Force*. London: BBC. Available at: http://www.newsbbc.co.uk (accessed 10 October 2006).

Brooks, L. (2006) *The Story of Childhood, Growing up in Modern Britain*. London: Bloomsbury.

Carvel, J. (2005) Commission urges workshops for parents on raising children. *The Guardian*. London/Manchester: Guardian Unlimited. Available at: http://www.guardian.co.uk.

Children Act (1989) London: HMSO.

Children Act (2004) London: Crown Copyright.

de Mauser, L. (ed.) (1974) *The History of Childhood*. London: The Psychohistory Press.

Department of Health (2000a) *Protecting Children, Supporting Parents. A Consultation Document on the Physical Punishment of Children*. London: Department of Health.

Department of Health (2000b) *Protecting Children, Supporting Parents: Responses to the Consultation on Physical Punishment of Children*. Available at: http://www.dh.gov.uk (accessed 20 August 2007).

Durrant, J. (2000) *A Generation without Smacking: The Impact of Sweden's Ban on Physical Punishment*. London: Save the Children.

Education and Skills (Department of) (2003) *Every Child Matters*. London: Education and Skills.

Education and Skills (Department of) (2006a) *Working Together to Safeguard Children. A Guide to Inter-Agency Working to Safeguard and Promote the Welfare of Children*. HM Government. London: Crown Copyright.

Education and Skills (Department of) (2006b) *Information Sharing: Practitioners' Guide. Integrated Working to Improve Outcomes for Children/Young People*. HM Government. London: Crown Copyright.

Education and Skills (Department of), Department of Health (2004) *National Service Framework for Children, Young People and Maternity Services. Standard 5 – Safeguarding and Promoting the Welfare of Children/Young People*. London: Education and Skills, Department of Health.

Education and Skills (Department of) (2007) *Section 58 Consultation*. Available at: section58.consultation @dfes.gsi.gov.uk (accessed 20 August 2007).

Human Rights Act (1989) London: Crown Copyright.

Hollingshead, I. (2005) Whatever happened to. . . smacking? *The Guardian*. London/Manchester: Guardian Unlimited. Available at: http://www.guardian.co.uk (accessed August 2007).

Leach, P. (1993) Should parents hit their children? *The Psychologist* 6(5): 216–220.

Laming, L. (2003) *The Victoria Climbé Inquiry. Report of an Inquiry by Lord Laming*. London: Crown Copyright.

Newson, J., Newson, E. (1989) *The Extent of Physical Punishment in the UK*. London: Approach.

Royal College of Nursing (2004) *Child Protection, Every Nurse's Responsibility*. London: Royal College of Nursing.

Shipman, M. (1972) *Childhood, a Sociological Perspective*. Windsor: NFER Publishing Company.

The Observer (2003) *History of Punishment*. 4 May 2003.

33 The Health of Children/Young People in Care

Cathy Sheehan

NSF

The National Service Framework (NSF) for children, young people and maternity services (Education and Skills, Department of Health, 2004) discusses the importance of promoting the physical and mental health needs of children/young people who are *looked after* in care. The standards with most relevance to this client group include – standard 1: promoting health and well-being; standard 4: growing up into adulthood; standard 8: disabled children, young people and those with complex needs; and standard 9: the mental health and psychological well-being of children/young people.

Introduction

Growing up fit and healthy both physically and emotionally is important if children/young people living away from home are to benefit from the care and education provided for them. Children/young people who are looked after in care are often amongst the most socially excluded of groups. In England and Wales, for example, there are some 60 900 children/young people who are in the care of the local authority. This is a decrease of less than 1% from the previous year but an increase of 3% from 2001 (Office of National Statistics, 2005).

The number of children/young people looked after could almost fill Wembley stadium. In real terms, this means that 1 in every 200 children each year experiences local authority care (in England and Wales).

Children/young people who are looked after are by definition those that are cared for by the local authority. The term *looked-after* children/young people is related to the following:

- Accommodated under a voluntary agreement with their parents' consent or own consent if aged between 16 or 17 years of age.
- In care on a care order or interim care order.
- Accommodated – remanded to local authority care.
- On an emergency protection order.

The largest placement for children/young people who are looked after is in foster care. Foster care accounts for 68% of all placements. The number of foster care placements has increased by 9% since 2001, but a gap still remains. There are too many children/young people cared for within residential units. Residential units care for approximately 15% of placements (Education and Skills, 2007). These placements may be far from children's/young people's homes or local neighbourhoods, giving rise to feelings of loneliness and alienation. In cultures of poor care the alienation of children/young people may be further reinforced by low expectations amongst staff and residents.

The health of looked-after children/young people can be challenging, as they move placements and their health records get misplaced. They sometimes refuse health assessments. Practitioners become confused over issues such as consent and confidentiality. Health is the responsibility of all. It is important that all practitioners work together to achieve robust and timely health advice and action when needed for children/young people looked after in care.

The policy context of children who are in care

The aspirations for all children/young people are outlined in the consultation document *Building a Strategy* for children/young people (Children's/Young People's Unit, 2001), which is set clearly in a context of both combating *social exclusion* and *promoting good outcomes*, including health. The hope is that children/young people will develop healthy lifestyles in a context of high-quality preventive and treatment services, if and when they need them. Children/young people should develop the ability and emotional well-being that allows them to play, learn and relate to other people (Children's/Young People's Unit, 2001).

The policy context for public services is moving rapidly, and it is an exciting time for children's policy development in the United Kingdom (UK). There have been a number of policy initiatives in recent times that have identified children/young people in care as a vulnerable client group at risk of the greatest inequalities in health, education and future opportunities. These include both Children Acts (1989, 2004), *People Like Us* (Department of Health, 1997a), *Quality Protects Programme: Transforming Children's Services* (Department of Health, 1998), *Promoting the Health of Children Looked After Children* (Department of Health, 2002), *Every Child Matters* (Education and Skills, 2003), *National Service Frameworks for Children, Young People and Maternity Services* (Education and Skills, Department of Health, 2004), *Looked After Children Strategy – Consultation* (Education and Skills, 2006), *Our Health, Our Care, Our Say* (Department of Health, 2006) and more recently *Care Matters:*

Time for Change (Education and Skills, 2007). All have highlighted the high level of health neglect, unhealthy lifestyle and emotional health needs that characterise children/young people in care.

The NSFs (Education and Skills, Department of Health, 2004) and *Every Child Matters* (Education and Skills, 2003) are both grounded in local Government policy and have set standards for all children's/young people's services. This includes children/young people in special circumstances, such as those who are in the care of the local authority. The outcomes framework of *Every Child Matters* will highlight where partnership working is making good progress and also identify gaps in service provision.

Improving the life chances of all looked-after children/young people, ensuring their safety and promoting their well-being is an essential part of delivering the agenda for *Every Child Matters* (Education and Skills, 2003). Promoting the emotional well-being as well as the physical health of this small, but very vulnerable, group of children/young people is a priority. They need to be supported to achieve good health outcomes. Planning care for vulnerable children/young people benefits from a sense of purposeful foresight, seeing each child within the long-term context of her/his growth and potential (Caan, 2004).

Why are looked-after children different? The main reason is that once they have been removed from their family of origin, looked-after children/young people become the responsibility of a capable but deeply fragmented corporate parent (Dunnett et al., 2006). This is further borne out in the literature; it suggests that the health of children/young people in local authority care is often poor in comparison to that of their peers. They experience higher levels of substance misuse (Department of Health, 1997b), significantly higher rates of teenage pregnancy (Brodie et al., 1997; Corlyon and McGuire, 1997) and a greater prevalence of mental health problems (Bramford and Welkind, 1988; Arcelus et al., 1999; Buchanan, 1999; Richardson and Joughlin, 2000).

The rate of self-harm and high-risk behaviour among those in the care setting is another indicator of poor mental and emotional well-being (Shaw, 1998). This is particularly noticeable among young people in residential care and secure accommodation.

The principle mechanism to safeguard the health of children/young people in local authority care has been the health assessment, with an appropriate health care plan. The statutory health assessment is an opportunity to assess, safeguard and promote health. Although, following examination, there is actually little systemic research evidence to recommend its quality.

The *Healthy Care Programme* provides a multi-agency framework to improve the health of looked-after children/young people in England. The Government has funded the National Children's Bureau to develop the Healthy Care Programme over 4 years. The Healthy Care Programme has been developed in response to the document – *Promoting the Health of Looked After Children* (Department of Health, 2002). A key principle identified in this guidance is the direct involvement of children, young people and their carers. The document states to be successful in improving the health outcomes of this group *partnership working*, which builds on the views of children/young people themselves, is a priority.

The Healthy Care Programme provides a practical tool. The Healthy Care framework coordinates and addresses the issues that affect the health and well-being of children/young people, especially those identified as most vulnerable. It intends to do this through partnership working. Implementing the programme will ensure that care settings will provide a healthy and caring environment, quality provision of health assessments, as well as health care and treatment.

The Healthy Care Programme provides information about the following:

- It provides a programme to promote the health and well-being of looked-after children/young people.
- The National Healthy Care Standard describes the entitlements of looked-after children/young people and the outcomes that will help to measure the progress towards achieving a healthy care environment.
- Healthy Care can help to provide evidence for inspection processes and other reviews.
- Healthy Care audits to develop and implement Healthy Care action plans. All the tools and resources are provided through the Healthy Care Programme.

As it stands currently, promoting the health of looked-after children/young people holds statutory status amongst local authorities but is non-statutory for the NHS (Department of Health, 2002). In order to promote better joint working and to remove any inconsistency in the application of the guidance, the Government will do the following:

- Re-issue the guidance paper – *Promoting the Health of Looked After Children* (Department of Health, 2002) in 2008 on a statutory footing for both local authorities and health care bodies.
- Use the statutory guidelines to strengthen protocols and agreements within NHS bodies and update regulations as necessary.
- Address the need for coordination within health care bodies to meet the needs of looked-after children/young people.

This should all help the care of children/young people who are looked after.

The role of the primary health care team

The primary care team, mainly the general practitioner, health visitor and school nurse, will provide the basic aspects of child health and development in terms of prevention and promotion for all children/young people. Children/young people who are looked after will have the same health needs as any child/teenager. Due to the nature of the child/young person having a disadvantaged early life and becoming looked after, some of this basic care may be missing, including routine immunisations and health/development checks, for example.

The primary care team has a pivotal role to play in supporting the health of looked-after children/young people. In some instances, they will provide continuity of care, providing services before, during and after the child is looked after (Dunnett et al., 2006). At times of transition, which can be numerous for some looked-after children/young people as they experience placement changes, multi-agency working becomes even more important. The role of primary care becomes especially important when children/young people are placed back within their family unit, and when young people go into aftercare/leaving care services.

The actions of local authorities and health care bodies in addressing the health of looked-after children/young people are currently informed by the NSFs (Education and Skills, Department of Health, 2004) along with the guidance paper – *Promoting the Health of Looked After Children* (Department of Health, 2002). The guidance paper sets out roles and responsibilities of local authorities and health care bodies as follows:

- To act as advocates for the health of looked-after children/young people.
- Ensure timely and sensitive access to an appropriate member of the primary care team.
- Ensure referrals to specialist services are timely to address the inequalities of looked-after children/young people.
- Maintain a record of the health assessment and contribute to any action or recommendation as the health care plan indicates.
- Ensure that case notes identify the status of the looked-after child/young person, so that her/his particular health needs can be acknowledged and addressed.
- Regularly review the clinical records and contribute information to each review of the health care plan.

The NHS is constantly evolving. This is evident in the role of health visitors and school nurses. They are already at the forefront of early detection and intervention in the physical, emotional and mental health needs of children, young people and their families. Identification of looked-after children/young people ensures that school nurses and health visitors can support their foster carers, are able to transfer case notes as necessary, and also provide an awareness of when health and developmental needs have not been met. It is vital that all these practitioners work in partnership to meet the holistic health needs of this small but very vulnerable group of children/young people, to ensure better health outcomes for them.

The health of unaccompanied asylum-seeking children

Unaccompanied asylum-seeking children are a growing number of children/young people within the looked-after population. They frequently have additional health care needs compared to the indigenous looked-after population. Asylum seekers come from all areas of the world. These children/young people can become estranged from their families en route, and have sometimes experienced harrowing journeys in their efforts to reach safety.

Unaccompanied asylum-seeking children/young people are under the age of 18 years, who are separated from both parents and have left their country of origin. They are not being cared for by an adult who by law has the responsibility to do so. They apply for recognition as a refugee and await the decision about their future. The health needs of this group are monitored by looked-after health teams, and supported by primary care teams, in the same way as other looked-after children/young people.

Important consideration about this category of looked-after children/young people is language, age assessment and their legal status. To ensure that a full and holistic health history is obtained from these children/young person, it is important that a suitable interpreter is used. For reasons of confidentiality and impartiality, the interpreter should have no previous connection with the child/young person (Leverson and Shama, 1999). Ideally for cultural reasons, the interpreter should be the same gender as the child/young person, in order to discuss sensitive issues such as sexual health and lifestyle issues.

Many arrive in this country with no more than the clothes on their back. In some cases they have no legal documentation, and they can be uncertain about their age. Doctors are being asked more and more to give an opinion on age, especially in assessing if a young person is under the age of 18 years. The use of growth measurements and stages of puberty as an estimate may be made, but there can be a margin of error in this assessment of 2–5 years either side. Poor nutritional health and illness may delay puberty, thus making it more difficult to define age. Dental development may be another way of assessing age, but again there is a margin of error. According to guidance from the Royal College for Paediatricians, as the margin of error is wide, the best clinical judgement may be in terms of whether a child is probably, likely, possibly or unlikely to be under the age of 18 years (Leverson and Shama, 1999).

Legal status is quite complicated and is decided on an individual basis. When an unaccompanied asylum-seeking child/young person comes to the notice of the authorities, frequently by the police, the Home Office assesses the child's legal status. As it stands presently (at the time of writing), such a child/young person will have the same rights as a child/young person born in the UK. Children's services need to promote the health of this group and work with specialist and local services to improve their health and well-being.

The difficulties this group of looked-after children/young people experience is enormous. They will feel the loss of their family, loss of things familiar, loss of cultural norms, and perhaps be grieving over family and friends who may have died by violent means. These traumatic life events will impact on their physical, mental and emotional health needs. It is essential that a holistic health assessment is undertaken to ensure their health issues are dealt with sensitively and appropriately.

Conclusion

This chapter has looked at the policy context of children/young people who are looked after. The role of the primary health care team with this group has been discussed, particularly relevant at this time, the health needs of unaccompanied asylum-seeking children/young people. Nurses need to work hard to both promote and meet the needs of these vulnerable children/young people. The chapter has perhaps helped to raise nurses' awareness about why it is so important to help looked-after children/young people, whose needs are after all significant.

Resources

Policy documents and guidance on looked-after children/young people are the following:

- *Promoting the Health of Children Looked After* (Department of Health, 2002).
- *Every Child Matters* (Education and Skills, 2003).
- *Keeping Children Safe: The Government's Response to the Victoria Climbé Inquiry Report and Joint Chief Inspectors Report Safeguarding Children* (Department of Health, Education and Skills, Home Office, 2003).

- *National Service Framework for Children, Young People and Maternity Services* (Education and Skills, Department of Health, 2004).
- *Care Matters: Time for Change* (Education and Skills, 2007).

References

Arcelus, D., Bellenby, T., Vostenus, P. (1999) A mental heath service for young people in the care of the local authority. *Clinical Child Psychology and Psychiatry* 4(2): 233–245.

Bramford, F., Welkind, S. (1988) The physical and mental health of children in care. In: *Research Needs*. London: ERSC.

Brodie, I., Berridge, D., Beckett, W. (1997) The result of looked after children by local authorities. *British Journal of Nursing* 6(7): 386–391.

Buchanan, A. (1999) Are care leavers significantly dissatisfied and depressed in adult life? *Adoption and Fostering* 23(4): 35–40.

Caan, W. (2004) Framework shows a new vision of health in life. *British Medical Journal* 329: 1239.

Children Act (1989) London: HMSO.

Children Act (2004) London: Crown Copyright.

Children's and Young People's Unit (2001) *Building a Strategy for Children and Young People*. London: Children's and Young People's Unit.

Corlyon, J., McGuire, C. (1997) *Young Parents in Public Care*. London: National Children's Bureau.

Department of Health (1997a) *People Like Us. The Report of the Review of the Safeguards for the Children Living Away from Home*. London: Department of Health.

Department of Health (1997b) *Substance Misuse and Young People, the Social Services Response*. London: HMSO.

Department of Health (1998) *Quality Protects Programme: Transforming Children's Services*. London: Department of Health.

Department of Health (2002) *Promoting the Health of Looked After Children*. London: HMSO.

Department of Health (2006) *Our Health, Our Care, Our Say: A New Direction for Community Services*. London: TSO.

Department of Health, Education and Skills (Department of), Home Office (2003) *Keeping Children Safe: The Government's Response to the Victoria Climbé Inquiry Report and Joint Chief Inspectors Report Safeguarding Children*. London: HMSO.

Dunnett, K., White, S., Butterfield, J., Callowhill, I. (eds) (2006) *Health of Looked after Children and Young People*. Dorset: Russell House Publishing.

Education and Skills (Department of) (2003) *Every Child Matters*. London: Education and Skills.

Education and Skills (Department of) (2006) *Looked after Children Strategy – Consultation*. London: Education and Skills.

Education and Skills (Department of) (2007) *Care Matters: Time for Change*. London: Education and Skills.

Education and Skills (Department of), Department of Health (2004) *National Service Framework for Children, Young People and Maternity Services, Standards – 1 (Promoting Health and Wellbeing), 4 (Growing Up into Adulthood), 8 (Disabled Children and Young People and Those with Complex Health Needs), 9 (The Mental Health and Psychological Wellbeing)*. London: Crown Copyright.

Leverson, R., Shama, A. (1999) *The Health of Refugee Children: Guidelines for Paediatricians*. London: Royal College of Paediatricians and Child Health.

Office of National Statistics (2005) Available at: http://www.statistics.go.uk (accessed May 2007).

Richardson, J., Joughlin, C. (eds) (2000) *The Mental Health Needs of Looked After Children*. London: Gaskell.

Shaw, C. (1998) *Remember My Messages*. London: Who Cares? Trust.

Theme 10

Teenage Health Issues

Chapter 34 Health Promotion Course – Living with Teenagers

Chapter 35 Promoting Sexual Health to Young People

Chapter 36 Preventing and Managing Substance Misuse

Chapter 37 Smoking Cessation

Health Promotion Course – Living with Teenagers

Joanna Livingstone

NSF

The National Service Framework (NSF) through its different standards sets out the need for practitioners to support parents, provide family-centred care, and particularly support young people as they grow into adulthood (Education and Skills, Department of Health, 2004) (standards 2, 3 and 4). The Living with Teenagers health promotion initiative aims to meet these needs through its work with parents/carers and their teenage children.

Introduction

This chapter, *Living with Teenagers* (LWT), looks at promoting adolescent health through the development of a parenting course. The chapter explores the important role that parents/carers have in adolescent health. The course is an example of good practice, which illustrates how parents/carers of teenagers can be supported within their parenting role.

LWT is part of a series of parenting courses which have been operating in an area of the East Midlands for over 12 years. Other courses in this series include *Living with Babies* and *Living with Children*. Details about Living with Babies feature in Chapter 27.

Theory

Evidence has shown that good parenting contributes significantly to the self-esteem and long-term achievement of children/young people, for example, in education and employment (Liabo et al., 2004). The effect of poor parenting is felt to contribute to a greater propensity towards crime, drug abuse, teenage pregnancy and sexually transmitted diseases (Moffit et al., 1996; Rutter et al., 1998). The LWT course addresses these issues by enabling improved parenting skills so parents/carers are better able to support their teenagers, so there is less likelihood of inappropriate behaviours developing.

Evidence in the field of parenting teenagers suggests that developmentally adolescents move into a different phase during which time it is a natural process for them to detach or distance themselves from their parents/carers (Glasper and Richardson, 2006). This process is shown in a tendency for teenagers to feel embarrassed at being around their parents/carers and to feel more strongly drawn towards the influence of their peers. These behaviours and the subsequent immaturity of brain development also mean that teenagers are more likely to indulge in high-risk behaviours and experimental phases. This might include drinking, drug taking and sex. Recent research carried out by Straunch (2003) suggests that changes within the teenage brain may actually be as significant as those referred to in younger children, and are equally important developmentally.

Previously Begley (1996) and Balbernie (1999) indicated that children's experiences within the first 3 years of life were found to alter the structure of the brain and influence *neural circuitry*, which in turn had an effect on skills and abilities developed for life. New research regarding the teenage brain indicates that at the adolescent stage the brain is being remodelled during a significant growth spurt. During childhood the *grey matter* in the brain continues to thicken and develops extra connections. Adolescence is felt to be a time when this process peaks. A *pruning* process then occurs within the brain where the grey matter thins out and uneccessary brain connections are discarded. This process is thought to have an effect on the development of inhibitions and memory, which are fine-tuned during the later stages of teenagehood (Straunch, 2003). Many teenage behaviours, therefore, which may seem incomprehensible to their parents/carers, such as defiance and impulsiveness, can actually be explained as the effect of processes going on at a much deeper, unseen level. Many parents/carers do not understand the normality of these processes and therefore may find such changes difficult to deal with as their child moves into a different phase in her/his life. As parents/carers see their role in protecting and providing for their children, relinquishing this role can be a very difficult for them, and may contribute towards difficulties in the already widening gap between parent and child.

The LWT programme aims to address issues that affect both parents/carers and their teenagers, at this time of change. It is hoped by addressing issues that concern them all, as well as the developmental changes taking place; it will ease any actual or potential frictions in their relationship.

Evidence looking at the effects of parenting indicate that the way children/young people are brought up can have a significant impact on them throughout life. Riesch et al. (2006) indicate that *communication* is a key component within families. They suggest that open communication and general satisfaction with family life, including the ability to manage conflict effectively, can have a positive effect on teenagers. Riesch et al. (2006) believe this can actually reduce behaviours which have a negative impact on health. In support of this work, Resnick et al. (1997) state that families who are *con-nected*, who communicate well with each other, may protect their teenagers from indulging in such behaviours. Costa et al. (1989) suggest that families have an important part to play in acting as *role models* for their children in terms of behaviour, and are therefore able to communicate their expectations to their children, with consequent effect.

The effect of these feelings of connectedness within families, general satisfaction, the ability to communicate effectively, learning to problem-solving and manage conflict are felt to have a profound influence on teenage behaviour. The impact of effective use of communication within families is thought to reduce the early onset of sexual activity, reduce drug and alcohol use, improve ability to have successful intimate relationships later in life, and reduce the risk of self-harm/suicide (Riesch et al., 2006).

Such evidence is supported both in the field of parenting skills and in recent Government documentation relating to children and families. The NSFs (Education and Skills, Department of Health, 2004) place a strong emphasis on both supporting parents and young people. The 11 standards relating to these groups tie in with the 5 outcomes from *Every Child Matters* (Education and Skills, 2003) where children/young people are supported to:

- be healthy;
- stay safe;
- enjoy and achieve;
- make a positive contribution;
- achieve economic well-being.

Standard 2 in the NSF (Education and Skills, Department of Health, 2004) requires that parents/carers will have access to services which enable them to support and manage their children/young people from babyhood and throughout their time at school. This standard also refers to access for parents/carers to manage any behavioural issues via a range of interventions, one of which could be through a parenting skills group, which may also signpost parents/carers on to services that are specific to their individual needs.

Similarly, standard 4 (Education and Skills, Department of Health, 2004) supports the notion of the changing needs of young people as they grow up, and for services to be shaped and respond to these needs. This standard refers to the importance of promoting the health of young people, in particular the need to reduce teenage pregnancies as well substance misuse, sexually transmitted infections and suicide. Such issues are covered within the LWT parenting skills programme, where parents/carers are encouraged to help their teenagers make a safe transition into adulthood through strategies designed to meet young people's needs.

In addition, standard 3 (Education and Skills, Department of Health, 2004) refers to the provision of high-quality services for children and families in response to their *felt needs*. This standard also refers to the provision of children's centres and extended schools where such services can be provided within local communities. These innovative services offered by children's centres and extended schools represent a real opportunity to provide *accessible* services for families. Parenting skills programmes are just one of the services which will be provided within these settings.

Practice

A key objective of the LWT programme is to raise parental self-esteem, and thus enable them to raise the self-esteem of their teenagers (North Eastern Derbyshire Primary Care Trust, 2006). Sessions facilitate this process by looking at communication and listening skills, setting boundaries/discipline and conflict resolution. Parental awareness is also raised through sessions covering sex and relationships and drugs education. Some parents/carers do not want to acknowledge that their teenagers are involved in sexual relationships and in the experimental use of alcohol or drugs. However, evidence suggests that early onset of sexual relationships may be prevented through greater, more accurate knowledge of issues concerning sex, knowledge of contraception and sexually transmitted infections (Chambers and Licence, 2005). Improvement of communication on these issues and an open attitude may actually deter teenagers from taking risks, if they feel they are able to be honest and open with their parents/carers. The LWT programme therefore aims to foster better relationships in families through skills learned by parents/carers on the course.

The overall objective of the LWT programme addresses needs identified by both national and local

policies. These policies focus on prevention (rather than crisis intervention) and the importance of family and child health. These include *Supporting Families* (Home Office, 1998, 1999), *Every Child Matters* (Education and Skills, 2003), the NSFs (Education and Skills, Department of Health, 2004), *Choosing Health* (Department of Health, 2004a) and *Chief Nursing Officer Review of Nursing and Midwifery and Health Visiting* (Department of Health, 2004b).

Evidence in the field of parenting programmes suggests that prevention is six times more effective when based in the community than individual programmes provided in the clinical setting (Cunningham et al., 1995). Such programmes are felt also to be more cost-effective at an average cost of £600 per child in comparison with costs of processing a young offender through the criminal justice system, which could cost between £1000 and £7000. This cost however does not take account of the implications and costs for their families.

The LWT programme aims to encourage parents/carers to access a course to help them, depending on their child's/young person's development and needs, which could be from 9 years of age upwards. The course aims to facilitate parents/carers ability to access information which is pertinent to their own families' needs. Similarly, by providing a group setting in conjunction with other parents, they can share their experiences and develop workable strategies, which can be used at home. The provision of an 8-week programme means that parents/carers can try strategies at home and refer back to the group for further support each week.

The Living with Children (LWC) service was already a successful and well-established parenting programme for parents/carers of children. However, the LWC team were increasingly receiving requests to provide a similar programme for parents/carers of teenagers, a service which was not yet on offer. Consequently, the LWC service worked in conjunction with Health Promotion's Healthy Schools Team to devise and pilot a suitable programme – the LWT programme. The initial pilot took place with funding obtained via the Children's Fund. This successful pilot was subsequently expanded within the area and rolled out to other areas within the East Midlands.

By making the parenting programme (LWT) available to parents/carers of teenagers, we aimed to improve the overall health and well-being of these families across the area. By expanding the course it helped to improve equity of service, making the course accessible to more families.

The following will outline the content of the course. The LWT programme consists of eight sessions, delivered once per week, lasting 3 hours (including lunch). The sessions provide a chance for parents/carers to consider issues affecting teenagers and to think about ways of dealing with situations at home. The course is free to participants at the point of access.

Areas covered by the course are the following:

- Building self-esteem.
- Expectations and challenges.
- Listening and problem-solving.
- Setting boundaries and parenting styles.
- Discipline.
- Sex and relationships education.
- Drugs education.

Session 1

The opening session aims to introduce the course and develops good group dynamics and feelings of trust within the group. The session begins with a *group round*, acknowledging participants' hopes and fears for the course. This method is used at the beginning and end of each week to enable participants to identify anything which needs to be clarified and as a means of ongoing evaluation. Participants' feelings regarding their parenting role are evaluated through completion of a self-esteem scale, which is reassessed at the end of the course.

The setting of clear *ground rules* from the outset aims to enable participants to feel safe sharing their own feelings and experiences with others. Participants may therefore gain the maximum amount from the course within a confidential setting.

Through the use of a group activity using pictures of teenagers and the *what's it like to be a teenager?* Activity, the session, aims to encourage participants to step into their teenagers' shoes and to empathise with how life is for modern-day teenagers. The session also looks at building up a toolkit of parenting skills that can be identified and built upon over 8 weeks of the course. This is in order that partic-

ipants can tailor the course to their own needs. A parent booklet given out each week assists with this process.

The final activity in the session encourages parents/carers to focus on self-esteem and the more positive aspects of the relationship with their teenager. Parents/carers are asked to think about five things they like about their teenager, as well as five things they do well as a parent/carer.

Session 2

Session 2 looks at being a *good enough parent* and aims to build parents'/carers' self-esteem, establish realistic expectations of themselves and encourage them to take *time out* regularly. The session begins with the parent *job description* (Box 34.1) which is a humorous reminder to parents/carers about the demands of their role.

Box 34.1 Parent job description.

A full-time opportunity exists – for person with commitment and dedication. Offers varied and demanding employment. No specific qualifications required but all-round skills desirable. No training given, job learnt by trial and error. Managerial, counselling and diplomacy skills useful at all times. Stamina, energy and ability to work night shifts desirable. Rest days: nil, pay: nil, prospects of promotion: low, minimum length of service: 18 years.

The next activity uses statements cards which refer to things that a good enough parent might do. For example, a parent:

- is there when your child needs you;
- cooks the tea every night;
- is honest about the mistakes they made as a teenager.

Group members are asked to place the cards along a continuum which has *agree* at one end and *disagree* at the other. The purpose of this activity is to promote discussion amongst participants and consider how opinions might differ, rather than a definitive list of answers.

The session moves on to look at self-esteem both for parents/carers and teenagers. Scenarios are used to enable parents/carers to look at the kind of responses they use with their teenagers, and those which will build self-esteem. The session ends with facilitators asking participants to identify some personal time during the coming week in order to build their own self-esteem through an activity such as buying a magazine, going for a walk or having a peaceful bath with no disturbances.

Session 3

Session 3 looks at *listening skills* and aims to enable participants to recognise both verbal and non-verbal means of communication, to reflect upon and improve listening skills. They need to consider how these could be effectively utilised at home. Participants are encouraged to identify *helpful* and *unhelpful* types of listening. The significance of voice tone and non-verbal means of communication are emphasised in order that participants can reflect upon the effect these may have on communication.

A carousel activity is used where participants take turns at being the teenager or parent/carer, using scenarios and range of different listeners, both good and bad. The exercise enables participants to experience at first hand what it feels like when someone does not listen properly, or is distracted whilst doing something else.

The session goes on to discuss the use of different types of listening, for example, silent and reflective listening. Role-play is used in order that participants can practise away from the home setting. Participants are encouraged to try their new skills with their teenagers at home.

Session 4

Session 4 covers *parenting styles*, boundary setting and conflict resolution, and aims to look at the effects of different parenting styles on teenagers. The purpose is to develop an understanding regarding boundary setting/conflict resolution and to consider how methods of communication that may assist this process. A group activity is used to ascertain participants' own knowledge of boundaries and to

find out what type of boundries they are using with their teenagers currently.

The session begins by looking at different parenting styles, both those used with teenagers and those that were used on participants themselves, when they were growing up. These include the following:

- Jellyfish/laid back parent.
- Brick wall/controlling parent.
- Backbone/negotiating parent.

The effect these parenting styles might have on teenagers' self-esteem is considered.

The session moves on to examine how different types of communication may influence interactions with teenagers. Participants are encouraged to familiarise themselves with the use of *I feel* messages. This is an assertiveness technique which enables parents/carers to get their concerns over to teenagers without being interpreted as negative or blaming.

Finally, participants are asked to work through a common problem they might have with their teenager using the *5-step process* of conflict resolution. The process encourages parents/carers and teenagers to listen to the views of the other and negotiate mutually agreeable solutions with a review date being set to discuss progress. Participants are encouraged to try this technique at home as problems arise.

Session 5

Session 5 looks at *discipline*. The aim is to introduce the topic by examining where parents'/carers' ideas about discipline came from, and to help them develop a sense of self-discipline in their teenagers. An activity is used which aims to check participants' understanding of the term discipline. Participants are encouraged to think about positive discipline, as a way for their teenager to reach her/his potential, rather than as punishment for bad behaviour. Participants reflect on how they were disciplined as children through a group activity. More importantly, how this made them feel. Methods of discipline which are really effective in encouraging teenagers to comply, are considered, which participants can add to their parenting toolkit. The effects of more negative types of discipline are discussed, and the impact this might have on teenagers' self-esteem.

Session 6

Session 6 aims to examine participants' experiences of sex and relationships education and to build parents'/carers' confidence in talking to their teenagers about the subject without embarrassment. Participants are split into small groups and a paper carousel activity is used, with headings at the top of each piece of flip chart paper, which are rotated around each group. The questions ask how participants learnt about sex and relationships, whether these experiences were positive or negative, and how these experiences would influence discussion on similar issues with their teenagers.

A subsequent activity asks participants to consider what their worries and hopes are for their teenagers in light of their own experiences. These elements of the session aim to enable participants to reflect upon and gain insight from their own experiences for the benefit of their teenagers. The message is one of honest open discussion within families and to promote more responsible and informed choices for teenagers.

The session ends with a discussion about local sexual health services that teenagers can access. Leaflets are also available for parents/carers to take home, which may prompt discussion within their families.

Session 7

Session 7 aims to inform participants about drug use – to reflect upon their own experiences of drug use/risk-taking behaviour, and to differentiate between problem and non-problem drug use. An activity is used to define what participants think a drug is and similar or differing reasons why adults and teenagers take drugs. This activity is consolidated by looking at a model of drug use, where the differences between experimental, recreational and problem drug use are discussed. The aim is to get participants to question any preconceived ideas they may have regarding drugs, and to consider how they may use drugs themselves such as alco-hol, caffeine and prescription medications for similar reasons to their teenagers.

The session goes on to explore the notion of risk, through a card game where participants place various risky activities, which include drug use and other pursuits such as sport and motor vehicle use, on a continuum according to their perception of risk. The aim is for parents/carers to think about the risks involved in all these activities, and what can be done to reduce the risks, for example, safety measures. The session may also involve a guest speaker from a local drug education agency, who helps to educate participants about drug facts. A quiz is available to test participants' knowledge afterwards.

Session 8

Session 8 aims to enable participants to reflect on and consolidate their learning throughout the course and to signpost them on to other relevant services. Participants are encouraged to reflect upon the difference in their responses compared to earlier in the course.

Evaluation of the course is carried out using the self-esteem scale, which was completed in week 1, so participants can see how they have progressed. Comments on parents'/carers' feelings regarding the course and what they have gained from it are also part of a more general evaluation (Figure 34.1) and are fed back into the ongoing evaluation process.

The group is then divided into smaller groups and an activity looking at local sources of support is explored, and then fed back into the larger group. The session ends with *rosy-glow* activity, which aims to bring participants back to the recurring self-esteem theme established in week 1. Participants are asked to make a positive comment about each group member on a sheet of paper. The papers are passed around the group to facilitate this. The final product is a list of compliments for each participant to take home to refer to when self-esteem takes a dip.

The session closes with a final group round where participants are encouraged to look at the *hopes and fears* identified in week 1 and consider whether these have any relevance now. Participants are encouraged to continue with any informal support networks they may have established within the group for ongoing support.

Tell us about the course

When you have completed LWT, please answer all the questions. Feel free to comment, we are keen to make improvements in the course that we offer to parents.

Which of the following sessions have you found most interesting and which more practical?	Interesting	Practical
Week 1: Self-esteem	☐	☐
Week 2: Nobody's perfect – good enough parenting	☐	☐
Week 3: Listening skills	☐	☐
Week 4: Setting boundaries, parenting styles and conflict resolution	☐	☐
Week 5: Discipline	☐	☐
Week 6: Sex and relationships	☐	☐
Week 7: Drugs	☐	☐
Week 8: Closing session	☐	☐

What would you have liked to have spent more time on?	Would have liked more time
Week 1: Self-esteem	☐
Week 2: Nobody's perfect – good enough parenting	☐
Week 3: Listening skills	☐
Week 4: Setting boundaries, parenting styles, conflict resolution	☐
Week 5: Discipline	☐
Week 6: Sex and relationships	☐
Week 7: Drugs	☐
Week 8: Closing session	☐

(a) What did you expect to get out of the course? Please comment.

(b) Has the course met your expectations? Please tick one box.

Yes	No	Partly
☐	☐	☐

Please tick one box for each statement:

(c) I have gained a great deal from the LWT course

(d) I think promoting self-esteem in children is important

(e) I have enjoyed meeting other parents on this course

(f) I would recommend this course to a friend

(g) I think this course is too long

(h) I feel more positive about the way I deal with my children at home

(i) The facilitators on the course were very helpful

Response format for each statement

Strongly disagree	Disagree	Neither agree nor disagree	Agree	Strongly agree
☐	☐	☐	☐	☐

Many thanks for completing our questionnaire. Your comments are really valued.

Figure 34.1 Living with teenagers evaluation form.

They are also informed about a further evaluation that will be carried out in coming months by post or phone.

The process

Funding to deliver the programme was a successful bid via the Neighbourhood Renewal Fund. A designated project worker was employed for 4 days per week in order to effectively deliver the programme across the community.

The community was chosen due to an identified need to support parents in an area with high levels of health inequalities (Department of Health, 2006; Payne, 2006). The LWT programme was aimed at all parents/carers in the community with teenagers, with resources particularly being targeted at those most in need of support.

The programme contributed towards wider community safety and youth offending strategies by targeting parents/carers in need of support through a multi-agency referral process. Local agencies such as health, youth offending team, social services and voluntary services were incorporated in this *partnership* approach. Interestingly, over the 2 years of the programme, a number of other agencies became involved. This increased partnership enabled LWT to be more widely known about, and therefore a greater number of parents/carers became involved in the programme.

Initially, the number of parents/carers on the course was low. Subsequently, we adjusted the way the course was *publicised*. Local press releases, local networking events and services accessed by the community such as doctors' surgeries were all targeted. Strong links were developed with schools by regularly attending parents' evenings, and health promotion events, in order to have direct contact with parents of teenagers. Additionally, we organised a school *leaflet drop* prior to each course so that all parents of years 7, 8 and 9 pupils received a flyer with details about the course. There are now a consistently high number of parents/carers who attend LWT.

In order to promote *accessibility* of the course to parents/carers, the LWT course offered free lunch, transport and child care costs to all parents/carers who attended. This is a key element of the programme's philosophy, where we wish to promote equity of access to all families.

Benefits of the programme are thought to include the following:

* Improved health and well-being of families.
* Support for parents/carers to develop their own self-esteem and building social networks.
* Practical strategies for dealing with parenting issues within the home.
* Promotion of a multi-agency approach by working in partnership with youth offending team, social services, local authority and voluntary sector.

Further potential developments have included opportunities to address the public health agenda through a reduction in teenage pregnancy, reduction in health inequalities, reduction in crime and youth offending, as well as promotion of health in children, young people and their families. LWT has also provided the opportunity for practitioners to participate in community development work, through its implementation, and to cascade their newly acquired knowledge and skills across the target area.

Through use of a community-based venue, the sessions were able to assist development of *social networks* amongst parents/carers, which have continued beyond the 8 weeks of the programme. Such networks also encouraged participation in other activities, such as adult education and employment, thus promoting sustainability within the local community, through participation in the course. Each LWT programme has a maximum of 15 participants. Evaluation has been continuous over the year to enable adaptation of course content to cater for local needs.

Evaluation

Over the pilot period for the programme, eight courses and two training events were delivered. The LWT intervention had an impact on 74 parents/carers, as well as the practitioners who delivered the programme.

The evaluation demonstrated that there was an improvement in parenting skills. This encompassed an increase in parents'/carers' self-esteem, and an improvement in family relationships for those attending the course, as well as an improvement in quality of life. These improvements were reflected in comments made by parents/carers on their course evaluations, and follow-up sessions conducted 3 months after course completion.

Comments included the following:

- The course has helped me to understand my teenager and me.
- We have been able to share problems on the course.
- I guess I always knew there were no quick fixes, but it has been useful to talk through various strategies in a positive and encouraging setting.
- Facilitators are very informed. Thoroughly enjoyed the course. I would recommend it.

The overall aim of the course was to help improve family communications by providing parenting support. In some cases the course might have even prevented crisis intervention from services such as social services and adult mental health services.

Practitioners indicated that they had benefited from both an increase in knowledge and skills through facilitating the course. In addition, the specialist training and support available to them through the LWT service had been beneficial.

Comments from LWT facilitators included the following:

- I have found the course content to be very nurturing for families. I wish I had known about it when bringing up my own children.
- It is great to see the participants working well together and supporting each other. The course seems to be having a positive impact on family relationships. I am hopefully more prepared myself as a parent to teenagers.
- Participants are able to gain support from each other, as well as being signposted towards other agencies if needed.

The ever increasing number of multi-agency workers joining the LWT programme is a particularly good example of *partnership* working, and ties in well with local and national priorities which advocate working in this way in order to improve health outcomes for children/young people. Practi-

tioners benefited both from the time spent working together and gaining insight and into each other's roles. Networks were established which will enable them to work more effectively together in the future.

The LWT programme also aimed to have an impact on local health targets. This included reducing health inequalities, reducing teenage pregnancy and the promotion of health for children/young people and their families. A reduction in crime and youth offending was hoped for too.

Teenage pregnancy – some parents/carers initially found this a difficult subject area to address. However, many indicated that it had been useful in terms of being able to speak more freely to their teenagers on the subject. Having acquired these skills, parents/carers are better able to discuss contraception, information on sexually transmitted infections and positive sex and relationships education. We hope that this greater knowledge will result in a reduction of teenage pregnancy and sexually transmitted infections. Future data may hopefully reveal this.

Crime reduction and youth offending – the project has made strong links with both the community safety partnership and youth offending team. Parents/carers have been referred to LWT through these services and have successfully completed the LWT course, some of whom were on parenting orders. Parents/carers along with practitioners reported a significant impact of the programme in relation to improved communication and resolution of family conflict. Practitioners hope where communications have improved within families with young offenders that this may in turn help to prevent siblings from offending.

The future

Amongst mainstream service providers, there is a willingness to provide in-kind costs, through enabling their staff to facilitate LWT courses. This has been a major influence on the programme's success. There is considerable recognition locally of the importance to support parents through parenting skills courses. In addition, a high regard exists for the LWT programme. This should influence the future sustainability of the LWT programme.

The LWT team plan to continue to deliver their courses across the target area, and in particular look at new ways to involve *hard to reach families* and communities. Current considerations include how we could provide some kind of preparatory work for families who find it difficult to access the group setting currently provided.

The programme received an innovation award from the local PCT in 2005, in the category *Improving the Health of Local People*. This award has been beneficial in promoting the service to a wider audience.

References

Balbernie, R. (1999) Infant mental health: how events wire up a baby's brain. *Young Minds Magazine* 39: 17–18.

Begley, S. (1996) Your child's brain. *Newsweek*, 19 February, 57–62.

Chambers, R., Licence, K. (2005) *Looking After Children in Primary Care: A Companion to the Children's National Service Framework*. Oxford: Radcliffe Publishing.

Costa, P., Jessa, R., Donovan, J. (1989) Value on health and adolescent conventionality: a construct validation of a new measure in problem behaviour theory. *Journal of Applied Social Psychology* 19: 841–861.

Cunningham, C., Bremner, R., Boyle, M. (1995) Large group community-based parenting programs for families of preschoolers at risk of disruptive behaviour disorders: utilisation, cost effectiveness and outcome. *Journal of Child Psychology and Psychiatry* 36(7): 1141–1159.

Department of Health (2004a) *Choosing Health*. London: Department of Health.

Department of Health (2004b) *Chief Nursing Officer Review of Nursing Midwifery and Health Visiting*. London: Department of Health.

Department of Health (2006) *Choosing Health – Making Healthier Choices Easier, Health Profile for Bolsover 2006*. London: Crown Copyright.

Education and Skills (Department of) (2003) *Every Child Matters*. London: Education and Skills.

Education and Skills (Department of), Department of Health (2004) *National Service Framework for Children, Young People and Maternity Services – 2 (Supporting Parenting), 3 (Child, Young Person and Family-Centred Services), 4 (Growing up into Adulthood)*. London: Education and Skills, Department of Health.

Glasper, A., Richardson, J. (2006) *A Textbook of Children's and Young People's Nursing*. London: Churchill Livingstone Elsevier.

Home Office (1998) *Supporting Families – Consultation Document*. London: The Stationary Office.

Home Office (1999) *Supporting Families – Summary of Responses to the Consultation Document*. London: The Stationary Office.

Liabo, K., Gibbs, J., Underdown, A. (2004) *Group-Based Parenting Programmes and Reducing Children's Behaviour Problems*. Highlight No. 211. London: National Children's Bureau Library and Information Service.

Moffit, T., Caspi, A., Dicksen, N., Silva, P., Stanton, W. (1996) Cited In: Liabo, K., Gibbs, J., Underdown, A. (2004) *Group-Based Parenting Programmes and Reducing Children's Behaviour Problems*. Highlight No. 211. London: National Children's Bureau Library and Information Service.

North Eastern Derbyshire Primary Care Trust (2006) *Living with Teenagers Facilitators Training Pack*. Derbyshire: NEDDC.

Payne, N. (2006) *A Directory of the Health of the People in Bolsover. Tables from the Derbyshire Health Profile and Commentary about the Health of the People of Bolsover*. Derbyshire: Bolsover District Council.

Resnick, M., Bearman, P., Blum, R. (1997) Protecting adolescents from harm. *Journal of the American Medical Association* 278: 823–832.

Riesch, S., Anderson, L., Krueger, H. (2006) Parent-child communication processes: preventing children's health risk behavior. *Journal for Specialists in Pediatric Nursing* 11(1): 41–56.

Rutter, M., Giller, H., Hagell, A. (1998) *Antisocial Behaviour by Young People*. Cambridge: Cambridge University Press.

Straunch, B. (2003) *Why Are They So Weird? What's Really Going on in a Teenager's Brain?* London: Bloomsbury.

35 Promoting Sexual Health to Young People

Barbara Richardson-Todd

NSF

This chapter links most closely with standard 4 of the National Service Framework (NSF) for children, young people and maternity services, which asserts that all children should have access to age-appropriate services, which are representative of their specific needs as they grow into adulthood (Education and Skills, Department of Health, 2004).

Introduction

The purpose of this chapter is to raise awareness on some of the current issues concerning sexual health, the challenges and what is needed to develop a successful service for young people using the *five A's approach*. The issue of confidentiality with young people under 16 is considered, and a practice example of taking sexual health services into educational institutions is given. The aim of this chapter is to help nurses feel able to raise the issue of sexual health with young people, by offering advice, support and guidance during this crucial, bewildering and often risk-taking stage of their lives.

Current issues

Teenage pregnancy rates have decreased over the past 20 years in most Western European countries.

However, the rates in the United Kingdom (UK) are still high. UK rates are twice those of Germany, three times those of France and six times those of Holland (Council of Europe, 1997).

Table 35.1 shows conception data for under 16-year-olds in England, Scotland and Wales. There is minimal data available for Northern Ireland, as terminations are only legal in certain circumstances and often women travel to England to have a termination. However, there were 1395 teenage births (under 20 years), a rate of 21.7% per 1000 of 15- to 19-year-olds in 2005.

In England, for example, the data show the rate of conceptions in the under 16 years increased slightly in 2005 compared to 2002 and 2004 (provisional statistics for 2005, Office of National Statistics, Teenage Pregnancy Unit, 2007).

High teenage pregnancy and sexually transmitted infection (STI) rates are closely associated. The UK has the highest rate of STIs among teenagers in Western Europe (Nicoll et al., 1999). Chlamydia is the most commonly diagnosed STI, with rates increasing fivefold since 1995. An estimated 10% of sexually active teenagers have the infection, potentially leading to pelvic inflammatory disease, ectopic pregnancy and in some cases infertility (Health Protection Agency, HPA, 2004).

The incidence of chlamydia, gonorrhoea and genital warts continues to rise among young people, which may be linked to them not having the

Table 35.1   Under 16 years conceptions in England, Scotland and Wales.

England	Number of conceptions	Conception rate per 1000 females aged 13–15	Percentage leading to legal abortion
2005	7462	7.8	57.4
2004	7181	7.5	57.6
2002	7395	7.9	55.7
1998	7855	8.8	52.9
Scotland (includes miscarriages managed in hospital, as well as registered births and abortions)			
2003/2004	706	7.5	58.3
2002/2003	703	7.5	57.0
2001/2002	692	7.3	54.7
1998/1999	841	9.0	50.3
Wales (National Assembly for Wales)			
2005	455	7.8	50.8
2004	434	7.5	49.3
2002	480	8.3	53.5
2000	495	8.8	46.5

Sources: Teenage Pregnancy Unit (2007)
http://www.everychildmatters.gov.uk/resources/
ISD Scotland (2008) http://www.isdscotland.org/isd
National Assembly for Wales (2006) http://www.statswales.gov.uk

information they need and/or complacency that STIs will not happen to them (HPA, 2004). Young women aged 16–24 years have the highest rates of chlamydia (HPA, 2006).

In the UK there has been a 3% increase in STIs rising from 751 282 to 790 387 between 2004 and 2005 (HPA, 2006), reflecting increases in unprotected sex (HPA, 2005). Table 35.2 shows the rates of sexually transmitted infections between 1995 and 2004.

Why are rates in the UK so high?

There is no single factor for the high rates of teenage pregnancies and STIs, but there are a number of im-

Table 35.2   Rates of sexually transmitted infections 1995–2004 (HPA, 2005).

STI	1995	2004	Increase
Chlamydia	32 288	104 155	300%
Gonorrhoea	10 580	22 335	200%
Genital warts	60 247	79 618	32%
Genital herpes	16 479	18 923	15%
Syphilis	141	2252	1497%
HIV	2500	7000	300%

portant considerations. These include the following:

- Young people's lack of knowledge about contraception and STIs.
- What to expect in relationships, and what it means to be a parent.
- Access to advice and support.
- Level of emotional well-being.
- Expectations teenagers have about their future prospects of employment and educational attainment.
- Cultural and peer group influences, including mixed messages from the media.

The net result is not less sex, but less protected sex (Social Exclusion Unit, SEU, 1999). Table 35.3 highlights factors associated with early sexual initiation.

Policy drivers

There has been a plethora of policies concerning sexual health and teenage pregnancy in recent years. Government targets aim to half the rate of conceptions in the under 18 years and to reduce the

Table 35.3 Factors associated with early sexual initiation, contraceptive use and teenage pregnancy.

Individual	Family	Educational	Community	Socio-economic	Contraceptive
Knowledge	Parent/child communication	Academic attainment, educational goals	Social norms/sexual activity	Poverty	Contraceptive services
Self-esteem	Mother or sister teenage pregnancy history	Truancy	Peer influence	Employment prospects	Awareness
Skills base	Family structure including single-headed families	Sex education	Cultural and religious influences	Housing and social conditions	Availability
Cognitive maturity		Media influences	Accessibility		
Experimental behaviour		Child abuse			

From NHS Centre, Effective Health Care (1997).

number of conceptions in the under 16 years by 2010 (SEU, 1999). There are also targets to increase teenage mothers in education or training by 60% (SEU, 1999). Public Service Agreements and Local Delivery Plans are also working towards these targets, as well as reducing the spread of STIs.

The Department of Health has published key policies prioritising the improvement of sexual health; these include *Choosing Health: Making Choices Easier* (Department of Health, 2004); *Delivering Choosing Health: Making Healthy Choices Easier* (Department of Health, 2005). In 2001 the first national strategy for sexual health detailed actions for improvements – better prevention, better services, better sexual health: the national strategy for sexual health and human immunodeficiency virus (HIV). In 2003 the national strategy for sexual health and HIV implementation plan was published (Department of Health, 2003). The NSFs for children, young people and maternity services (Education and Skills, Department of Health, 2004) set out standards for children/young people. The documents emphasise the need to encourage open communication between young people and their parents/carers, especially around sexual health issues.

The five key outcomes of *Every Child Matters* (Education and Skills, 2003) have almost become a mantra to health practitioners:

- Being healthy.
- Staying safe.
- Enjoying and achieving.
- Making a positive contribution.
- Achieving economic well-being.

Sexual health cuts across all of these outcomes. The youth green paper – *Youth Matters* (Education and Skills, 2005) – aims to give choices and empowerment to young people, somewhere to go, something to do and someone to talk to.

The *Healthy Schools* initiative, a joint venture between Education and Skills and Department of Health (2005), aims to encourage schools to develop a holistic view of health and help young people to develop healthy lifestyles. The *Extended Schools* and the *Extended Services* initiative will provide onsite health advice or make speedy referrals to the local services (Education and Skills, Department of Health, 2007).

The National Institute for Health and Clinical Excellence (NICE, 2007) guidelines – *Preventing Sexually Transmitted Infections and Reducing Under 18 Conceptions* – offer strategies for advancing the sexual health of young people. Looked-after children are extremely vulnerable and the Government's green paper – *Care Matters* (Education and Skills, 2006a) – sets out how to achieve better outcomes.

Two documents, *Teenage Pregnancy Next Steps* and *Accelerating the Strategy to 2010* (Education and Skills, 2006b, c), look at areas where there have been significant decreases in teenage conception rates, and examines the underlying causes in areas where the rates are high.

Good practice is described in the toolkit – *Teenage Pregnancy: Working towards 2010* (Education and Skills, Department of Health, 2006d). It states that young people need to be involved in setting up and monitoring the services, as well as ensuring that young men are included. A clear confidentiality statement needs to be made with a full range of contraceptive services available. Services must be *highly visible* and promoted. All services relating to sexual health should be working in partnership, including general practitioner (GP) services, sexual health clinics, reproductive health services and pharmacies.

The Sexual Offences Act (2003) does not prevent health practitioners from giving confidential advice and treatment to young people under 16 if acting to protect the young person from STIs, pregnancy, protecting the physical safety of the young person or promoting their emotional well-being. Even if under 16, a young person still has the right to confidential advice on contraception, condoms, pregnancy and abortion.

Why is sexual health important?

Sexual health has been outlined by the World Health Organization (WHO, 1975) as the integration of physical, emotional, intellectual and social aspects of a sexual being, in ways that are positively enriching. Sexual health is important. With knowledge and support many of the problems experienced by young people can be avoided, leading to better health outcomes for them, both physically and emotionally.

Early-age sex can involve risks. These risks can include STIs, which may lead to more chronic health issues (Department of Health, 2001). For example, viral illnesses hepatitis B and C or HIV can lead to chronic ill health. Additionally, bacterial illnesses such as chlamydia or gonorrhoea can also have more chronic consequences.

There is of course the obvious risk of pregnancy. Becoming a mother when more mature and in a loving relationship can be a wonderful experience, but being pregnant while still at school can have a detrimental effect on life opportunities.

Unintended teenage pregnancy may lead to abortion, with possible long-term physical and mental health consequences. Alternatively, keeping the baby may lead to underachieving and continuing the cycle of deprivation (Education and Skills, 2006b, c).

What does sexual health mean to young people? Unfortunately, the all encompassing WHO definition (above) does not appear to be totally applicable to young people today. Sexual health requires a positive and respectful approach to sexuality and sexual relationships, as well as the possibility of having pleasurable and safe sex, free from coercion, discrimination and violence. For sexual health to be attained and maintained, the sexual rights of all persons must be respected.

For many young people sex is often not enriching and may have little to do with love. Many teenagers wish they had waited, and sometimes sex is unwanted or forced. All too often teenage sex is a risk-taking behaviour.

Greenhouse (1994) has outlined sexual health as the enjoyment of sexual activity of one's choice without causing any harm to others. Interestingly, research by Watson (2001) revealed that young people's definition of sexual health was

- not getting an STI,
- getting sex often,
- not getting caught,
- not getting pregnant,
- not getting lectures from adults
- and finding the right precautions to use.

Watson (2001) concludes that having *accessible* and *user-friendly* sexual health services alongside interagency working is the answer to improving the sexual health of our young people.

Barriers

Although sexual health services are provided at reproductive health centres, GP surgeries and some local hospitals, statistics show that not all young people access these services (Gleeson et al., 2002; Sherman-Jones, 2003). This is mainly because of difficulties associated with access, availability and lack of awareness of these services (Gleeson, 2001). The focus of many services, especially those for young people, is often on avoiding pregnancy. However, young people may be relatively uninformed about STIs. A service that helps reduce the negative consequences of sexual activity will improve the health of young people.

The most effective way to reduce teenage pregnancies is a multifaceted approach. This should include helping young people to resist pressure to have early sex, to improve sex and relationships education in schools, to link school-based sex education with appropriate local services, to improve access to effective contraceptive advice services and support parents/carers in talking to their children (NHS, 1997).

Increasing evidence shows that many teenagers fail to seek health advice when they need it, particularly about sensitive issues such as contraception, sexual health, abuse and domestic violence. Although most parents/carers would like their children/young people to talk to them, and to visit the GP where necessary, many appear reluctant to attend a GP's surgery to seek advice. A combination of self-consciousness and fears about confidentiality seem to be the main reasons why young people will not visit their GP. Other reasons cited are stigma, language, discrimination, embarrassment, previous bad experiences, social exclusion and poverty (Richie, 2006). In addition, there are always some young people who feel unable to confide in their teachers, parents/carers or friends.

Young people want services that are sensitive and responsive to their needs. They want them to be non-judgemental, confidential, accessible, acceptable and friendly.

Practice

The following section looks at practice. There are essential elements for a successful service, which is illustrated through the *Five A's*. Confidentiality is also discussed.

Essential elements for a successful service (five A's)

This is the five A's approach:

- Awareness.
- Availability.
- Accessibility.
- Attitude.
- Approach.

Awareness

Young people need to be aware that a service exists for them. They need to know where it is placed, how to find it, what the service offers and what to expect. There needs to be clear advertising, written in language that the young people can easily read and understand. The information also needs to be written in languages other than English for non-English speaking young people. Some young people may not be aware of the terms used such as *contraception*, and feel that emergency contraception is only for the *morning after* due to mis-naming in previous years.

Availability

Services have to be open at times that are convenient. Although lunchtimes are convenient for office workers, it may not be for a young person in school, unless the service is in, or located very near to the school. Young people may have to attend when their parents/carers will not be suspicious of their absence. Twilight times from 3 pm until 6 pm, Saturdays and even Sunday lunchtimes may be more appropriate.

Accessibility

A young person's use of a service is influenced by the distance they have to travel, particularly in deprived areas. Young people are more likely to access services within 1 km of their home. Services therefore need to be local, based in the community, in order for the young people to access them. More than a quick bus ride away is too far. Young people do not have the money to travel far, nor do they have the time, especially if they do not want their parents/carers to know. Drop-in sessions in places where young people spend their time, such as leisure centres, the football club, neighbourhood centres, youth clubs, schools and local supermarkets or stores, would be beneficial. This is particularly important for boys and young men, who are less likely to access advice and services in the traditional settings of surgeries and clinics.

Attitude

Young people face barriers to reproductive health services because most are designed for adults and do not always have the capacity to meet the special needs of adolescents. A reason for this might be that young people are not clearly understood. Some adults may hold uncompromising attitudes toward adolescent sexual behaviour. A nurse must be non-judgemental in the information that she/he provides.

Approaches

Young people do not like to explain to a receptionist the reasons why they need to see the nurse. Some surgeries have provided credit card size smart cards which the young person shows and then does not have to offer an explanation when attending. Young people usually want to see a nurse quite quickly, and this is where drop-in services without the need for appointments would be favoured. Services need to be using a positive, quality, youth-oriented, holistic sexual health approach. The approach should not simply be one of pregnancy prevention and disease. Services also need to be youth friendly, male friendly and gender sensitive. They should promote *empowerment* and the rights of young people.

Using the five A's approach can promote sexual health services for young people. When working with young people, confidentiality is important, as the following outlines.

Confidentiality

Confidentiality is a huge issue for young people. Some young people will risk pregnancy rather than seek contraceptive advice and yet they are all entitled to advice on sexual health. The issues about confidentiality must be explained clearly and simply to young people to allay any concerns. The duty of confidentiality owed to a person under 16 is as great as that owed to any other person. If a young person is under 16, issues of confidentiality and consent may need to be looked at more closely. All too often, young people mistakenly fear that the nurse or their GP cannot respect their confidentiality and so do not attend a GP surgery. It is worth remembering that competent young people, regardless of age, can independently seek medical advice and give valid consent to medical treatment (British Medical Association, 1994) (Box 35.1).

Nurses have a duty of confidentiality when working as a registered nurse under the Nursing and Midwifery Council (NMC, 2004) rules. For young people, the assurance that what they say to a nurse is confidential is an important factor, as this is the basis for a trusting relationship. It is most important to explain the policy on confidentiality to young people when they use the service. This needs to be undertaken simply and clearly, for example:

> Sometimes a person might talk about a situation where they have been harmed by someone. If this happens, we may need to talk to someone else, especially if it is something that is still happening to you, or if the person who harmed you may still be hurting someone else. Apart from that, we will be careful not to share what you say with anyone else; we would want to be able to agree with you what should be done, and who should be told.
>
> (Richardson-Todd, 2006a)

It is equally important for the nurse to encourage the young person to involve their parents/carers and make every effort to inform them with the young person's consent. However, when consent is refused, the nurse is bound by the code of professional practice, which states that confidentiality must be maintained unless there are concerns about safeguarding issues. The nurse needs to recognise that the duty of confidentiality for a person under 16 years is as great as that given to any other person, unless there are reasons to the contrary (British Medical Association, 1994).

The duty of confidentiality has practical implications for setting up and maintaining a confidential system for recording consultations and keeping documentation for legal and ethical requirements. This includes collection and storage of data needed for monitoring and evaluating the service. These issues need to be discussed with management to ensure that correct policies are followed and secure storage for documents and data is provided.

Case study: sexual health services in a school setting

Educating young people about relationships throughout their school years, before they become

Box 35.1 Fraser Guidelines.

- The young person can understand the advice and has sufficient maturity to understand what was involved in terms of the moral, social and emotional implications.
- The doctor or nurse cannot persuade the young person to inform their parents/carers to allow him/her to inform them that contraceptive advice was being sought.
- That the young person would very likely to begin, or to continue having sexual intercourse with or without contraceptive treatment.
- That, without contraceptive advice or treatment, the young person's physical or mental health, or both, would be likely to suffer.
- That the young person's best interest required them to give contraceptive advice, treatment or both without parental consent.

Issued in 1985 by Lord Fraser following the House of Lord's ruling in the case of Victoria Gillick vs West Norfolk and Wisbech Health Authority (Hadley, 1998).

sexually active, can promote a mature attitude to sexual health. One of the most effective ways of reducing teenage pregnancy is to link sex and relationship education in personal social health and citizenship education (PSHCE) classes in schools. This is encouraged within the Healthy Schools initiative.

For many years school nurses have been involved with PSHCE sessions in schools, delivering sex education. School nurses can also be involved in open access *drop-in* services in high schools. Other agencies can be involved, forming a regular multi-agency drop-in service. Young people have access to a whole range of practitioners who are able to inform, guide and support them (Richardson-Todd, 2006b). Although it may be seen to be controversial by including sexual health services in schools (Bloxham, 1997), this *one-stop-shop* approach enables young people to access a variety of services without stigma. Young people can get advice on contraception and sexual health, obtain condoms, guidance on relationships and peer pressure, have a pregnancy test, obtain emergency contraception and be screened for chlamydia, if appropriate. They may also see, if appropriate and available, Connexions personal adviser, a youth worker, a counsellor, young carers' officer, a mental health worker and perhaps a GP or practice nurse. Basically, whoever may be part of the partnership can be accessed by young people.

Aim

The aim of a school-based drop-in service is to ensure that young people have access to professional advice and support on a variety of health, relationships and emotional issues. This may include advice on avoiding self-harm, eating disorders, bullying, depression, relationships, drugs, alcohol, acne as well as sexual health. The advice should be free, confidential, non-judgemental, and open access service for young people.

The drop-in must be based on the principle that the interests and welfare of young people are paramount. There may be differences in individual and agency philosophies with respect to maintaining confidentiality. Issues around confidentiality need to be discussed and understood. It is vital to ensure protocols and guidelines are in place beforehand, so that staff involved are aware of the nurse's position regarding issues around safeguarding, confidentiality and accountability (Richardson-Todd, 2006a).

Objectives

Objectives can include the following:

- To improve young people's access to health services, information, advice and support.
- To provide a confidential service for young people.

- To provide a non-judgemental environment in which a young person can feel safe.
- To allow the young person to discuss worries, concerns or problems however trivial they may seem.
- To improve young people's sexual health and help make informed choices.
- To give young people an opportunity to take responsibility for their own behaviour, health care and lifestyle.
- To improve general health and well-being of young people (Crowe, 2000).
- To attempt to influence behavioural change.
- To listen, to act upon and promote the views of the young people.
- To improve, develop and promote the services provided.
- To signpost or refer to other services as necessary.

The role of the nurse when providing a drop-in service

It has been found that the provision of young person focused sexual health services, which are trusted by young people and well known by practitioners, have the greatest impact on reducing teenage pregnancy (Education and Skills, 2006b). The service offered needs to be young person friendly, confidential, trusted and in a safe environment. It needs to be accessible and acceptable to young people, so they can visit without embarrassment to see the nurse in private.

Young people may attend in small groups or with a friend. They may attend for several visits without disclosing the main reason for their visit, as young people like to build a trusting relationship beforehand. Once trust has been established, they are more likely to interact. Young people need time to feel comfortable and feel able to talk about their concerns. The drop-in should provide a safe and supportive environment. Boxes 35.2 and 35.3 demonstrate posters that can be displayed at the drop-in, which may encourage people about the safety and trusting nature of the service.

Safeguarding issues must always be at the forefront of a nurse's mind when dealing with young people. Training needs to be kept updated on safeguarding issues.

Box 35.2 A Safe environment.

THIS IS A SAFE ENVIRONMENT
It's OK. . .
To expect confidentiality
To be yourself
To ask questions and say if you don't understand
To have feelings
To expect respect
We expect . . .
Respect for ourselves
Respect for our property
Respect for the rights of others
To help you – we don't know everything
You to work with us and not against us

Box 35.3 Confidentiality poster.

CONFIDENTIALITY
What you tell a nurse is
CONFIDENTIAL
that means it is private between the two of us.
I will not tell anyone
(including your parents/carers and teachers)
that you have been to see me
or what we have discussed
UNLESS
you wish me to do so,
or what we have discussed has or may put either you
or someone else
at risk of significant harm.

Nurses need to ensure they are competent, have appropriate training, knowledge and skills with a genuine interest to develop a channel of communication and liaison with young people. Nurses need to feel confident in discussing sex and relationships, which will help young people make informed and positive choices about their future.

Group work sessions can be offered to give young people the opportunity to explore issues such as refusal and negotiation skills, communication within relationships, and to improve their self-esteem. Research suggests that these concerns are not discussed as much as could be within the classroom situation (Hudson and West, 1996). Such discussions can help young people to feel more informed and confident.

Young men are half the problem and half the solution (SEU, 1999) and much work needs to be undertaken with them, as they are often forgotten. Having a male worker included in the drop-in can provide a much-needed positive role model.

The nurse needs to offer free, informal advice, information and support networks to young people on all health issues. Clear and unambiguous information needs to be given as well as including some interpersonal development such as negotiation and refusal skills. Interventions need to be age appropriate and timely such as discussing future contraception and STI testing when a young person receives a negative pregnancy test result. The nurse needs to check that interventions and services signposted or where referrals are made are accessible to young people (Figure 35.1, drop-in poster). Networking to join up with other services and partners in the community is important. A local culture where discussion of sex, sexuality and contraception is permitted needs to be encouraged (Teenage Pregnancy Unit, 2000).

The success of a multi-agency school-based drop-in is more likely if school staff, parents/carers and particularly the young people themselves are involved right from the beginning. Those involved need to draw up an agreement to ensure commitment and consistency in such aspects as confidentiality and data sharing.

Promoting the drop-in

Appropriate and adequate advertising and promotion of the drop-in service is essential in the initial stages of setting it up. Some tips on how to promote the drop-in are the following:

- Getting young people involved in designing and producing posters and leaflets, giving a sense of ownership.
- For a drop-in clinic to be successful, the service has to be well publicised at regular intervals.
- Don't forget that word of mouth is the most economical, efficient and effective form of advertising the service.

Meeting the challenge

Although less than a third of young people are sexually active by the time they are 16, half of all those who are use no contraception the first time. It appears that most young women wish that they had waited, and for quite a few girls, sex is forced or unwanted. Young people who do not use contraception have a 90% chance of conceiving in 1 year. Those who do not use condoms are also exposed to a range of sexually transmitted infections. Half of young women pregnant at under 16 years and more than a third of those pregnant at 16 and 17 years old opt for an abortion (SEU, 1999; Education and Skills, 2006b,c,d).

The number of teenage pregnancies and STIs could be reduced through the following:

- Improved access to sexual health services, for example, school drop-in services.
- Clear messages to young people – boys as well as girls, on the negative consequences of having sex at an early age. This would include information on the increased risk of unplanned pregnancies and STIs, and the poorer health and education outcomes for teenage parents and their children. Details about the high levels of regret experienced by young people themselves should not be forgotten.
- Young people should be provided with the knowledge, skills and confidence to prevent pregnancy and how to manage their sexual health.
- Improving access to advice and support on contraception and sexual health.
- Helping to facilitate open discussions between parents/carers and their children on sex and relationships.
- To ensure that advice on contraception is an integral part of the support provided to young women who have experienced a prior conception (either leading to an abortion or birth), to avoid the risk of second and subsequent conceptions (Education and Skills, 2006c).

The school nurse, practice nurse, emergency department nurse, nurse practitioner, children's nurse, family planning/reproductive health nurse, midwife or health visitor or any nurse who comes into contact with young people can use the opportunity to raise the issue of sexual health. Practice nurses when carrying out the booster immunisations for school leavers have an ideal

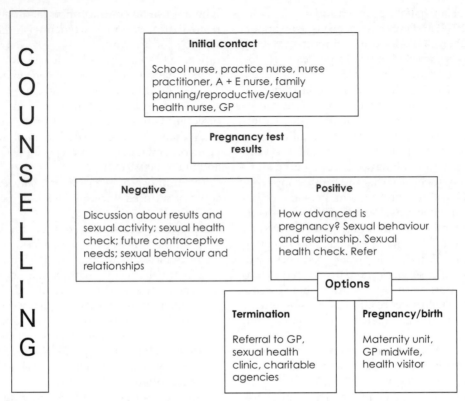

Figure 35.1   I think I'm pregnant.

opportunity to discuss all aspects of health with the young people. School nurses have many opportunities to engage young people on the subject, especially through a school drop-in service.

Conclusion

This chapter has discussed meeting the challenge of educating our young people to be sexually healthy. We can achieve this by synergy, working together to produce an effect greater than the sum of individual effects. Better outcomes can be achieved by joint working and joined-up working, engaging and unifying the relevant agencies, media, parents/carers and most importantly – young people themselves. Perhaps if this were to happen, young people would not have to encounter the trauma of an unplanned pregnancy or STI.

Resources

http://www.likeitis.org.uk
http://www.ypsh.net
http://www.lifebytes.gov.uk
http://www.ruthinking.co.uk
http://www.there4me.com
http://www.18r.uk.nt/go/home
http://www.mindbodysoul.gov.uk
http://www.need2know.co.uk/health
http://www.teenagehealthfreak.org
http://www.embarrassingproblems.com
http://www.kidshealth.org
http://www.condomessentailwear.co.uk
http://www.playingsafely.co.uk/
http://www.thesite.org
http://www.takecare.co.uk
http://www.coolsexinfo.org.uk
http://www.sexplained.com
http://www.fpa.org.uk
http://www.brook.org.uk
http://www.avert.org/yngindex.htm

http://www.youthinformation.com
http://www.sexualhealthprofessional.org.uk/teenage-pregnancy-policy/
http://www.dfes.gov.uk/teenagerpregnancy/
http://www.opsi.gov.uk/ACTS/acts2003/20030042.htm

References

Bloxham, S. (1997) The contribution of interagency collaboration to the promotion of young people's sexual health. *Health Education Research* 12(1): 91–101.

British Medical Association (1994) *Confidentiality and People Under 16*. Guidance issued jointly by the BMA, HEA, Brook Advisory Centres, FPA and RCGP, January 1994. London: BMA.

Council of Europe (1997) *Recent Demographic Developments in Europe*. Strasbourg: Council of Europe.

Crowe, A. (2000) Providing a drop-in centre in partnership with young clients. *Community Practitioner* 73(10): 796–798.

Department of Health (2001) *Better Prevention, Better Services, Better Sexual Health: The National Strategy for Sexual Health and HIV*. London: The Stationery Office.

Department of Health (2003) *National Strategy for Sexual Health and HIV Implementation Action Plan*. Available at: http://www.dh.gov.uk (accessed 25 February 2007).

Department of Health (2004) *Choosing Health: Making Choices Easier*. London: Department of Health.

Department of Health (2005) *Delivering Choosing Health*. London: Department of Health.

Education and Skills (Department of) (2003) *Every Child Matters*. London: Education and Skills. Available at: http://www.everychildmatters.co.uk (accessed February 2007).

Education and Skills (Department of) (2005) *Youth Matters*. London: Education and Skills.

Education and Skills (Department of) (2006a) *Care Matters*. London: Education and Skills.

Education and Skills (Department of) (2006b) *Teenage Pregnancy Next Steps: Guidance for Local Authorities and Primary Care Trusts on Effective Delivery of Local Strategies*. London: The Stationery Office. Available at: http://www.everychildmatters.gov.uk (accessed 25 February 2007).

Education and Skills (Department of) (2006c) *Teenage Pregnancy: Accelerating the Strategy to 2010*. London: The Stationery Office. Available at: http://www.everychildmatters.gov.uk (accessed 25 February 2007).

Education and Skills (Department of) (2006d) *Teenage Pregnancy: Working Towards 2010 – Good Practice and Self-Assessment Toolkit*. Available at: http://www.everychildmatters.gov.uk/ete/extendedschools/ (accessed 24 February 2007).

Education and Skills (Department of) (2007) *Under-16 Conception Statistics 1998–2005*. Available at: http://www.everychildmatters.gov.uk/teenagepregnancy/ (accessed 25 February 2007).

Education and Skills (Department of), Department of Health (2004) *National Service Framework for Children, Young People and Maternity Services*. London: Education and Skills, Department of Health.

Education and Skills (Department of), Department of Health (2005) *National Healthy School Status*. London: Crown Copyright.

Education and Skills (Department of), Department of Health (2007) *Extended Schools: Improving Access to Sexual Health Advice Services*. Available at: http://www.everychildmatters.gov.uk/ete/extendedschools/ (accessed 25 February 2007).

Gleeson, C. (2001) Children's access to school health nurses. *Primary Health Care* 11(9): 33–36.

Gleeson, C., Robinson, M., Neal, R. (2002) A review of teenagers' perceived needs and access to primary health care: implications for health services. *Primary Health Care Research and Development* 3(3): 184–193.

Greenhouse, P. (1994) A sexual health service under one roof: setting up sexual health services for women. *Journal of Maternal and Child Health* 19: 228–233.

Hadley, A. (1998) Teenage sexual health. *Practice Nursing* 9(15): 26–30.

Health Protection Agency (HPA) (2004) HIV and other sexually transmitted infections in the United Kingdom in 2003. *HPA Annual Report*, November. London: HPA.

Health Protection Agency (HPA) (2006) *Epidemiological Data – Sexually Transmitted Infections*. Available at: http://www.hpa.org.uk/infections/topics (accessed 7 August 2006).

Health Protection Agency, (HPA) and The UK Collaborative Group for HIV and STI Surveillance (2005) *Mapping the Issues. HIV and Other Sexually Transmitted Infections in the United Kingdom*. London: Health Protection Agency.

Hudson, F., West, J. (1996) Needing to be heard: the young person's agenda. *Education and Health* 14(3): 43–47.

ISD Scotland (2008) *Sexual Health*. Available at: http://www.isdscotland.org/isd (accessed September 2008).

National Assembly for Wales (2006) *Teenage Conceptions in Wales*. Statistical Bulletin. Available at: http://statswales.gov.uk (accessed September 2008).

National Institute for Health and Clinical Excellence NICE (2007) *Preventing Sexually Transmitted Infections and Reducing Under-18 Conceptions*. Available at: http:// www.nice.org.uk/page (accessed 25 February 2007).

NHS Centre for Reviews and Dissemination, University of York (1997). Preventing and reducing the adverse effects of unintended teenage pregnancies. *Effective Health Care* 3(1): 1–12.

Nicoll, A., Catchpole, M., Cliffe, S., Hughes, G., Simms, I., Thomas, D. (1999) Sexual health of teenagers in England and Wales: analysis of national data. *British Medical Journal* 318(7194): 1321–1322.

Nursing and Midwifery Council (NMC) (2004) *The NMC Code of Professional Conduct*. London: NMC. Office of National Statistics. Available at: http://www.statistics.gov.uk (accessed 2007).

Richardson-Todd, B. (2006a) Setting up a school nurse drop-in clinic. *School Health* 2: 35–37.

Richardson-Todd, B. (2006b) Sexual health services in school: a multi-agency drop-in. *Journal of Family Health Care* 16(1): 17–20.

Richie, G. (2006) Strategies to promote sexual health. *Nursing Standard* 20(48): 35–40.

Sexual Offences Act (2003) Available at: http://www.opsi.gov.uk/ACTS/ and http://www.opsi.gov.uk/acts/acts2003/December 2008.

Sherman-Jones, A. (2003) Young people's perceptions of and access to health advice. *Nursing Times* 99(30): 32–35.

Social Exclusion Unit (SEU) (1999) *Teenage Pregnancy*. London: SEU.

Teenage Pregnancy Unit (2000) *Best Practice Guidance on the Provision of Effective Contraception and Advice Services for Young People*. Available at: http://www.dfes.gov.uk/teenagepregnancy (accessed February 2007).

Teenage Pregnancy Unit (2007) Available at: http://www.dfes.gov.uk/teenagepregnancy (accessed February 2007).

Watson, P. (2001) Sexual Health – an integrated approach to care. *Primary Health Care* 11(5): P16–17.

World Health Organization (WHO) (1975) Education and treatment in human sexuality: the training of health practitioners. A report from a WHO meeting. *WHO Technical Report* Series No. 572. Available at: http://www.who.int/reproductivehealth/publications/sexualhealth/index.htl(accessed December 2008).

36 Preventing and Managing Substance Misuse

P.C. John Graham, Janet Savage, Karen Moyse, Jimi Poyser and Donnamarie Donnelly

NSF

The National Service Framework (NSF) for children, young people and maternity services advocates *listening* to young people and *involving* them in their own care (Education and Skills, Department of Health, 2004).

Introduction

Preventing substance misuse considers a variety of health promotion strategies and teaching methods which are aimed at discouraging young people from becoming involved in substances that may cause them harm – such as smoking, alcohol and drug misuse. Janet looks at drama in education as a teaching method that can be used to discourage smoking. Equally, this teaching method can be applied to health promotion activities on preventing alcohol or drugs misuse. Drug Abuse Resistance Education (DARE) is a health promotion programme aimed at discouraging young people from becoming involved in substance misuse, with the use of life skills training. DARE is examined through the eyes of P.C. John Graham, a DARE officer.

Nurses can help to prevent young people from becoming caught up with substances that may be harmful to their health. At a community level nurses can help through health promotion campaigns or at an individual level working directly with young people themselves. School nurses can particularly be involved by working closely with pupils in school and collaborating with other agencies such as DARE.

Preventing substance misuse is one of five key health promotion areas highlighted as important for young people in the NSF. Others include nutrition, sexual health, mental health and injury prevention (Education and Skills, Department of Health, 2004).

Substances such as cigarettes, alcohol and drugs can potentially lead to serious risks to health. They can create dependency, making it difficult for a young person to stop. Long-term morbidity and mortality can be affected. Young people can come to depend on these substances which may potentially have consequence for the rest of their lives.

Young people and their development

Adolescence is a time of change and transition; young people want to try new things, enjoy being involved with friends, and perhaps psychologically move away from some of the more familiar things in their lives. They may want to try smoking, drinking or taking drugs perhaps. However, there are risks associated with becoming involved in these substances, which young people need to be informed about.

It would seem that a variety of different influences determine if a young person becomes involved in substance misuse. This can include the influence of family, friends and culture, as well as factors about the individual. Evidence has shown that the family is particularly influential. For example, with smoking, if a child grows up in a household where adults smoke, the child may grow up with the belief that she/he will do the same as other adults in the family. Tassoni (2007) points out that a child growing up in a household where both parents smoke is three times more likely to become a smoker herself/himself, than if parents do not smoke at home.

Role models can be influential too, as Bandura (1977) has highlighted. The behaviour of celebrities in the media, for example, smoking or taking illegal substances, may unwittingly promote certain behaviours. Young people may admire them and want to replicate their behaviours. With today's culture of celebrity pushed so strongly through the media, young people may not be able to disassociate themselves from what is portrayed before them, and thus think it is *cool* to undertake similar behaviours.

Furthermore, psychological factors about the individual can contribute to a young person becoming involved in substance misuse. Tassoni (2007) describes psychological factors such as an individual feeling vulnerable, who may not feel part of her/his own family, unsupported and looking towards something else to fill that gap. That gap might be filled with substance misuse, which gives the individual a sense of belonging to a particular group, who together engage in similar behaviours.

Physiological development during adolescence may have a bearing too. It has been known for some time that the brain undergoes critical periods of development during the early years. Recently, however, evidence has been produced which demonstrates that certain regions of the brain continue to develop during adolescence (Blakemore, 2007). The parts of the brain associated with these changes are those involved in social cognitive processes, such as understanding the behaviour of others (Blakemore, 2007). Young people do not function as well as adults in areas of social cognitive development (Blakemore, 2007). This aspect of understanding develops later and may be one reason why young people may misunderstand others, and do not see the risks in certain situations and relationships, which would be more obvious to adults.

It would seem that there are a variety of different factors which influence whether young people become involved in substance misuse. Nurses need to be aware of these influences if they want to help young people. Importantly, Government strategy on the treatment of young people with problems of substance misuse recommends a thorough assessment of all their needs to be able to help them effectively (National Treatment Agency, 2007). Looking at the different factors involved in an individual's life may help the nurse to understand why particular young people go on to misuse certain substances, such as drugs, alcohol or cigarettes.

Smoking

Smoking can be seen as a trendy thing to do when you are young. Some young people try it but find that it is not for them. Others smoke for a white, perhaps while mixing with a particular group of friends, but ultimately give up. Meanwhile, others go on to become hooked. Nicotine (contained in cigarettes) is an addictive substance, which can be difficult to give up.

Age and gender are relevant factors with regard to smoking. Figures indicate that there is a sharp increase in smoking with age; 1% of 11-year-olds smoke regularly compared with 22% of 15-year-olds (Department of Health, 2004). Smoking appears to be more prevalent amongst girls than boys (Department of Health, 2004). Smoking is an important health issue; it can be the cause of long-term health problems such as diseases of the circulatory system and cancers.

Recently, there have been a number of legislative changes related to smoking. The age at which young people can purchase cigarettes has changed; it is illegal to buy cigarettes under the age of 18 years. Smoking in public places has now become illegal too. There are now more legal and social barriers in place to smoking than ever before.

The Government has proposed a number of ways to discourage young people from becoming interested in smoking through the use of the following strategies:

- Increase the choice and availability for young people to engage in positive activities in their spare time.
- Increase the accessibility and relevance of health advice that is available to young people.
- Build on *Every Child Matters* (Education and Skills, 2003) by ensuring that all young people are able to access expert advice, particularly those at risk of experiencing poor health outcomes.
- Develop new ways of supporting parents of teenagers (Department of Health, 2004).

Putting in place such strategies may in some cases help prevent young people from starting to smoke.

Strategies particularly need to be in place for those young people who want to give up smoking. In Chapter 37, Roger Kirkbride discusses some of these strategies in more depth, and highlights a range of services that are available, which young people can access.

Teaching techniques

When teaching young people about avoiding substance misuse, drama techniques can be a useful method. Young people can participate themselves, engaging in the behaviours and feelings of the characters involved or simply observe the actions of others. Janet presents some ideas in relation to discouraging young people from smoking. Health promotion through the use of drama can have a powerful impact.

Using *theatre in education* techniques for discouraging smoking

The issue of giving up smoking was addressed as part of a drama performed with young people. The pupils were given a letter that was addressed to an agony aunt. The letter set a scenario; the leading character had experienced some problems since she had started at senior school.

Once the letter had been read the pupils created still images of the scenario. Still images are the creation of an image using a group of people to capture a particular moment, as in a photograph or video freeze-frame. Thought tracking was then used. Thought tracking links in with still images.

After the pupils had created a realistic image the school nurse asks them, whilst they are still frozen, what their characters were thinking and feeling. The aim is to reinforce an understanding of the image they have created.

Further into the session the school nurse then takes on the part of the leading character (pupil at senior school), and is interviewed by the pupils. This method is known as hot seating. It provides an opportunity to highlight the main character's motivations and feelings about smoking. The intention is that the technique will increase pupils' awareness of the feelings and behaviours of others. Pupils can go on to develop an understanding of how the views of others may differ from their own on smoking.

To conclude the session pupils are asked to imagine themselves as the agony aunt. How would they reply to the main character? Pupils can come up with some really good strategies for not starting to smoke or refusing cigarettes.

Another method that can be used is forum theatre. It involves the school nurse acting as a facilitator and encouraging young people to change the drama from within. Forum theatre is undertaken by splitting the class into groups and asking them to prepare a short scene that ends in a crisis. Each scene is performed in front of the class. Once the pupils have watched all scenes, they then go on to observe them a second time. On the second occasion pupils are invited to stop the action at any point where they would have reacted differently. Pupils can either tell the performers what they would have said, or even take on the role of a character themselves, thus altering the course of action. Forum theatre can be beneficial for older groups. A scenario of being offered a cigarette can be undertaken and differing techniques for refusing could be explored and discussed together.

Alcohol and drugs

As with smoking, there are similarities with drug and alcohol use. In a Department of Health survey recently, drug and alcohol consumption amongst young people increased with age, rising steadily from 11 to 15 years. Cannabis was found to be the most commonly used drug (Tassoni, 2007). There are concerns about cannabis, as it is seen as a gateway drug. From here young people may go on to explore other drugs (Tassoni, 2007). A survey published in 2003 highlighted that 21% of pupils (12–19 years) had taken drugs in the last year (Education and Skills, Department of Health, 2004).

Alcohol consumption shows that young people are interested in a variety of different drinks. Girls are now beginning to consume as much as boys. In a survey for the Department of Health recently, it showed that 22% of 11- to 15-year-olds had drunk alcohol in the last week. A growing culture of binge drinking is frequently portrayed in the media amongst some groups of young people. Binge drinking imposes risks to health, with both short- and long-term consequences.

Some of the signs of alcohol and drug misuse to look out for have been outlined by Bootzin and Acocella (1988):

- Moodiness.
- Poor concentration.
- Tiredness.
- Behaviourally less cautious.
- Withdrawal from family and friends.

The accompanying risks of dependency must not be forgotten.

Health promotion strategies

Drug and alcohol awareness education, including the teaching of *life skills*, can be an effective way to teach young people about the dangers. Tassoni (2007) maintains that young people need to be given accurate information. The message that all drugs are bad is simply not an effective strategy. The NSF supports young people engaging in the development of life skills (Education and Skills, Department of Health, 2004).

The NSF (Education and Skills, Department of Health, 2004) also advocates a number of other strategies:

- Listening to young people, listening to their concerns.
- Information available for young people so they can make informed decisions.
- The NSF advocates seeking to inform and engage parents/carers in drug education.

The risks of substance misuse need to be dealt with, *not* in isolation, but in the context of other behaviours (Education and Skills, Department of Health, 2004). As explored earlier in this chapter, there are complicated reasons and influences on why young people engage in substance misuse. Issues need to be handled with care. Underlying factors need to be fully explored. Support can be invited from family too.

Literature is available through health promotion units, particularly a wide range of leaflets, which may provide a useful starting point. There is a very helpful website – *Frank*, the national drugs information campaign (National Drugs Information, 2007; http://www.talktofrank.com), which provides information, as well as a helpline (Education and Skills, Department of Health, 2004).

Youth services work with young people on alcohol and drug misuse. Connexions advisors may also be able to help, supporting young people with advice on health and social care issues.

Specialist support must be available for those who have complex needs (Education and Skills, Department of Health, 2004). There are specialist services available in many communities which can help support young people who have difficulties with substance misuse. Local primary care trusts will be able to help, as the section 'Managing Substance Misuse' later highlights.

The NSF importantly points out that adult treatment services will not be appropriate for young people, tailor-made support, which is fully integrated with the wider provision for young people should be available (Education and Skills, Department of Health, 2004).

Age-appropriate, accessible services are the key.

DARE – life skills

DARE provides life skills training for young people, helping them to develop positive attitudes and behaviours, helping them with the strength of character to make good decisions in life.

DARE is a Drug Abuse Resistance Education programme for children/young people. It works as a partnership between the police, education, health and other agencies. DARE was first started in America, coming to the United Kingdom (UK) in the early 1990s. The police have always taken a leading role with the delivery of DARE in the UK. However, at the current time of writing, this is about to change.

The DARE programme aims to deliver, over a period of 10 weeks, for 1 hour each week, life skills to enable children/young people to make healthy life choices. These healthy choices are particularly aimed at providing children/young people with knowledge and understanding about the impact of drugs, alcohol, smoking and other substances, that may be harmful to their health.

DARE equips children/young people with the skills to resist *peer pressure*. As previously discussed, friends are particularly important to children/young, the teenage years especially so, when young people may hold others in high esteem, finding their behaviours and attitudes especially influential and persuasive.

The DARE programme is delivered to children/young people between the ages of 9 and 11 years. This is just the age when children/young people might begin to become tempted by their peers into trying out new things, which may be harmful to them. As they enter adolescence, young people may begin to engage in risk-taking behaviours. DARE tries to prevent and discourage adolescents from embarking upon a path where risk-taking behaviours involve substance misuse.

Experiences with DARE

This is a personal account written by John Graham, who has worked both as a police officer and with children/young people in school as an officer for DARE.

I was an operational policeman for 34 years. Thirty of those years were spent in the traffic department dealing with both serious and fatal road accidents. Some of those accidents had been caused by drivers who had been drinking.

For 10 of those years with the police force, I was working as a trained firearms officer, with a police force in the Midlands, frequently travelling in an armed response vehicle. Retiring in 2001, I left at a time when I was still very much enjoying the job. At this time DARE was looking for retired police officers to go into schools to help maintain the DARE programme. Police officers were undertaking the role as part of their normal duties, but were finding this increasingly difficult due to the demands of their work.

So after a short period of training, I found myself going into schools. I had undertaken school visits before as a police officer, but this was with a patrol car, usually dealing with situations of conflict. Undertaking the DARE programme with children/young people was quite a different approach.

I have now undertaken the DARE programme for over 4 years. During this period of time I have been amazed how positively children/young people respond to the programme. The contrast is incredible. Instead of dealing with situations of conflict, as I did on a routine basis as a police officer, I now find that children/young people respond to the DARE programme with smiles and genuine enthusiasm for lessons.

The DARE programme seems to offer children/young people something quite special. I find that teachers too are very interested in the programme too. It is different from the normal curriculum. The DARE programme seems to bring a personal, individual approach, which children/young people enjoy and appreciate. They respond positively and fully engage themselves in the processes that are happening within the classroom.

About the programme

The DARE programme aims to reach children/young people with information and life skills to assist them in making healthier choices. Content of the programme includes sessions on the following:

- Self-esteem.
- Peer pressure/how to deal with a dilemma.
- Tobacco. ⎤
- Cannabis ⎥ risks of.
- Alcohol. ⎦
- Awarding of certificates.

DARE provides the opportunity for children/young people to develop decision-making skills. As part of the work on peer pressure, the programme focuses on the management of disagreements and how to deal with antisocial behaviour.

The programme looks at issues surrounding tobacco, alcohol, cannabis and other volatile substances. The children/young people are given a decision-making dilemma to deal with. As part of this they are required to do the following:

- D = Define the problem.
- A = Assess, what the choices might be.
- R = Response, making a decision.
- E = Evaluating that decision.

The approach taken with this exercise will not only help children/young people with their DARE lessons, but will also help them to make well thought-out decisions during their lives.

To conclude, I am amazed how popular the programme has become. I have seen hundreds of children/young people graduate from the programme. The content of the programme, I feel, enables children/young people to develop qualities of self-esteem and respect for others, as well as themselves.

Perhaps the acquisition and further development of these life skills not only helps children/young people to enhance their relationships with peers, but also is useful in other areas of their lives.

The role of the nurse

This section will look at different ways the nurse can help children/young people with issues that surround drug misuse: informing them about the risks, helping them to develop the strength to say NO and supporting those who have concerns. Work in these areas can be undertaken individually and on a group basis. Nurses have a particularly valuable role in supporting the emotional health of children/young people as the following outlines.

Nurses may find themselves involved with DARE, particularly in the future. Involvement might consist of inviting a DARE officer along to present the programme to children/young people in school. Or perhaps, nurses might go on to deliver aspects of the DARE programme themselves. I attended a number of DARE workshops myself recently, which certainly helped in understanding what DARE is trying to achieve with young people. The work of DARE also fits well with the *Healthy Schools* programme. Healthy Schools are about helping children/young people to develop healthy behaviours. The Government believes that by focusing on physical and emotional health in schools,

this will promote healthier lifestyles (Department of Health, 2005). The work of DARE is particularly about promoting the emotional health of children/young people, helping them to be more confident and developing strength of character. This is an area where school nurses may want to develop their role, working collaboratively with their school and DARE. In doing so they would be helping to promote the emotional health of children/young people.

For the Healthy Schools programme to be effective, the Government realises and encourages practitioners from external agencies to be involved within the school curriculum, particularly the PSHE (Personal, Social and Health Education), and citizenship curriculum. The Government believes that involvement from practitioners, such as school nurses, and drug education advisers can help to improve knowledge and skills within schools (Department of Health, 2005). This is an important area for both DARE education officers and school nurses.

School nurses need to be available to support the curriculum, but additionally they have an important role in supporting children/young people emotionally on an individual basis. School nurses providing children/young people with the opportunity to discuss health issues that may concern them, such as questions about the risks of drugs, for example, may help to increase understanding and direct them on to other services. Children/young people may feel confident about talking with their school nurse, a familiar face who will listen to their concerns.

A leaflet is available for children/young people which outlines details on the role of a school nurse. It also includes details about how children/young people can contact their school nurse. The leaflet discusses how school nurses link with the Healthy Schools programme (Department of Health, Education and Skills, Healthy Schools, and National Children's Bureau, 2006). The leaflet can be obtained via the website – http://www.wiredforhealth.gov.uk (Education and Skills, 2007). This is the official website for the Healthy Schools programme. The Wired for Health website is useful for accessing a range of materials. It provides details of other useful websites too.

Nurses have a valuable role to play individually beyond school. Nurses working in hospitals may be able to support young people with emotional problems. For example, a children's nurse can help a young person who comes into hospital with emotional problems, and has resorted to substance misuse as a way of getting through a bad experience. The children's nurse can guide the young person towards appropriate sources of help, support and advice. Simply listening may be a useful starting point.

Nurses have a role to play at a community level too, becoming involved with local campaigns and strategies. This might include putting on a number of events within the local community to raise awareness about different sources of help, with the use of posters, leaflets and local community involvement. Think about the places that young people regularly attend, and how nurses might be able to become involved.

To be able to provide appropriate help and support for young people, nurses need to ensure that they are trained to do so. If substance misuse is a field of particular interest, find out what courses you can access that will help. Courses on adolescent health may be a useful starting point. If particularly interested in improving the service you provide to young people, access:

- *Getting It Right for Teenagers in Your Practice.* Royal College of General Practitioners and Royal College of Nursing (2002), http://www.rcn.org.uk.

This information will provide some useful pointers.

Managing substance misuse

Nottinghamshire Healthcare
NHS Trust
Positive about mental health and learning disability

Jimi and Donnamarie look at how substance misuse is managed in the community, through the work of *Face It*, an organisation located in Nottinghamshire.

There are young people's drug and alcohol services based both within the NHS and the voluntary sector. Face It – Young Persons Drug and Alcohol Service – is one example of such a service within the NHS.

Face It is provided by Nottinghamshire Healthcare NHS Trust. The service provides confidential drug and alcohol advice, information, treatment

and support for young people under 18 years and care leavers up to the age of 21 years. The service is provided within communities throughout Nottinghamshire County.

Face It aims to provide a high-quality range of services for young people *at risk of using* or *using* substances. Services provided are young person centred and specific, with the highest regard to confidentiality and safeguarding.

All interventions and interactions are appropriate to the maturity and level of development of each individual young person. The needs, lifestyle, gender, ethnicity and beliefs of the young person are respected. The service is provided to young people on an equitable basis and in a non-discriminatory way.

The approach used is within the ethos of harm reduction, empowering young people with accurate, up-to-date information to enable them to make informed choices about their lives, which will reduce the harm caused by substance use to them as individuals, their families and their communities.

Face It offers their services in line with *Every Child Matters* (Education and Skills, 2003), *Essential Elements* (National Treatment Agency, 2005) and Integrated Children's Services.

Approaches used with a young person

Approaches used with a young person will vary. This can include the following:

- Detached contact.
- Group work.
- One-to-one intervention.

Detached contact

The focus on detached work is to offer proactive prevention and education. This takes place within environments where young people gather such as parks, the streets and young people's events. The aim of detached work is to introduce the services offered by Face It to young people, developing a familiarity where trust can be developed to enable the service to offer non-appointment support, allowing ease of access should the young person want/need further individual intervention.

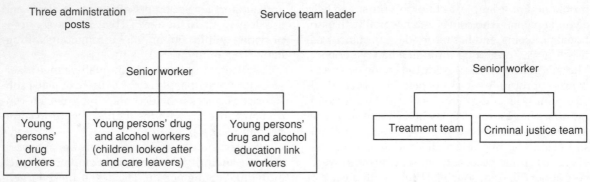

Figure 36.1   Face it, the structure of the service.

Group work

The focus of group work is targeted intervention with young people at risk of using or misusing drugs/alcohol. This is an educative approach again based on harm minimisation. Group work can be one of or part of a planned programme. This takes place with young people at risk of exclusion or who are excluded from education, with young offenders, children looked after/care leavers and young people who are classified as homeless.

One-to-one intervention

This can be brief intervention, crisis intervention, risk assessment, full assessment, pharmacological intervention, acupuncture and care planned treatment programmes. Intervention is assessed according to the young person's needs and wants.

Face It has a free phone for young people as well as a text-messaging facility. There is an open door policy for receipt of referrals. Self-referral is preferred; however, referrals are accepted from practitioners with the young person's knowledge and consent. Referrals are also accepted from the Youth Justice Services where the young person's substance use is linked to their offending behaviour and may form part of a mandatory order from court.

Partnership work is essential in ensuring the best outcome for young people and the service ensures links are made to other young people's provision, for example, youth services, education, connexions, housing, child and family health service.

The opportunities for the best outcomes to be achieved with young people are when the young person, services and the family work together.

In order to meet the needs of the young people in contact with the service, there are specialist

workers. The structure of the service is shown in Figure 36.1.

Conclusion

This chapter has focused on strategies and teaching methods that aim to help young people to be informed about substances that may be harmful to their health, and develop the skills to say No. The use of life skills training has been examined through the DARE programme. Drama in education has been presented by Janet, as a useful teaching method to discourage smoking.

Strategies outlined within the NSF advocate the importance of listening and providing young people with information, so they can make informed life choices, along with support from their parents/carers (Education and Skills, Department of Health, 2004). The school nurse has a particularly valuable role to play in listening and providing information to young people.

The chapter has also explored how strategies to manage the misuse of substances needs to be approachable for young people. In line with this the work of Face it has been discussed.

Young people, as they become older progressing into adulthood, may decide to smoke and drink. But this may be at an age where they are less vulnerable to the influences of others and are in a better position to make informed choices about their health. If they have been able to access health information and develop life skills when young, they will be able to understand the risks they are taking, and how to avoid some of those risks by imposing their own limits upon drinking and smoking, for example.

Resources

http://www.nottinghamshirehealthcare.nhs.uk
http://www.drugs.gov.uk
http://www.nata.nhs.uk
http://www.drugmisuse.isdscotland.org
http://www.wales.gov.uk
http://www.healthpromotionagency.org.uk/work/drugs/menu.htm

References

Bandura, A. (1977) *Social Learning Theory*. New Jersey: General Learning Press.

Blakemore, S. (2007) The social brain of a teenager. *The Psychologist* 20(10): 600–602.

Bootzin, R., Acocella, J. (1988) *Abnormal Psychology, Current Perspectives*. New York: McGraw-Hill Publishing Company.

Department of Health (2004) *Making Healthy Choices Easier*. London: Crown Copyright.

Department of Health (2005) *National Healthy Schools Status*. London: Crown Copyright.

Department of Health, Education and Skills (Department of), Healthy Schools, and National Children's Bureau (2006) *What School Nurse?* London: Crown Copyright.

Education and Skills (Department of) (2003) *Every Child Matters*. London: Crown copyright.

Education and Skills (Department of) (2007) *Healthy Schools Programme*. Available at: http://www.wiredforhealth.gov.uk (accessed November 2007).

Education and Skills (Department of), Department of Health (2004) *National Service Framework for Children, Young People and Maternity Services. Standard 4 – Growing up into Adulthood*. London: Crown Copyright.

National Drugs Information (2007) *Talk to Frank*. HM Government. Available at: http://www.talktofrank.com (accessed November 2007).

National Treatment Agency (2005) *Young People's Substance Misuse Treatment Services. Essential Elements*. Available at: http://www.nta.nhs.uk (accessed 28 January 2008).

National Treatment Agency (2007) *Young People's Specialist Substance Misuse Treatment Plan 2008/9*. London: Crown Copyright.

Royal College of General Practitioners and Royal College of Nursing (2002) *Getting It Right for Teenagers in Your Practice*. London: Royal College of General Practitioners and Royal College of Nursing. Available at: http://www.rcn.org.uk

Tassoni, P. (2007) *Child Development, 6 to 16 Years*. Oxford: Heinemann from Harcourt.

37

Smoking Cessation

Roger Kirkbride

NSF

Young people need services that are tailor-made to their needs (Education and Skills, Department of Health, 2004).

Introduction

The adverse effects of smoking on health are well known. Figures produced by Peto et al. (2006) suggest that smoking kills around 114 000 people in the United Kingdom (UK) every year – one in five deaths. It has been estimated that approximately 364 000 hospital admissions each year are due to smoking-related diseases (Action on Smoking and Health, 2006a).

Many more people suffer from long-term conditions that are caused or exacerbated by smoking. Most people who smoke in their adult life start as teenagers. Some of the most lasting effects of smoking can be experienced by children exposed to environmental tobacco smoke. Smoking through pregnancy and passive smoking in childhood can have profound effects on small children, effects which may continue throughout their lives.

The effects of passive smoking on young children are avoidable, and the effects of smoking on older children and teenagers can be substantially mitigated, by not smoking. Lader and Goddard (2005)

report that over 70% of people who smoke claim they want to give up with 88% of them citing a health reason for wanting to quit. However, these are generally personal health reasons. Only 15% of people want to stop smoking because they are concerned about the health of their children. The intent to give up smoking is even higher; 75% of people claim that they intend to stop smoking with more than 55% intending to give up within the next year.

Why, then, is smoking still so prevalent? Stopping smoking is hard; nicotine, the principle active drug in tobacco, is addictive; and the habits of smoking are difficult to break. Smokers are realistic about their chances of stopping. A minority are confident that they will quit within a year.

This chapter primarily focuses on teenagers; how nurses and other services can work together to help them give up smoking. Help needs to be provided before smoking takes a hold on their lives, impacting on their own health, and that of their children, as they go on to have families of their own. Services need to be geared to their specific needs, as the NSF highlights (Education and Skills, Department of Health, 2004).

Young people and smoking

Action on Smoking and Health (2006b) cites peer pressure and advertising as being influential in young people taking up smoking. However, these factors are much less significant than the presence of other smokers in the household; an older sibling or a parent who smokes trebles the chances that a child will take up smoking as they approach their teenage years.

The Government regularly surveys the rate of smoking among young people; a report produced by The Information Centre (2006a) revealed that by the age of 11, approximately one in seven young people have smoked, although only a very small percentage class themselves as regular or occasional smokers. By the age of 15, approximately 64% of young people have personal experience of smoking and 31% class themselves as regular or occasional smokers. Girls are more likely to smoke than boys; by the age of 15 years, 25% of girls are regular smokers and 12% are occasional smokers; the figures for boys are 16% and 9% correspondingly.

Young people who smoke are more prone to coughs and increased phlegm, wheeziness and shortage of breath; they take more time off school and they are less fit than non-smokers. 80% of adults who smoke started as young people, and the long-term risks of smoking (for example, cancer and heart disease) are initiated at this stage.

Young people find it easy to buy cigarettes from shops and other outlets. In an attempt to make it harder, the UK Government has (with effect from 1 October 2007) made it illegal to sell tobacco products to people below the age of 18 (previously 16). It is anticipated that increasing the minimum age of purchase to 18 may reduce the consumption of cigarettes among 11- to 16-year-olds by 14% (Department of Health, 2007)

Smoking cessation

All drug addictions carry a risk of physical symptoms on withdrawal, and nicotine is no exception. According to Action on Smoking and Health (2005), people stopping smoking may experience all or some of the following:

- Cravings for tobacco   70%
- Increased appetite   70%
- Depression   60%
- Restlessness   60%
- Poor concentration   60%
- Irritability/aggression   50%
- Night-time awakenings 25%
- Light-headedness   10%

These effects wear off over a relatively short period of time; all but increased appetite lasts less than 4 weeks.

There are a number of ways in which people may choose to get through the period where they are experiencing these effects. There is no one clear methodology for stopping smoking that works well for everyone, and many techniques have no clear clinical evidence of effectiveness. Techniques include the following:

- Cold turkey – stopping without any kind of aid. Most people give up smoking using this method.
- E-mail or text motivation messages (via mobile phones) – provision of messages designed to reinforce the individual's motivation according to the reasons why they have selected for wanting to stop. Young people are keen users of digital media, and may find this kind of support particularly useful.
- NHS Stop Smoking Helpline – a telephone helpline that acts as a source of information and advice.
- NHS Stop Smoking Services – a variety of locally available services provided in each Primary Care Organisation.
- Nicotine replacement therapy – preparations including chewing gum, lozenges, nasal sprays, inhalators and transdermal patches are all now licensed for use by adolescents over 12 years of age. These preparations reduce the craving for cigarettes by providing an alternative source of nicotine.

All can be used successfully – but only if the individual's motivation is high enough. The model of change developed by Di Clemente et al. (1991) identifies five stages of change:

- Pre-contemplation.
- Contemplation.
- Preparation.
- Action.
- Maintenance.

Until an individual reaches the action stage, behavioural change will not be effected; support may be required to help people move between stages. Even at the action or maintenance phases, support may be necessary to prevent relapse.

A review of NHS smoking cessation services (The Information Centre, 2006b) suggests that a combination of techniques that includes nicotine replacement therapy supported by one-to-one or group support is the most successful at achieving good rates of stopping smoking. However, even when adequately supported, less than one-third of people can be shown to have quit at 4 weeks after they commenced their smoking cessation programme.

The role of the nurse

Standard 4 of the NSF discusses how young people should have access to services that are geared to helping them with specific problems (Education and Skills, Department of health, 2004). It also suggests a number of other ways services can help:

- Young people are entitled to accurate information and support.
- Adult services do not work for young people; they need tailor-made support.
- Specialist support should be available to those that have complex needs.

These are all key points outlined in the NSF (Education and skills, Department of Health, 2004), which should guide the development of services for young people, including smoking cessation services.

Nurses can play a central and vital role in reducing the harm that can be caused through smoking. Nurses have contact with teenagers in school. Often teenagers are more willing to listen or seek help from a school nurse, rather than their parents/carers who may be more judgemental and less supportive.

Nurses have a role to play too, where young people have started families of their own. Midwives are in contact with young mothers throughout pregnancy and have the opportunity to support them to stop smoking. The NSF states that mothers need to have access to high-quality maternity services which are designed to support their individual needs (Education and Skills, Department of Health,

2004). Support can be provided to help them to stop smoking. Nurses can also be influential with young mothers in the early months of their children's lives, when health visitors have access to all the family, encouraging them to stop smoking for the benefit of all, particularly their young children. This may be a time when family members are a little more receptive to health advice.

However, the greatest impact that nurses may have is within a well coordinated programme utilising the skills of all health care practitioners with multiple opportunities to promote smoking cessation. Nurses can act as educators, providing a source of impetus to the health promotion programme and delivering smoking cessation services.

Collaborative working

In the Midlands, for example, the smoking cessation service – *New Leaf* – utilises a multidisciplinary, multifaceted approach. The health promotion strategy recognises that no single way of communicating with smokers will be effective and no single service will be effective at helping young people to quit. It engages general practitioners, nurses, pharmacists, health promotion, community workers and counsellors in promoting the smoking cessation message. Services are provided where and how they are most convenient to the patient. These include brief interventions, groups or clinics, or one-to-one interventions. They are provided in locations varying from traditional health care locations to community-based facilities – libraries, colleges, schools, family centres.

Training for practitioners includes information on the safety and effectiveness of nicotine replacement therapy in pregnancy. Training is also provided on how to use the patient group direction to help mothers obtain free nicotine replacement therapy.

During pregnancy, for example, young mothers would be asked to asses their own readiness to give up smoking. They are asked to indicate where they sit on the Cycle of Change (Di Clemente et al., 1991), and whether they would like to receive help to quit smoking. If yes, the smoking cessation team are informed, and the team make contact to ascertain what support young mothers may need to stop smoking. Typically, they come from less advantaged backgrounds. They have partners or family that smoke in the household, who may be very reluctant to give up smoking.

Schools

All schools are required to promote healthy lifestyles, and the school nurse can be integral in designing and delivering health promotion programmes. According to a survey conducted on behalf of the Royal College of Nursing (2005), 98% of school nurses working in State sector schools in England are involved in health promotion activity; 75% develop health policies for schools and two-thirds provide substance (including tobacco) misuse services.

The average State school nurse has over 2700 pupils under her/his care. It is impractical for school nurses to deliver all activities and services directly. A range of practitioners working alongside school nurses will help. This brings a range of complementary skills that enable services to be tailored to the needs of young people and the specific communities in which they live.

Each Primary Care Organisation working with schools will have their own system for promoting healthy lifestyles and for helping young people to deal with health issues including smoking. At primary school level few children smoke and the focus of activity is in promoting healthy living.

Once young people reach the age of 11 and move up through the school system, the range of services on offer to young people increases. Under the *Healthy Schools* programme, all schools should have a no smoking policy by September 2007 (Department of Health, 2005). Health promotion activities may include taught modules, group sessions, drop-in centres, clinics and one-to-one counselling. Nurses work alongside teachers, health care assistants, counsellors and other health care practitioners to design and deliver services. These examples indicate the range of nurse-led services offered to young people:

- In an area within the North of England, for example, nurses are able to supply nicotine replacement therapy to young people aged 12 or over, under a patient group direction. The nurses provide nicotine replacement therapy patches to young people with an addictive habit and monitor their usage very closely.

- In the Midlands some school nurses organise group workshops over a 10-week period to support pupils and staff who want to stop smoking. An overall framework is used for the workshops which include the health implications of smoking and the benefits of quitting, techniques for resisting cravings and avoiding peer pressure. Each session is planned on a weekly basis to take account of feedback.
- In the South of England, school nurses, who have been trained as smoking cessation advisors, work alongside teachers, a school counsellor and a substance misuse worker to provide services to pupils at secondary schools. Pupils are recruited to one-to-one friendship pairs or larger groups for each of the six sessions. Nurses either run their own sessions or support teachers in delivering the programme.

In each case the school nurses have been successful in helping young people to quit or reduce the amount they smoke. However, there are difficulties in providing services through school; often services cannot be delivered during curriculum time and this makes them less popular with pupils; school nurses have little time to devote to these services – other services having greater immediate call on their time. Most school nurses would like to spend more time on such health promotion activities, but are prevented from doing so by competing workloads.

Conclusion

The health impact of tobacco smoke on young people is serious and profound, but is avoidable. Nurses can be crucial in supporting young people to stop smoking. They can help design services to meet the specific needs of young people, being both supportive and non-judgemental. Importantly, to be really effective, nurses need to work with or alongside other practitioners in the provision of such services for young people, as some of the practice examples have illustrated.

Resources

http://www.ash.org.uk
http://gosmokefree.nhs.uk/

References

Action on Smoking and Health (2005) *Fact Sheet No. 11 – Stopping Smoking: The Benefits and Aids to Quitting*. Action on Smoking and Health. Available at: http://www.ash.org.uk (accessed October 2006).

Action on Smoking and Health (2006a) *Fact Sheet No. 2 – Smoking Statistics Illness and Death*. Action on Smoking and Health. Available at: http://www.ash.org.uk (accessed October 2006).

Action on Smoking and Health (2006b) *Fact Sheet No. 3 – Young People and Smoking*. Action on Smoking and Health. Available at: http://www.ash.org.uk (accessed October 2006).

Department of Health (2005) *National Healthy Schools Status*. London: Crown Copyright.

Department of Health (2007) *Explanatory Memorandum to the Children and Young Persons (Sale of Tobacco Etc.) Order 2007 No. 767*. Available at: http://www.opsi.gov.uk (accessed 11 May 2007).

Di Clemente, C., Prochaska, J., Fairhurst, S., Velicer, W., Velasquez, M., Rossi, J. (1991) The process of smoking cessation: an analysis of precontemplation, contemplation, and preparation stages of change. *Journal of Consulting and Clinical Psychology* 59(2): 295–304.

Education and Skills (Department of), Department of Health (2004) *National Service Framework for Children, Young People and Maternity Services. Standard 4 – Growing Up into Adulthood*. London: Education and Skills, Department of Health.

Lader, D., Goddard, E. (2005) *Smoking-Related Behaviour and Attitudes*. London: Office for National Statistics.

Peto, R., Lopez, A., Boreham, J., Thun, T. (2006) *Mortality from Smoking in Developed Countries 1950–2000*, 2nd edn. Oxford: Oxford University Press.

Royal College of Nursing (2005). *School Nurses: Results from a Census Survey of RCN School Nurses in 2005*. London: Royal College of Nursing.

The Information Centre (2006a) *Drug Use, Smoking and Drinking among Young People in England in 2005*. London: Government Statistical Service.

The Information Centre (2006b) *Statistics on NHS Stop Smoking Services in England, April to June 2006*. London: Government Statistical Service.

Theme 11

Evaluating Health Promotion

Chapter 38   Evaluating Health Promotion

38 Evaluating Health Promotion

Karen Moyse

Introduction

This chapter explores evaluation and its importance for health promotion activities, courses and services. An example from practice will be presented, which demonstrates a research-based approach used to evaluate a health promotion service – the Sure Start community children's nursing (CCN) service.

Why evaluate and how to go about it?

This section explores why evaluation is important and how to go about it. The section provides a general introduction to the process of evaluation.

Importance and benefits

As nurses working with children/young people and their families, we need to know exactly how our health promotion activities (courses or services) are impacting upon their health. Importantly, evaluation should be central to all health promotion activities undertaken.

What is evaluation?

Daines and Graham (1992) maintain that evaluation should be seen as simply a way of working. It can involve a continuous process of observing, asking questions and then offering explanations based on the evidence explored. From this process changes to practice can then take place. Daines and Graham (1992) also provide a further perspective, which involves looking at a learning event, with a view to determining if it is achieving something of value. Value can be considered in terms of *quality*, but also in terms of *cost*. Health promotion activities can be considered as learning events for those participants taking part.

Why do we need to know the impact of our health promotion activities?

Knowing exactly what impact our health promotion activities are having on children/young people and their families will inform practice. Importantly, is that impact what we set out to achieve in the beginning? At a broad level that impact has to be influencing the health of children/young people in a very positive way. However, at a more specific level, we need to know exactly what is being achieved. Parahoo (1997) suggests that one way to do this is to examine the objectives/outcomes of the activity in some detail, to see if they are being achieved.

Evaluation is central

Evaluation should be central to all health promotion activities undertaken. By ensuring that evaluation is central, the process can be so much easier. Reid (1988) even goes as far as to advocate evaluation as being central to every aspect of practice.

In setting up the Sure Start CCN service, for example, the team leader wanted to ensure that evaluation strategies were firmly in place from the very outset of the project. Evaluation strategies were thus devised at the same time as the service was being developed.

Parahoo (1997) states that evaluation can sometimes be an afterthought. By making evaluation a priority, it then becomes central to the health promotion process. Evaluation is not suddenly something that has been thrown together shortly before it is due to be presented to those funding it. Having an evaluation process firmly in place, which has been clearly thought out and is appropriate to the needs of that health promotion activity, can make the daunting process of evaluation so much easier.

From experience a well-planned evaluation can also be influential to the success or otherwise of a new initiative. In a climate of short-term funding, it can make the difference between success and failure. Will the service be able to continue for a further year, or will funding no longer be provided, bringing the initiative to an abrupt end?

Other issues to consider

- There is no purpose in repeatedly undertaking the same health promotion activities if they are not helping those for which they are intended.
- Cost has important implications within the National Health Service.
- Evaluation can be invaluable; it can be the catalyst for change. By exploring the views of others, it can tell you what needs changing to make things better.

In summary, evaluation is essential. As highlighted, evaluation can have a number of benefits, particularly if well planned.

What needs to be evaluated?

It is useful to evaluate most things. As a nurse or nurse researcher, one is then in a good position to demonstrate the impact of health promotion activities being delivered. Evaluation might involve evaluating one-to-one contacts, for example, through sessions, courses and services.

Daines and Graham (1992) maintain that evaluation should take place all the time. However, there are times when this may not be appropriate. For example, if a nurse is doing a large number of similar health promotion activities, it may not be necessary to evaluate each one, but a random selection might be equally as effective.

As highlighted, evaluation frequently gets left until the end of a health promotion activity or course. In some cases this may be too late. The opportunity to improve things for some participants has been lost. By evaluating during the activity or course, as Daines et al. (1993) suggest, the nurse is in a better position to improve things for participants. A further evaluation can always take place at the very end.

The results of evaluations can be fed into future health promotion activities or courses, improving the activities for participants. However, it is useful to remember that what suits one group may not always suit the next. To help with evaluation, it is often helpful to find out at the beginning what each group would like to see included in the activity or course. If it is possible and appropriate include it, so participants' needs are really being met. Daines and Graham (1992) advocate checking participants' views periodically to see if the health promotion activity is providing what they need.

Once you have established what is going to be evaluated, how to evaluate then needs to be considered.

How to evaluate?

Objectives (outcomes)

Objectives/outcomes can be essential for evaluation. They can provide the basis for an evaluation.

As mentioned in earlier chapters, the aim outlines the purpose of your health promotion activity. However, it does not specify what learning should be taking place (Daines et al., 1993). The objectives/outcomes identify exactly what our participants should be learning (Daines et al., 1993).

For example, an aim for the Sure Start CCN service in providing children's minor illness and minor injury service is specified below.

Aim – to advance parents'/carers' knowledge and skills in the management of young children's minor illnesses/injuries, so they feel more confident in caring for their young children.

Some of the objectives/outcomes are set out below. The objectives/outcomes in this example depended on what was actually wrong with the child, as well as needs of the child and family, so would be individual to each family. The example below illustrates the objectives/outcomes where a child has a fever, for instance.

Parents/carers will be able to:

- recognise when their child has a high temperature;
- care for their child appropriately when her/his temperature rises.

Objectives/outcomes can be demonstrated through the behaviours people undertake, and attitudes/feelings which people hold, as well as knowledge they have gained (Daines et al., 1993). For example, the Sure Start CCNs were able to observe changes in behaviours and attitudes of parents/carers in the management of their young children's illnesses, following advice received from the service.

The service needed to be able to systematically assess if these objectives/outcomes were being achieved, not just from observation alone. The objectives/outcomes acted as the basis for this assessment. The Sure Start CCNs assessed the achievement of these objectives/outcomes with the use of a questionnaire designed for the purpose.

Objectives/outcomes are widely used within nurse education, as well as in practice. They are used to measure individual change (Daines et al., 1993). One particular learning outcome you might be familiar with is *competence* (Daines et al., 1993). This is specific to a learning outcome related to *doing*, which also embraces the knowledge and skills

needed *to do*. To be competent means to be able to perform at a particular level, in line with certain standards (Daines et al., 1993).

Sure Start wanted parents/carers to feel themselves that they were competent to care for their children when unwell with a minor illness or minor injury; to feel competent to manage minor illnesses such as colds and stomach upsets, for example. But at the same time, Sure Start wanted parents/carers to feel confident to call for help when needed. Particularly, if they felt their child's health was deteriorating.

Objectives/outcomes can help identify what needs to be evaluated. However, there are other ways evaluation can be approached, as the following outlines.

Other approaches to evaluation

There are other aspects of a health promotion activity or course, as well as the achievement of learning objectives/outcomes, that can be evaluated. The basis of evaluation work can also centre on the following:

- Assessing participants' views.
- Peer evaluation.
- Self-evaluation or reflection.
- Health data – local, national.
  These will be discussed further.

Participants' views – find out at the beginning what each group would like to see included in the activity or course. Daines and Graham (1992) advocate checking participants' views periodically to see if their needs are being met. Participants' views can then be used to form the basis of an evaluation.

Peer evaluation is another approach. It can be undertaken by colleagues who can observe and provide feedback. Daines et al. (1993) suggest that you first identify particular aspects that your colleagues need to focus on, for which they provide feedback. With the Sure Start CCN evaluation, peer evaluations were sought from other practitioners involved with the same families. They were able to provide a further perspective on how the service was being received by these families and what kind of impact it was having.

Self-evaluation or reflection is another approach, which has been discussed by Schon (1983).

Reflecting on one's experiences can help to advance practice, by helping the nurse to learn from those experiences. Parahoo (1997) states that a nurse can evaluate her/his practice by reflecting on or thinking about what she/he does. The difference between reflection and evaluation, he states, is that evaluation is a systematic appraisal which uses different research methods. However, reflection alone will not provide sufficient insights for an evaluation. Although, at an individual level it will inform one's practice. In our example, the CNNs reflected on their activities with families, when young children were unwell.

Looking at *health data*, and examining changes, can demonstrate if health promotion activities are meeting important targets. For example, with the Sure Start CCN evaluation, examining acute hospital admission data for young children living in the area was able to inform Sure Start if there had been a reduction in hospital admissions associated with the Sure Start (2003/4) target, since the introduction of the CCN service.

With health data it can sometimes be difficult to access the data that you need. It is worth being persistent. It is useful to be able to draw comparisons with the data, so you may want to request data at different time intervals.

This section has identified how the process of evaluation might be approached. A number of different approaches have been suggested. In addition, the importance of evaluation has been discussed.

Simple methods of evaluation

Simple methods of evaluation will be discussed here. Some important points that need to be considered when evaluating with children/young people will be outlined.

When considering small health promotion activities or courses, simple evaluation methods are beneficial. Evaluation can be undertaken with the use of a questionnaire, which individual group members can complete. An alternative is as a group discussion. Or a combination of these methods might be useful, providing a broader perspective. Parahoo (1997) states that there is value in combining methods. A group discussion, for example, can help stimulate ideas that individuals may not have considered, but could go on to explore when completing their own questionnaire.

There are a number of other methods that can be used. These can include the following:

- Questioning.
- Exercises.
- Group participation.
- Quiz.

There is no reason why these have to be bland. They can be made fun and interesting, as well as achieving the aim of evaluation.

Example of a simple evaluation form

A common approach to the evaluation of a health promotion activity is the use of a simple evaluation form, used in the middle or towards the end of an activity or course. It can include a number of simple questions for participants to complete. Evaluation forms can be made easy, both for those participants completing them and for the nurse collating them. Where response formats for questions are already provided, such as *yes*, *no*, *not sure*, participants will find these formats easy to complete. However, bear in mind they might not provide you as the nurse researcher, with enough information.

If using a written evaluation form, ensure that all your participants are going to be able to read it and understand it. You do not want to cause embarrassment.

Daines et al. (1993) advocate that when using an evaluation form some of the following questions are useful, as outlined in Box 38.1.

Box 38.1 Daines et al.'s (1993) ideas on questions to include in an evaluation form.

Daines et al. (1993) suggest asking participants to identify the following:

- One of the most valuable aspects of the course (so far).
- One of the least valuable aspects of the course (so far).
- The thing I like best about coming on this course.
- If I could change the course, I would.
- I should like to say that.

From undertaking a number of health promotion evaluations, other useful questions to include centre around content and the resources used. It is particularly important to find out if participants were able to understand that information in the way, it was presented. It needs to be presented at the right level for them. Presenting concise information in a clear way, enhanced with the use of effective visual aids, will help participants' understanding. Too much information serves only to confuse. Box 38.2 presents some additional questions that might be useful to include in an evaluation form.

Box 38.2 Questions to include in evaluation form.

Please spend a few minutes writing a sentence or two in response to the following questions:

- Did you find the information clear?
- Do you think the content will be useful to you? If useful, in what ways?
- Did you find that the visual aids helped your learning?
- Would you like to make any other comments about what you have learnt?

Thank you. Your comments will be used to inform future activities.

Try to make the layout inviting to those who are going to complete the form. Always thank participants for their comments. Consider how you are going to categorise the responses will the results, and how be presented. These are all important issues to consider when putting together even the simplest of evaluation forms.

Children/young people evaluating

When evaluating the views and learning of children/young people, a number of specific issues need to be considered. The process should be made easy, interesting and fun. Obviously permission to evaluate with them must be sought first.

Any forms that are specifically designed need to be put together in a way that will enable children/young people to clearly understand what is being asked of them. The response formats should be made interesting and fun. Their age and cognitive abilities must always be considered.

For young children a good example of this can be found with the pain-rating scales that are commonly used in hospitals, such as Wong and Baker's (1988) *happy/sad pain-rating scale.* Children point to the image which depicts how they feel. Children are able to understand how to use it, and are able to respond appropriately. This tool can be used with children as young as 3/4 years of age (Smith, 1995).

Rosch et al.'s (1976) work on categories provides useful insights into the cognitive abilities of young children. They found that 4-year-old children were able to categorise quite well at a basic level. Starkey (1981) demonstrates that the foundation of this cognitive process begins to emerge earlier in childhood. By middle childhood (8 years old) the ability to categorise becomes more defined; the ability to create categories increases (Inhelder and Piaget, 1964).

Categorisation is a simple concept that can be applied to the design of forms. Children from the age of 4 to 5 years could be asked to group items into simple categories of two or three groups. From the age of 8 to 9 years a few more categories can be added.

Categorisation might be used in relation to a session on *healthy eating*, for example, as a means of assessing children's learning following the session. Children (4 to 5 years old) could be asked to put foods into particular categories; simple categories to start with such as healthy foods/not sure/unhealthy foods.

As children become older (8 to 9 years old), a few more categories can be introduced, such as asking children to put foods into different food groups.

Categorisation is a useful concept. It can be used for evaluation purposes to assess children's learning, as well as their views.

Other ways to evaluate children's views and learning includes observing their behaviour during a health promotion activity, and also asking them at the end of that activity about their thoughts. Children can be amusingly honest in their replies. Hopefully, you will be able to observe their enthusiasm as they participate.

Experiences of evaluating with a group of 7-year-olds undertaking a first-aid session were recently enlightening. A short interactive session on first-aid with a group of 12 children was undertaken at a local school. It was evaluated by observing their behaviour and asking them at the end what they thought about it. As the nurse I could see from the enthusiastic way they joined in and the questions they asked that it was enjoyable and of interest to them. Learning of new information was clearly evident; they demonstrated the skills they had learnt. At the end children said what they thought about the session, and wanted to know when we would be doing the next one mentioned.

With young people you could adopt some of the other strategies earlier in the chapter. They may find the interaction and competitive nature of a quiz appealing, for example.

The views of children/young people can be sought in the evaluation of a service too, although this can be a little more difficult. Children, like adults, have to be protected as participants in research (Royal College of Nursing, 2004). Obviously, permission from children/young people, parents/carers will all be needed, as well as those of the service provider. Ethical agreement will need to be sought from the local ethics committee. Careful attention will need to be paid to the wording of any evaluation tools.

Jennings (1994), for example, in her evaluation of a hospital-at-home service, asked children for their views about the service, compared to hospital care. Children from the age of 6 years were consulted. The response rate was small – 47% of the sample. Most of the children surveyed said they would choose home care again. An established questionnaire was used for the survey. This meant that Jennings (1994) did not have the time-consuming task of designing and validating her own research tool.

Some general points in relation to undertaking simple evaluations have been discussed. Some ideas have been provided about evaluating with children/young people. The following sections look at the use of research within evaluation.

A research-based approach to evaluation

Why research?

A more *complex* approach to evaluation can be undertaken, as demonstrated through the work of the Sure Start CCN service. Sure Start identi-

fied that a systematic research-based approach was needed to evaluate its brand new children's nursing service.

There were lots of questions that needed asking, as outlined below:

- Was it helping families, and if so, how was the service helping them?
- Was it helping other health practitioners in their support of families?
- How did the CCNs feel about the way the service was working?
- What impact was the service having, if any, on local health statistics, in relation to preventing young children (0–5 years) from being admitted to hospital?
- How did the service relate to guidelines/ standards of good practice? For this the NSF (Education and Skills, Department of Health, 2004) was used as an essential guide. A variety of research methods were thus employed.

A research-based approach to evaluation would provide an evidence base upon which to build the service.

Evidence-based care is said to assume great importance (Parahoo, 1997). Evaluative studies tend to focus on a particular aspect of practice, policy or an event (Parahoo, 1997). In this situation it was a particular aspect of practice – the Sure Start CCN service.

Parahoo (1997) states that research has the potential to improve quality of care, as it provides nurses with the opportunity to ask questions. The Sure Start CCN service was fundamentally about improving the quality of care for young children (0–5 years) locally. Evaluation would hopefully demonstrate that the service was doing this. Evaluation would also provide guidance on how the service could be further developed for local families.

What is research?

Research has been defined as a systematic attempt to discover the principles governing a phenomenon (Chaplin, 1985). Perhaps a more practical way for nurses to consider research is that it provides the tools necessary to systematically evaluate their health promotion practice, so they can demonstrate if practice is achieving its objectives. There is obviously more to research than this, but this may provide a useful starting point.

Using research for evaluative purposes can be quite daunting, particularly the first time one uses it. Importantly, think about – what do you want to know, and how best can you find this out? There will not be one answer, but undoubtedly several options.

When trying to decide on the most appropriate research design and research methods to use with your evaluation, remember to consider carefully the advantages, as well as the limitations that they offer. What research methods will be the most helpful?

Below is a brief list of research texts that nurses may find helpful to consult when considering research. These include the following:

- *The Practice of Nursing Research, Conduct, Critique and Utilization*, by Burns and Grove.
- *Evaluating Health Interventions*, by Øvretveit.
- *Nursing Research, Principles, Process and Issues*, by Parahoo.
- *Research, Methods, Appraisal, and Utilization*, by Polit and Hungler.

The reader may also find articles in the *Journal of Advanced Nursing* and *Nurse Researcher* helpful.

Nurses will need to consult research text to gain a better understanding of what research is about and the processes involved. This chapter simply talks about the evaluation of one health promotion initiative to develop a service for sick children. The chapter explains the research methods used, so that nurses can gain a better understanding of how evidence-based practice can be developed.

Research methods

A variety of different research methods were used in the Sure Start CCN evaluation. The main design of this evaluation was a *survey design*. One particular research method that will be looked at in some depth therefore will be *questionnaires*, as they are a particular feature of survey designs, and were used in the Sure Start CCN evaluation.

Three different surveys were used:

- Minor illness/injury survey (for parents/carers).
- Parent's/carer's satisfaction survey.
- Health practitioners' survey.

A research proposal

A research proposal has to be completed before the research can begin. Burns and Grove (1997) describe this as a written plan that identifies the major elements of the research. It outlines the purpose of the research, as well as methods that will be used. A research proposal may need to be submitted to the local ethics committee, service provider and also potential funders, depending on the circumstances of the evaluation.

Aims and objectives

Parahoo (1997) maintains that the *aims and objectives* should provide the benchmark against which the success of an activity or service can be measured. The aims and objectives of the Sure Start CCN service were used to formulate research aims and objectives for the evaluation. One of the research aims is included below:

To evaluate the Sure Start CCN service to find out if it is able to *empower* parents/carers, so they feel more knowledgeable and skilled in the management of their young children's minor illnesses/injuries.

Research questions were formulated, using the research aims and objectives to inform the development of these questions.

Ethics

Obtaining ethical permission was one of the first considerations. The local ethics committee was approached with the research proposal. They wanted assurances that the views of individuals participating within the study would remain anonymous. These guarantees were provided. It is important that individuals who are participating in research are able to provide their views freely. As the Royal College of Nursing (2004) states participants should be safeguarded.

Anonymity was achieved by ensuring that the questionnaires individuals were given to complete were identified by number and not by name. Individuals were informed of this, so they would feel more confident about sharing their views. The ethical principals of *anonymity* and *confidentiality* (Beauchamp and Childress, 1994) helped to guide the research.

Quantitative and qualitative approaches

The approach one takes with research needs to be considered. The quantitative and qualitative approaches to research are commonly used and are based on different research paradigms.

Quantitative is commonly associated with the positivist paradigm. It examines things in terms of cause and effect, objective measurement, which can be made by reducing things down to a specific number (Parahoo, 1997).

Qualitative is associated with naturalistic observation and focuses on the experiences of people. It stresses the uniqueness of the individual, as well as the cultural/social factors which influence behaviour (Parahoo, 1997).

Whatever approach is used, whether it is quantitative or qualitative, it will have strong implications for the research methods used (Polit and Hungler, 1997).

The Sure Start CCN evaluation adopted mainly a quantitative approach, but also incorporated some qualitative methods. Quantitative methods were used when number analysis was more pertinent. Qualitative methods were applied where the data seemed more relevant to this type of approach, particularly where parents expressed their feelings.

Sampling

Sampling – *purposive* sampling was used. Burns and Grove (1997) describe this as the researcher consciously selecting certain individuals to be included within the research. It is judged as not being as rigorous as some sampling methods (Polit and Hungler, 1997). To use another sampling method, such as randomised sampling, for example, which is considered to be the most rigorous (Burns and Grove, 1997), would not have provided enough parents/carers or health practitioners for the study.

The survey was taking place at a particular moment in time – a set time interval. Parents/carers who used the service within this time interval were surveyed.

The sample for each questionnaire was as follows:

- 25 parents/carers (minor illness/injury questionnaire).
- 25 parents/carers (satisfaction survey).
- 11 health practitioners – general practitioners, health visitors and Sure Start colleagues (health practitioners' questionnaire).

Obviously, a key part of the evaluation involved looking at the views of others, the users of the service – parents/carers, as well as health practitioners who worked with the same families. However, looking at the views of others can be problematic. A drawback of this approach, as Polit and Hungler (1997) maintain, is that people's views change over time. However, in this context, it was felt appropriate to examine the views of users and practitioners, as they could best describe how the service was working for them at that time, which was both relevant and important. Researching the views of users is actually an approach which is advocated by Sure Start (2000).

Design and questionnaires

Specific *research tools* had to be designed to access the data. Sure Start was not aware of any research tools available that would specifically meet the needs of this evaluation. The design of research tools was a time-consuming process. Once designed, they had to be tested for validity and reliability.

Fink and Kosecoff (1985) describe a survey design as a method of collecting information from people in the form of a questionnaire (or interview). The Sure Start CCN had previous experience of designing research tools, particularly questionnaires. There were a number of different advantages that appealed about using questionnaires. Large amounts of data could be collected within a relatively short space of time (Parahoo, 1997). With a sample group of 25 parents/carers this seemed an appropriate method, allowing a number of different views to be collated fairly quickly. The questionnaire designed for health practitioners could be self-administered. An advantage of using this type of questionnaire meant that the health practitioners could complete the questionnaire at their own convenience, as part of their normal working practice.

Critics of the questionnaire say that bias can be introduced due to non-response (Crossby et al., 1989). Typically, questionnaire response rates are within the range of 25–30% (Gordon and Stokes, 1989). To prevent this happening, a strategy was introduced to boost the response rate. This included reminding everyone when the questionnaires would be coming out and then again when they needed to be returned.

All this contact was aimed at achieving a high response rate for the survey. It did seem to impact on the final result. The minor illness/injury questionnaire achieved a response rate of 100% ($n = 25$), and so too did the satisfaction survey (100%, $n = 25$). The health practitioners' questionnaire was a little less successful, achieving 81% ($n = 9$, from a sample of $n = 11$). Statistical analysis was used to analyse the results of all the questionnaires.

Example: Evaluating the Sure Start CCN service

The following provides a summary of the evaluation. The evaluation was undertaken over a 14-month period. It explored families' and practitioners' views about the service. It also examined referrals received during the evaluation period (Moyse, 2005).

Evaluation was felt to be central to the development of the service. Sure Start and the local PCT needed to know if the service really was helping to improve the care of children's health locally. Interestingly, Øvretveit (1998) states that evaluation is about examining if services are able to improve people's health, and the results of which can then be used to improve practice. Nurses are thus able to develop services based on clear evidence (Øvretveit, 1998).

The NSFs (Education and Skills, Department of Health, 2004) actually identify evidence-based care as a *marker of good practice* for children's services. By undertaking the evaluation, it would seem that Sure Start was taking positive steps towards improving the standards of care for children locally.

Research questions

The process of enquiry involved formulating research questions, as previously highlighted:

- Is the Sure Start CCN service able to promote the health of young children living in a deprived community, by advancing parents' knowledge and skills in the management of children's minor illnesses and injuries?
- Is the service able to reduce the number of young children admitted to hospital as an emergency with gastroenteritis, respiratory infection and injuries, as required by the Sure Start (2003/4) target?

The following outlines the data required for collection. The research tools used are included within brackets:

(1) Parents'/carers' knowledge and skills on young children's minor illness/injury management (minor illness/injury questionnaire).
(2) Parent's/carer's satisfaction survey (questionnaire).
(3) Health practitioners' views about the service (questionnaire).
(4) Evaluation of first-aid and minor illness courses (simple evaluation questionnaire).
(5) CCN reflective diary (diary).
(6) Examination of health data in relation to the Sure Start (2003/4) target (information from PCT Health Informatics department).
(7) Examination of referrals to the service (audit tool).
(8) Comparisons with *markers of good practice* contained within the NSFs (Education and Skills, Department of Health, 2004).

Results

(1) Minor illness/injury survey – on most of the variables presented, parents/carers felt that their knowledge and skills on children's minor illness/injury management had improved, since accessing support and care from the service.
(2) Satisfaction survey – all the parents/carers were very satisfied with the service. All wanted

the service to be extended into an *out of hours* service.

(3) Health practitioners felt that the service was very supportive to families, and where children were very ill, helped children access hospital services more easily.

(4) The first-aid and minor illness courses were always well attended, and parents/carers reported that the information was very useful.

(5) Diary observations – the CCNs were able to observe at first hand an improved level of confidence in the nursing of sick children, with mothers particularly and sometimes even grandparents.

(6) Health data obtained from the PCT Health Informatics department allowed a comparison between *yearly hospital admission figures*. Acute hospital admissions figures for the 2 years since the Sure Start CCN service had been introduced were compared with the previous 2 years, when the service had not been available. There was a reduction in young children being admitted to hospital suffering from the target illnesses and injuries, since the service had been in place. A particular reduction was noted in admissions associated with respiratory infections. Most of the referrals to the service were received from families with children suffering respiratory illnesses.

(7) Referrals – 160 referrals were received during the evaluation period and were examined. The most common referrals were children with high temperatures, gastroenteritis and, of course, from respiratory illnesses.

(8) The NSFs (Education and Skills, Department of Health, 2004) *markers of good practice* were examined in relation to standard 6 (children who are ill) and standard 10 (medicines for children).

The Sure Start CCN service clearly met some of these *markers of good practice*:

- Children with minor illness and injuries need ready access to local services (standard 6).
- Children should receive services close to home (standard 6).
- Access to medications for children needs to be improved (standard 10).

- Parents/carers should receive up-to-date information on the safe use of medicines (standard 10).

The service provides an easily accessible service in the home for young children who are unwell with minor illnesses and injuries. The service therefore meets standard 6.

The CCNs are also able to provide prescriptions (if appropriate) for young children when ill. Nurse prescribing was not implemented until following the evaluation, so therefore was not included in the evaluation process.

Nurse prescribing, once in place, the Sure Start CCNs could see, was making a difference to young children with the accessibility of medication, as standard 10 indicates. For each prescription written, the Sure Start CCN always provide information on the safe use of medicines for children, as recommended by standard 10 (NSFs, Education and Skills, Department of Health, 2004). This provides a brief summary of the results for the evaluation.

Recommendations

The results of that evaluation have demonstrated that the Sure Start CCN service is able to support and empower families when their children are ill. Any future developments to the service can now be based on direct evidence-based practice, produced by this evaluation.

The service has helped the care of sick children locally, resulting in less need for children to attend their general practitioners and A + E departments, able to be cared for at home (where appropriate). Parents/carers feel more knowledgeable and skilled in their own management of children's minor illnesses/injuries, as they have identified themselves. The service has also helped to reduce the number of young children admitted to hospital as an emergency in line with the Sure Start (2003/4) target.

However, there is a need to continue this important work. The service could be extended, so that it is more *accessible* to families. This could be achieved by making the service into an *out of hours* service, which is currently not available to families.

Dissemination

Dissemination is an essential part of the research process. Ewles and Simnett (1987) suggest writing up health promotion work and circulating the results to colleagues. This provides colleagues and others with the opportunity to learn from your work and experiences.

Too often good pieces of work sit on a shelf gathering dust, when others could be benefiting from the insights they offer. With the Sure Start CCN service, it was felt that this experience and knowledge should be shared. A number of presentations on the evaluation were undertaken locally. An article was also published in *Paediatric Nursing* – Walmsley and Moyse (2006), discussing the development of the service. Further dissemination will take place with the evaluation.

Awards are another way to showcase good practice. The Sure Start CCN service was entered for two local awards and one national award. It won a local PCT award in 2004 *modernisation in health care*, and in 2005 it was a finalist for both a local and national award.

Conclusion

The chapter has examined evaluation and its importance. Suggestions on how evaluations might be undertaken have been considered. An example of a research-based evaluation is explored through the work of the Sure Start CCN service.

References

Beauchamp, T., Childress, J. (1994) *Principles of Biomedical Ethics*, 4th edn. Oxford: Oxford University Press.

Burns, N., Grove, S. (1997) *The Practice of Nursing Research*, 3rd edn. London: W. B. Saunders and Company.

Chaplin, J. (1985) *Dictionary of Psychology*. New York: Laurel Books.

Crossby, F., Ventura, M., Feldman, M. (1989) Examination of a Survey. *Nursing Research* 38(1): 56–58.

Daines, J., Daines, C., Graham, B. (1993) *Adult Learning, Adult Teaching*, 3rd edn. Nottingham: Department of Adult Education.

Daines, J., Graham, B. (1992) Supporting and developing adult learning, reviewing learning. *Adults Learning* 3(7): 172–178.

Education and Skills (Department of), Department of Health (2004) *National Service Framework (NSFs) for Children, Young People, and Maternity Services*. London: Department of Education and Skills and Department of Health.

Ewles, L., Simnett, I. (1987) *Promoting Health, a Practical Guide to Health Education*. Chichester: John Wiley & Sons Ltd.

Fink, A., Kosecoff, J. (1985) *How to Conduct Surveys*. Newbury Park: Sage.

Gordon, S., Stokes, S. (1989) Improving response rate to mailed questionnaires. *Nursing Research* 38(6): 375–376.

Inhelder, B., Piaget, J. (1964) *The Early Growth of Logic in the Child*. New York: Harper & Row.

Jennings, P. (1994) Learning through experience: an evaluation of hospital at home. *Journal of Advanced Nursing* 19: 905–911.

Moyse, K. (2005) *Sure Start Community Children's Nursing: Evaluating the Service*. Derbyshire: Sure Start Creswell, Langwith/Whaley Thorns and Shirebrook, North Eastern Derbyshire Primary Care Trust.

Øvretveit, J. (1998) *Evaluating Health Interventions*. Buckingham: Open University Press.

Parahoo, K. (1997) *Nursing Research, Principles, Process and Issues*. Hampshire: Macmillan Press Ltd.

Polit, D., Hungler, B. (1997) *Essentials of Nursing Research, Methods, Appraisals and Utilisation*, 4th edn. Philadelphia: Lippincott.

Reid, N. (1988) The Delphi technique: its contribution to the evaluation of professional practice. In: Ellis, R. (ed.) *Professional Competence and Quality Assurance in the Caring Professions*, 2nd edn. London: Chapman & Hall.

Rosch, E., Mervis, C., Gray, W., Johnson, D., Boyes-Braem, P. (1976) Basic objects in natural categories. *Cognitive Psychology* 8: 382–439.

Royal College of Nursing (2004) *Research Ethics*. London: Royal College of Nursing.

Schon, D. (1983) *The Reflective Practitioner*. New York: Basic Books.

Smith, F. (with Nottingham Children's Nurses) (1995) *Children's Nursing in Practice, the Nottingham Model*. London: Blackwell Science.

Starkey, D. (1981) The origins of concept formation: object sorting and object preference in early infancy. *Child Development* 52: 489–497.

Sure Start (2000) *Sure Start: A Guide for 2nd Wave Programmes*. London: Sure Start.

Sure Start (2003/4) *Sure Start Aim and Objectives*. London: Sure Start.

Walmsley, C., Moyse, K. (2006) Sure Start community children's nursing: setting up a minor illness and injury service for children up to 5 years of age. *Paediatric Nursing* 18(3): 30–33.

Wong, D., Baker, C. (1988) Pain in children: comparison of assessment scales. *Paediatric Nursing* 14(1): 9–17.

Theme 12

Health Promotion in Context

Chapter 39   Health Promotion in Context

39 Health Promotion in Context

Vicky Grayson

NSF

The National Service Framework (NSF) for children/young people and maternity services talks about the importance of promoting children's health (Education and Skills, Department of Health, 2004).

Introduction

How do practitioners deliver health promotion to children/young people within the different contexts in which they work? *Hospital*, *community*, *nurseries*, as well as *schools* are four different contexts where health promotion with children/young people takes place. This chapter explores health promotion in these different settings. Examples from practice will be presented. Some are based on my own experiences of practice. In all practice examples presented, names and places have been altered to maintain patient confidentiality, as outlined in the Nursing and Midwifery's Council code of professional conduct (Nursing and Midwlfery Council, 2004).

It is recognised that health promotion for children/young people is achieved in all sorts of contexts, youth clubs and sports clubs, for example. However, these contexts and others will not be ex-

amined within the scope of this chapter. Having worked as a children's nurse both in hospital and community settings, I have encountered a variety of ways health promotion can be achieved with children/young people, which this chapter aims to explore.

Hospital

Health promotion in the hospital setting is possibly the most difficult to explain, because it is not obvious; it is implicit within nursing care. Whilst nurses are undertaking their normal duties, health promotion advice is continually being given. For example, when a child's temperature is being taken, parents/carers will be receiving advice about temperature management from the nurse.

Children's/young people's wards

Health promotion is undertaken in the ward setting in a variety of different ways, as the following demonstrates. Sometimes nurses find it difficult to explain how they provide health promotion advice as nurses do not distinguish it from their other nursing duties. Health promotion should be seen as part of the care received by all children, young people and their family in the ward setting.

Communication

As discussed in earlier chapters, good communication skills are essential for effective health promotion (Ewles and Simnett, 2002). On a children's ward verbal communication is the main method used for giving health promotion advice. It is undertaken from admission through to discharge. The following outlines an example.

Jimmy, a 14-month-old boy, was admitted to his local hospital following a febrile convulsion. On admission to the ward the nurse explained to Jimmy's parents how to care for him during his stay by preventing his temperature from rising again, which might cause a further febrile convulsion. Health promotion advice was given on what medication to use, and how it should be given, as well as other methods they could use to keep Jimmy cool.

During a child's stay in hospital, the nurse could be seen as a role model, demonstrating to parents/carers how to care for their ill child (Whiting, 2001). Through observing and questioning the nurse, parents/carers are able to learn. In Jimmy's case, for example, parents observed the actions of the nurse, asked questions, and went on to undertake Jimmy's care themselves, replicating the behaviours of the nurse.

The public perceive children's nurses as being knowledgeable about the care of children/young people. Children's nurses therefore play an important role in educating the general public on issues relating to children's/young people's health. In the Midlands, a children's ward recently supported *National Accident Prevention Week*. Nurses joined police officers to promote children's safety in cars. They went out with the police to supermarket car parks to check and advise parents/carers on car seat safety for their children. All involved with this initiative felt the presence of children's nurses had a greater impact than the police alone. Joint working between agencies in this way provided parents/carers with a broader perspective on children's safety.

Written information

It is good practice to provide written information to support any verbal health promotion advice given. Some hospitals have developed their own health promotion leaflets on common childhood illnesses, which parents/carers can take away. In the case of Jimmy, for example, an easy-to-read leaflet on tem-perature control and preventing febrile convulsions was given on discharge from hospital.

There are also other ways of obtaining reliable evidence-based knowledge for health practitioners and parents/carers to use. The National Health Service (NHS) provides several sources for accessing information: NHS Direct, NHS Direct Online and Prodigy. They all provide leaflets which can be given to parents/carers to help when caring for a child who is unwell.

Giving recognised and evidence-based information is important. Parents/carers are naturally concerned when their child is unwell and usually require additional information and support. Providing reliable up-to-date health promotion information in a written form can be useful to them.

Display boards

Display boards are used on children's/young people's wards to present health promotion information. In a study by Whiting (2001), it was found that display boards were common practice on a children's ward.

Information is often displayed relevant to the care of children/young people on that particular ward. An ENT (ears, nose and throat) ward, for example, might display material on what to expect when caring for a child following a tonsillectomy.

Wards will also display material on national campaigns which focus on children's health. To find out when to display appropriate material associated with national health promotion campaigns, access the website – http://www.dh.gov.uk/assetRoot/ (Department of Health, 2005). Local health promotion units will also provide details. The list below presents an example of key dates for national campaigns held during May 2007:

- 1 May – National Asthma Day.
- 13–19 May – National Breastfeeding Awareness Week.
- 13 May to 12 June – National Smile Month (dental health).
- 21–25 May – National Allergy Week.
- 21–27 May – Cancer Prevention Week.
- 21–25 May – Walk to School Week.
- 31 May – World No Tobacco Day.
- May – Save a Baby Month.

Display boards can be used to highlight health promotion relating to seasonal topics too, such as sun safety.

The highly dependent/critically ill child

When children/young people are seriously ill, health promotion remains important. One aspect of health promotion might include information on maintaining children's/young people's hygienic needs. As the Department of Health (2003) maintains, personal and oral hygiene are essential. Importantly, practitioners need to share best practice on hygiene to achieve quality care for those they are nursing.

Involving parents/carers with washing their child provides them with opportunities to be part of their child's care. Having a nurse present when the child is being washed is also useful, as it allows for a full assessment of the child's needs. Observing the skin for red and sore areas should be undertaken. The skin protects; it is a barrier to infection and regulates the body temperature. Incontinence, perspiration, poor nutrition and obesity all influence the ability of the skin to protect, which if not cared for appropriately, can lead to pressure sores (Geraghty, 2005).

Health promotion issues to consider when nursing the highly dependent/critically ill child are the following:

- Provide support and advice to parents/carers about their child's care.
- Demonstrate and provide health promotion information to parents/carers on ways that can assist in their child's care.
- Allow the parents/carers time to spend with their child, so they can talk, play or provide their child with the opportunity to listen to music.
- Regular turning of the child to prevent pressure sores.
- Regular washing of the child to prevent the skin from breaking down.
- Mouth care, including brushing the child's teeth.
- Keeping the child's eyes and nose moist to prevent sores and cracks.
- Providing the child with appropriate nutritional support which has been recommended by the dietician.

Information on all these different aspects of care can be discussed with parents/carers, so they can be involved and understand their child's needs at a time of critical illness.

For example, Alison, a 12-year old, was critically ill in hospital. Her mother helped in her care by giving Alison oral sponges to keep her mouth moist. The nurse explained to her mother the purpose and importance of this to Alison's care.

Accident and emergency department

The accident and emergency department (A & E) is frequently the first place where children/young people are examined when entering hospital. A quarter of attendances at A & E are children/young people and the most common reason why they attend is trauma (Evans, 1999).

After an accident may be a useful time to provide health promotion information. Whiting (2001) maintains it is important that this information is given in a light-hearted manner, and discourages practitioners from lecturing children/young people about their health.

Bradley, an 8-year-old boy, attended A & E after sustaining a head injury following a fall from his bike. The nurse examined Bradley's injury and questioned how he had injured himself. In a good-humoured way, the nurse suggested to Bradley that he wore a cycle helmet in the future.

A & E is a busy department and sometimes children/young people may not be given all the relevant health promotion advice (Evans, 1999). Many hospitals have a liaison health visitor who is responsible for informing health visitors and school nurses in the local community about children/young people who have attended the hospital. Liaison health visitors relay information that may need to be given to the family. The child's health visitor or school nurse can then follow up the case and provide any additional health promotion advice.

Outpatient department

Outpatient departments provide health promotion by organising clinics for specific conditions such as constipation, diabetes and enuresis. The clinics allow a variety of health practitioners to all come together to see the child/young person and their family. For example, at a diabetic clinic a diabetic nurse, the doctor, and a dietician will see the child and her/his family. Some clinics for conditions such as constipation and enuresis are even nurse led.

Clinics have resources available which are child/young person friendly. Puzzles, computer programmes and books can all be used to promote health. For example, at a constipation clinic a nurse may use a computer programme which explains what constipation is and why children need to attend clinic. The programme will be fun and easy to understand, allowing children to learn more about their condition, and what they can do to help themselves.

Display boards and health promotion leaflets are often located throughout areas of the outpatient department. Having accessible information where families are waiting can encourage them to read leaflets and display materials more easily.

Outpatient departments often have access to the internet. This can be particularly useful where a child/young person has just been diagnosed with a specific condition. Information can be accessed immediately for the child and family.

Health Promotion Hospital

An additional point to consider in relation to health promotion and hospital is the concept of the health promotion hospital. Here, we are considering health promotion from a policy perspective, rather than working directly with the individual, although policy will obviously impact on the individual's care. The ethos of the health promoting hospital, as highlighted by World Health Organization (2008), is that health promotion can be considered as a core quality dimension of hospital services.

The concept of health promoting hospitals is not new. In 1989 the first model project was set up in Austria. The evaluation demonstrated an enhanced protection of patients' health by reducing hospital infections (Berger et al., 1998).

Berger et al. (1998) outlined some of the core principles of health promoting hospitals to include promoting human dignity, acknowledging differences in needs and values of different population groups, improving quality of care, realisation of

the potential in becoming a learning organisation, using hospital resources efficiently and forming close links with the community. It may be a concept worth considering more in relation to hospital practice.

This section has explored some of the ways health promotion information can be delivered in the hospital setting. Display boards and information leaflets are commonly used in many settings. Most importantly, however, nurses are continually giving health promotion advice, whilst undertaking all aspects of nursing care.

Community

In the past, health promotion has predominately been viewed as a community-based activity (Bollard, 2003). General practitioners, health visitors and school nurses have often been perceived as the practitioners who promote healthy lifestyles. However, the development of the NSF (Education and Skills, Department of Health, 2004) has made it clear that health promotion is the responsibility of all health practitioners working with children/young people and their families. The following illustrates health promotion examples from community practice.

Health visitors and the Child Health Promotion Programme

Health visitors work in the community and promote family health, particularly with families who have young children. The work of health visitors is guided by the Child Health Promotion Programme (Hall and Elliman, 2003). The settings in which health visitors undertake their practice include clinics, community groups and visiting families at home.

Health promotion advice to families can include the following:

- Providing advice about child health and development.
- Establishing groups for mothers and their babies as a way of helping to promote emotional health.

- Advice about public health matters, such as immunisations, which may include the giving of immunisations.
- Providing advice and support on a variety of family health matters.

An example from practice is presented. *Sally had her first baby 4 months ago. She was happily married but her husband worked away and she had no family living in the area. Sally contacted her health visitor because her baby, Sophie, was often upset in the evenings and cried inconsolably. The health visitor visited Sally at home and gave her some advice on what to do when Sophie was unsettled. During the visit the health visitor noticed that Sally seemed quite low. Sally expressed feelings of isolation. The health visitor invited her to attend a local mother and baby group. This Sally did each week, and got to know other mothers and their babies.*

Providing families with emotional support is an important part of a health visitor's role. Prodigy (2006) outlines that one in ten mothers suffer from post-natal depression. In Sally's case attending the group helped her to feel part of the community, and as a result she felt happier. Taking action like this can help mothers feel emotionally supported, and perhaps less likely to develop post-natal depression.

Childhood immunisation plays an important part in structuring the Child Health Promotion Programme. Immunisation is an important way of preventing serious diseases in childhood (Education and Skills, Department of Health, 2004). In recent years concerns have been raised about the MMR (mumps, measles and rubella) vaccine, resulting in some parents/carers failing to have their children immunised. The NSF (Education and Skills, Department of Health, 2004) states that at least 95% of the population need to be immunised against diseases such as measles or an outbreak can occur, exposing children to the disease and its potential side effects. Health visitors can help to promote this vaccine, thus reducing unnecessary risks to children's health.

An example from practice is presented. *Brandon, 2-year old, visited the health centre for his 2-year assessment. During the assessment the health visitor discovered Brandon had never been given his MMR vaccine. The health visitor discussed with Brandon's mother the importance of MMR vaccine and recommended that Brandon should have it. His mother was anxious about possible side effects from the vaccine. The health visitor discussed the benefits of the vaccine, as well as any potential risks. Written health promotion material was given in the form of a health promotion leaflet. Brandon's mother had a long discussion with her family and visited baby clinic several times to discuss the matter further with her health visitor. The following month Brandon had his MMR vaccine.*

Support groups

Health promotion activities also take place within support groups. In the community some families can feel isolated due to their child having a long-standing illness or disability. Developing support groups for these families can enable them to feel supported, and provides the opportunity for them to meet with other families.

At a Sure Start centre in the Midlands, for example, a playgroup has developed for children with disabilities. A specialist nursery nurse, experienced in the care of young children with disabilities, organises the group. Special toys and equipment are available to encourage development. Parents/carers who attend the group find it emotionally supportive and it allows them to meet other families.

Bookstart

Bookstart (Booktrust, 2006) is a national programme aimed at encouraging children to look at books. The programme is funded at present by the Government. Each child should receive a Bookstart pack, which contains several books, along with details about joining the local library. Young children usually receive three Bookstart packs, from as early as 8 months of age, right through to 4 years. Bookstouch is available for children who are blind or partially sighted. Books can be used as a method of promoting children's health, parents/carers and children reading, looking or discussing books together.

Accessible health services

Designated children's centres allow for many community health services to be in one place, providing easy access for local families.

Sure Start centres provide a range of services for families with young children. In one deprived area in the Midlands, there are a number of villages each with their own Sure Start centre. Some of the services provided by the centres are outlined below:

- Play groups.
- Summer holiday events for preschool and school-age children.
- Education courses for parents/carers, which include health promotion courses, such as children's first-aid, children's behaviour management and communicating with children. To make it easier for parents/cares to attend crèche facilities are also available for young children.
- Health visitors and community nursery nurses are all based within the centres.
- A respiratory support group is available for parents/carers with children who have respiratory problems such as asthma.
- In some centres a dentist is available.
- Dental nurses organise sessions on dental health promotion and healthy eating.
- Self-help support groups are available for parents/carers, such as the *Stop Smoking* campaign. Parents/carers meet together, obtain patches to help them stop smoking and gain support from each other.
- For practitioners the centres provide health promotion updates.

This section has focused on a variety of different ways young children's health can be promoted in the community, along with that of their families. Health visitors and other practitioners such as community nursery nurses and community children's nurses all have a key role to play.

Nursery schools

In modern cultures it can be the norm for both parents to be employed. Young children (0–5 years) can receive care during the day from either a nursery or a childminder, or cared for by a member of the extended family (grandparent), while parents work.

The United Kingdom (UK) Government has recognised that early education is fundamental. Families are provided with a contribution towards nursery costs for their child, if aged 3 and 4 years

(Department of Work and Pensions, 2003). These funds can be used in a variety of ways, as outlined:

- Nursery schools – this can include private nurseries, day nurseries and nurseries attached to primary schools.
- Voluntary preschools and playgroups.
- Primary school reception classes for 4-year-olds.
- Accredited childminders who provide early education.
- Groups delivered by children's centres.

The Foundation Education Curriculum is regulated by the Office for Standards in Education, similar to schools.

Play

Preschool children are at a critical stage in their development. Children aged 3–5 years rapidly develop socially, intellectually, physically and emotionally. Piaget (1896–1980) spent much of his life studying how children think and learn (Smith et al., 2003). Piaget strongly believed that young children learn differently from adults. Adults can learn by being told information. Young children can effectively learn from seeing and doing, interacting with the world around them. Piaget recommended that teachers and nursery staff need to create scenarios to allow young children to learn, so they can visualise the concepts that are being taught.

Play is vital in the development and learning process for children (Smith et al., 2003). Curriculum guidance for foundation stage learning recognises this and agrees play sessions allow children to explore by trying to make sense of the world (Qualification and Curriculum Authority and Department for Education and Employment, 2000). Structured play as well as ordinary play sessions can aid health promotion.

The following outlines an example from practice. *Hattie is 4 years old. Today at nursery she was taught about crossing the road. The nursery staff set up the nursery so that it represented a road scene. Toy cars and bikes were brought in from the outside area to make the scene appear realistic. The nursery staff structured the session so that children were able to explore the dangers of crossing the road. On Hattie's way home that evening she told her father all about learning to cross the road and insisted on leading him across all the roads along the way.*

A further example is presented. At a local hospital a member of the play team from the children's ward regularly visits local nurseries and primary schools to prepare children for hospital admission. A video is shown about a child's trip to hospital. Equipment such as syringes and bandages are taken for children to explore and experiment with through play. Children who have participated in these sessions seem less worried about going into hospital, because they have been prepared for the experience.

Both these examples from practice highlight how young children can learn from experiential learning. Children, young children especially, can learn from experiences, such as role-play scenarios and interacting with relevant tools and resources.

Books and puppets

Story time is often an ideal opportunity to examine a particular health promotion issue with children. Nutbrown (2006) argues stories are essential to human experiences as they allow children to develop new knowledge, and explore their thinking and emotions. Stories can also be enhanced with the use of puppets.

There are various resources available for nurseries to purchase, related to health promotion activities. These include books on hygiene, healthy eating and going into hospital, for example.

The British Dental Association has a list of books they recommend for educating children on dental health, for example. Encouraging good dental health is essential in preschool. The NSF states that 39% of 5-year-olds have one decayed, missing or filled tooth (Education and Skills, Department of Health, 2004). Health promotion activities can help to instil dental health practices that may prevent dental problems in later life.

Jack, a 4-year old, did not like brushing his teeth, so his mother brought him a special toothbrush and toothpaste. Jack used them, but still he did not want to clean his teeth. At quiet time the teacher read the class a story about a crocodile called Colin. Colin did not like brushing his teeth. He ate lots of sweets and cake, until eventually some of his teeth fell out. Colin then started to find eating difficult, so he began brushing his teeth. Colin, the crocodile, never missed brushing his teeth again. Jack started to clean his teeth more regularly after hearing this story.

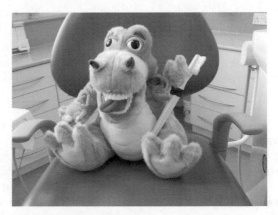

Figure 39.1 Colin the crocodile.

Using a story like this allows children to see the importance of brushing their teeth. Children are able to relate to the main character, Colin the crocodile. Figure 39.1 is a picture of a crocodile puppet, which is taken into nurseries and schools by dental nurses to educate young children about dental hygiene.

In many nursery schools toothbrushes are kept in the cloakroom, so after meals and snacks children can brush their teeth. This allows children to get into a routine and the activity can be reinforced at home. For this daytime tooth brushing routine to continue through childhood, it would be ideal for children to be able to take their toothbrush to school.

Health promotion libraries often have storybooks and puppets for hire. There are a wide variety of stories that relate to health promotion. Puppets can be used to act out the story and allow children to develop their thinking (cognitions). Encouraging children to participate in the stories helps their imagination too.

Cultural and ethnic differences can be investigated during these story sessions. There are many puppets available, which represent different ethnic origins. Different religious beliefs and celebrations can be incorporated into stories, using puppets. One example could be the celebration of the Chinese New Year in January. Different healthy foods could be explored.

Nurseries can use a variety of different and cognitively appropriate health promotion methods for young children to learn about their health. The use of puppets and storybooks has been explored here, but other methods might include nursery rhymes, puzzles and games, for example.

Schools

The World Health Organization (WHO, 1999) states that an effective school health programme is one of the most important and cost-effective ways a nation can develop. Encouraging a healthy lifestyle from a young age reinforces good habits and creates an environment where learning is beneficial (Education and Skills, 2005).

In the UK, health promotion is part of the school curriculum. The Government has developed the National School Health Programme (NSHP) (Education and Skills, 2005). The NSHP is a framework that local education authorities provide to schools in assisting them to become healthier organisations. The NSHP has four sections:

- Healthy eating.
- Physical activity.
- Personal, social and health education (including sex and relationship education, and drug education).
- Emotional health and well-being.

The Government's aim is for all schools to achieve the NSHP status by 2009 (Education and Skills, 2005).

Healthy eating

In recent years it has been well publicised that Britain has an increasing obesity problem. Junk food combined with a lack of exercise has contributed to this growing problem. Obesity is problem for children/young people, as well as adults. For example, in England between 1995 and 2002 the number of children/young people who were overweight and obese rose by 25% (Education and Skills, Department of Health, 2004). The NSF indicates that 28% of girls and 22% of boys are overweight or obese between the ages of 2 and 15 years (Education and Skills, Department of Health, 2004).

The Child Health Promotion Programme (Hall and Elliman, 2003) reinforces the need for children/young people to receive a healthy diet. Schools are often one of the first places where children/young people choose food and drink which is not prepared for them by their parents/carers.

Schools can therefore play an important role in educating about healthy eating.

Schools can explore food and drink in a variety of ways:

- Health promotion sessions, exploring factual information about food.
- Health promotion displays.
- Designing healthy eating leaflets.
- Cooking – baking bread and experimenting with healthy recipes in cookery classes (supervised).
- Food-tasting games can be developed. Primary school children can pick out foods (healthy/unhealthy) using a pillowcase, containing various foods. The children can take turns to choose a food. They then identify the food, taste it, and describe what it is like and why it is healthy or unhealthy. (Check for allergies first.)

Allowing children/young people to explore different foods is important. In the school setting they observe their peers trying different foods. This may have a positive impact and encourage them to experiment with foods which they have not previously considered.

The Government has responded to concerns about rising obesity by launching the *5 a Day* campaign, where everyone is encouraged to eat five portions of fruit and vegetables each day (Department of Health, 2004). As part of the 5 a Day campaign all 4- to 6-year-olds are entitled to a piece of fruit each day at school. Schools are provided with information and recipes, along with details about how they can make the fruit more enticing to eat.

An information leaflet is also available for families. The leaflet explains the campaign and ways to encourage 5 a Day at home are explored.

Schools may want to structure health promotion sessions, using the fruit as a basis for healthy eating. Places where the fruit grows and how it grows can be discussed for interest.

Physical activity

In line with healthy eating, children/young people also need to exercise frequently. The NSF (Education and skills, Department of Health, 2004) has set two targets, initially, to increase the uptake of physical activity to at least 30 minutes three times a week with all children/young people under 16 years. The second target is to increase opportunities for children/young people to undertake sporting activities within and beyond the curriculum.

The Health Development Agency (2006) outlines examples from practice, one is presented here. A member of staff at a primary school in the South East of England incorporates mathematics lessons with physical education lessons, using a digital skipping rope. When the pupil makes a full rotation with the skipping rope, the monitor moves along one number, but when the rope is rotated backwards, the monitor deducts one number. This activity encourages children to experiment with the skipping rope. As a project the children were asked to count how many skips they could achieve in 1 minute. In the mathematics class they then produced charts and graphs to illustrate their achievements.

The school found introducing the skipping ropes greatly improved the children's numerical skills and encouraged them to look at their own physical performance. Skipping became a popular activity in the playground for both boys and girls (Health Development Agency, 2006).

The Health Development Agency (2006) also cites an example of a school in the Midlands. The school introduced the *SmartCATZ scheme*. The scheme aims to encourage pupils to cycle or walk to school. The area surrounding the school is a car-free zone so even pupils who are driven to school still have to walk the final part of the journey. Pupils have a travel card to promote the scheme. Every time they walk or cycle outside the zone, they receive a point. Prizes are given to those who have achieved the most points each month (Health Development Agency, 2006).

Personal, social and health education

Personal, social and health education (PSHE) includes learning about being healthy, becoming a confident and happy person, as well as respecting other people's feelings and ideas. PSHE is a subject taught independently as part of the curriculum (Qualification and Curriculum Authority, 2006). This section will discuss some of the subjects presented in PSHE.

Road safety

Road safety skills are essential for children/young people to learn. Traffic is the biggest single cause of accidental death in young people between the ages of 12 and 16 years (Department for Transport, 2005). The Department for Transport (2005) has estimated that 22 000 children/young people are injured on the road every year. Educating them on road safety is therefore vital. Some schools have been encouraged to set up school cycle routes and walk ways. Children/young people going to and from school using these routes are therefore much safer.

In primary schools, road safety can be taught in a variety of ways. Role-play, for example, can be used to educate children about traffic and crossing the road safely. Videos and practical sessions can also be organised.

A practice example is outlined. *Tom is 10 years old. At school a police officer provided some sessions on road safety. Tom loves to ride his bike and so he attended the sessions. Every Friday he took his bike to school and attended an hour-long session with the police officer. Tom learnt about the importance of cycling safely by watching a video, studying some worksheets and practising what to do by using the school playground as a pretend road. After 6 weeks Tom took his cycling proficiency test which involved some questions and a practical test. Tom passed the test and was awarded a cycling proficiency certificate in assembly.*

Drug and solvent misuse

It is important to educate children/young people about the effects of drugs and solvent abuse. Playgrounds are common places for addicts to gather, causing items such as needles and syringes to be left around for children/young people to find.

An example from practice is presented. *Millie was 9 years old. Her mother took her to the park, but whilst Millie was playing she discovered some needles and syringes. Millie knew not to touch them.*

A few weeks earlier in school assembly, the school nurse had talked to the children about drug awareness. A session following assembly provided children with the opportunity to draw and colour items they might find in a park, which should not be touched. Glass, aerosol cans, syringes and needles were some of the items children drew and discussed. Due to these sessions Millie knew she was not to touch the needles and syringes that she found in the park that day. Millie let her mother know what she had found.

Sexual health

The UK has the highest teenage pregnancy rate in Western Europe with some of these pregnancies ending in abortion (Education and Skills, Department of Health, 2004). The NSF advises that young people who speak openly about sexual activity are less likely to engage in risk-taking behaviour, resulting in a lower chance of teenage pregnancy (Education and Skills, Department of Health, 2004). Open discussions and teaching about sexual health are encouraged.

A practice example is outlined. *Natalie, 15-year old, attends her PSHE classes. As part of her course a baby doll is given to each boy and girl. The doll simulates a real baby; therefore, the young person has to attend to their doll's every need, responding to its cries, night or day. Natalie was initially excited about the project, but after having the doll for one night, she quickly changed her mind. The experience was both tiring and demanding. Natalie had not realised how demanding taking care of a baby could be.*

Simulation can help young people to learn how certain life experiences may impact on their future lives. Simulation may influence young people to think carefully before taking certain actions.

Emotional health and well-being

The Scottish Executive Education Department (2006) maintains that promoting mental and emotional health is essential for children/young people. Qualification and Curriculum Authority (2006) suggests teachers should respond sensitively and appropriately when examining emotional health.

As children/young people grow and develop, they may have difficulties in coping with feelings and thoughts in relation to particular experiences. Demands at school, friends, family and media can create pressure or stress for some children/young people.

Schools feel that it is important to encourage children to voice their thoughts about health issues (Health Development Agency, 2006). In some schools, school council representatives are elected by each class to pass their thoughts on to teachers. Seeking children's views allows teachers to be more aware of their feelings. Any issues can be sensitively dealt with by each class teacher.

However, sometimes children need to speak individually with either a teacher or a school nurse on a matter that may concern them personally. School nurses can particularly help on health matters.

A practice example is presented. *Michelle was 12 years old. Michelle's main carer was her father since her mother had left the family when she was a baby. The previous week in PSHE they had been discussing periods and menstruation. Michelle did not want to talk to her father about such matters. The school nurse taught the PSHE lesson. At lunchtime Michelle made an appointment to see her. The school nurse was able to talk with Michelle individually. Michelle was able to ask questions about periods and menstruation. She had not felt comfortable about asking questions whilst in class. The school nurse provided Michelle with some samples of sanitary towels and invited her to contact the school nursing service again.*

A one-to-one conversation can be really helpful for some children. Asking questions in front of fellow classmates can sometimes be quite embarrassing, particularly if the issue is a sensitive or personal one.

For some children/young people health issues go much deeper. The NSF (Education and Skills, Department of Health, 2004) recognises that mental health issues can develop in adolescence. Psychoses, eating disorders (anorexia nervosa and bulimia) and self-harm are some of the more common disorders which emerge. Adolescence can be a difficult time where an individual's body is changing both physically and emotionally. There are sometimes pressures in making the transition from being a dependent child to becoming an independent young person. In addition, making career choices and developing relationships can often be difficult. Many young people respond well to the pressures of modern society, but others do not. They will need extra help and support. Nurses need to look out for any signs of difficulty. By being available to talk and listen to children/young people, nurses can provide them with the opportunity to voice their concerns.

This section has explored the school setting; how health can be promoted by nurses in school, as well as other practitioners. There have been many health promotion initiatives recently put in place by the Government to encourage schools to be more proactive in promoting healthy lifestyles. As mentioned earlier, the WHO (1999) believes having a school health programme is an effective way of improving the nation's health.

Conclusion

This chapter has examined health promotion in context, looking at a number of different settings where nurses work, how they, along with other practitioners, can promote children's/young people's health. Four settings have been explored: hospital, community, nursery and schools. Each setting is able to provide health promotion information in a variety of different ways, according to the needs of children/young people who attend. The NSF (Education and Skills, Department of Health, 2004) gives clear guidelines on the health promotion issues where children/young people are most likely to need support. Several examples from practice have been presented, illustrating how health promotion information can help children/young people.

Personally, a real health concern regarding Britain's children/young people is obesity. Junk food and minimal exercise all contribute to increasing health problem. As a health practitioner it is important that a holistic approach to tackling childhood obesity is taken, looking at all aspects of children's/young people's lives. Practitioners too all need to work together – hospital, community, nursery and school – to reduce the problem of childhood obesity.

Importantly, to provide health promotion information effectively, children/young people need to be listened to, as well as being involved with the planning of any initiatives. From experience they are more likely to respond to health promotion initiatives if they have been consulted and their views considered. Finally, it is important to remember that children/young people are the next generation – it is essential they are healthy. Nurses promoting their health in a variety of different contexts can help.

References

Berger, H., Krajic, K., Paul, R. (eds) (1998) Health promoting hospitals in practice: developing projects and networks. In: *Proceedings of the 6th International Conference, April/May 1998*. Germany: G. Conrad Health Promotion Publications.

Bollard, M. (2003) Health promotion and learning disabilities. *Nursing Standard* 16(27): 47–53.

Booktrust (2006) Bookstart. Available at: http://www.bookstart.co.uk (accessed 13 September 2006).

Department of Health (2003) *Essence of Care: Patient-Focused Benchmarks for Clinical Governance*. London: Department of Health.

Department of Health (2004) *5 a Day*. Available at: http://www.5aday.nhs.uk (accessed 7 August 2006).

Department of Health (2005) *Health Events 2007*. Available at: http://www.dh.gov.uk/assetRoot/ (accessed 25 April 2007).

Department for Transport (2005) *Teenagers*. Available at: http://www.thinkroadsafety.gov.uk/usergroups/teenagers (accessed 10 May 2006).

Department of Work and Pensions (2003) *United Kingdom Employment Action Plan: A Report on the Principal Measures Undertaken by the UK to Implement Its Employment Policy in Line with Article 128(3) of the EN Treaty*. Available at: http://www.dwp.gov.uk/publications/ (accessed 3 December 2006).

Education and Skills (Department of) (2005) *National Healthy School Status*. London: Department of Health.

Education and Skills (Department of), Department of Health (2004) *The National Service Framework for Children, Young People and Maternity Services. Core Standards*. London: Education and Skills, Department of Health.

Evans, K. (1999) Emergency services for children and young people. *Nursing Standard* 13(32): 38–41.

Ewles, L., Simnett, I. (2002) *Promoting Health. A Practical Guide*, 5th edn. London: Balliere Tindall.

Geraghty, M. (2005) Nursing the unconscious patient. *Nursing Standard* 20(1): 54–64.

Hall, D., Elliman, D. (2003) *Health for All Children*, 4th edn. Oxford: Oxford University Press.

Health Development Agency (2006) *Case Studies by Theme*. Available at: http://www.wiredforhealth.gov.uk (accessed 15 September 2006).

Nursing and Midwifery Council (2004) *The NMC Code of Professional Conduct: Standards for Conduct, Performance and Ethics*. London: NMC.

Nutbrown, K. (2006) *Threads of Thinking: Young Children Learning and the Role of Early Education*. London: Paul Chapman Publishers.

Prodigy (2006) *Postnatal Depression*. Available at: http://www.patient.co.uk/ (accessed 2 December 2006).

Qualification and Curriculum Authority (QCA) and Department for Education and Employment (2000) *Curriculum Guidance for Foundation Stage*. London: QCA.

Qualification and Curriculum Authority (QCA) (2006) *About Personal, Social and Health Education*. Available at: http://www.qca.org.uk/7835.html (accessed 23 September 2006).

Scottish Executive Education Department (2006) *Emotional Wellbeing*. Available at: http://www.healthpromotingschools.co.uk/ (accessed 23 September 2006).

Smith, P., Cowie, H., Blades, M. (2003) *Understanding Children's Development*, 4th edn. Oxford: Blackwell Publishing.

Whiting, L. (2001) Health promotion: the views of children's nurses. *Paediatric Nursing* 13(3): 27–31.

World Health Organization (1999) *Improving Health through Schools. National and International Strategies*. Available at: http://www.who.int/schoolyouth health/media (accessed 24 September 2006).

World Health Organization (2008) *Health Promoting Hospitals*. Available at: http://www.eurowho.int (accessed September 2008).

Theme 13

National Perspectives

Chapter 40   National Perspectives

40 National Perspectives

Carolyn Neill, Kate McPake, Susan Anne Jones, Nicola Lewis and Karen Moyse

---

NSFs

The National Service Framework (NSF) for children, young people and maternity services (Education and Skills, Department of Health, 2004) advocates promoting the health of all children/young people in the UK.

Introduction

This is an opportunity to view children's health promotion activities from a national perspective; looking at a variety of different activities taking place in each of the four countries that make up the UK – Northern Ireland, Scotland, Wales and England.

Carolyn Neill provides insights on activities in Northern Ireland, while Kate McPake provides information on activities in Scotland. The Welsh perspective is examined by Susan Anne Jones and Nicola Lewis. Finally, the English perspective is provided by Karen Moyse.

Each perspective looks at different health promotion initiatives for children/young people. The influence of the Government policies is also considered within each perspective, and importantly the contributions of the NSFs for children, young people and maternity services (Education and Skills, Department of Health, 2004) are acknowledged.

The NSFs are vital to the future development of health promotion initiatives taking place across the UK. Of course, the involvement of children/young people themselves (and their families) in any new initiative is essential.

Recently announced by the Government is a new initiative on child poverty. A new unit is to be set up to battle against child poverty. The Government wants to half the number of children living in poverty by 2010 (Hain, 2007, Work and Pensions Secretary). Child poverty is a key determinant of health, which influences the health of children/young people in all four countries of the UK.

Why is it so important to look at national perspectives? Studying national perspectives is important when promoting health, as it draws attention to health issues that are not only relevant nationally, but will also have relevance locally. It can encourage nurses to make comparisons between their local community and the country. Nurses can then identify if their local community is doing better or worse than the national evidence suggests.

Have a look at your local health profile. Find out about the health issues that are particularly relevant in your area. This might help when putting together health promotion activities, health reports and those all-important assignments. Contact your local community primary care trust who might be able to provide further information. Other useful sources of information include the clinical medical

Activity

As part of the Health Profile for England (Department of Health, 2006a), for example, details are included on local health profiles. These are available from http://www.communityhealthprofiles.info

officer's annual report on public health and data from the Office of Population and Statistics.

Northern Ireland

Introduction

The latest estimate of the size of Northern Ireland population is 1.7 million people of whom 380 141 are children aged under 16 years (approximately 22% of the population) and 432 014 are under 18 years (Northern Ireland Statistics and Research Agency, 2006).

This section addresses the following major health-related challenges which are being faced by children/young people in Northern Ireland today:

- Healthy eating.
- Obesity.
- Dental health.
- Road safety.
- Smoking, drugs and alcohol.
- Mental health.

Key facts are summarised together with examples of health promotion actions, which are being undertaken to address the main issues.

Healthy eating

Research conducted by the Health Promotion Agency for Northern Ireland (HPANI, 2001) has highlighted concerns regarding the eating patterns of children/young people aged 5–17 years. Important findings include the following:

- A low intake of fruit and vegetables across all age and socio-economic groups.
- A high intake of fizzy drinks.

- Frequent consumption of snack products high in fat and/or sugar.

Two groups are of particular concern:

- Girls aged 12–17 years – overall, many of the dietary intakes for this group are less favourable than for other age and gender groupings.
- Children from manual households – these children regularly eat more meat products and fried foods than those from non-manual groups.

Action

The *Fresh Fruit in Schools* initiative was developed by the Investing for Health Team at the Department of Health, Social Services and Public Safety Northern Ireland (DHSSPSNI), HPANI and four health action zones, with the aim of providing one free piece of fresh fruit to primary 1 and 2 children within selected schools. Evaluation of the first 2 years of this project (2002–2004) indicates that greatest improvements in fruit consumption involve those whose intake was poor to start with (HPANI, 2005). Further evaluation of the scheme in 2006 found that to ensure effectiveness, it needs to be incorporated into a whole school approach on the issue of food in school (HPANI, 2007).

Further significant action will include allocation of additional funding to ensure that new nutritional standards for school meals are effectively introduced (DHSSPSNI, 2005).

Obesity

Levels of obesity among children in Northern Ireland are increasing yearly with 1:5 boys and 1:4 girls being overweight or obese in primary one (DHSSPSNI, unpublished data). Furthermore, the Young Hearts study indicates that among 12- to 15-year-olds living in Northern Ireland, the levels of overweight and obesity have increased by more than a quarter in the past decade (Watkins et al., 2005).

The issue of obesity is so significant that the DHSSPSNI has identified the following population health outcome as part of its Investing for Health Strategy (DHSSPSNI, 2002): 'Harm will (also) be avoided by stopping the increase in levels of obesity in children by 2010 and reducing it by 50% by 2025' (p. 13).

Action

Fit Futures: Focus on Food, Activity and Young People is a cross-departmental taskforce set up by the DHSSPSNI in 2004 to examine the options for preventing a rise in the levels of overweight and obesity in children/young people. The taskforce was also charged with the responsibility of making recommendations for priorities for action. In their executive summary (DHSSPSNI, 2006a), the taskforce concluded that policies and strategies to tackle obesity should consider the role of families in establishing and supporting good nutrition. Particular attention must also be paid to children/young people from low-income families and to those with a disability, as they face additional barriers to healthy eating and active living. It was also highlighted that health practitioners need to work together to tackle obesity.

Dental health

Dental decay in children is a significant problem in Northern Ireland. Compared to other parts of the UK, 12-year-olds in this region have almost three times the level of decay (DHSSPSNI, 2006b). Freeman et al. (2001) conclude that this reflects the socio-economic deprivation and poor dietary habits among children in the region.

Action

Initiatives to address poor oral health in Northern Ireland include the Dental Caries Reduction Programme (DHSSPSNI, 2006b). The programme consists of 11 schemes across Northern Ireland and involves community dental service staff visiting schools, nurseries and homes. Toothbrushes, toothpaste and dental advice are provided to children from birth to 5 years, living in the most deprived areas.

A second initiative entitled the *Smart Snacks Scheme* has been developed in the Western Health and Social Services Board where numbers of decayed, missing and filled teeth are among the worst in the province. The scheme was established in 1998 and targets school children in the primary, special and nursery school sector. Between 2002 and 2003, over 220 schools were involved whereby at mid-

morning break time, only milk or water and/or fruit or vegetables were allowed. Evaluation of the initiative indicated that the primary schools showed an improvement in their dental health and a significant improvement in the number of children who were caries free (O'Neill and O'Donnell, 2003). A similar project developed in the Southern Health and Social Services Board entitled *Boost Better Breaks* also achieved a positive evaluation (Freeman et al., 2001).

Road safety

It is estimated that the introduction of seat belt legislation and the use of child restraints has halved the level of fatalities on Northern Ireland's roads since the mid-1970s (Office of the First Minister and Deputy First Minister (OFMDFM), 2006a). However, Northern Ireland has more road deaths per 100 000 people than any other region in the UK (Department of the Environment for Northern Ireland, DoENI, 2002). In 2006/2007, 8 children under 16 were killed on Northern Ireland roads, 128 were seriously injured and 847 were slightly injured (Police Service for Northern Ireland, 2007).

The Northern Ireland Road Safety Strategy (2002–2012) (DoENI, 2002) includes the goal of achieving a 50% reduction in the numbers of children killed or seriously injured on Northern Ireland's roads each year from the 1996 to 2000 average of 250 to fewer than 125 by 2012. If this is achieved, it is estimated that the lives of 50 children will have been saved and 700 fewer children will have been seriously injured in road traffic collisions.

Action

The DoENI's children's road safety campaign entitled *Stop, Look, Listen, Live* was launched in March 2005. Central to the initiative is a television advertisement which aims to raise awareness of the dangers encountered on the roads and to advise young people how to keep themselves safe.

Approximately £65 million is spent annually on school transport for pupils in Northern Ireland, which is more than in the rest of the UK. One example of significant financial investment is the OFMDFM's announcement in September 2006 of a school bus safety boost including provision of more school buses fitted with seatbelts (OFMDFM, 2006b).

Smoking, alcohol and drugs

The young persons' behaviour and attitudes survey (NISRA, 2003) uncovered the following statistics pertaining to the participants aged 11–16 years living in Northern Ireland:
  Smoking

- 33% had smoked.
- 54% of those who had smoked started before the age of 12 years.

  Drugs and solvents

- 23% had used either drugs or solvents.
- The average age at which young people started to use drugs or solvents was 12.5 years.

  Alcohol

- 60% of the respondents had consumed alcohol.
- The average age of first taking alcohol was 11.9 years.

Action

A key goal identified in the Investing for Health Strategy (DHSSPSNI, 2002) emphasises that action must be taken to increase the percentage of young people who do not smoke from 86.9 to 95% by 2025.

The New Strategic Direction for Alcohol and Drugs (2006–2011) is a 5-year plan aimed at reducing alcohol and drug-related harm in Northern Ireland (DHSSPSNI, 2006c). It includes the goal of developing treatment and support services for children/young people at local and regional level.

Resources developed by the HPANI include a website entitled *Up-2-You* (http://www.hpani.org) which provides information for young people on smoking, alcohol, drugs and mental health. A booklet about drugs called *Your Body, Your Life, Your Choice* has been devised for 14- to 17-year-olds (HPANI, 2006). A similar booklet is available for 11- to 13-year-olds (HPANI, 2004).

Mental health

Despite a lack of epidemiological studies of child mental health in Northern Ireland, it has been proposed that children/young people in this region experience more mental health problems and disorders than in other parts of the UK (Bamford, 2006). This conclusion is underpinned by the following facts:

- Northern Ireland has a higher level of socio-economic deprivation than in England.
- The province has suffered from 30 years of civil conflict.
- There is increasing awareness of the effects of the 'troubles' on children/young people.
- There is a higher prevalence of mental health problems in the Northern Ireland adult population than in England.

A significant problem which contributes to mental health difficulties is that of bullying. In a study involving 120 schools in Northern Ireland, 40% of primary children and 30% of secondary pupils reported that they had been bullied recently (Department of Education for Northern Ireland, 2002).

Action

Key targets of the *Promoting Mental Health Strategy and Action Plan 2003–2008* (DHSSPSNI, 2004) involve the development of policies and resources for the promotion of the mental health of children/young people.

The Northern Ireland Commissioner for Children/Young People has specified bullying as one of its key priorities for action (http://www.niccy.org). Initiatives include a *Stop Bullying Guidance Pack* for schools and a curriculum focusing on bullying for early years settings aimed at preschool children.

The *Vision of a Comprehensive Child and Adolescent Mental Health Service* (Bamford, 2006) highlights the need for a range of statutory, voluntary and community services to work together to safeguard the mental health of children/young people in Northern Ireland.

Rising to the challenges at the Royal Belfast Hospital for Sick Children

It is recognised that the needs of children/young people are best served in an environment which is genuinely children/young people centred. In Northern Ireland this has been a key influence in the plans for the new Royal Belfast Hospital for Sick Children which will open in 2016. In order to provide high-quality care for children/young people, the current upper age limit for a patient to be admitted to the accident and emergency department will increase from the child's 13th birthday to the age of 16 years.

Over recent years, there has already been a significant increase in the number of children/young people attending the hospital, having used drugs/solvents or who have consumed excessive amounts of alcohol. Children/young people who have self-harmed also present more frequently. The raising of the upper age limit will present new challenges as the number of young people being treated will increase.

Nursing staff at the Royal Belfast Hospital for Sick Children recognise the need to develop new skills, and therefore training programmes and relevant policies are being devised in order to prepare staff to meet the changing needs of their patient population.

Conclusion

There is clearly a huge amount of work being undertaken throughout Northern Ireland with the aim of improving the health of children/young people and this must surely be of interest to children's nurses and other nurses working with children/young people in our endeavour to provide holistic care.

Scotland

Since Devolution in 1998 the Scottish Executive has made the promotion of health for children/young people one of its top priorities. In 1999 the Scottish Executive Health Department pledged £15 million to support four national health demon-stration projects, two of which relate to children/young people, namely child health and young people's sexual health (Ross and de Caestecker, 2003).

The NSF for children, young people and maternity services core standards (Education and Skills, Department of Health, 2004) states that there are areas in the lives of children/young people where making healthy choices can make a real difference to their life chances. *Delivering for Health* (Scottish Executive, 2005) is the Scottish document, which identifies how these core standards will be met. The document states that this is a fundamental shift in how we work, tackling the causes of ill health and providing care which is quicker, more personal and closer to home.

The child health project is called *Starting Well* and commenced with a pilot project in two areas of Glasgow, namely Gorbals, Govanhill, North Toryglen and Greater Easterhouse (Greater Glasgow NHS Board, 2006). It was evaluated independently by Glasgow University (McKenzie et al., 2005), and is currently in phase two of its implementation. It will be instituted in all five community health partnerships in Glasgow. The aim of the project is to improve the immediate and long-term health of families with young children via a coordinated programme of intensive support.

It had four approaches:

(1) An intensive home visiting programme
(2) Development of community support services
(3) Improved links between home visiting and community interventions
(4) Links to other policy initiatives aimed at improving the health of families with young children.

The aim of Starting Well's (Greater Glasgow NHS Board, 2006) second phase is to demonstrate that child and family well-being, for vulnerable and disadvantaged children and families, can be enhanced. This can be achieved through an integrated and cohesive multidisciplinary and multi-agency approach.

The health visitor-led teams are multi-agency and consist of nursery nurses, health support workers, administrative assistant, social care workers, along with speech and language therapists. Phase 2 aims to extend the team by including education and social work colleagues.

The practitioners offer home visits for a limited period where a need for intensive support has been identified within a family. A positive parenting programme and referral to appropriate agencies in the community are offered to meet the needs of families. The support workers provide practical help in the home such as organising washing and shopping or care of the children. In providing this support, the main objective was to enable and empower the mothers through education.

The evaluation of the first phase of Starting Well showed that amongst the practitioners there has been improved team working. The skill mix model of care was successful and services used evidence-based protocols.

The family health outcomes were measured using a baseline mother report questionnaire around the time of her baby's birth, again when the baby was 6 months old, and once again when the baby was 18 months old. The results showed that there were short-term benefits in the psychological health of mothers involved in the study (at 6 months postnatal). There were also longer-term developmental benefits for the children in the study (as measured at 18 months). It is hoped that a further evaluation will explore whether this intensive home visiting approach will have an effect on more general skills, such as readiness of children for school entry.

While support for mothers in the immediate postnatal period has proved to be positive, there are other areas of health promotion where national and local initiatives are having an impact. The consultation document *Health and Healthcare of Children/Young People in Lothian* (NHS Lothian, 2006) identifies specific targets for health promotion over the next 5 years. These include the following:

- Encourage all young people to have five portions of fruit or vegetables per day.
- 50% of all 11- to 15-year-olds taking vigorous exercise three times a week.
- Keep children safe in their homes.
- 60% of all 5-year-olds free from dental disease.
- Reduce pregnancy among 13- to 15-year-olds by 20% from the level in 1995.

Practical health promotion projects have been initiated in different areas of Scotland. Nurses have worked in conjunction with other practitioners in an attempt to change the health levels of children/young people addressing these issues.

Through the Health Promoting and Nutrition (Scotland) Bill (Scottish Executive, 2006), the education minister proposed to ensure the following:

- Food and drink in schools meets strict nutritional standards.
- Councils promote the uptake and benefits of school meals and free school meals.
- The stigma associated with free school meals will be reduced.
- Councils to have the power to provide healthy snacks.
- Place health promotion at the heart of school activities.

Schools can work towards accreditation as *Health Promoting Schools*. Highland Council along with NHS Highland has been the first region in Scotland to accredit all of their schools in June 2006 (Halliday, 2006).

The *Free Fruit* (Health Promoting Schools, 2006) initiative was launched in 2003, and in Edinburgh and Glasgow there are schemes for the delivery of fruit to schools (http://www. healthpromotingschools.co.uk). All primary 1 and 2 pupils receive fruit three times a week in order to encourage children to try new tastes and to impact on their eating habits. This is a popular and successful project. During visits to schools and to children's homes, I have observed how fruit has replaced sugary snacks. Children really enjoy it.

The *Eat Well to Play Well* game has been developed for nursery-aged children. It is a physical activity and nutrition game, which was developed by dieticians. Pre-5 staff and a physical activity co-coordinator from the *Have a Heart Paisley* national demonstration project are involved. The game stimulates discussions about food and health among very young children through a matching game that uses colour, a large food mat and models of food. The game aims to teach children about the basics of healthy eating. Further developments in Inverclyde have linked the game to a parents' cooking workshop, and there are plans to create a play based on the game.

Lack of exercise in children/young people is not only a Scottish problem but the *Scottish Health*

Survey (1998) showed that one in three primary school-aged girls and one in four primary school-aged boys did not achieve the minimum levels required (Burns, 2006). From the age of 4 years, girls exercise less than boys and by the age of 16 years, two in three girls and one in three boys do not reach the minimum recommended levels of activity (Reilly et al., 2004).

The World Health Organization supports a guideline of at least 1 hour of moderate activity a day to provide direct health benefits. To encourage this from an early age, parents/carers in Fife teach their children gross motor skills through an interactive movement and play programme called *play@home*. The programme has three books and these guide parents/carers through progressive activities that are appropriate for children's development from birth to 5 years. The books are handed out by health visitors to families with new babies and later at 1 year and 3 years of age.

In older girls, a project, which is supported by Sportscotland, the Youth Support Trust and Scottish Health Promoting Schools is the *Nike Girls in Sport* project which will offer teenage girls the opportunity to take part in specially devised workshops, 80 are planned. The aim is to encourage habits of exercise, which will be sustained throughout life.

In Edinburgh there is a project called *Staysafe*, which seeks to reduce childhood accidents at home by providing free and subsidised safety equipment to families of low incomes. Small items of safety equipment such as socket covers and cupboard locks are given free at baby clinics and large items such as safety gates are available at a small charge through vouchers. The vouchers are issued by NHS Lothian and then redeemed at Argos.

The National Dental Inspection Programme reported in 2004 that 50.7% of all primary 1 (P1) school children had no dental decay. This represents a considerable improvement on the 2003 figure of 45% (Burns, 2006). The target by 2010 is to achieve no dental decay in 60% of all children starting school. This is an area where education, health, the voluntary sector and statutory sectors of nursery provision all work together. In areas of deprivation a great impact has been made on preventing premature tooth loss.

Dental packs are available for babies of 4 months old at child health clinics, visits to nurseries by practitioners, along with the encouragement of good

dental hygiene in crèches, and mother and toddler groups, has been very influential. In the Greater Glasgow area between 1995/1996 and 2003/2004, there has been a drop from 63 to 50% of all children starting school with signs of dental decay (Burns, 2006). While there is room for improvement, the targeting of deprived areas does seem to have reduced from 75 to 58% of all P1 children having no signs of tooth decay.

Conclusion

In all of these initiatives nurses have been crucial to the success of projects. Their work has helped improve the health of Scotland's children/young people. Undoubtedly, nurses will continue to work hard to promote the health of the next generation.

Wales

National perspective for Wales

Health promotion aimed at children/young people in Wales is addressed by a wide variety of nurses both in the acute sector, but also in the primary and public health sectors. Education programmes to support the learning needs of children's nurses in these areas are well supported by the Welsh Assembly Government (WAG).

Midwifery services in Wales begin the task of health promotion for children by educating pregnant women in antenatal classes on how to care for their baby. Health visitors assume responsibility from the midwife until a child reaches school age. In many areas of Wales, care is then handed to school health nurses (SHNs). The role of SHN will be discussed in more detail. This section will begin by highlighting the work of specialist nurses and hospital nurses in Wales.

Many local health boards (LHBs) and National Health Service (NHS) trusts employ specialist children's nurses in areas including diabetes, epilepsy and respiratory disease. They offer expert support, advice and interventions in the hospital and home settings aimed at controlling the effects of these conditions on their young clients. These nurses aim to ensure that hospital admissions are minimised and that children/young people are fully informed about, and are involved in decisions which affect their health. This information is provided in an age-appropriate way, helping to ensure that children's/young people's rights are fully met (United Nations, 1989; Department of Health, 2004a; National Assembly for Wales, NAW, 2005).

In many regions across the principality specialist nurses are supported by and work closely with community children's nursing teams (CCNs). CCNs work with children/young people with complex health needs. Hospital children's nurses fulfil an essential role by working with acutely ill children in the paediatric ward. Practice nurses run specialised support clinics, particularly for chronic conditions such as asthma, in the primary care setting. All these nurses undertake health promotion activities, as well as ongoing support for children/young people and their families by working closely with many and varied multidisciplinary colleagues.

The NSF for children, young people and maternity services in Wales (NAW, 2005) has provided many challenges to the way services are delivered for Welsh children. Of particular significance to children's nurses are the core aims that children/young people should enjoy the best possible health, be listened to, have their views respected, and be provided with a range of learning opportunities.

The identified need within the NSF for nurses to work more closely with parents/carers has raised the profile of SHNs. It has been suggested that their role is to keep the healthy in good health for the future, and that being involved in school policy development and the local community will help to serve this aim (Bartley, 2004).

Health promotion is the bread and butter of public health practice and is centrally concerned with empowering people to take control of and responsibility for their own health (World Health Organization, 1986, 1996; Department of Health, 1999; Wanless, 2002). The SHN is nationally identified as a key practitioner in this area (DeBell and Jackson, 2000; Hall and Elliman, 2003; Naidoo and Wills, 2005; Department of Health, 2006c). It is recognised that school health nursing is a complex field of practice that has developed into a well-defined speciality (Gleeson, 2004), within public health.

In Wales the unique position of the SHN in public health nursing, working across the health and education divide, linking with the families of children on their caseload (DeBell and Jackson, 2000), is

becoming highly valued. It is recognised that their role enables them to implement health promotion directly linked to reforming social structures and policies that contribute to the health of individuals in their own community (Whitehead, 2003).

Recent and successive national Government documents that support the SHN role have returned them to their original domain of public health (Department of Health, 1997, 2001, 2004b, 2006c), and placed the emphasis of their child-centred role in health promotion (Croghan et al., 2004).

As a result most trusts in Wales now have school health nurse teams with many SHNs accessing the specialist community public health practitioner academic route at university (Earles, 2005). Although they study alongside health visitor colleagues, they qualify as distinct and autonomous specialist community practitioners. The target set, for every school having a named nurse, has generally been achieved. So far the necessary changes to practice for facilitating this have been made within existing resource. It is widely expected that a consultation document, which is being drawn up for the national assembly, will result in radical reform in the future (In Brief, 2007).

There are many examples of excellent SHN evidence-based practice across the principality in all areas of health promotion relevant to children/young people. Of particular note is the support afforded to their colleagues in education with the provision of sex and relationships education (SRE) in line with Government and WAG policy (Department for Education and Employment, DfEE, 2000; NAW, 2002a). A draft parenting action plan disseminated for consultation by the Welsh Assembly Government (WAG, 2005a) highlights parents discussing SRE with their children to be one of four key areas where parents need advice and support.

The literature has identified issues for teachers and parents/carers that compromise the delivery of effective SRE. It is suggested that SHNs can be a key agent of change in this area. They have a significant role in facilitating multidisciplinary collaborative working and coordinating programmes, as well as providing a consistent approach to involving the wider community (Day and Lane, 1999; Cotton et al., 2000; Cooper, 2005). It is suggested that SHNs can be effective in engaging parents/carers to work in collaboration with them and the schools for children's/young people's benefit (Harrison, 2005).

Wainwright et al. (2000) carried out a systematic review for Health Promotion Wales focusing on work published in the 1990s regarding the SHN role. They identified that a majority of 79% of all schools already utilise the SHN as a guest speaker. Coupled with this is evidence of highly successful examples of multidisciplinary working between SHNs, local education authorities and LHBs and essentially the National Public Health Service.

SHNs in many areas play an important part in the success of the school's *Healthy School Scheme* (HSS) (DfEE, 1999) providing support in all areas of the curriculum. This includes health promotion sessions on hygiene, which involve discussions on hand washing and personal hygiene, as well as sessions on diet and exercise. The SHN manager is often a member of the steering group for the HSS locally, and many SHNs are also working in partnership with multidisciplinary colleagues as accreditors for the scheme.

In many regions, because they are dually qualified as contraception and sexual health nurses, the SHN teams also provide individual sexual health promotion advice. Opportunities exist for this via either drop-in sessions at school or confidential sessions offered outside school hours in venues accessible to young people. The venues include youth clubs and clinics, with many SHNs providing, where appropriate, contraception and sexual health services in line with WAG recommendations (NAW, 2001).

Along with all these interventions, the SHNs in Wales continue to deliver the National Public Health Service programmes of vaccinations in school and carry out height, weight and vision screening programmes; some are also involved in hearing screening. SHNs are currently being consulted by the Assembly Government regarding a way forward to tackle the acknowledged problem of childhood obesity.

The need for effective health promotion activities aimed at children/young people is evidenced by the recently published *Health Needs Assessment 2006* (Lester, 2007). The latest available figures included in this document identify that 15% of girls and 17.8% of boys in Wales are pre-obese at age 13 years. As a result the WAG has sanctioned a pilot study in three trust areas, led by SHNs, to record and col-late the height and weight of children in reception class at age 5 years, and again in year 6 at age 11 years. The data generated will be used to establish an up-to-date baseline of statistics. The results will be used to plan a long term strategy and focused health promotion activities, which will help to prevent obesity.

Lester (2007) identifies that the prevalence of smoking at 21.5% of girls at age 15 years is higher than in both England and Scotland. Although at 12.1%, the figure for boys of the same age who smoke is actually lower. It remains an area of great concern for the future health of the principality's young people. Smoking is an issue often highlighted by schools as an identified aim they chose to address when working towards achieving accreditation under the HSS initiative.

One initiative utilised with children aged 8–11 years in primary schools is the *Smoke Bugs programme*. This WAG initiative trains comprehensive school pupils to deliver a programme to primary school children who can also sign up to a newsletter which maintains the momentum of the health messages that are delivered.

Although historically higher than in England, the conception rate in the under 16 years in Wales has reduced in recent years to 7.8% per 1000 and now compares closely with English statistics. It is suggested that this decrease has been achieved at least in part by improved SRE in schools, the provision of drop-in clinics for young people and the advice offered by specially trained youth workers who sign-post young people to relevant services for advice and contraception. Many of these interventions and service provisions are as a direct result of the policy included in Government and WAG documents (DfEE, 2000; NAW, 2001, 2002b).

However, the incidence of 54.4% of girls and 58% of boys aged 15 years who consume alcohol on a weekly basis remains higher than that in either England or Scotland. In an effort to address this issue, many schools utilise a guest speaker from their local drug and alcohol abuse service to provide factual information and advice via school-based personal and social education lessons. In Wales young people also have access to the WAG-funded web-based *Cliconline* site, which is aimed at 11- to 25-year-olds. This website provides information on many topics relevant to their lives including health issues and the facts about drugs, alcohol, and their effects.

The SHN service, by being involved in relevant initiatives, has a huge potential to impact positively on the health of the future generation. This can in turn reduce the need for costly acute and long-term interventions. Health promotion that is evidence based provides the necessary information to facilitate informed and healthy lifestyle choices and can empower children/young people to assume responsibility for their own lives. By meeting this identified need, the SHN is also directly meeting the Wanless (2002) recommendation, which states that communities must be empowered to assume responsibility for their own health.

Community children's nursing – the Welsh perspective

All children/young people who are sick or who have a chronic condition do have the right to be cared for at home by appropriately qualified nurses, wherever possible. The CCN is well placed to provide this care and support to children/young people and their families, helping to promote their health.

The development of CCN services has increased gradually over the past 20 years. In 1987 there were 150 teams (Royal College of Nursing, RCN, 2002) compared to the 239 in 2006 (RCN, 2006a) with significant developments in Wales. There are currently 16 CCN services throughout Wales.

Eaton (2001) described 6 models of CCN practice throughout Wales, and it is fair to state that the current 16 services use an eclectic mix of these models to provide a service to meet the needs of their individual localities. There is a need, however, to further expand the current provision of CCN services to provide better provision for children/young people and their families. This will enable children/young people to receive more equitable and accessible services.

Government legislation has widely documented the need for trusts and LHB to develop CCN services throughout the decades (Ministry of Health, 1962, 1971; Department of Health and Social Security, 1976; House of Commons Health Select Committee, 1997; NAW, 2005; WAG, 2005b).

In Wales in 2003, practitioners were encouraged by the Welsh Assembly Government's chief nursing officer (CNO) for a review of children's services in Wales, where her findings clearly indicated a gap in CCN services throughout Wales. The CNO identified that developed services were struggling to meet the changing needs of children, young people and their families. The CNO stated that CCN development was to be seen as an area of main concern for the future. Further to this the NSF for children, young people and maternity services in Wales (NAW, 2005) has now importantly set as one of its targets, the following: 'A CCN service is available to meet the local needs in every area in Wales' (NSF – NAW, Chapter 7, p. 65).

Challenges facing CCN service development

There are several challenges that Welsh CCNs encounter as part of their service development:

- Recognition of the CCN role.
- Continuing care and respite for sick and disabled children.
- Funding.
- Acute CCN service development.

Recognition of the CCN role

The role of the CCN is to provide a skilled nursing service for children/young people and their families in the community. This consists of supporting families in the nursing care of their child and the provision of health promotion advice. The aim is to help empower parents/carers, so they feel more confident in caring for their child at home (RCN, 2002). Further evaluation and audit of services is essential to highlight the good work of CCN practitioners.

Continuing care and respite for sick and disabled children

CCN and LHB in Wales do not use a common assessment document. It is the aim of the Welsh CCN forum to develop an All Wales Continuing Care Strategy for children/young people, including those in transition to adult services. The aim is to have a common assessment, criteria and documentation, further enhancing the theory of equity across the country, and thus meeting the NSF (NAW, 2005) target that is expected.

Health and Social Services Committee Review of Services for Children/Young People with Special

Needs (NAW, 2002c) advocated that services should be flexible to meet the needs of this client group and their families. A comprehensive respite service should be available for all from an early age.

Funding

Many trusts in Wales have used reallocation of monies and nursing posts to develop CCN services, and LHBs have commissioned respite services. CCN services are cost-effective, reduce hospital admissions and promote early discharge, yet there is little evidence at present to justify their existence. An effective audit tool is essential (Eaton and Thomas, 1998) to provide both qualitative and quantitative data to enhance business cases for future service development.

Acute CCN service development

As well as caring for children with longer term conditions, CCNs are well placed to care for children who are acutely ill, suffering from childhood illnesses (see Chapter 11) or recovering from acute illness. The *Health of Children in Wales* (NAW, 1997) document advocated that health authorities and local authorities should develop home care services for sick children. CCNs are best placed to provide this role. They can provide an advisory health promotion role as well as hands-on clinical care to support parents/carers. CCNs have a high degree of knowledge and skills that would transmit confidence to children/young people and the families they are caring for with acute illnesses. As Whiting (1998) states some parents/carers find it stressful caring for a sick child, CCNs can help.

Some of the benefits of an acute CCN service can be as follows:

- Facilitation of early discharge from hospital.
- Prevention of hospital admission for acute paediatric illnesses, such as otitis media, upper respiratory tract infections, urinary tract infections, high temperatures and gastroenteritis.
- Reduction in ward attendees and need for a paediatric outpatient review appointment for urinalysis, blood sampling requests by general practitioners, constipation advice and management.
- Reduction in the incidence of hospital-acquired infections.

- Supporting day case surgery by promoting early discharge.
- A decrease in children's/young people's anxiety, as they have the opportunity to receive care within their own home environment. A reduction in parental/carer anxiety too.
- Preventing disruption to normal family life.
- An effective use of limited health service resources especially within the climate of cost improvement and the NHS modernisation agendas.

Many Welsh trusts have used the reallocation of nursing posts where acute hospital beds have been closed to develop an acute CCN service. Many are adopting to utilise a CCN in paediatric assessment/ambulatory care units.

The development of acute CCN service provision should be planned in a systematic way, ensuring there is a balance in providing services which are responsive to local needs. These developments must be consistent and equitable throughout Wales and who best to provide this service – a CCN. Such a service can prevent hospital admissions and promote health for children/young people.

Welsh CCNs are encouraged by the NSF (NAW, 2005) and feel that it has given them motivation to assess the needs of their own localities, which are known to be greater than the services they are currently providing. With the use of a good audit tool, they will be able to produce evidence to the trusts, LHB and WAG that further investment is required. It is important to ensure that children/young people and their families in Wales receive a CCN service. CCN services should be equitable across Wales.

England

England – a country of diversities.
– Office for National Statistics (ONS, 1999)

Introduction

Under the theme of *diversity* this section on national perspectives looks at two issues which are highly relevant to the health of children/young people living in England at this time: *child poverty*, and *population diversity*. England has health promotion initiatives in place focusing on these issues.

As a country England demonstrates much diversity. Parts of England are quite affluent, while other places are considerably less so, with deprivation clearly evident. Deprivation continues to impact on the lives of children/young people as it has done historically. Tackling deprivation has been highlighted within the *Health Profile of England* (Department of Health, 2006a), as needing further action. Child poverty, an effect of deprivation, will thus be discussed.

Diversity is also present in terms of the population. England is home to people from many different countries and from diverse cultural backgrounds. Immigration seems to be an increasing concern; an ever present discussion in the media. It therefore warrants attention, as it impacts on the role of nurses as they come into contact with more and more children/young people from different countries.

There is also much diversity in terms of the health issues that affect children/young people. Nurses working both in hospital and community contexts come across a wide range of different health issues; some of them associated with social and environmental problems. In some cases the social and environmental problems can be linked back to both deprivation and immigration.

Child poverty

Deprivation continues to impact on the lives of children/young people in England (Department of Health, 2006a). Historically, documents have highlighted deprivation as an issue that impacts upon children's health – the Black report (Townsend and Davidson, 1982), for example. For less affluent communities deprivation and child poverty are significant issues. The Department of Health (2006a) expresses concern about the persistence of deprivation and child poverty in England.

Deprivation is related to many factors: geography, ethnicity and socio-economic status, as well as age and gender (Department of Health, 2006a). Deprivation influences the cause of many health problems. The Government sometimes refers to deprivation as one of the determinants of health (Department of Health, 2006a).

Child poverty is an issue which this Government has always placed high on its agenda. Baroness Jay in 1997, then Shadow Labour Minister, highlighted concerns about child poverty, and what might be achieved to tackle it (Jay, 1997). Child poverty is a theme which continues within Government policy today. Encouraging more parents back to work has and continues to be one approach taken by Government. Another approach is action on parenting, which will be discussed further.

The Government feels that parenting has an overwhelming influence on the health and education of future generations. Parenting has been targeted as a way of helping children living in poverty to achieve better health and education, thus improving their long-term prospects.

Parenting is important for the emotional health of children, as well as their physical health. Parenting can lay the foundations for later-life relationships. Parenting can also influence the health behaviours of children, perhaps encouraging them to adopt healthy lifestyles. Education is seen as a way of progressing in life, getting out of the so-called *poverty trap*. The Government (Department of Health, 2007) believes that a healthy start, influenced by parents, can provide better opportunities for children.

Parenting may hold the key, as the Government suggests. There is no doubt that parents can influence the health of their children. Indeed, some parents would welcome greater parenting support, so they can spend more time influencing the health behaviours of their children. Mothers particularly have much to contend with, bringing up a family, running a home, as well as trying to hold down a job in some cases. Juggling so many different things, it is not surprising that something may slip occasionally. Some parents find it hard to influence their children, particularly when they do not have enough time to spend with them. Conversely, other parents might not welcome what they could see as interference in family life from Government. These are some of the mixed views that exist among parents in England.

Action taken so far by the Government on parenting includes developing many Sure Start centres around the country in areas of deprivation, which provide services for families with young children. The Department of Health (2007) believes in developing many similar centres for children (children's centres), where families can receive advice on parenting. Children's centres will act as focal points for families, providing access to health, and parenting support (Department of Health, 2007). Extended schools have also been developed, where parenting groups and parent support advisors are available (Lindsay et al. 2008), for those families with older children.

From experiencing Sure Start at first hand, it can help and support families. In the past not all areas were able to access Sure Start services. Services were developed for families with young children (those under 5 years of age) in very deprived areas. However, more families will have the opportunity to access the range of services that children's centres will offer, due to Government proposals to develop more such centres. In time children's centres will be able to provide services for children of varying ages (not just the under 5s), in different areas.

England is also a country where there are high rates of crime, particularly in areas of deprivation. Crimes are being committed by young people, and some of them are quite violent crimes. The Government is focusing on the early influences of crime. Here again, parenting is thought to be highly influential. Future Government plans include helping families with the parenting of troubled young people. The hope is that young people will grow up to feel responsible for their own behaviour, and thus not commit crimes. One proposal put forward is for a scheme of *Supernannies* to support such families (BBC Radio 4, 2007) in the future.

There is definitely much more focus on the role of parenting in England today than there has ever been in the past, particularly as a way of helping children out of poverty, to improve their long-term health.

Nurses are very much involved in undertaking parenting work with families in Sure Start and children's centres, in schools, and in hospitals too. They are all working hard to support parents and promote children's health.

Population diversity (cultural health promotion)

Diversity is also an issue which reflects itself in terms of England's population. Over the years England has welcomed people from many different countries, resulting in communities growing up with varied cultural backgrounds. Over past decades people from the Indian and Asian subcontinents settled here. More recently, with the development of greater ties with Europe, families from Eastern Europe are coming to live in England.

Diversity in population poses particular challenges for nurses, who need to learn about the different cultural backgrounds of families, so they are able to meet their health needs effectively. Awareness of such issues as customs and traditions, as well as religion and cultural beliefs, need to be considered. The status of women and expectations on cultural dress, as well as family structures, are all significant matters that have relevance to the health promotion advice given by nurses.

An important health issue that needs to be considered closely in a multicultural community is immunisation. When children/young people are coming into this country from abroad, their immunisation status needs to be examined, in an effort to prevent ill health. Health visitors, school nurses or practice nurses can look at what immunisations children/young people might need. The NSF (Education and Skills, Department of Health, 2004) advises that immunisation information should be available in different languages, allowing families to make informed choices about immunisation. These materials are usually available via health promotion units, as well as the internet.

Currently, many asylum seekers are coming to live in England. England's children's commissioner has expressed concern about the care of asylum seeker children/young people (RCN, 2006b). Asylum seekers are individuals seeking sanctuary in this country. They may have experienced terrifying events before coming here, as well as having to leave family and friends behind. They find themselves in a place where they do not know anyone, and may not be able to speak English. Children may feel confused about where they are. Health care services are an important source of support for these families and their children.

There are patient-held health records for asylum seekers and their families, which can be downloaded from the internet via the Department of Health website. The records provide information in many languages.

Nurses need to find out more by reading and attending conferences, on how to meet the health care needs of children/young from abroad who settle here. The Government has produced a very useful resource – *Meeting the Health Needs of Refugee and Asylum Seekers in the UK, an information and resource package for health workers* (Burnett and Fassil, 2002). The book provides key information and guides nurses towards many useful resources.

Working with families, certainly in the initial stages, will require time. Time is a resource nurses do not have in abundance. However, to enable these children/young people to settle, a little extra care and attention in the early stages can be of enormous benefit.

Importantly too, for families of different nationalities, services need to be accessible. The Department of Health (2006b) provides examples where community nurses have set up services in community centres where adults from particular cultures regularly attend. Perhaps the same needs to be considered for children/young people, where nurses may experience difficulties accessing some families. Nurses need to develop relationships within these communities in an effort to promote children's health.

General health

When studying the Health Profile of England (Department of Health, 2006a), the diversity of health issues that can affect children/young people really comes across. The document disappointingly shows a rise in childhood obesity, along with rising rates of diabetes, and high rates of teenage pregnancy. However, on the positive side the document does show that the infant mortality rate is at its lowest level ever, and the number of road deaths and serious injuries related to traffic flow have fallen, along with improvements in dental health (Department of Health, 2006a). This data shows improvements for the health of children/young people in England, but still more work needs to be achieved by nurses through health promotion activities and campaigns, to help England's children.

Close

The evidence for England shows that there are improvements in children's/young people's health, but there is still much more to be achieved. Child poverty and issues surrounding population diversity, as well as childhood obesity and teenage pregnancy, are all areas of high priority. Nurses need to think carefully about what health promotion initiatives might help children/young people locally. Team working with other practitioners may provide some interesting collaborative initiatives. This may be particularly feasible where Sure Starts or children's centres are linked to local schools, or hospitals, for example.

The NSFs for children, young people and maternity services (Education and Skills, Department of Health, 2004) provide important guidance for the development of any new initiatives. The NSFs emphasise the need for all nurses working with children, young people and their families to actively promote the health of the next generation. This is as important in England, as it is in the other countries of the United Kingdom.

Conclusion

This chapter has looked at health for children/young people in the following countries:

- Northern Ireland.
- Scotland.
- Wales.
- England.

There are some health issues which are similar. Obesity and dental health are significant health issues for all. However, there are differences in priorities too as can be seen from the text. There are many health promotion initiatives taking place all around the UK for children/young people. Nurses have an important role to play in these activities.

Studying national perspectives has provided some useful insights into the development of different health promotion initiatives taking place across the UK. Importantly, nurses have been able to share their knowledge and experiences. Nurses working collaboratively in this way may encourage others to develop opportunities for children's/young people's health in their area, in line with the NSFs.

Acknowledgements

I would like to thank all the contributors to this chapter, who have enabled different perspectives from across the UK to be presented.

Resources

Bunton, R., McDonald, G. (1992) *Health Promotion Disciplines, Diversity and Developments*, 2nd edn. London: Routledge.

Community Health Profiles. *Health Profile of England*. Available at: http://www.communityhealthprofiles.info (accessed August 2007).

Department of Health. *Patient-Held Records for Asylum Seekers and Refugees*. Available at: http://www.dh.gov.uk/en/Policyandguidance/International/asylumseekers-Andrefugees/ (accessed 22 August 2007).

Johnston, L. (2006) *Reducing Health Inequalities in Early Years*. Edinburgh: NHS Lothian.

Laverock, G. (2004) *Health Promotion Practice and Empowerment*. London: Sage.

Malam, S. (2005) *Health Education Population Survey Accidents and Safety 1996–2004*. Edinburgh: NHS Scotland, RoSPA.

Office of National Statistics. Available at: http://www.ons (accessed August 2007).

Pike, S., Forster, D. (eds) (1995) *Health Promotion for All*. Edinburgh: Churchill Livingstone.

Scottish Executive (2003) *Improving Health in Scotland – the Challenge*. Edinburgh: Scottish Executive.

Scriven, A., Orme, J. (eds) (2001) *Health Promotion – Professional Perspectives*. Hampshire: Palgrave.

Tones, K., Green, J. (2004) *Health Promotion. Planning and Strategies*. London: Sage.

World Health Organization (1996) *The Ottawa Charter for Health Promotion*. Geneva: WHO. Available at: http://www.healthpromotingschoolsunit@LTScotland.org.uk (accessed 11 October 2006).

References

Bamford, D. (2006) *Vision of a Comprehensive Child and Adolescent Mental Health Service*. Belfast: DHSSPSNI.

Bartley, J. (2004) Health promotion and school nurses: the potential for change. *Community Practitioner* 77(2): 61–64.

BBC Radio 4 (2007) *Supernannies*. News report. 14 September.

Burnett, A., Fassil, Y. (2002) *Meeting the Health Needs of Refugee and Asylum Seekers in the UK, An Information and Resource Pack for Health Workers*. London: Crown Copyright.

Burns, H. (2006) *Health in Scotland 2005*. Edinburgh: Scottish Executive.

Cooper, P. (2005) A co-ordinated school health plan. *Educational Leadership* 63(1): 32–36.

Cotton, L., Brazier, J., Hall, D., Lindsay, G., Marsh, P., Polnay, L., Williams, T.S. (2000) School nursing: costs and potential benefits. *Journal of Advanced Nursing* 31(5): 1063–1071.

Croghan, E., Johnson, C., Aveyard, P. (2004) School nurses: policies, working practices, roles and value perceptions. *Journal of Advanced Nursing* 47(4): 377–385.

Day, P., Lane, D. (1999) Sex education: lessons to be learnt from going Dutch. *Community Practitioner* 72(8): 259–260. London: McMillan-Scott.

DeBell, D., Jackson, P. (2000) *School Nursing within the Public Health Agenda. A Strategy for Practice*. London: MacMillan-Scott.

Department for Education and Employment (DfEE) (1999) *National Healthy School Standard*. Nottingham: DfEE Publications.

Department for Education and Employment (DfEE) (2000) *Sex and Relationships Education Guidance*. Nottingham: DfEE Publications.

Department of Education for Northern Ireland (2002) *Bullying in Schools: A Northern Ireland Study*. Bangor: DENI.

Department of Health (1997) *The New NHS: Modern, Dependable*. London: HMSO.

Department of Health (1999) *Making a Difference*. London: TSO.

Department of Health (2001) *Public Health Practice Development Document for School Nurses*. London: Department of Health.

Department of Health (2004a) *Children Act*. London: Department of Health.

Department of Health (2004b) *Choosing Health*. London: Department of Health.

Department of Health (2006a) *Health Profile of England*. London: Crown Copyright.

Department of Health (2006b) *Our Health, Our Care, Our Say: A New Direction for Community Services*. London: Crown Copyright.

Department of Health (2006c) *School Nurse: Practice Development Resource Pack. Specialist Community Public Health Nurse*. London: Department of Health.

Department of Health (2007) *Delivering Health Services through Sure Start Children's Centres*. London: Crown Copyright.

Department of Health and Social Security (1976) *Fit for the Future. The Report of the Committee on Child Health Services*. The Court Report. London: DHSS.

Department of Health, Social Services and Public Safety Northern Ireland (DHSSPSNI) (2002) *Investing for Health*. Belfast: DHSSPSNI.

Department of Health, Social Services and Public Safety Northern Ireland (DHSSPSNI) (2004) *Promoting Mental Health Strategy and Action Plan 2003–2008*. Belfast: DHSSPSNI.

Department of Health, Social Services and Public Safety Northern Ireland (DHSSPSNI) (2005) *Health of the Public in Northern Ireland*. Report of the Chief Medical Officer. Belfast: DHSSPSNI.

Department of Health, Social Services and Public Safety Northern Ireland (DHSSPSNI) (2006a) *Fit Futures. Focus on Food, Activity and Young People. Executive Summary*. Belfast: DHSSPSNI.

Department of Health, Social Services and Public Safety Northern Ireland (DHSSPSNI) (2006b) *Your Health Matters. The Annual Report of the Chief Medical Officer for Northern Ireland*. Belfast: DHSSPSNI.

Department of Health, Social Services and Public Safety Northern Ireland (DHSSPSNI) (2006c) *The New Strategic Direction for Alcohol and Drugs*. Belfast: DHSSPSNI.

Department of the Environment for Northern Ireland (DoENI) (2002) *The NI Road Safety Strategy 2002–2012*. Belfast: DoENI.

Earles, C. (2005) *A Survey of School Health Nurses in Wales Regarding their Public Health Role*. Health Professions Wales research fellowship.

Eaton, N. (2001) Models of community children's nursing. *Paediatric Nursing* 13(1): 32–36.

Eaton, N., Thomas, P. (1998) Community children's nursing service an evaluative framework. *Journal of Child Health Care* 2(4):170–173.

Education and Skills (Department of), Department of Health (2004) *National Service Framework for Children, Young People and Maternity Services*. London: Crown Copyright.

Freeman, R., Oliver, M., Bunting, G., Kirk, J., Saunderson, W. (2001) Addressing children's oral health inequalities in Northern Ireland: a research-practice-community partnership initiative. *Public Health Report* 116(6): 617–625.

Gleeson, C. (2004) School health nursing – evidence-based practice. *Primary Health Care* 14(3): 38–41.

Greater Glasgow NHS Board (2006) *The Starting Well Health Demonstration Project*. Glasgow: NHS Scotland.

Hain, P. (2007) *New Unit to Tackle Child Poverty Announced*. Department of Work and Pensions. London: Crown Copyright.

Hall, D., Elliman, D. (2003) *Health for All Children*, 4th edn. Oxford: Oxford University Press.

Halliday, W. (2006) *Health Promoting Schools Newsletter* (Issue 2 June). Dundee: Scottish Health Promoting Schools Unit.

Harrison, S. (2005) Under 12s have sex one night and play with Barbie dolls the next. *Nursing Standard* 19(39): 14–16.

Health Promotion Agency for Northern Ireland (HPANI) (2001) *Eating for Health? A Survey of Eating Habits among Children and Young People in Northern Ireland*. Belfast: HPANI.

Health Promotion Agency for Northern Ireland (HPANI) (2004) *What Do You Know About Drugs? Your Body, Your Life, Your Choice*. Belfast: HPANI.

Health Promotion Agency for Northern Ireland (HPANI) (2005) *Fresh Fruit in Schools Evaluation 2002–2004: Summary Report*. Belfast: HPANI.

Health Promotion Agency for Northern Ireland (HPANI) (2006) *Your Body, Your Life, Your Choice*. Belfast: HPANI.

Health Promotion Agency for Northern Ireland (HPANI) (2007) *Fresh Fruit in Schools. Summary Report 2002–2006*. Belfast: HPANI.

Health Promoting Schools (2006) *Free Fruit*. Health Promoting Schools. Available at: http://www.health-promotingschools.co.uk (accessed 11 October 2006).

House of Commons Health Select Committee (1997) *Health Services for Children and Young People in the Community – Home and School*. London: The Stationery Office.

In Brief (2007) *Nursing Standard* 21(24): 6.

Jay, M. (1997) *Shadow Labour Minister*. Speech at the School Nurse conference. Royal College of Nursing.

Lester, N. (2007) *Health Needs Assessment 2006. Children and Young People*. Wales: National Public Health Service for Wales.

Lindsay, G., Band, S., Cullen, M., Cullen, S. (2008) *Parenting Early Intervention Pathfinder Evaluation. Additional Study of the Involvement of Extended Schools*. Centre for Educational Appraisal and Research. University of Warwick. Department for Children, Schools and Families. Warwick: Crown Copyright.

McKenzie, M., Shute, J., Berzins, K., Judge, K. (2005) *Starting Well Executive Summary Independent Evaluation*. Scotland: University of Glasgow, Edinburgh Scottish Executive.

Ministry of Health (1962) *A Hospital Plan for England and Wales*. London: HMSO.

Ministry of Health (1971) *Hospital Facilities for Children*. London: HMSO.

Naidoo, J., Wills, J. (2005) *Public Health and Health Promotion, developing practice*, 2nd edn. London: Bailliere-Tindall.

National Assembly for Wales (NAW) (1997) *The Health of Children in Wales*. Cardiff: NAW.

National Assembly for Wales (NAW) (2001) *A Strategic Framework for Promoting Sexual Health in Wales*. Cardiff: NAW.

National Assembly for Wales (NAW) (2002a) *Sex and Relationships Education in Schools. Circular No: 11/02*. Cardiff: NAW.

National Assembly for Wales (NAW) (2002b) *Too Serious a Thing. A Review to Safeguard Children and Young People Treated and Cared for by the NHS in Wales. The Carlile Review.* Cardiff: NAW.

National Assembly for Wales (NAW) (2002c) *Health and Social Services Committee Review of Services for Children with Special Health Needs.* Cardiff: NAW.

National Assembly for Wales (NAW) (2005) *National Service Framework for Children, Young People and Maternity Services in Wales.* Cardiff: NAW.

NHS Lothian (2006) *Health and Healthcare of Children and Young People in Lothian.* Consultation document. Edinburgh: NHS Lothian.

Northern Ireland Statistics and Research Agency (NISRA) (2003) *Young Persons' Behaviour and Attitudes Survey.* Belfast: NISRA.

Northern Ireland Statistics and Research Agency (2006) *Registrar General Annual Report.* Belfast: NISRA.

O'Neill, M., O'Donnell, D. (2003) Smart Snacks Scheme: A healthy breaks initiative in the school environment. *Education and Health* 21(1): 9–13.

Office for National Statistics (1999) *Britain 2000, the Official Yearbook of the United Kingdom.* London: Stationery Office.

Office of the First Minister and Deputy First Minister (OFMDFM) (2006a) *Our Children and Young People – Our Pledge. A Ten-Year Strategy for Children and Young People in Northern Ireland 2006–2016.* Belfast: OFMDFM.

Office of the First Minister and Deputy First Minister (OFMDFM) (2006b) *Eagle Announces 37 Million School Bus Safety Boost. News Release.* Belfast: OFMDFM.

Police Service for NI (2007) *Injury Road Traffic Collisions and Casualties. 1st April 2006–31st March 2007.* Belfast: PSNI.

Reilly, J., Jackson, D., Montgomery, C. (2004) Total energy expenditure and physical activity in young Scottish children: mixed longitudinal study. *Lancet* 363(9404): 211–212.

Ross, M., de Caestecker, L. (2003) The starting well health demonstration project: the best possible start in life? *International Journal of Mental Health Promotion* 5: 5–12.

Royal College of Nursing (RCN) (2002) *Community Children's Nursing. Information for Primary Care Organisa-*tions, Health Authorities and All Professionals Working with Children in Community Settings. London: RCN.

Royal College of Nursing (RCN) (2006a) *Directory of Community Children's Nursing Services.* London: RCN.

Royal College of Nursing (RCN) (2006b) Commissioners voice concern over asylum seekers. *News.* London: RCN.

Scottish Executive (2005) *Delivering for Health.* Edinburgh: Scottish Executive.

Scottish Executive (2006) *Health Promoting and Nutrition (Scotland) Bill.* Edinburgh: Scottish Executive.

Townsend, P., Davidson, N. (eds) (1982) *The Black Report.* London: Crown Copyright.

United Nations (1989) *Convention on the Rights of the Child.* Geneva: UN.

Wainwright, P., Thomas, J., Jones, M. (2000) Health promotion and the role of the school nurse: a systematic review. *Journal of Advanced Nursing* 32(5): 1083–1091.

Wanless, D. (2002) *Securing Our Future Health: Taking a Long Term View.* Final Report. London: UK Government.

Watkins, D.C., Murray, L.J., McCarron, P., Boreham, C.A.G., Cran, G.W., Young, I.S., McGartland, C., Robson, P.J., Savage, J.M. (2005) Ten year trends for fatness in Northern Irish adolescents: the young hearts projects, repeat cross-sectional study. *International Journal of Obesity* 29: 579–585.

Welsh Assembly Government (WAG) (2005a) *Parenting Action Plan. Supporting Mothers, Fathers and Carers Raising Children in Wales. Draft for Consultation.* Cardiff: WAG.

Welsh Assembly Government (WAG) (2005b) *National Service Framework for Children, Young People and Maternity Services in Wales.* Cardiff: WAG.

Whitehead, D. (2003) Evaluating health promotion: a model for nursing practice. *Journal of Advanced Nursing* 41(5): 490–498.

Whiting, M. (1998) Expanding community children's nursing services. *British Journal of Nursing* 3(4): 183–190.

World Health Organization (1986) *Ottawa Charter for Health Promotion.* Geneva: WHO.

World Health Organization (1996) *Health Promoting Schools.* Geneva: WHO.

Index

Note: Italicised page numbers refer to boxes, figures, and tables.

5 a Day campaign, 8, 73–4, 214*f*, 283, 374

accident and emergency department, 369
accident prevention, 101–110
    activities for children/young people,
        109–110
    garden safety campaigns, 106–107
    home safety campaigns, 102–103
    priority areas, 6–7
    road safety, 104–106
    role of nurses in, 101–102
    session for parents/cares, 107–109
    sources of information, 102–103
accidents, 101, 103–104
Action on Smoking and Health, 346–347
acute pain, 250
acutely ill child, 115
addiction, 253
adjuvants, 253
adolescence, 49
adolescents, 55–56
    alcohol use in, 339–340
    drug use in, 339–340
aims, 14–15
alcohol use, 339–340
    in adolescents, 339–340
    in childhood cancer survivors, 206–207
    North Ireland, 383–384
allergy, 196
ambulatory care, 164–165
amitriptyline, 253
Anti-bullying alliance, 297
anti-inflammatory medication, 186
antipyretics, 124, 253

anxiety, in childhood cancer survivors, 207
Area Child Protection Committees, 39
aspirin, 253
asthma, 181–190
    action plans, 188
    attacks, 188–189
    breathing test, 183
    causes of, 182
    definition of, 181
    diagnosis of, 183
    health promotion, 189
    medical history, 183
    physical examination, 183
    prevalence of, 181–182
    resources, 189–190
    symptom monitoring, 183
    symptoms of, 182–183
    treatment of, 185–189
        anti-inflammatory medication, 186
        bronchodilators, 185–186
        combination therapy, 186–187
        delivery devices, 187
        leukotriene receptor antagonists, 187
        self-management, 187–188
    triggers of, 183–185
        cigarette smoke, 185
        excitement, 184–185
        exercise, 184–185
        house dust mite, 184
        pets, 184
        respiratory infections, 184
    worsening, 188
asylum-seeking children, unaccompanied, 310–311
attention, 50

auditory learning, 26–27
autonomy, 48–49

babies, health promotion activities for, 29
baby club, 281–286
    aims of, 281
    description of, 283–284
    mum's experience of, 284–285
    planning, 281–282
    Solihull approach, 282
    stimulating babies in, 282–283
baby massage, 259–264
    benefits of, 261
    bonding in, 260
    cautions, 263–264
    positive touch in, 259–260
baby play, 272–280
    aim of, 273–274
    case study, 278–279b
    equipment, 274–276
        balls, 274
        books, 275
        bubble blowing, 276
        hats, 276
        home-made rattles, 275
        margarine tubs, 275
        pans and spoons, 275–276
        pull along toy, 276
        safety mirror, 274–275
        stacking cups, 275
        treasure basket, 276
    evaluation of, 279–280
    history of, 273
    leaflets, 279f
    overview, 272
    practice, 273
    preparing for group, 277
    starting sessions, 277–278
    theory, 272–273
    venue, 277
baby yoga, 259–264
    bonding in, 160
    cautions, 263–264
    emotional benefits of, 262–263
    overview, 259
    physical benefits of, 263
    positive touch in, 259–260
balls, 274
basal cell carcinoma, 96
Black Report, 4
books, 275, 373
Bookstart, 371
breastfeeding, 71–73
    benefits of, 71–72
    family support in, 72
    NSF standards, 72–73
breathing test, 183
British Lung Foundation, 190
British National Formulary for Children (BNFC), 41
bronchodilators, 185–186

bubble blowing, 276
bullying, 293–299
    books and resources, 297
    cyberbullying, 298–299
    description of, 293–294
    government strategies, 295–296
    health promotion unit, 296
    helplines, 296
    location of, 294
    nurses' role in helping victims, 297–298
    overview, 293
    psychological factors, 294–295
    signs of, 295
    victims of, 294
Bumps and Babes groups, 72–73

carbamazepine, 253
car-safety seats, 104–105
case studies, 32
categorisation, 50
child development, 45–56
    adolescence, 49
    communication in, 51–53
    learning in, 50–51
    overview, 45
    puberty, 49–50
    theories, 45–49
Child Health Promotion Programme, 370–371
child poverty, 392–394
child-centred services, 155–158
    aims of, 119
    family-centred care, 156
    information sharing in, 158
    play in, 157–158
    preoperative assessment, 156–157
childhood cancer survivors, 202–208
    alcohol use in, 206–207
    anxiety in, 207
    drug use in, 206–207
    emotional health of, 207
    health behaviours in, 202–208
    health promotion in, 204
    long-term follow-up, 204–206
    model of care for, 203
    obesity in, 206
    sex and fertility, 207
    short stature of, 206
    smoking in, 206–207
    survival rate, 202
    survivors, 202
childhood diabetes, 220–226
    children/young people in school, 223–224
    documents and recommendations, 221–223
        Every Child Matters, 221
        National Service Framework, 222–223
        NCC-WCH, 221–222
    health promotion, 224–226
        dental health, 225
        immunisation, 225
        sexual health, 225–226

overview, 220–221
    screening recommendations, *225b*
childhood obesity, 70–81
    definition of, 70
    in England, 395–396
    and growth, 75
    overview, 69–70
    prevention, 70–71
        books, 75
        breastfeeding, 71–73
        children's TV programmes, 75
        cookery lessons, 75
        dinner menu, 74
        food in schools, 73–74
        healthy eating, 80–81
        physical activity, 76–80
        toolkits, 74–75
ChildLine, 296
children. *See also* adolescents; young people
    asylum-seeking, 310–311
    bullying in, 293–299
    causes of mortality in, 5–6
    communication in, 60–61
    diabetes in, 220–226
    disabled, 40, 228–231
    discipline of, 304–305
    fever management in, 124–133
    growth monitoring, 61–63
    health promotion activities for, 29–30
    length and height, 62
    looked-after, 307–311
    minor illnesses in, 134–143
    obesity in, 70–81
    safeguarding, 300–305
    weight, 61–62
Children Act (2004), 34, 301–304
Children Are Unbeatable Alliance, 305
children in hospital, 40
    play, 53–56
    pre- and postoperative care, 155–161
children's outpatient department, 53–54
children's TV programmes, 75
child/young person-centred services, 37–38
chronic pain, 250
cigarette smoke, 185
clinical interview, 46
codeine, 253
cognitive development, stages of, 46
cognitive processes, 20–24
    attention, 22
    communication, 23–24
    memory theories, 22–23
    motivations, 20–21
    senses, 22
cold turkey, 347
combination inhalers, 186–187
communication, 23–24
    asking questions, 52
    in children, 60–61
    and children's independence, 52

listening to children/young people, 51
    special time, 51
community children's nursing, 116–117, 389–391
comparative need, 14
concrete operational stage, 47
constipation, 209–218
    and behaviour, 217
    in children, 210
    diagnostic criteria, 210
    facts about, 211
    government policy, 217
    health promotion, 212–216
        drinking, 212–213
        eating, 212
        exercise, 213–214
        potty training, 214–216
        toilet training, 214–216
    Hirschsprung's disease, 211
    history and assessment, 211–212
    medicine management, 216–217
    overview, 209–210
    physical factors, 210
    psychological factors, 210
    signs and symptoms, 210
    social factors, 210
    and soiling, 210
    and withholding, 210
content, 14–15
corporal punishment, 302–303
corticosteroids, 186
cough, 182
creativity, 25–32
    differentiation in, 28–32
    learning, 26–28
    overview, 25
    skills to teach health promotion, 25–26
cyberbullying, 298–299
cycle safety, 105–106

DARE (Drug Abuse Resistance Education), 340–343
    description of, 341–342
    experiences with, 341
    overview of, 340–341
    role of nurse in, 342–343
day surgery, *171t*
demonstrations, 16
dental check-ups, 89
dental health promotion, 83–94
    children with special needs, 85
    community practice, 91–92
    cultural factors in, 85
    dental health surveys, 84–85
    and dental problems, 86
    deprived areas, 85
    development of teeth, 83–84
    and diabetes management, 225
    government policy, 86–87
    hospital practice, 93–94
    key messages, 87–89
        avoiding fizzy drinks, 88–89

dental health promotion (*cont.*)
    dental check-ups, 89
    diet, 88
    fluoride, 87–88
    regular tooth brushing, 87
    North Ireland, 382–383
    resources, 89–91
        assessment of learning, 91
        books, 90
        campaigns, 89–90
        interactive website, 90
        models, 90
        quiz, 91
        samples and stickers, 90
        songs and poems, 91
    tips for young people, 84
dermatitis, 197
Diabetes Control and Complications Trial (DCCT), 224–226
diabetes in children, 220–226
    children/young people in school, 223–224
    documents and recommendations, 221–223
        Every Child Matters, 221
        National Service Framework, 222–223
        NCC-WCH, 221–222
    health promotion, 224–226
        dental health, 225
        immunisation, 225
        sexual health, 225–226
    overview, 220–221
    screening recommendations, *225b*
diclofenac, 253
diet. *See also* obesity in children
    and dental health, 88
    healthy eating, 374
dinner menu, 74
disabled children/young people, 228–231
    case study, 229–231
    needs, 228–229
    NSF standard, 40
    nurses' practice, 229
    overview, 228
    play and development programme for, 229
discharge
    complex, 174
    information, 167–168
    nurse-led, 170
    preparing for, 166–167
discharge planning, 169–176
    checklist for day surgery, *171t*
    child protection, 174
    complex discharges, 174
    complex health needs, 174–175
    complex mental health conditions, 174
    follow-up and support, 173–174
    information for parents/carers, 171–172
    medication, 172–173
    and minor illnesses, 169–170
    overview of, 169
discipline of children, 304–305
discussions, 16–17

dissemination, 363
doubt, 48–49
drinks, 212–213
drop-in service, school-based, 331–334
    aim, 331
    counsellor, 331
    objectives, 331–332
    promotion of, 333
    role of nurses in, 332–333
    services, 333–334
drug use. *See also* alcohol use
    in adolescents, 339–340
    in childhood cancer survivors, 206–207
    health promotion, 375–376
    North Ireland, 383–384
dust mite, 184
dyslexic children, 29
dyspnoea, 182

Eat Well to Play Well, 386
eating habits, and constipation, 212
eczema, 197–200. *See also* skin conditions
    allergy testing, 200
    atopic, 197
    bandaging and wet wrapping, 200
    seborrhoeic, 197
    special diets, 200
    steroid creams for, 198–200
    treatment instructions, 198
Education for Health, 190
egocentrism in children, 46
e-mail motivation messages, 347
emergency department, 369–370
emotional health, 376
empowerment, 12–13, 59, 267, 327, 330
England, 391–396
    childhood obesity, 395–396
    childhood poverty, 392–394
    diversity in health issues, 391–392
    population diversity, 394–395
episodic memories, 50
Erikson, Erik, 48–49
evaluation, 19–20
evaluation of health promotion, 353–363
    central to health promotion activities, 354
    children/young people evaluating, 357–358
    focus of, 354
    importance and benefits, 353
    issues to consider, 354
    objectives, 354–355
    participant's views, 355
    peer evaluation, 355
    research-based, 358–363
    self-evaluation, 356
    simple evaluation form, 356–357
    simple methods, 356
Every Child Matters, 35, 221, 327
excitement, 184–185
exercise, 184–185, 213–214
expressed need, 14

Face It, 343–344
 detached contact, 344
 group work, 344
 one-to-one intervention, 344
 overview of, 343–344
family-centred service, 119, 156
felt need, 14
fertility, 207
fever, 124
 first-dose medication for, 131
 reason for, 125
 and serious illnesses, 125–126
 signs of, 126–127
fever management, 124–133
 combined approaches, 129
 documentation, 131
 importance of, 124–125
 leaflets/advice sheet, 130
 managing high temperature, 131–132
 non-pharmacological approaches, 127–128
 clothing, 127
 fluids, 127
 at home, 127
 tests, 127–128
 pharmacological approaches, 128–129
 ibuprofen, 128–129
 paracetamol, 128
 practice interventions, 129–131
 prescribing, 129
fizzy drinks, avoiding, 89
fluoride, 87–88
food allergy, 197
formal operational stage, 47
forum theatre, 81
Fraser guidelines, *331b*
Free Fruit, 386
Fresh Fruit in Schools, 382
fungal infections, 196

gabapentin, 253
garden safety campaigns, 106–107
gastroenteritis, 136–137
government policy, 33–42
 child-related, 34–35
 Every Child Matters, 35
 National Service Frameworks, 35–42
 overview of, 33
 understanding, 33–34
growth monitoring, 61–63
 head circumference, 62
 interpreting results, 62–63
 length and height, 62
 measurement techniques, 61–62
 recording and plotting, 62
 weight, 61–62
guilt, 49

happy/sad pain-rating scale, 357
hats, 276
head circumference, 62

head lice, 195–196
health behaviours, 11–12
Health for All Children, 58–65
 communication, 60–61
 growth monitoring, 61–63
 health promotion, 59–60
 major issues, 59
 overview, 58–59
 Sure Start centres, 64–65
health inequalities, 3–4
 infant mortality, 5
 mortality in children and young people, 5–9
 and social classes, 4–5
health promotion, 367–377
 asthma management, 189
 for childhood cancer, 202–208
 in childhood diabetes, 220–226
 in children's minor illnesses, 132–143
 in community, 370–372
 accessible health services, 371–372
 Bookstart, 371
 Child Health Promotion Programme,
  370–371
 health visitors, 370–371
 support groups, 371
 consistency in, 60
 evaluation of, 353–363
 fever management, 124–132
 in hospitals, 367–370
 accident and emergency department, 369–370
 children's/young people's wards, 363–370
 communication, 368
 display boards, 368–369
 highly dependent/critically ill child, 368–369
 outpatient department, 370
 written information, 368
 in minor illnesses, 134–143
 in minor injuries, 144–150
 in nursery schools, 372–373
 books, 373
 play, 372–373
 puppets, 373
 planning, 11–24
 activities, 12
 elements of, 13–14
 empowerment approach, 12–13
 positive health behaviours, 11–12
 for postoperative care, 155–161
 for preoperative care, 155–161
 responsibility in, 59–60
 in schools, 374–376
 drug and solvent misuse, 375–376
 emotional health, 376
 healthy eating, 374
 personal, social and health education, 375
 physical activity, 374–375
 road safety, 375
 sexual health, 376
 scope of, 60
 sexual health, 325–334

health promotion (*cont.*)
  skills to teach, 25–26
  in surgical wound healing, 155–161
Health Promotion and Nutrition Bill, 386
health visitors, 370–371
Healthy Care Programme, 309
healthy eating
  North Ireland, 381–382
  promotion of, 374
height, 62
Hirschsprung's disease, 211
home safety campaigns, 102–103
home-made rattles, 275
hospitals, 367–370
  accident and emergency department, 369
  children's/young people's wards, 363–370
  communication in, 368
  display boards, 368–369
  highly dependent/critically ill child, 368–369
  outpatient department, 369–370
  play in, 53–56
    adolescents, 55–56
    children's outpatient department, 53–54
    functions of play, 53
    overview of, 53
    paediatric intensive care unit, 54–55
    pre- and postoperative care, 157–158
  written information, 368
house dust mite, 184

ibuprofen, 128–129
identity, versus role confusion, 49
ill child, 39–40
immunisation, 225
independent prescribing, 243
industry, versus inferiority, 49
infant mortality, 5
infection, prevention of, 165–166
infectious diseases, preventing, 142–143
inferiority, 49
initiative, versus guilt, 49
injury prevention, 6–8
interactive teaching, 14–15
iron deficiency anaemia (IDA), 63–64
  causes of, 63–64
  effects of, 63
  signs and symptoms, 63

junior school children, health promotion activities for, 29–30

Kidscape, 296–297
kinaesthetic learning, 26–27

laxatives, 216
Lazy Town (television show), 75
learning, 26–28
  auditory, 26–27
  kinaesthetic, 26–27
  style and rapport in, 27–28
  visual, 26–27

lectures/talks, 16
leukotriene receptor antagonists, 187
lifestyle, 8–9
listening to children, 51–52
Living with Babies (LWB), 266–271
  course content, 268–269
  evaluation of, 269
  future developments, 269
  health promotion, 267
  implementation of, 269
  overview of, 266–267
  partnership with Sure Start, 268
  teaching styles, 268
Living with Teenagers (LWT), 315–324
  benefits of, 322
  evaluation form, *321f*
  evaluation of, 322–323
  future directions, 322–323
  practice, 315–320
  process, 322
  sessions, 318–320
  theory, 315–317
long-term memory, 22
looked-after children/young people, 307–311
  asylum-seeking children, 310–311
  definitions of, 307
  overview, 307–308
  policy context, 308–309
  role of primary health care team, 309–310

malignant melanoma, 96
margarine tubs, 275
massage, baby, 259–264
  bonding in, 160
  overview, 259
  positive touch in, 259–260
maternity services, 41–42
medicines management, 235–245
  access to medicine, 242–243
  collaboration, 243–244
  definition of, 235–236
  and discharge planning, 172–173
  independent prescribing, 243
  need for, 236
  NSF standard, 41, 236–242
    compliance with medication regime, 238
    concordance with medication regime, 238–239
    monitoring and reviewing, 241–242
    optimising medication regime, 236–238
    organising supply and administration, 239–241
  nurse prescribers' formulary, 243
  overview, 235
  patient group directions, 243
  patient-specific directions, 242
  principles, 236
  supplementary prescribing, 243
memory, 50–51
meningitis, 140–142
mental health, 40–41, 384
mild upper respiratory infections, 137–140

minor burns, 145–149
  first-aid management, 147
  follow-up, 148
  health promotion campaigns, 146
  incidence of, 145
  infection control, 148
  injury assessment, 148
  pain assessment, 147
  wound care, 148
minor illnesses, 134–143
  course development, 135–136
  discharge planning, 169–170
  gastroenteritis, 136–137
  health promotion in, 134–143
  mild upper respiratory infections, 137–140
  preventing infectious diseases, 142–143
minor illness/injury service, 115–123
  community children's nursing service in, 116
  coping with sick children in, 115–116
  developing, 116–122
  Sure Start community children's nursing, 116–122
minor injuries, 144–150
  definition of, 144–146
  health promotion, 144–150
    courses, 149
    leaflets, 149
    literature sources, 149
    for older children, 150
    for parents/carers, 149
  health promotion in, 144–150
  minor burns, 145–149
  nurses' role in managing, 144–146
  overview, 144
mistrust, 48
mites, 194
morphine, 253
mortality, 5–6
  in children and young people, 5–6
  infant, 5–6
mother and baby drop-in group, 73

naproxen, 253
National Association of Hospital Play Staff, 53
National Collaborating Centre for Women's and Child
    Health (NCC-WCH), 221–222
National Electronic Library for Health, 19
National Service Frameworks (NSFs) for children, 35–42
  for children/young people, 223
  for diabetes, 222
  main purpose of, 36
  main themes, 36
  for maternity services, 223
  overview of, 35–36
  standards, 36–42
    children in hospital, 40
    child/young person-centred services, 37–38
    disabled children/young people, 40
    growing into adulthood, 38
    health promotion, 36–37
    ill child, 39–40

maternity services, 41–42
  medicines management, 41
  mental health, 40–41
  supporting parents/carers, 37
  welfare of children and young people,
      39
National Smile Month, 89–90
needs, 14
Neighbourhood Renewal Fund, 322
nerve pain, 253
nettle rash, 196
neuropathic pain, 253
NHS Direct, 19
NHS Stop Smoking Helpline, 347
NHS Stop Smoking Services, 347
nicotine replacement therapy, 347
Nike Girls in Sport, 386
non-steroidal anti-inflammatory drugs (NSAIDs),
    253
normative need, 14
North Ireland, health promotion in, 381–384
  alcohol use, 383–384
  dental health, 382–383
  drugs and solvents, 383–384
  healthy eating, 381–382
  mental health, 384
  obesity in children, 382
  overview of, 381–382
  road safety, 383
  smoking cessation, 383–384
nurse prescribers' formulary, 243
nurse-led discharge, 170
nursery schools, health promotion in, 372–373
  books, 373
  play, 372–373
  puppets, 373
nut allergy, 197

obesity in children, 70–81
  childhood cancer survivors, 206
  definition of, 70
  and growth, 75
  North Ireland, 382
  overview, 69–70
  prevention, 70–71
    books, 75
    breastfeeding, 71–73
    children's TV programmes, 75
    cookery lessons, 75
    dinner menu, 74
    food in schools, 73–74
    healthy eating, 80–81
    physical activity, 76–80
    toolkits, 74–75
objectives, 14–16
Oliver's Vegetables (book), 75
ordered antics, 32
outcomes, 14–15
outpatient department, 369–370
overflow soiling, 210

paediatric intensive care unit (PICU), 54–55
pain, 250–251
　acute, 250
　assessment of, 250–251
　chronic, 250
　physiological aspects of, 250
pain management, 249–254
　community perspective, 254
　definition of pain, 250
　distraction, 251
　drugs in, 252–253
　　ibuprofen, 253
　　local anaesthetics, 253
　　opioids, 253
　　paracetamol, 252
　environmental methods, *251–252b*
　importance of, 249
　non-drug, 251
　NSF standard, *249–250b*
　overview, 249
　sucrose, 252
　in surgical wound healing, 165
pans and spoons, 275–276
paracetamol, 128, 252
parenting, 287–288
Parentline Plus, 297
participant's views, 355
patient group directions, 243
patient-specific directions, 242–243
peak expiratory flow rate (PEFR), 183
peer evaluation, 355
personal, social and health education (PSHE), 375
pets, 184
Piaget, Jean, 45–46
piroxicam, 253
planning, elements of, 14–20
　aims, 14–15
　content, 14–15
　evaluation, 19–20
　needs, 14
　objectives, 14–16
　outcomes, 14–15
　resources, 18–19
　teaching methods, 15–18
play in hospital, 53–56
　adolescents, 55–56
　children's outpatient department, 53–54
　functions of play, 53
　overview of, 53
　paediatric intensive care unit, 54–55
　pre- and postoperative care, 157–158
play in nursery schools, 372–373
positive parenting, 287–291
　definition of, 287
　evaluation of, 291
　practicing, 288–289
　relationship, 288
　supporting families in, 290
　teaching parents, 290–291
　techniques, 289–290

postoperative care, 155–161
　child-centred services, 156–158
　clinical governance, 158–159
　emotional safety, 160
　equality of care, 159
　overview, 155–156
　pain assessment and management, 159
　physical safety, 160
　quality and safety of, 158–159
　quality of setting and environment, 160–161
potty training, 214–216
poverty trap, 393
praises, 23, 51
pregnant women, diabetes management in, 226
pre-operational stage, 46–47
pre-operative care, 155–161
　child-centred services, 156–158
　clinical governance, 158–159
　emotional safety, 160
　equality of care, 159
　fluids and nutrition in, 160–161
　overview, 155–156
　pain assessment and management, 159
　physical safety, 160
　quality and safety of, 158–159
　quality of setting and environment, 160–161
preschool children, health promotion activities for, 29
prescribing, 129
presentations, 14
puberty, 49–50
pull along toy, 276
puppets, 373
pyrexia, 124

qualitative method, 360
quantitative method, 360
questioning techniques, 17
questionnaires, 360–361
questions, 52

rattles, 275
recommendations, 362
research, 358–363
　aims and objectives, 359
　definition of, 358–359
　design and questionnaires, 360–361
　dissemination, 363
　ethics, 359–360
　methods, 359
　proposal, 359
　qualitative approach, 360
　quantitative approach, 360
　reasons for, 358
　recommendations, 362
　sampling, 360
resources, 18–19
respiratory infections, 184
rewards, 23, 51
road safety, 104–106
　car-safety seats, 104–105

cycle safety, 105–106
education on, 105
and health inequalities, 8
health promotion, 375
North Ireland, 383
reduced driver speed, 104
traffic-calming systems, 104
role models, 337–338
role-play, 17
Royal Belfast Hospital for Sick Children, 384

safeguarding children, 300–305
corporal punishment, 302–303
discipline, 304–305
overview, 301
safety gates, 103
safety mirror, 274–275
sampling, 360
Sarcoptes scabiei, 194
scabies, 193–195
school dinners, 74
school health nurses, 387–389
school-based drop-in service, 331–334
aim, 331
counsellor, 331
objectives, 331–332
promotion of, 333
role of nurses in, 332–333
services, 333–334
schools, health promotion in, 374–376
drug and solvent misuse, 375–376
emotional health, 376
healthy eating, 374
personal, social and health education, 375
physical activity, 374–375
road safety, 375
sexual health, 376
Scotland, health promotion in, 385–387
search, 17–18
seborrhoeic eczema, 197
sensorimotor stage, 46
septicaemia, 140–142
sexual health, 325–334
barriers, 328
and diabetes management, 225–226
importance of, 329
policy drivers, 326–328
promotion of, 325–334, 376
sexual health services, 329–334
accessibility of, 329
availability of, 329
awareness of, 329
case study, 330–331
confidentiality of, 330
Fraser guidelines, *331b*
practice, 329
school-based drop-in service, 331–334
aim, 331
counsellor, 331
objectives, 331–332

promotion of, 333
role of nurses in, 332–333
services, 333–334
sexually transmitted infection (STI), 325–326
shame, 48–49
short-term memory, 23–24
skin cancer, 96–100
health promotion, 97–100
resources, 99
sun damage, 97
sun protection, 97–98
sun protection factors, 98–99
sunscreens, 98–99
incidence of, 96
overview, 96
risk factors, 97
types of, 96–97
skin conditions, 192–200
assessing new patient, 192–193
atopic eczema, 197
eczema, 197–200
examination of, 193
family history, 193
food or nut allergy, 197
fungal infections, 196
general advice, 192–193
giving health information, 193
head lice, 195–196
history, 193
overview, 192
scabies, 193–195
seborrhoeic eczema, 197
tests and investigations, 193
urticaria, 196–197
viral rashes, 193
small group work, 17
smoke alarms, 104
Smoke Bugs programme, 389
smoking. *See also* substance misuse
in childhood cancer survivors, 206–207
and young people, 346–347
smoking cessation, 346–349
collaborative working, 348–349
North Ireland, 383–384
overview, 346–349
role of nurse in, 348–349
schools, 349
stage of change, 347–348
techniques, 347
withdrawal symptoms, 347
social classes, 4–5
social identity, formation of, 48–49
soiling, 210
Solihull approach, 282
solvent misuse, 375–376, 383–384
special time, 51
squamous cell carcinoma, 96
stacking cups, 275
Starting Well, 385
steroid creams, 198–200

still images, 81
substance misuse, 337–344
    and adolescence, 337–338
    alcohol, 339–340
    drugs, 339–340
    health promotion strategies, 340–344
        DARE, 340–343
        Face It, 342–343
    overview of, 337
    role models, 337
    smoking, 338–339
sucrose, 252
sun protection factors (SPFs), 98–99
sunscreens, 98–99
Sunsmart, 99
supplementary prescribing, 243
support groups, 371
Sure Start community children's nursing, 115–123
    action plan, 120–121
    aims of services, 118–119
    evaluation of, 361–363
    future developments, 122
    home visiting for sick children, 121
    objectives of, 117–118
    overview of, 64–65
    pain management in, 254
    parents' perspectives, 121–122
    partnership with Living with Babies, 268
    principles, 119
    services, 372
surgical wound healing, 163–168
    ambulatory care, 164–165
    children's care in hospital, 163–164
    discharge information, 167–168
    health promotion, 163
    pain relief, 165
    preoperative preparation, 164–165
    preparation for discharge, 166–167
    prevention of infection, 165–166
    teaching wound care, 166
swimming, 79–80

talks, 16
teaching methods, 15–18
    healthy eating, 80–81
    interactive, 14–15
    presentations, 14
teaching plans, 20
teenage pregnancy, 325–326
teeth, 83–86. *See also* dental health promotion
    decay, 86
    development of, 83–84
    erosion, 86
    and gum disease, 86
    injuries to, 86
    structure of, 83, *84b*
temperature, 124

text motivation messages, 347
thermometers, 130
toddlers, health promotion activities for, 29
toilet training, 214–216
tooth brushing, 87
traffic-calming systems, 104
treasure basket, 276
trust, 48

urticaria, 196–197

viral rashes, 193–200
visual learning, 26–27
visually impaired children, 29
Vygotsky, Lev, 47–48

Wales, 387–391
    community children's nursing, 389–391
    health promotion in, 387–389
    school health nurses, 387–389
weight, 61–62
Welfare Food scheme, 74
wheeze, 182
Why Your Child's Weight Matters (leaflet), 75
window safety, 103
withholding, 210
wound healing, 163–168
    ambulatory care, 164–165
    children's care in hospital, 163–164
    discharge information, 167–168
    health promotion, 163
    pain relief, 165
    preoperative preparation, 164–165
    preparation for discharge, 166–167
    prevention of infection, 165–166
    teaching wound care, 166

yoga, 77–79
    benefits of, 78
    for older children, 78–79
    for young children, 77–78
yoga, baby, 259–264
    bonding in, 160
    emotional benefits of, 262–263
    overview, 259
    physical benefits of, 263
    positive touch in, 259–260
YogaBugs, 77
young children (0–5 years), fever management in, 124–133
young people. *See also* children
    causes of mortality in, 5–6
    disabled, 40, 228–231
    health promotion activities for, 30–32
    looked-after, 307–311
    sexual health in, 325–334
    smoking in, 346–347